J. G. TOPLISS

Quantitative
Structure–Activity
Relationships of Drugs

MEDICINAL CHEMISTRY

A Series of Monographs

A complete list of titles in this series appears at the end of this volume.

Quantitative Structure–Activity Relationships of Drugs

Edited by

John G. Topliss

Warner-Lambert/Parke-Davis
Pharmaceutical Research Division
Ann Arbor, Michigan

1983

ACADEMIC PRESS

A Subsidiary of Harcourt Brace Jovanovich, Publishers

New York London
Paris San Diego San Francisco São Paulo Sydney Tokyo Toronto

ACADEMIC PRESS, INC.
111 Fifth Avenue, New York, New York 10003

United Kingdom Edition published by
ACADEMIC PRESS, INC. (LONDON) LTD.
24/28 Oval Road, London NW1 7DX

Library of Congress Cataloging in Publication Data

Main entry under title:

Quantitative structure-activity relationships of drugs.

(Medicinal chemistry series)
Includes index.
Contents: Introduction / C. John Blankley -- Synthetic anti-infective agents / M.S. Tute -- Semisynthetic antibiotics / Yvonne C. Martin and Elizabeth W. Fischer -- Antitumor agents / W.J. Dunn III -- [etc.]
1. Structure-activity relationship (Pharmacology)
I. Topliss, John G. II. Series.
QP906.S75Q36 1983 615'.7 82-25280
ISBN 0-12-695150-0

PRINTED IN THE UNITED STATES OF AMERICA

83 84 85 86 9 8 7 6 5 4 3 2 1

Contents

Contributors

Numbers in parentheses indicate the pages on which the authors' contributions begin.

V. Austel (437), Department of Chemistry, Dr. Karl Thomae GmbH, Biberach an der Riss, West Germany

Joel G. Berger (329), Schering-Plough, Research Division, Bloomfield, New Jersey 07003

C. John Blankley (1), Warner-Lambert/Parke-Davis, Pharmaceutical Research Division, Ann Arbor, Michigan 48105

Richard D. Cramer III (253), Research and Development Division, Smith, Kline and French Laboratories, Philadelphia, Pennsylvania 19101

W. J. Dunn III (137), College of Pharmacy, Department of Medicinal Chemistry and Pharmacognosy, University of Illinois, Chicago, Illinois 60612

Elizabeth W. Fischer (77), Department of Chemistry, Barat College, Lake Forest, Illinois 60045

James Y. Fukunaga (329), Schering-Plough, Research Division, Bloomfield, New Jersey 07003

Peter Gund (285), Merck Sharp & Dohme, Research Laboratories, Rahway, New Jersey 07065

Norman P. Jensen (285), Merck Sharp & Dohme, Research Laboratories, Rahway, New Jersey 07065

E. Kutter (437), Department of Chemistry, Dr. Karl Thomae GmbH, Biberach an der Riss, West Germany

Philip S. Magee (393), Chevron Chemical Company, Agricultural Chemicals Division, Richmond, California 94804

Yvonne C. Martin (77), Abbott Laboratories, Abbott Park, North Chicago, Illinois 60064

John G. Topliss (497), Warner-Lambert/Parke-Davis, Pharmaceutical Research Division, Ann Arbor, Michigan 48105

M. S. Tute (23), Central Research, Pfizer Ltd., Sandwich, Kent, England

Stefan H. Unger (177), Syntex Research, Palo Alto, California 94304

*Manfred E. Wolff** (351), Department of Pharmaceutical Chemistry, School of Pharmacy, University of California, San Francisco, California 94143

*Present address: Allergan, Irvine, California 92713.

Preface

Some eighteen years have elapsed since the landmark publications of Hansch and Fujita and of Free and Wilson ushered in the era of quantitative methodology analyzing the structure–activity relationships of drugs, or QSAR as it is commonly known. Over this period there has been an increase in the sophistication, depth, and number of methods available. A range of statistical methodologies has now been tapped. Cluster analysis, discriminant analysis, and principal component and factor analysis have been employed beyond the original use of multiple regression analysis. In addition to the linear free-energy based method, others such as pattern recognition, topological methods, and molecular modeling have come into use, and there has been continued development of quantum mechnical methods.

It might be asked, What has all this accomplished? Previous books in the QSAR field have concentrated on methodology; discussions of the principles and theories underlying the different methods and descriptions of how to apply these methods to actual problems have been provided. The objective of this book is to critically review applications of various QSAR methodologies in different drug therapeutic areas and examine the results in terms of their contribution to medicinal chemistry. There is now a sufficient body of accumulated information on this subject so that an undertaking of this kind appears timely and should shed some light on the question of how useful QSAR is in the broad context of medicinal chemistry.

A broad definition of QSAR has been used here so that applications of all methods that employ some type of quantitative measure have been included. Also, the term "drug" will be interpreted in its broadest sense as meaning a biologically active substance. An attempt has been made to standardize the way equations are presented. Many different formats and levels of statistical information have appeared over the years so that a completely uniform presentation is not possible. The statistical significance of equations and of individual terms in them should be considered adequate unless stated otherwise by the chapter author.

Not every published paper on QSAR applications is mentioned. The intent is to cover the most significant work and to be analytical and critical as opposed to encyclopedic. Where possible, information and conclusions from different papers have been integrated in an attempt to provide new insight and generalizations.

It is hoped that after reading this book, medicinal chemists will have a better understanding of just what QSAR has contributed to the field of medicinal chemistry and what it might reasonably be expected to contribute in the future.

Finally, I would like to express my gratitude to all of the chapter authors whose expertise and hard work have made this book possible and to other fellow scientists who have provided valuable comments and advice.

1

Introduction: A Review of QSAR Methodology

C. JOHN BLANKLEY

I. INTRODUCTION

Before embarking upon a critical examination of the applications of quantitative structure–activity relationships (QSAR) in biology, it is nec-

QUANTITATIVE STRUCTURE–ACTIVITY
RELATIONSHIPS OF DRUGS

ISBN 0-12-695150-0

essary to review what methods have been used to obtain QSAR. The purpose of this chapter is to gather together in one place and describe briefly the various procedures, the results of which will be discussed in the subsequent chapters of the book. Some reviews that cover the same ground in other contexts may also be consulted (*119,120,132*).

II. FREE ENERGY MODELS

A. The Hansch Equation

First and foremost among the QSAR methods is the model proposed by Hansch and co-workers (*67,68,72*). It was the seminal contribution of this group to propose that the early observations of the importance of relative lipophilicity to biological potency (*51,125,133*) be incorporated into the useful formalism of linear-free energy relationships (LFER) (*104*) to provide a general model for QSAR in biological contexts. As a suitable measure of lipophilicity, the partition coefficient, log P, between 1-octanol and water was proposed, and it was further demonstrated that this was roughly an additive and constitutive property and hence calculable in principle from molecular structure (*56,84*). Using a probabilistic model for transport across biological membranes, Hansch derived Eq. (1a) (Eq. 1b is an alternate form), which is now known by his name (*68*).

$$\log(1/C) = -k\pi^2 + k'\pi + \rho\sigma + k'' \qquad (1a)$$

$$\log(1/C) = -k(\log P)^2 + k'(\log P) + \rho\sigma + k'' \qquad (1b)$$

C is the molar concentration (or dose) that elicits a constant biological response (e.g., ED_{50}, MED, IC_{50}), π is the substituent lipophilicity, log P is the partition coefficient, σ is the substituent electronic effect of Hammett (*49*), and k, k', ρ, and k'' are the regression coefficients derived from the statistical curve fitting. The reciprocal of the concentration reflects the fact that higher potency is associated with lower dose, and the negative sign for the π^2 or $(\log P)^2$ term reflects the expectation of an optimum lipophilicity, designated π_0 or $\log P_0$.

The statistical method used to determine the coefficients in Eq. (1) is multiple linear regression (*33,40,176*). A number of statistics are derived in conjunction with such a calculation, which allow the statistical significance of the resulting correlation to be assessed. The most important of these are s, the standard error of the estimate (in many papers called simply the standard deviation), r^2, the coefficient of determination or percentage of data variance accounted for by the model (r, the correlation coefficient is also commonly cited), F, a statistic for assessing the overall significance of the derived equation (statistics table list critical values for the appropriate number of degrees of freedom and confidence level), and *t* values (also compared with statistics tables) and confidence intervals (usually 95%) for the individual regression coefficients in the equation. Also very important in multiparameter equations are the cross-correlation coefficients between the independent variables in the equation. These must be low to assure true "independence" or orthogonality of the variables, a necessary condition for meaningful results.

The applicability of Eq. (1) to a broad range of biological SAR has been convincingly demonstrated by the Hansch group and many others in the years since 1964 (*15,69,70,73*). The success of this model led early to its generalization to include additional parameters. In attempts to minimize the residual variance in such correlations, a wide variety of physicochemical parameters and properties, structural and topological features, molecular orbital indices, and, for constant but theoretically unaccountable features, indicator or "dummy" (1 or 0) variables have been employed (*119,140,173*). In fact, the widespread use of Eq. (1) has provided an important stimulus for the review and extension of established scales of substituent effects (*18*), and even for the development of new ones (*2,48,76,109,174*). It should be cautioned, however, that the general validity or, indeed, the need for these latter scales has not been established.

Lipophilicity in particular, as reflected in partition coefficients between aqueous and nonaqueous media, most commonly water (or aqueous buffer) and 1-octanol after the initial suggestion of Fujita *et al.* (*56*), has received much attention (*74,105,142–144*). Log *P* for the octanol–water system has been shown to be approximately additive and constitutive and hence schemes for its *a priori* calculation from molecular structure have been devised using either substituent π values or substructural fragment constants *f* (*74,143,144*). A computer adaptation of the method of Leo *et al.* (*74*) has recently been reported (*20*). The approximate nature of any partition coefficient calculation has been frequently emphasized (*17,74,143*), and indeed, some of the structural features that cause unreliability have been identified and accommodated (*142*). Other complications such as steric effects (*36*), conformational effects (*135,136*), and substitution at the active positions of heteroaromatic rings (*162,164,181*) have been observed but cannot as yet be accounted for systematically. Theoretical (*79,145*), statistical (*43,53*), and topological (*128*) methods to approach some of these problems have been reported. The observations, originally by Collander (*23*), of linear relationships among partition coefficients between water and various organic solvents have been extended and qualified (*105,143*). New methodology for the more convenient measurement of log *P* or relative lipophilicity by thin-layer chromatography

(TLC) (*87,163*) or high-pressure liquid chromatography (HPLC) (*87, 120,129,130,171,172*) procedures has been reported. Parameters other than partition coefficients have been proposed as measures of relative lipophilicity, but apart from the chromatographically derived R_m values, these have not as yet been widely used. In several of the cited reviews these are discussed (*69,73,119,120,132,173*).

It is not the present purpose to review all of the other parameters that have been employed in Hansch correlations because these have been adequately discussed elsewhere (*15,74,119,120,132,173*). Several compilations of the most commonly used substituent constants in QSAR work have been published (*18,50,74,113,119,131,171*). The fact that the values listed in these tables do not always agree simply underlines the need for caution in accepting any "critical" collection of constants as definitive.

Another consequence of the empirical and statistical nature of the Hansch model, especially with the proliferation of variables that have been used to seek correlation of biological data, has been the heightened awareness of statistical requirements and constraints. Problems with multicolinearity or cross correlation of independent variables have been noted and discussed (*13,24,114,115*). The potential for chance correlation when too many variables are surveyed to correlate too few data has been pointed out (*166,169*). Misleading results due to "cluster correlation" (*111*) or inappropriate scaling of parameters (*112*) have recently been discussed. The effect of error in the independent variables on the reliability of the regression results has been scarcely mentioned (*52,61,119*) and not at all studied, even though it is an important assumption of regression analysis that the independent variables have minimal error (*33*). "Overfitting" the data, that is obtaining standard deviations lower that the experimental error of the biological measurements, should arouse suspicion (*61*). It is very important, but also difficult to evaluate properly, that any statistically derived equation make good chemical and/or biological sense. This has been urged before (*170,171*), and one study of the steric effects of alkyl groups (*38*) is particularly instructive in this connection.

B. Other Free Energy Models

The success of Hansch in demonstrating that free energy correlations can be successfully applied to biological processes has prompted many workers to reexamine the derivation of the Hansch equation. Using the principles of theoretical pharmacology (*1,60*) or pharmacokinetics (*147,148,153,154*), they have sought to provide improved theoretical models to accommodate more complex relationships between biological activity and chemical structure or properties, or to broaden the scope of

Eq. (1) to include, for example, ionizable compounds. Excellent discussions of these models have been provided by Martin (*119,120*) and Kubinyi (*101*). With one exception, these models have not as yet been tested to a degree that would permit a reasonable evaluation of them to be made. The semiempirical "bilinear" model of Kubinyi (*94,97,99–101*) is a more flexible version of Eq. (1) that still allows for an optimum log P but provides linear ascending and descending portions of the curve with separately determinable slopes. The bilinear model is given by Eq. (2),

$$\log(1/C) = a \log P - b \log(\beta P + 1) + c \tag{2}$$

where C and log P have the same meaning as in Eq. (1), and a, b, β, and c are the coefficients derived by nonlinear regression analysis (*99*).

III. FREE–WILSON MATHEMATICAL MODEL

The idea that substituents ought to contribute constant increments or decrements to biological activity in an analog series has probably been a long-held intuition of medicinal chemists trained in organic chemistry. However, very few solid demonstrations of this can be found in the literature prior to 1964 (*9,11,182*). The existence of linear Hansch correlations is one verification of this idea. However, at about the same time that the Hansch model was proposed, Free and Wilson demonstrated a general mathematical method both for assessing the occurrence of additive substituent effects and for quantitatively estimating their magnitude (*55*). According to their method, the molecules of a drug series are structurally decomposed into a common moiety or core that is variously substituted in multiple positions. A series of linear equations of the form

$$BA_i = \sum_j a_j X_{ij} + \mu \tag{3}$$

are constructed where BA is the biological activity, X_j is the jth substituent with a value of 1 if present and 0 if not, a_j is the contribution of the jth substituent to BA, and μ is the overall average activity. All activity contributions at each position of substitution must sum to zero. The series of linear equations thus generated is solved by the method of least squares for the a_j and μ. There must be several more equations than unknowns and each substituent should appear more than once at a position in different combinations with substituents at other positions. Craig (*25*) and Purcell *et al.* (*82,140*) have discussed in detail the requirements and constraints of the Free–Wilson model as originally formulated. The attractiveness of this model, also referred to as the de novo method, is fourfold:

(1) any set of quantitative biological data may be employed as the dependent variable, (2) no independently measured substituent constants are required, (3) the molecules of a series may be structurally dissected in any convenient manner, and (4) multiple sites of variable substitution are easily accommodated. There are also several limitations: a substantial number of compounds with varying substituent combinations is required for a meaningful analysis; the derived substituent contributions give no reasonable basis for extrapolating predictions outside of the substituent matrix analyzed; and the model will break down if nonlinear dependence on substituent properties is important or if there are interactions between the substituents.

Fujita and Ban (*57*) suggested two modifications of the original formulation. First, the biological activity should be expressed as $\log(1/C)$ or an equivalent measure proportional to a free energy change so that the derived substituent constants might be compared with other free energy related parameters, and second, that μ, the overall average, become analogous to an intercept, that is the calculated activity of the unsubstituted or reference compound of the series. This obviates the need for the cumbersome symmetry or restriction equations of the original method. The Fujita–Ban modification is the form of the Free–Wilson method in common use today. Simplified methods for calculating (*98*) or estimating (*146*) solutions to this model have been reported.

The mathematical implications of the Free–Wilson model have been discussed on several occasions (*14,58,150,151,156*), and the relationship of it to the Hansch model has been noted. Kubinyi (*93,95,96*) has provided the definitive discussion of the interrelationship between the two models. These may be pictured as opposite extremes of the same multiple regression model, the Hansch equation using continuous independent variables and the Free–Wilson model using only discrete (1 or 0) variables. The use of indicator variables in a Hansch equation or of $(\log P)^2$ or π^2 terms to accommodate nonlinearity in a Free–Wilson model, as suggested by Kubinyi, illustrates a mixed model (*95*).

IV. OTHER STATISTICAL MODELS

A. Discriminant Analysis

In many cases of interest the biological measurements available are only semiquantitative or qualitative in nature, and activity assessments such as highly active (+++), moderately active (++), slightly active (+), or inactive (0), or simply active/inactive, must be evaluated. Such data may arise from measurements with inherent imprecision, subjective evaluation of behavioral or response observations, or a combination of several criteria of interest into a single index. Passing over the question of to what extent data of this type are suitable for correlation in free energy models, it is nevertheless interesting to try to obtain some insight into the operative properties or structural parameters responsible for the variations in such data. Discriminant analysis has been proposed to deal with this type of problem (*119,120*). This method seeks a linear combination of parameters, called a linear discriminant function, that will successfully classify the observations into their observed or assigned categories. Parameters are added or deleted as needed to improve discrimination, and the results are judged by the number of observations correctly classified. Martin *et al.* (*118,119*), Bock *et al.* (*10*), and Prakash and Hodnett (*138*) all discuss the background of the method as well as provide examples of its use.

B. Principal Components and Factor Analysis

One of the statistical concerns in multiple regression analysis noted above is cross correlation between the independent variables under consideration. This can be simply assessed by examination of the correlation matrix of the parameters. Further manipulations can be performed on this matrix or on the variance–covariance matrix including the dependent variable. By methods of linear algebra such a matrix may be transformed by prescribed methods into one containing nonzero elements only on the diagonal. These are called the eigenvalues of the matrix, and associated with each of these is an eigenvector that is a linear combination of the original set of variables. Eigenvectors, unlike the original set of variables, have the property of being exactly orthogonal, that is the correlation coefficient between any two of them is zero. If a set of variables has substantial covariance, it will turn out that most of the total variance will be accounted for by a number of eigenvectors equal to a fraction of the original number of variables. A reduced set containing only the major eigenvectors, or "principal components," may then be examined or used in various ways. It should be noted that the determination of how many eigenvectors may be reasonably ignored is a subjective decision and depends to a large degree on the purpose of the analysis.

This method is most often used as a preprocessing tool. If only the principal components are considered, new orthogonal variables can be constructed from the eigenvectors, and hence the dimensionality of the parameter space can be reduced while most of the information in the original variable set is retained. This is particularly useful in the multidimensional methods of the pattern recognition variety (see following section). It has also been recommended as a preliminary step in series design (*121,158*) or in multiple regression analysis of the Hansch variety (*54,115*). Darvas *et al.* (*35*) used the principal component method to analyze the antibacterial activity of several series of structurally related γ-pyridonecarboxylic acids against a spectrum of bacterial strains. It was concluded that two major physiological mechanisms were involved in the activity of this type of compound.

Factor analysis involves other manipulations of the eigenvectors and is aimed more at gaining insight into the structure of a multidimensional data set. Weiner and Weiner (*177*) first proposed a use of this technique in biological SAR and illustrated this with an analysis of the activities of 21 diphenylaminopropanol derivatives in 11 biological tests of CNS effects. More common use of this method has been made in trying to determine the "intrinsic dimensionality" of certain experimentally determined chemical properties, that is the number of "fundamental factors" required to account for the variance. Of particular interest for QSAR work are studies of liquid state properties by Cramer (*28*) and aromatic log P values by Franke *et al.* (*53*).

C. Cluster Analysis

Cluster analysis is simply a method to group entities, for which a number of properties or parameters exist, by similarity. Various distance measurements are used, and the analysis is performed in a sequential manner, reducing the number of clusters at each step. Such a procedure has been described for use in drug design as a way to group substituents that have the most similarity when various combinations of the parameters π, σ, F, R, and MR are considered (*71,74*).

D. Combined Multivariate Analyses

Some or all of the above-described methods may be used to analyze a given set of biological data. Because many of the methods are complementary, it seems likely that their combined use will be a major trend in future QSAR work. A study of the QSAR of quinazoline inhibitors of tetrahydrofolate dehydrogenase (dihydrofolate reductase) and thymidylate synthase used cluster analysis, factor analysis, discriminant analysis, and finally, multiple regression analysis to examine the data from various viewpoints (*19*). Lewi has outlined a technique called spectral mapping in which the biological profile and potencies of closely related compounds may be analyzed by a combination of cluster and principal components analyses (*106–108*). Perhaps the most impressively integrated multivariate statistical model yet proposed is the MASCA system of Mager (*115,116*). The whole battery of biometric statistical methods has been combined into a total system for the analyses of biological assay results, pharmacokinetic information, and series design, as well as structure–activity relationships.

V. PATTERN RECOGNITION

That branch of computer science that is optimistically called Artificial Intelligence contains an ensemble of techniques that go by the general name of pattern recognition. As they have been applied to QSAR, these methods comprise yet another approach to examining structural features and/or chemical properties for underlying patterns that are associated with differing biological effects. Accurate classification of untested molecules is again the primary goal. This is carried out in two stages. First, a set of compounds, designated the training set, is chosen for which the correct classification is known. A set of molecular or property descriptors (features) is generated for each compound. A suitable classification algorithm is then applied to find some combination and weight of the descriptors that allows perfect classification. Many different statistical and geometric techniques for this purpose have been used and compared (*22,86,91,92,157*). The derived classification function is then applied in the second step to compounds not included in the training set to test predictability. In published work these have generally been other compounds of known classification also. Performance is judged by the percentage of correct predictions. Stability of the classification function is usually tested by repeating the training procedure several times with slightly altered, but randomly varied, training sets.

The two pattern recognition systems that were used earliest in QSAR work were that of Kirschner and Kowalski, called ARTHUR (*91*), and that of Stuper and Jurs, named ADAPT (*159,160*). The generally abstract structural descriptors used by these programs make the interpretation of a successful training vector difficult to impossible in terms useful to a drug designer. Two other methods described later attempt in different ways to address this problem. One is the SIMCA system of Wold *et al.* (*44–46,179*). This method makes use of principal components analysis to provide structure and limits to the classification groups so that not only can group membership be determined, but also the level of activity within each group. The published applications of this method have tended to use physicochemical parameters as molecular descriptors in preference to the structural features relied upon by the earlier methods.

Cammarata and Menon have proposed a different approach (*16,123*). Here the principles of principal components and factor analysis are applied to structural codings derived by superimposing molecules on a composite or "hypermolecule" template, recording the presence or absence of groups at designated positions of highest variation, and weighting these by the molar refractivity of the atom or group present. After factor analysis of the resulting matrix, the major eigenvectors are used as axes to graph the data points. Compounds with similar types of action are then expected to cluster together in different areas of the plot. Henry and Block (*75*) have proposed to modify this method by using the molecular connectivity indices of Randic (*141*), as developed by Kier and Hall (*90*), in place of molar refraction as weighting factors. Henry and Block also report results with a variety of alternate classification methods applied to the Cammarata–Menon approach.

Another pattern recognition method called adaptive least squares (ALS) has been reported by Moriguchi *et al.* (*126,127*). This is related to discriminant analysis.

A proposal for still a different sort of pattern recognition based on substructure frequencies was made by Cramer *et al.* (*26*). This is meant to be used with a large file of structures and associated biological activities, which also has a substructure coding system for the compounds. The frequency of the association of any given substructure with a given activity can readily be calculated. Comparison of this with the frequency of the substructure in the total set tested for that activity gives a probability measure for activity. For a set of untested compounds the probabilities associated with each substructure present can be summed and averaged. The compounds with the highest mean scores might be hoped to have a better chance of showing activity than those with low mean scores. This expectation has no support from theoretical chemistry. Even from the purely probabilistic viewpoint, there are severe problems of intrinsic bias, not only in the data file itself, but in the compound selection. Hodes *et al.* (*77,78*) have suggested a more refined method based on the same thinking but using a different scoring method and including inactivity frequencies as well.

VI. TOPOLOGICAL METHODS

The importance of molecular shape in influencing biological activity, especially where enzymes or receptors are involved, is universally conceded. However, whereas size or bulk is a scalar quantity for which several measures are conceivable and accessible, the distribution of bulk (i.e., shape) is a vectorial quantity. The problem of finding the mathematical means to express differences in such a geometric feature in an adequate manner for use in developing QSAR functions has been a continuing challenge in the field. Several approaches have been examined.

The first has been to find parameters suitable for use in a Hansch equation. Taft's E_s parameter or its variants derived from the acid and base hydrolysis rates of aliphatic esters has been most widely used (*119,132*), in spite of doubts about its theoretical propriety for this purpose. Some later work on the nature of the E_s values has helped to sort out some of the factors underlying this parameter, and hence provides a sounder basis for its use and interpretation (*5,38,42,110,134*). Shape dependencies can be probed crudely by simply evaluating E_s contributions from various positions of substitution independently in a related set of molecules, for example ortho, meta, and para positions of a benzene ring (*102*).

Verloop *et al.* (*174*) have proposed to treat the problem of directionality of steric effects by the direct expedient of modeling a substituent and calculating its extension in five orthogonal directions. The resulting set of STERIMOL parameters for each substituent consists of L, the length along the axis connecting the group to the substituted moiety, and B_1–B_4, width measurements perpendicular to this axis in four rectilinear directions, with B_1 the shortest measurement. Recalculated values for some of these have been reported (*11a*).

Kier and Hall (*90*) have adapted the molecular connectivity index χ, a number derived originally by Randic (*141*) from graph theoretical principles to express the relative topology of variously branched hydrocarbon isomers, for QSAR correlations. Many χ terms can be calculated for a given molecule, differing in the number of atoms taken together ($^n\chi$), and these may ignore or include ($^n\chi_v$) weightings for the specific atom or bond types present. The various terms for the molecules of a series may be tested as parameters in the usual multiple regression correlation model. A comparison of the performance of E_s, STERIMOL, and χ parameters in QSAR application has been reported (*161,175*), and also an attempt has been made to relate $^n\chi$ to E_s (*129*).

An alternate approach to expressing topological differences has been taken by Simon and co-workers (*6,155*). In the minimal steric difference (MSD) method, a natural substrate molecule or the most active compound in a series is assumed to fit optimally to a receptor. This molecule is then used as a template upon which to superimpose the other members of the series. The number of noncoincident atoms is counted and this constitutes the MSD in the simplest version of the method. This can be viewed as a crude measure of how much a member of a series deviates from "ideal" geometry and is used in LFER equations to express the steric or shape component. A refinement of this method to remove some of the arbitrariness in the choice of a reference molecule and to include the possibilities that an occupied vertex may either contribute positively, negatively, or be irrelevant to activity is called the minimal topological difference (MTD) method. Balaban *et al.* (*6*) describe these methods in detail and also give examples of their use and comparison with alternate models.

All of the above-mentioned topological methods seek to reduce the geometric differences between molecules to one or a small number of parameters that can be used in a LFER equation of the Hansch type. Another method has been described that is more akin to the Free–Wilson model. The DARC/PELCO method of Dubois and co-workers (*41,124*), like the Free–Wilson method, analyzes a set of molecules into a focus, or common core, and various positions of substitution (directions of development). Also it determines additive increments, but unlike the Free–Wilson method, it does not associate these increments with whole groups or substituents but rather with "sites" and their associated atom types. The sites are generated in a progressive and ordered manner along each direction of development from the focus. If additivity is not found initially for the site contributions, interaction terms between sites are sought and added until the residual error of the analysis approaches the experimental error of the data. A topological map of activity increments is thus produced, important sites and site occupants are located relative to each other, and threshold or cutoff behavior becomes evident. Favorable or unfavorable interactions between sites may be identified. Although there have been few reported applications of this method, an interesting comparison has been made between Hansch, DARC/PELCO, and molecular connectivity analyses of the antimicrobial activity of a series of alkyl- and halogen-substituted phenols (*47,66,124*). The strikingly different predictions of the various results offer a means to assess the relative merits of these methods.

The computer software molecular modeling package CAMSEQ-II of Hopfinger has been used to generate shape descriptors for QSAR work (*7,80,81*). Still another topological approach is the distance geometry technique described by Crippen (*30–32*), which analyzes ligand-binding data in terms of points of molecular interaction, energies of interaction of the points, and distance relationships between them, all of which are used to predict relative receptor-binding energies for a series of compounds.

VII. EXPERIMENTAL DESIGN

The use of statistical or mathematical models in any experimental science brings with it certain requirements for structuring the experiments.

Hypotheses must be framed in terms of the parameters that are chosen to test them. The experimental data must then be designed to reflect an appropriate range and distribution of these parameters. High variance and low covariance of the independent variables should be assured so that definitive tests of statistical significance can be obtained from the results. For medicinal chemists this means that more care must be taken in choosing substituent or structural variations at the beginning of a new program than has heretofore been the rule. Several authors have discussed these problems and have offered guidelines for making such selections.

Craig (*24*) first pointed out the utility of a simple graphical plot of π versus σ (or indeed any two parameters of interest) to guide the choice of a substituent set with minimal covariance. Topliss introduced operational schemes (*165,167,168*) that are based on the assumption of a successful Hansch relationship being ultimately derived for a new series. The biological result at each step of the way in this method suggests the form of the eventual equation, and new substituents are indicated sequentially to narrow the remaining possibilities. Following the direction of increasing activity leads in theory to the optimum compounds in a relatively short time. Darvas (*34*) proposed a sequential simplex analysis of substituent space to arrive at the optimum member of a series quickly. This technique was elaborated further by Gilliom *et al.* (*59*). Alternatively, Fibonacci search has been advocated by Bustard (*12*) and Santora and Auyang (*149*). See Deming (*37*) for a caveat on this latter method.

All of the above methods can be applied without using a computer. More sophisticated analyses have been performed using a variety of statistical techniques for selecting suitable groups of substituents. Martin and Panas (*121*) give perhaps the best overview of the considerations involved. Hansch and co-workers have analyzed their own extensive database by cluster analysis using various combinations of parameters (*71,74*). Other schemes have been reported by Wooton *et al.* (*180*), Unger (*171*), Franke *et al.* (*39,158*), and most recently by Austel and Kutter (*3,4*).

VIII. QUANTUM MECHANICAL METHODS

Molecular orbital calculations have been applied in biological contexts independently of QSAR work for many years (*139*). In QSAR they have been adapted mainly for two general purposes, namely, to provide calculable parameters for LFER expressions with the aim of gaining insight at some "fundamental" level into possible mechanisms of action, or to calculate conformations of bioactive molecules as a basis for comparison with mimics or antagonists. Kier reviews some of this work in his book (*89*). Other reviews and examples of the application of these methods may also be consulted for details (*8,21,88,152,178*).

IX. MOLECULAR MODELING

Recent advances in the field of computer graphics have led to the development of methods for the visual display and manipulation of chemical structures. Atomic coordinates are obtained from X-ray crystal structures or are calculated by programs using molecular mechanics or quantum mechanical methods. Potential functions based on van der Waals radii are applied and the molecules are manipulated within these constraints. Although not strictly within the province of QSAR methodology as reviewed in preceding sections, these newer techniques offer the promise of complementing the mathematical and statistical models in precisely the area where these latter are weakest, namely, the conformational or three-dimensional aspect.

Thus pharmacophore identification is one of the challenges taken up by Marshall and co-workers using the MMS-X system at their disposal. Comparison of a series of similarly acting molecules by superposition allows the topography of a receptor binding site to be deduced from the compounds that bind at this site. Structurally similar but inactive compounds are found to protrude into portions of space not occupied by the active congeners, and the lack of activity is then presumed to be due to steric hindrance in these regions. Studies of inhibitors of *S*-adenosylmethionine synthetase, neuroleptic dopamine antagonists, and agonists of the glucose receptor of pancreatic β-cells are among the projects that have been reported (*83,117,160a*).

In a similar vein, the Merck Molecular Modeling System, developed by Gund and associates (*62,64,65*) has been used to propose a topographical description of how a variety of inhibitors of the cyclooxygenase step of prostaglandin biosynthesis can compete with the natural substrate, arachidonic acid, at the receptor site (*63*), among other applications.

The CAMSEQ-II molecular modeling package developed by Hopfinger and collaborators (*137*) has been used to compare and assess molecular conformations, especially as these are affected by various solvation shells. Some applications have already been noted above (*79,80*).

Perhaps the most sophisticated graphics capability to be demonstrated to date is found in the system reported by Langridge and co-workers (*103*). Macromolecules of the complexity of DNA or proteins are accommodated, connected atom or van der Waals surface representations are possible, color is available to highlight features of interest, and cross-sectional scans through the solid figures can be made, all of which allow detailed examination of the complementarity of intermolecular interactions. A report on an application of this system to the study of the thyroxine binding site on human prealbumin has appeared (*85*).

Descriptions and applications of still other approaches to computerized molecular modeling can be found in the volume cited in Christoffersen (*21*).

X. CONCLUSION

Several years have passed since the seminal papers of Hansch and Fujita on the one hand, and Free and Wilson on the other, initiated the full scale development of QSAR. The free energy model of Hansch and its elaborations has been by far the most widely used. This has been due not only to the many successful applications reported by the Hansch group, but also to its simplicity, its direct conceptual lineage to established physical organic chemical principles, and the ready availability of a database of substituent parameters. The mathematical model of Free and Wilson has not enjoyed nearly the popularity of the Hansch equation. Probably the restricted generality of a successful result, the severe constraints on substituent distribution and frequency, and the computationally more cumbersome procedure have contributed to this.

None of the other methods reviewed in this chapter have been widely used. Most require a considerable degree of mathematical or statistical background for proper application, or are dependent on complex computer software and/or hardware packages not commonly available to practicing medicinal chemists. Although this state of affairs may not be expected to continue, it has inevitably led to a new breed of specialist, the QSAR practitioner, who is conversant with all of the disciplines that provide knowledge of techniques relevant to the drug design process. One gauge of the relative importance and usefulness of the methods reviewed here can be had from the viewpoints on the practice of QSAR offered by Martin (*119,122*), Unger (*171*), and Cramer (*27,29*), three creative and successful contributors to the field who operate on an industrial rather than an academic basis. Two points of clear consensus that emerge are that retrospective QSAR analyses must usually be performed using a combination of methods to sort out reliably the underlying factors, and equally important, new projects should be subjected to what might be termed a prospective QSAR analysis so that information may be maximized and synthetic chemical effort minimized, or better, optimized.

It might be helpful in concluding this chapter to list a number of criteria by which a QSAR study might be evaluated or at least placed in proper perspective.

1. What is the purpose of seeking a quantitative correlation of the data? QSAR has developed primarily within the field of medicinal chemistry and hence drug design and the prediction of the activity of novel structures has always been in the forefront. Is it a matter then of lead generation or of lead optimization? Other goals of QSAR analyses have been to seek insight into mechanisms of action, to unravel pharmacokinetic behavior, to map receptors of enzyme active sites, or to summarize large collections of data on analog series concisely.
2. What is the nature of the biological data being employed, and its quality and precision?
3. Is the QSAR method that is chosen or proposed appropriate both to the nature and quality of the data and to the explicit or implicit purpose of the analysis?
4. Have the mathematical or statistical constraints and assumptions of the method chosen been properly understood and taken into account? Where applicable, have standard statistics been included for significance testing and have criteria for an acceptable level of significance been provided? Has due consideration been given to the possibility of chance correlation?
5. Are interpretations and speculations proportionate to the results obtained as well as to the original purpose of the analysis? Does the model implied by a statistically significant equation also make good chemical or biological sense? Have alternate models that are significant at the level judged acceptable been sought or considered? Is any attempt made to compare and/or reconcile a new result with other QSAR analyses on the same or related data or in the same biological system to provide perspective?
6. Finally, and most important, has any new knowledge or useful insight emerged as a result of the QSAR analysis, particularly any that would not likely have been found in the absence of such an analysis?

In the following chapters of this book, attempts are made to probe these questions with a review and analysis of QSAR studies in a number of important therapeutic areas published over the last 15 years.

REFERENCES

1. E. J. Ariens, "Molecular Pharmacology," Vol. 1. Academic Press, New York, 1964.
2. V. Austel, E. Kutter, and W. Kalbfleisch, *Arzneim.-Forsch.* **29**, 585 (1979).

3. V. Austel and E. Kutter, *in* "Drug Design" (E. J. Ariëns, ed.), Medicinal Chemistry, Vol. X, p. 1. Academic Press, New York, 1980.
4. V. Austel and E. Kutter, *Arzneim.-Forsch.* **31,** 130 (1981).
5. A. Babadjamian, M. Chanon, R. Gallo, and J. Metzger, *J. Am. Chem. Soc.* **95,** 3807 (1973).
6. A. T. Balaban, A. Chiriac, I. Motoc, and Z. Simon, *in* "Steric Fit in Quantitative Structure Activity Relations" (G. Berthier, ed.), Lecture Notes in Chemistry, Vol. 15, Springer-Verlag, Berlin and New York, 1980.
7. C. Battershell, D. Malhotra, and A. J. Hopfinger, *J. Med. Chem.* **24,** 812 (1981).
8. E. D. Bergmann and B. Pullman, eds., "Quantum and Molecular Pharmacology." Reidel Publ., Dordrecht, Netherlands, 1974.
9. K. Bocek, J. Kopecky, M. Krivacova, and D. Vlachova, *Experientia* **20,** 667 (1964).
10. P. R. Bock, B. Pollock, S. Schach, A. Fuchs, and R. Lohans, *Arzneim.-Forsch.* **26,** 1308 (1976).
11. T. C. Bruice, N. Kharasch, and R. J. Winzler, *Arch. Biochem. Biophys.* **62,** 305 (1956).
11a. T. Bultsma and G. J. Bijloo, *in* "Chemical Structure–Biological Activity Relationships. Quantitative Approaches" (F. Darvas, ed.), p. 205. Akadémiai Kiadó, Budapest, 1980.
12. T. M. Bustard, *J. Med. Chem.* **17,** 777 (1974).
13. A. Cammarata, R. C. Allen, J. K. Seydel, and E. Wempe, *J. Pharm. Sci.* **59,** 1496 (1970).
14. A. Cammarata, *J. Med. Chem.* **15,** 573 (1972).
15. A. Cammarata and K. S. Rogers, *in* "Advances in Linear Free Energy Relationships" (N. B. Chapman and J. Shorter, eds.), p. 401. Plenum, New York, 1972.
16. A. Cammarata and G. K. Menon, *J. Med. Chem.* **19,** 739 (1976).
17. A. Canas-Rodriquez and M. S. Tute, *in* "Biological Correlations—The Hansch Approach" (R. F. Gould, ed.), p. 41. Am. Chem. Soc., Washington, D.C., 1972.
18. See, e.g., M. Charton, *Prog. Phys. Org. Chem.* **13,** 119 (1981).
19. B.-K. Chen, C. Horvath, and J. R. Bertino, *J. Med. Chem.* **22,** 483 (1979).
20. J. T. Chou and P. C. Jurs, *J. Chem. Inf. Comput. Sci.* **19,** 171 (1979).
21. R. E. Christoffersen, *in* "Computer Assisted Drug Design" (E. C. Olsen and R. E. Christoffersen, eds.), p. 3. Am. Chem. Soc., Washington, D.C., 1979. (Several other relevant papers also appear in this volume.)
22. K. C. Chu, *Anal. Chem.* **46,** 1181 (1974).
23. R. Collander, *Acta Chem. Scand.* **5,** 774 (1951).
24. P. N. Craig, *J. Med. Chem.* **14,** 680 (1971).
25. P. N. Craig, *in* "Biological Correlations—The Hansch Approach" (R. F. Gould, ed.), p. 115. Am. Chem. Soc., Washington, D.C., 1972.
26. R. D. Cramer, III, G. Redl, and C. E. Berkhoff, *J. Med. Chem.* **17,** 533 (1974).
27. R. D. Cramer, III, *J. Med. Chem.* **22,** 714 (1979).
28. R. D. Cramer, III, *J. Am. Chem. Soc.* **102,** 1837, 1849 (1980).
29. R. D. Cramer, III, *CHEMTECH* p. 744 (1980).
30. G. M. Crippen, *J. Med. Chem.* **22,** 988 (1979).
31. G. M. Crippen, *J. Med. Chem.* **23,** 599 (1980).
32. G. M. Crippen, *J. Med. Chem.* **24,** 198 (1981).
33. C. Daniel and F. S. Wood, "Fitting Equations to Data." Wiley, New York, 1971.
34. F. Darvas, *J. Med. Chem.* **17,** 799 (1974).
35. F. Darvas, Z. Meszaros, L. Kovacs, I. Hermecz, M. Balogh, and J. Kardos, *Arzneim.-Forsch.* **29,** 1334 (1979).
36. J. C. Dearden and J. H. O'Hara, *Eur. J. Med. Chem.—Chim. Ther.* **13,** 415 (1978).
37. S. Deming, *J. Med. Chem.* **19,** 977 (1976).

38. D. F. DeTar, *J. Org. Chem.* **45,** 5166 (1980).
39. S. Dove, W. J. Streich, and R. Franke, *J. Med. Chem.* **23,** 1456 (1980).
40. N. R. Draper and H. Smith, "Applied Regression Analysis." Wiley, New York, 1966.
41. J.-E. Dubois, D. Laurent, P. Bost, S. Chamband, and C. Mercier, *Eur. J. Med. Chem.* **11,** 225 (1976).
42. J.-E. Dubois, J. A. MacPhee, and N. Panaye, *Tetrahedron* **36,** 919 (1980).
43. W. J. Dunn, III and S. Wold, *Acta Chem. Scand., Ser. B* **32,** 536 (1978).
44. W. J. Dunn, III, S. Wold, and Y. C. Martin, *J. Med. Chem.* **21,** 922 (1978).
45. W. J. Dunn, III and S. Wold, *J. Med. Chem.* **23,** 595 (1980).
46. W. J. Dunn, III and S. Wold, *Bioorg. Chem.* **9,** 505 (1980).
47. B. Duperray, M. Chasrette, M. C. Makabeth, and H. Pacheco, *Eur. J. Med. Chem.—Chim. Ther.* **11,** 323 (1976).
48. T. Esaki, *J. Pharmacobio-Dyn.* **3,** 562 (1980).
49. For a recent review of the Hammett equation, see O. Exner, *in* "Advances in Free Energy Relationships" (N. B. Chapman and J. Shorter, eds.), p. 1. Plenum, New York, 1972.
50. O. Exner, *in* "Correlation Analysis in Chemistry—Recent Advances" (N.B. Chapman and J. Shorter, eds.), p. 439. Plenum, New York, 1978.
51. J. Ferguson, *Proc. R. Soc. London, Ser. B* **127,** 387 (1939).
52. R. Franke, *in* "Biological Activity and Chemical Structure" (J. A. Keverling Buisman, ed.), Pharmacochemistry Library, Vol. II, p. 251. Elsevier, Amsterdam/New York, 1977.
53. R. Franke, S. Dove, and R. Kuhne, *Eur. J. Med. Chem.—Chim. Ther.* **14,** 363 (1979).
54. R. Franke, *Farmaco, Ed. Sci.* **34,** 545 (1980).
55. S. M. Free and J. W. Wilson, *J. Med. Chem.* **7,** 395 (1964).
56. T. Fujita, J. Iwasa, and C. Hansch, *J. Am. Chem. Soc.* **86,** 5175 (1964).
57. T. Fujita and T. Ban, *J. Med. Chem.* **14,** 148 (1971).
58. E. Gabler, R. Franke, and P. Oehme, *Pharmazie* **31,** 1 (1976).
59. R. D. Gilliom, W. P. Purcell, and T. R. Bosin, *Eur. J. Med. Chem.—Chim. Ther.* **12,** 187 (1977).
60. A. Goldstein, L. Aronow, and S. N. Kalman, "Principles of Drug Action—The Basis of Pharmacology," 2nd ed. Wiley, New York, 1974.
61. P. J. Goodford, *Adv. Pharmacol. Chemother.* **11,** 51 (1973).
62. P. Gund, *Prog. Mol. Subcell. Biol.* **5,** 117 (1977).
63. P. Gund and T. Y. Shen, *J. Med. Chem.* **20,** 1146 (1977).
64. P. Gund, *Annu. Rept. Med. Chem.* **14,** 299 (1979).
65. P. Gund, J. D. Andose, J. B. Rhodes, and G. M. Smith, *Science* **208,** 1425 (1980).
66. L. H. Hall and L. B. Kier, *Eur. J. Med. Chem.—Chim. Ther* **13,** 89 (1978).
67. C. Hansch, R. M. Muir, T. Fujita, P. Maloney, E. Geiger, and M. Streich, *J. Am. Chem. Soc.* **85,** 2817 (1963).
68. C. Hansch and T. Fujita, *J. Am. Chem. Soc.* **86,** 1616 (1964).
69. C. Hansch, *in* "Drug Design" (E. J. Ariëns, ed.), Medicinal Chemistry, Vol. I, p. 271. Academic Press, New York, 1971.
70. C. Hansch, *in* "Structure Activity Relationships" (C. J. Cavallito, ed.), Vol. 1, p. 75. Pergamon, Oxford, 1973.
71. C. Hansch, S. Unger, and A. B. Forsythe, *J. Med. Chem.* **16,** 1217 (1973).
72. C. Hansch, *J. Med. Chem.* **19,** 1 (1976).
73. C. Hansch, *in* "Correlation Analysis in Chemistry—Recent Advances" (N. B. Chapman and J. Shorter, eds.), p. 397. Plenum, New York, 1978.
74. C. Hansch and A. J. Leo, "Substituent Constants for Correlation Analysis in Chemistry and Biology." Wiley (Interscience), New York, 1979.

75. D. R. Henry and J. H. Block, *J. Med. Chem.* **22,** 465 (1979).
76. B. Hetnarski and R. D. O'Brien, *J. Med. Chem.* **18,** 29 (1975).
77. L. Hodes, G. F. Hazard, R. I. Geran, and S. Richman, *J. Med. Chem.* **20,** 469 (1977).
78. L. Hodes, *in* "Computer Assisted Drug Design" (E. C. Olsen and R. E. Christoffersen, eds.), p. 583. Am. Chem. Soc., Washington, D.C., 1979.
79. A. J. Hopfinger and R. D. Battershell, *J. Med. Chem.* **19,** 569 (1976).
80. A. J. Hopfinger, *J. Am. Chem. Soc.* **102,** 7196 (1980).
81. A. J. Hopfinger, *J. Med. Chem.* **24,** 818 (1981).
82. D. R. Hudson, G. E. Bass, and W. P. Purcell, *J. Med. Chem.* **13,** 1184 (1970).
83. C. Humblett and G. R. Marshall, *Annu. Rep. Med. Chem.* **15,** 267 (1980).
84. J. Iwasa, T. Fujita, and C. Hansch, *J. Med. Chem.* **8,** 150 (1965).
85. E. C. Jorgenson, R. Langridge, T. E. Ferrin, M. Connolly, and J. M. Blaney, *Abstr. Pap., Chem. Congr. North Am. Continent, 2nd, Las Vegas, Nev.* MEDI 63 (1980).
86. P. C. Jurs and T. L. Isenhour, "Chemical Applications of Pattern Recognition." Wiley (Interscience), New York, 1975).
87. R. Kaliszan, *J. Chromatogr.* **220,** 71 (1981).
88. J. Kaufman and W. S. Koski, *in* "Drug Design" (E. J. Ariëns, ed.), Medicinal Chemistry, Vol. V, p. 251. Academic Press, New York, 1974.
89. L. B. Kier, "Molecular Orbital Theory in Drug Research." Academic Press, New York, 1971.
90. L. B. Kier and L. H. Hall, "Molecular Connectivity in Chemistry and Drug Research." Academic Press, New York, 1976.
91. G. L. Kirschner and B. R. Kowalski, *in* "Drug Design" (E. J. Ariëns, ed.), Medicinal Chemistry, Vol. VIII, p. 73. Academic Press, New York, 1979.
92. B. R. Kowalski and C. F. Bender, *J. Am. Chem. Soc.* **94,** 5632 (1972).
93. H. Kubinyi and O.-H. Kehrhahn, *J. Med. Chem.* **19,** 578 (1976).
94. H. Kubinyi, *Arzneim.-Forsch.* **26,** 1991 (1976).
95. H. Kubinyi, *J. Med. Chem.* **19,** 587 (1976).
96. H. Kubinyi and O.-H. Kehrhahn, *J. Med. Chem.* **19,** 1040 (1976).
97. H. Kubinyi, *J. Med. Chem.* **20,** 625 (1977).
98. H. Kubinyi, *Arzneim.-Forsch.* **27,** 750 (1977).
99. H. Kubinyi, *Arzneim.-Forsch.* **28,** 598 (1978).
100. H. Kubinyi, *Arzneim.-Forsch.* **29,** 1067 (1979).
101. H. Kubinyi, *Prog. Drug Res.* **23,** 97 (1979).
102. E. Kutter and C. Hansch, *Arch. Biochem. Biophys.* **135,** 126 (1969).
103. R. Langridge, T. E. Ferrin, I. D. Kuntz, and M. Connolly, *Science* **211,** 661 (1981).
104. J. E. Leffler and E. Grunwald, "Rates and Equilibria of Organic Reactions." Wiley, New York, 1963.
105. A. Leo, C. Hansch, and D. Elkins, *Chem. Rev.* **71,** 525 (1971).
106. P. J. Lewi, *in* "Drug Design" (E. J. Ariëns, ed.), Medicinal Chemistry, Vol. VII, p. 209. Academic Press, New York, 1976.
107. P. J. Lewi, *Arzneim.-Forsch.* **26,** 1295 (1976).
108. P. J. Lewi, *in* "Drug Design" (E. J. Ariëns, ed.), Medicinal Chemistry, Vol. X, p. 308. Academic Press, New York, 1980.
109. D. J. Livingstone, R. H. Hyde, and R. Foster, *Eur. J. Med. Chem.—Chim. Ther.* **14,** 393 (1979).
110. J. A. MacPhee, A. Panaye, and J.-E. Dubois, *J. Org. Chem.* **45,** 1164 (1980).
111. H. Mager, P. P. Mager, and A. Barth, *Sci. Pharm.* **47,** 199 (1979).
112. H. Mager and A. Barth, *Pharmazie* **34,** 557 (1979).
113. P. P. Mager, H. Mager, and A. Barth, *Sci. Pharm.* **47,** 265 (1979).
114. P. P. Mager, H. Mager, and A. Barth, *Sci. Pharm.* **48,** 2 (1980).

115. P. P. Mager, *in* "Drug Design" (E. J. Ariëns, ed.), Medicinal Chemistry, Vol. IX, p. 187. Academic Press, New York, 1980.
116. P. Mager, *in* "Drug Design" (E. J. Ariëns, ed.), Medicinal Chemistry, Vol. X, p. 343. Academic Press, New York, 1980.
117. G. R. Marshall, C. D. Barry, H. E. Bosshard, R. A. Dammkohler, and D. A. Dunn, *in* "Computer Assisted Drug Design" (E. C. Olsen and R. C. Christoffersen, eds.), p. 205. Am. Chem. Soc., Washington, D.C., 1979.
118. Y. C. Martin, J. B. Holland, C. M. Jarboe, and N. Plotnikoff, *J. Med. Chem.* **17,** 409 (1974).
119. Y. C. Martin, "Quantitative Drug Design. A Critical Introduction." Dekker, New York, 1978.
120. Y. C. Martin, *in* "Drug Design" (E. J. Ariëns, ed.), Medicinal Chemistry, Vol. VIII, p. 1. Academic Press, New York, 1979.
121. Y. C. Martin and H. N. Panas, *J. Med. Chem.* **22,** 784 (1979).
122. Y. C. Martin, *J. Med. Chem.* **24,** 229 (1981).
123. G. K. Menon and A. Cammarata, *J. Pharm. Sci.* **66,** 304 (1977).
124. C. Mercier and J.-E. Dubois, *Eur. J. Med. Chem.—Chim. Ther.* **14,** 415 (1979).
125. H. Meyer, *Arch. Exp. Pathol. Pharmakol.* **42,** 109 (1899).
126. I. Moriguchi, K. Komatsu, and Y. Matsushita, *J. Med. Chem.* **23,** 20 (1979).
127. I. Moriguchi and K. Komatsu, *Eur. J. Med. Chem.—Chim. Ther.* **16,** 19 (1981).
128. W. J. Murray, L. H. Hall, and L. B. Kier, *J. Pharm. Sci.* **64,** 1978 (1975).
129. W. J. Murray, *J. Pharm. Sci.* **66,** 1352 (1977).
130. A. Nahum and C. Horvath, *J. Chromatogr.* **192,** 315 (1980).
131. F. E. Norrington, R. M. Hyde, S. G. Williams, and R. Wooton, *J. Med. Chem.* **18,** 604 (1975).
132. R. Osman, H. Weinstein, and J. P. Green, *in* "Computer Assisted Drug Design" (E. C. Olsen and R. C. Christoffersen, eds.), p. 21. Am. Chem. Soc., Washington, D.C., 1979.
133. E. Overton, *Z. Phys. Chem., Stoechiom. Verwandschaftsl.* **22,** 189 (1897).
134. A. Panaye, J. A. MacPhee, and J.-E. Dubois, *Tetrahedron* **36,** 759 (1980).
135. G. R. Parker, T. L. Lemke, and E. C. Moore, *J. Med. Chem.* **15,** 400 (1972).
136. G. R. Parker, *J. Pharm. Sci.* **67,** 513 (1978).
137. R. Potenzone, Jr., E. Cavicchi, H. J. R. Weintraub, and A. J. Hopfinger, *Comput. Chem.* **1,** 187 (1977).
138. G. Prakash and E. M. Hodnett, *J. Med. Chem.* **21,** 369 (1978).
139. B. Pullman and A. Pullman, "Quantum Biochemistry." Wiley (Interscience), New York, 1963.
140. W. P. Purcell, G. E. Bass, and J. M. Clayton, "Strategy of Drug Design: A Guide to Biological Activity." Wiley, New York, 1973.
141. M. Randić, *J. Am. Chem. Soc.* **97,** 6609 (1975).
142. R. F. Rekker, *in* "Biological Activity and Chemical Structure" (J. A. Keverling Buisman, ed.), Pharmacochemistry Library, Vol. II, p. 231. Elsevier, Amsterdam/New York, 1977.
143. R. F. Rekker, "The Hydrophobic Fragmental Constant." Elsevier, Amsterdam/New York, 1977.
144. R. F. Rekker and H. M. deKort, *Eur. J. Med. Chem.—Chim. Ther.* **14,** 479 (1979).
145. K. S. Rogers and A. Cammarata, *J. Med. Chem.* **12,** 692 (1969).
146. T. Rosner, R. Franke, and R. Kuhne, *Pharmazie* **33,** 226 (1978).
147. J. M. van Rossum, *Proc. Int. Pharmacol. Meet., 3rd, Sao Paulo, 1966* **7,** 237 (1968).
148. J. M. van Rossum, *in* "Drug Design" (E. J. Ariëns, ed.), Medicinal Chemistry, Vol. I, p. 469. Academic Press, New York, 1971.

149. N. Santora and K. Auyang, *J. Med. Chem.* **18,** 959 (1975).
150. L. J. Schaad and B. A. Hess, Jr., *J. Med. Chem.* **20,** 619 (1977).
151. L. J. Schaad, B. A. Hess, Jr., W. P. Purcell, A. Cammarata, R. Franke, and H. Kubinyi, *J. Med. Chem.* **24,** 900 (1981).
152. R. L. Schnaare, *in* "Drug Design" (E. J. Ariëns, ed.), Medicinal Chemistry, Vol. I, p. 251. Academic Press, New York, 1971.
153. J. K. Seydel, *in* "Drug Design" (E. J. Ariëns, ed.), Medicinal Chemistry, Vol. I, p. 343. Academic Press, New York, 1971.
154. J. K. Seydel and K.-J. Schaper, "Chemische Struktur und Biologische Activität von Wirkstoffen." Verlag Chemie, Weinheim, 1979.
155. Z. Simon, *Angew. Chem., Int. Ed. Engl.* **13,** 719 (1974).
156. J. A. Singer and W. P. Purcell, *J. Med. Chem.* **10,** 1000 (1967).
157. L. J. Soltzberg, C. L. Wilkins, S. L. Kaberline, T. F. Lam, and T. R. Brunner, *J. Am. Chem. Soc.* **98,** 7139, 7144 (1976).
158. W. S. Streich, S. Dove, and R. Franke, *J. Med. Chem.* **23,** 1452 (1980).
159. A. J. Stuper and P. C. Jurs, *J. Am. Chem. Soc.* **97,** 182 (1975).
160. A. J. Stuper and P. C. Jurs, *J. Chem. Inf. Comput. Sci.* **16,** 99, 105 (1976).
160a. J. Sufrin, D. A. Dunn, and G. R. Marshall, *Mol. Pharmacol.* **19,** 307 (1981).
161. G. Taillandier, M. Domard, and A. Boucherle, *Farmaco, Ed. Sci.* **35,** 89 (1980).
162. P. J. Taylor, personal communication (1978).
163. E. Tomlinson, *J. Chromatogr.* **113,** 1 (1975).
164. J. G. Topliss and M. D. Yudis, *J. Med. Chem.* **15,** 400 (1972).
165. J. G. Topliss, *J. Med. Chem.* **15,** 1006 (1972).
166. J. G. Topliss and R. G. Costello, *J. Med. Chem.* **15,** 1066 (1972).
167. J. G. Topliss and Y. C. Martin, *in* "Drug Design" (E. J. Ariëns, ed.), Medicinal Chemistry, Vol. V, p. 1. Academic Press, New York, 1974.
168. J. G. Topliss, *J. Med. Chem.* **20,** 463 (1977).
169. J. G. Topliss and R. P. Edwards, *J. Med. Chem.* **22,** 1238 (1979).
170. S. H. Unger and C. Hansch, *J. Med. Chem.* **16,** 745 (1973).
171. S. H. Unger, *in* "Drug Design" (E. J. Ariëns, ed.), Medicinal Chemistry, Vol. IX, p. 47. Academic Press, New York, 1980.
172. S. H. Unger and G. H. Chiang, *J. Med. Chem.* **24,** 262 (1981).
173. A. Verloop, *in* "Drug Design" (E. J. Ariëns, ed.), Medicinal Chemistry, Vol. III, p. 131. Academic Press, New York, 1972.
174. A. Verloop, W. Hoogenstraaten, and J. Tipker, *in* "Drug Design" (E. J. Ariëns, ed.), Vol. VII, p. 165. Academic Press, New York, 1976.
175. A. Verloop and J. Tipker, *in* "Biological Activity and Chemical Structure" (J. A. Keverling Buisman, ed.), Pharmacochemistry Library, Vol. II, p. 63. Elsevier, Amsterdam/New York, 1977.
176. W. Volk, "Applied Statistics for Engineers," 2nd ed. McGraw-Hill, New York, 1969.
177. M. L. Weiner and P. H. Weiner, *J. Med. Chem.* **16,** 655 (1973).
178. A. J. Wohl, *in* "Drug Design" (E. J. Ariëns, ed.), Medicinal Chemistry, Vol. I, p. 405. Academic Press, New York, 1971.
179. S. Wold, *Experientia, Suppl.* No. 23, p. 87 (1976).
180. R. Wooton, R. Cranfield, G. C. Sheppy, and P. J. Goodford, *J. Med. Chem.* **18,** 607 (1975).
181. E. Wulfurt, P. Bolla, and J. Matthieu, *Chim. Ther.* **4,** 257 (1969).
182. R. Zahradnik and M. Chrapil, *Experientia* **16,** 511 (1960).

2

Synthetic Antiinfective Agents

M. S. Tute

QUANTITATIVE STRUCTURE—ACTIVITY
RELATIONSHIPS OF DRUGS

ISBN 0.12-695150-0

I. INTRODUCTION

A. Scope

It has now been more than 100 years since Crum-Brown and Fraser (*33*) proposed that the physiological action of a molecule was a function of its chemical constitution. Since then, many theories have been developed as to the precise relationships that might be expected between biological effects and certain physicochemical parameters that characterize the constitution of a molecule.

Some of these theories have been highly successful in that they have enabled us to recognize the qualitative and quantitative significance of physicochemical properties or of structural characteristics of a molecule. When this recognition has come, it has enabled order to replace the apparent disorder of biological results, and stimulated the design of more effective drugs. In analyzing what contributions and insights have been provided by QSAR, it is appropriate to begin by surveying synthetic antiinfective drugs. The pioneering study by Bell and Roblin (*9*) of the relation between pK_a and antibacterial activity of sulfonamides; and the explanation by Albert (*1*) of the relation between pK_a, surface area, and antibacterial activity of acridines are classics of QSAR in the history of chemotherapy.

This chapter will highlight contributions of QSAR methodology to our understanding of drug action and to the rational development of new drugs by considering totally synthetic agents intended for use in the therapy of bacterial, fungal, viral, and other parasitic infections of man.

B. Expectations of QSAR

The complexity of the biological system is the most severe limitation on a successful QSAR study. If one can but eliminate pharmacokinetic factors, which include solubility, distribution, metabolism, protein-binding, etc. and study a series of molecules in a simplified (but never simple) system where the same rate-limiting event determines the response to each member of the series, then successful QSAR is probable. As the biological system increases in complexity, successful QSAR depends more and more on the degree of similarity between molecules in the series. With a highly congeneric series it is probable that all molecules will be similarly distributed and metabolized, and only the receptor interaction will vary and thus determine variation in observed response. Or alternatively, all will interact similarly with the receptor and response will vary according to distribution.

For use with a complex biological system and a series of low congenericity QSAR may be of no help in drug design because of the multiplicity of response-determining interactions. One solution to the problem of complexity is to study a very large number of compounds and to introduce several indicator variables. The study of Kim *et al.* (*77*) on 646 antimalarials acting against *Plasmodium berghei* in mice exemplifies this approach: an equation was developed having 14 terms, 9 of which are indicator variables.

An alternative solution is to develop QSAR for carefully selected subsets of compounds in isolated components of the biological system. Thus Seydel and co-workers have studied sulfonamides in a cell-free system to measure inhibition of the target enzyme, as well as inhibition of a bacterial population using both minimum inhibitory concentration (MIC) and growth rate as response and various pharmacokinetic parameters in animals. These elegant studies over the last 15 years illustrate what can be achieved by QSAR with careful attention to experimental design. Using good experimental design and appropriate physicochemical or mathematical modeling, successful QSAR can be generated.

But success is not merely the establishing of a correlation with a high regression coefficient. Success comes from recognizing the implications of the correlation or what may be termed its information content. Some QSAR publications fail to meet this criterion of success and will not be covered in this review. Successful QSAR supports, contradicts, or suggests a physicochemical mechanism for the response determining event. Interpolative prediction should be a feature of successful QSAR and may be used to suggest limiting the synthesis of unnecessary analogs predicted to have only modest activity. Extrapolative prediction is rarely accurate in a complex biological system, but the use of QSAR to make and test such predictions is surely going to further the development of the science of medicinal chemistry (*60*).

II. ANTIMICROBIAL ACTIVITY AND MEMBRANE DAMAGE

A. Optimum Log *P* and Mode of Action

A criterion of successful QSAR is that the relationship provides information of diagnostic or predictive value. The diagnostic information, particularly from model-based QSAR, is in terms of supporting or suggesting a mode of action for the drug series. When considering mode of action, drugs can be broadly categorized as "structurally specific" or "structurally nonspecific."

Drugs that are structurally specific will modify the activity of biopolymers (e.g., enzymes and nucleic acids) by interaction with specific sites on those biopolymers, known as receptors. Examples of such structurally specific antiinfective drugs are abundant, and they include antibiotics, sulfonamides, the dihydrofolate reductase inhibitors such as trimethoprim, the antimalarials quinine and chloroquine, and all potentially useful antiviral drugs. The major characteristics of such drugs, in addition to common structural features that are always present in a few compounds having the same effect, are high potency, commonly marked differences in potency between stereoisomers, and existence of competitive inhibition by related compounds.

Drugs that are structurally nonspecific also modify the activity of biopolymers, but do so either by changing the structure of the surrounding solvent without being attached to specific receptor sites, or by forming loose complexes with a variety of (rather than one particular) receptors. With such drugs activity is not sensitive to small changes in structure and is dependent on a relatively high concentration that is achieved in the biophase. Examples are anesthetics, sedatives, and hypnotics (which accumulate in nerve tissue) and many antiseptics, disinfectants, or preservatives, which appear to exert their effect by accumulating in microbial membranes. Characteristics of such drugs are that they are hydrophobic and that they are capable of making or breaking hydrogen bonds. Their effects are usually additive and never competitive.

It is of fundamental importance to distinguish between specific and nonspecific components of antimicrobial drug action, and QSAR can be used for this purpose.

Lien *et al.* (*92*) examined antibacterial data sets from 21 sources and compared the biological activity against seven gram-positive and four gram-negative bacteria with variation in hydrophobicity. From the statistically significant parabolic relationships found, a value for optimum log P, $\log P_0 = 6$ was suggested to be characteristic for structurally nonspecific agents that damage the cell membrane of gram-positive bacteria, and $\log P_0 = 4$ was suggested to be characteristic of such activity in gram-negative bacteria. The difference in $\log P_0$ between the two classes of bacteria indicated to the authors that micelle formation was not responsible for the downward trend in activity in the upper part of homologous series. If this were responsible, $\log P_0$ should depend on the type of compound and not on the organism; this is not the case.

Hansch and Clayton reviewed this work (*61*), and presented more equations for a total of 50 bacterial systems in which a parabola could best describe the activity–hydrophobicity relation. In 1977 Kubinyi (*85*) applied his bilinear model to many of the same data sets, and although his use of improved statistics allowed him to obtain rather lower log P_0 values, there is still clearly a significant difference between the two bacterial types.

In 1971 Hansch and Lien (*65*) published a lengthy analysis of 55 sets of antifungal data, again with the intention of using QSAR to distinguish nonspecific and specific activity. Some equations derived for the medicinally important fungus *Candida albicans* are of particular interest: Eq. (1)

$$\underset{\textbf{I}}{X{-}C_6H_4{-}NCS} \qquad \underset{\textbf{II}}{PhCH_2N(R)Me_2^+Cl^-} \qquad \underset{\textbf{III}}{RCO_2^-Na^+}$$

is related to the neutral substituted aryl isothiocyanates (**I**), Eq. (2) to quaternary *N*-alkyl-*N*,*N*-dimethylbenzylamines (**II**), and Eq. (3) to alkanoic acids (**III**). Log *P* in Eq. (2) refers to ion pairs and in Eq. (3) to anions. The log P_0 values are vastly different although the test system is the same. This underscores the fact that log P_0 depends to a degree on the type of compound and raises the question as to whether Eqs. (2) and (3) represent activity of a somewhat more specific kind. There are probably anionic receptors for the quaternary series and cationic receptors for the alkanoic acids.

$$\log(1/C) = 1.91 \log P - 0.19(\log P)^2 + (0.56 \pm 2.3) \qquad (1)$$

$$n = 10, \quad r = 0.936, \quad s = 0.104, \quad \log P_0 = 5.0\ (4.6\text{–}6.5)$$

$$\log(1/C) = 1.36 \log P - 0.26(\log P)^2 + (3.24 \pm 0.23) \qquad (2)$$

$$n = 11, \quad r = 0.978, \quad s = 0.199, \quad \log P_0 = 2.6\ (2.4\text{–}2.8)$$

$$\log(1/C) = -1.54 \log P - 0.64(\log P)^2 + (2.15 \pm 0.34) \qquad (3)$$

$$n = 6, \quad r = 0.991, \quad s = 0.090, \quad \log P_0 = -1.21\ (-1.3\text{–}1.0)$$

Comparing only neutral sets, Hansch and Lien (*65*) record 5.60 ± 1.0 for fungi, 5.7 ± 0.5 for gram-positive, and 4.4 ± 0.4 for gram-negative bacteria. On the basis of the "random-walk" kinetic model, the log P_0 differences between bacterial systems have been ascribed to difference in lipid content of the cell wall, which is outside the sensitive cell membrane, and is a possible permeability barrier. The gram-negative wall contains more lipid, hence was thought to be relatively more effective in slowing down the passage of highly lipophilic molecules (*92*).

In retrospect, the random-walk model is not a convincing one for most antimicrobial systems. The situation is probably better described as pseudoequilibrium, and certainly within the time span of most assays the compound will be equilibrated between compartments. The equilibrium model of Higuchi and Davis (*69*) is preferable, though no doubt too simplistic. The best model to date, judging by the quality of fit, is that of Kubinyi

(*85*). By any model, however, increased lipid content of any nonreceptor compartment would be expected to reduce the value of log P_0 if partitioning processes govern distribution.

But do partitioning processes alone govern equilibration in bacterial systems? The fine experimental work of Nikaido (*105*), who has investigated pathways for the diffusion of molecules across the outer membrane of gram-negative bacteria, has helped to provide the answer. Using mutants, Nikaido has shown that there is not only a "hydrophobic pathway," whereby a compound dissolves in the interior of the outer membrane and then crosses in accordance with the partition coefficient, but there is also a "hydrophilic pathway," whereby small hydrophilic molecules penetrate the membrane through water-filled pores. In a mutant organism with much reduced content of lipopolysaccharide in the outer membrane, sensitivity to relatively hydrophobic compounds such as phenol and the β-lactams nafcillin and oxacillin increased at least tenfold. Sensitivity to relatively hydrophilic compounds, including ampicillin, carbenicillin, and cephalothin remained the same or decreased slightly. Measurement of log P' (octanol:phosphate buffer, pH 7) showed that the hydrophobic pathway was associated with log $P' > -1.15$, and the hydrophilic pathway with log $P' < -1.7$. Any antimicrobial QSAR of compounds having log P in the region of $-1.4 + 1$ may be very severely compromised by the compounds of the set using two different routes to the receptor. The β-lactam antibiotics are clearly in this category.

B. The Relative Pharmacophoric Scale

Besides comparing log P_0 derived from parabolic or bilinear relationships, one may also compare the intercept from hydrophobicity equations. This allows direct comparison of potency between isolipophilic drugs of different type. Putting log $P = 0$ in Eqs. (2) and (3), for example, for an aryl isothiocyanate $\log(1/C) = 0.55$, whereas for a quaternary amine $\log(1/C) = 3.236$. The quaternary amine is about 500 times more potent. Using intercept values in this way, the intrinsic antifungal or antibacterial activity of different functions in isolipophilic molecules can be tentatively ordered on a logarithmic scale.

What is the significance and value of this work? Let us apply the criterion of successful QSAR: does it support or suggest a mechanism and is it in any useful way predictive?

In work with bacterial systems close parallels were observed between the equations for antibacterial activity and equations for hemolytic effect on red blood cells for the compounds listed in Table I (*62*). For those compounds there is independent evidence that antibacterial activity is a con-

TABLE I
Relative Pharmacophoric Scale

Function	Membrane perturbing ability[a]
R_4N^+	2.9 (3.2)
$RCOO^-$	2.8 (2.0)
$ROSO_3^-$	2.1
R_3NH^+, RNH_3^+	1.3 (2.0)
ROH, RCOOH, RCOOR, RCOR, ROR	0.0

[a] Figures in parentheses refer to antifungal data.

sequence of damage to the integrity of the cytoplasmic membrane (*88*), and it is fair to list average intercepts as relative membrane perturbing ability on a logarithmic scale. The average intercepts for many antifungal data sets are similar to those in Table I for antibacterial agents that perturb membranes. The QSAR strongly suggests that such fungicides bring about their action by membrane perturbation.

Some 2,4-bis(arylamino)pyrimidines have been shown to inhibit the growth of many gram-positive and gram-negative bacteria and fungi at very low concentrations. This breadth of spectrum might well indicate membrane damage. Analyzing the results of Ghosh (*53*) on Series (**IV**), Hansch and Lien (*65*) derived Eq. (4) correlating ED_{50} values against *Candida albicans:*

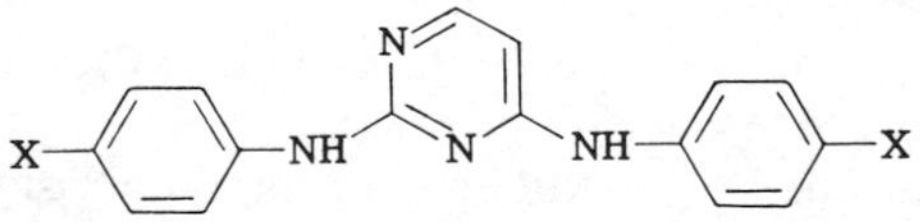

IV

$$\log(1/C) = (0.50 \pm 0.15) \log P + (4.15 \pm 0.35) \quad (4)$$

$$n = 8, \quad r = 0.957, \quad s = 0.223$$

In the light of the equations developed for compounds that act by perturbing membranes, the intercept for Eq. (4) is very high. The QSAR is therefore suggestive that the effect is not at the membrane and that a structurally specific drug effect is involved. Roy *et al.* (*116*) have provided evidence that the inhibitory activity of these compounds is exerted through interference with pyrimidine metabolism. This is an example of QSAR being used, not in isolation, but in conjunction with a framework of established QSAR in similar biological systems to suggest or support a mechanism.

These studies highlight the value of using established QSAR as a framework of reference in examining new data. There are, however, several pitfalls to such usage. First, the value of the intercept not only depends on intrinsic activity of the "function" or "pharmacophore" involved but is also sensitive to conditions of assay. Clearly the intercept will differ for different end points, for example, MIC or MBC (minimum bactericidal concentration), ED_{50}, or ED_{90}. Second, antimicrobial activity is frequently very sensitive to composition of the medium. Third, different strains of the same microorganism often exhibit wide variation in response to the same drug. Because of these variations in methodology and sensitivity, comparisons of QSAR equations must be made with great care, and interpretations from such comparison will always be tentative.

C. Case Studies

1. Cationic Detergents

Cationic detergents such as cetyltrimethylammonium bromide (**V**: R = $C_{16}H_{33}$) and cetylpyridinium chloride (**VI**: R = $C_{16}H_{33}$) are used as disinfectants and as active components of antiseptic throat lozenges. They apparently act by diffusing through cell walls, then associating with the negatively charged phospholipid components of the cytoplasmic membrane. Such association is strong, inasmuch as inhibition of bacterial growth by cationic materials cannot be reversed by washing following exposure, but washing does reverse the effect of anionic detergents (*46*). Accumulation of cationic detergent in the inner membrane leads to disorganization and lysis under osmotic stress (*88*).

Results from various QSAR studies on compounds of types **V** and **VI** do not add to our understanding of this picture of the mode of action. An optimum in chain length, or hydrophobicity, has generally been found (*61*). In many studies quaternary benzylammonium compounds have been employed. For compounds **VII**, a set in which the aromatic substituent is

$RN^{+}Me_3Br^{-}$

V

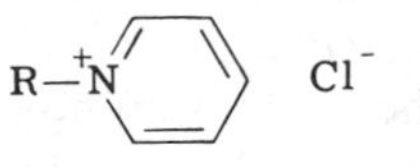

VI

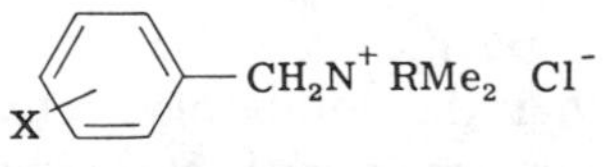

VII

varied as well as the length of chain, Murray *et al.* (*104*) compared regression of minimum killing concentration (MKC) for *Staphylococcus aureus* against log P (Eq. 5) and against first-order molecular connectivity (Eq. 6). In each equation a squared term was necessary.

$$\log(1/C) = (0.87 \pm 0.14) \log P - (0.17 \pm 0.03)(\log P)^2 + (2.93 \pm 0.16) \quad (5)$$

$$n = 45, \quad r = 0.884, \quad s = 0.306, \quad \log P_o = 2.62\ (2.45\text{–}2.82)$$

$$\log(1/C) = (4.58 \pm 0.32)\,\chi - (0.20 \pm 0.01)\,\chi^2 - (22.4 \pm 1.78) \quad (6)$$

$$n = 38, \quad r = 0.931, \quad s = 0.230$$

Statistically there is little to choose between the equations. But because the use of χ does not require the imagination of a particular physical mechanism, Eq. (6) suggests that size and shape—mirrored by χ—may be of importance in determining the limits of activity.

The studies of Tomlinson *et al.* (*127*) using benzylammonium quaternary salts and *Pseudomonas aeruginosa* are of interest. They examined micelle formation of the quaternary salts in deionized water and in simple bacterial growth media. This led them to suggest that use of high concentrations of salts in MIC tests will lower the effective concentration of the drug through micelle formation. This may be the explanation of parabolic relationships. The fact that log P_o for quaternary salts is considerably lower than that for neutral compounds disrupting membranes and that log P_o is about the same for both gram-positive and gram-negative organisms also accords with this explanation. To avoid such complications due to micelle formation, Brown and Tomlinson (*14*) later used deionized water, and studied growth inhibition by the benzylammonium quaternary salts (**VII**: X = H, R = C_{10}–C_{18}) in a series of stepwise polymyxin-resistant mutants of *Ps. aeruginosa*. Interestingly, they have now found a linear relation between alkyl chain length and the concentration required to reduce the colony count to 10% in 2 h. The authors speculated that in this system death was primarily due to damage to the outer membrane rather than the inner cytoplasmic membrane.

2. Phenols

Chlorinated phenols used in disinfectants such as "Lysol" and "Dettol" and in antiseptic soaps and shampoos are effective bactericides. At bactericidal concentrations membrane lysis occurs. At lower growth inhibitory concentrations a variety of biochemical effects occur and probably make it impossible for the bacterial cell to repair the damage to the membrane caused by higher concentrations (*28,74,88*).

Most QSAR studies of phenols have taken the data generated by Klarmann *et al.* (*78*) and expressed the phenol coefficient as PC. This is the molar concentration that is effective in killing bacteria following 10 min exposure, expressed relative to phenol. It is clearly a blunderbuss technique for compounds that have a multiplicity of effects, and one cannot expect very precise structural information to accrue by analysis of such results.

Lien *et al.* (*92*) applied QSAR to Klarmann's data on alkyl halophenols. For the lethal effect of alkyl bromophenols on *S. aureus* they derived the linear Eq. (7), and for that of alkyl chlorophenols on *S. aureus*, the parabolic Eq. (8).

$$\log PC = 0.85 \log P - 1.26 \tag{7}$$

$$n = 13, \quad r = 0.991, \quad s = 0.126$$

$$\log PC = 2.12 \log P - 0.17(\log P)^2 - 3.50 \tag{8}$$

$$n = 35, \quad r = 0.961, \quad s = 0.236, \quad \log P_0 = 6.36\ (5.98\text{–}6.94)$$

Though both equations appear to be statistically sound, we should not take them at their face value. On the argument advanced in Section II,B the intercepts can be compared and would suggest that for isolipophilic molecules a bromophenol should be about 200 times more active than a chlorophenol. Cursory examination of some data points does not support this.

Duperray *et al.* (*43*) analyzed the same data using two structural fragmentation methods, the Free–Wilson (with 31 variables) and the DARC/PELCO (with 27 topological structure descriptors). Both methods suffer from the need for an unusually large number of independent variables, and no useful conclusions can be drawn from these studies.

Hall and Kier (*57*) applied the molecular connectivity technique (*76*) to the same data set. Although 18 different variables were searched (different orders of χ and both connectivity and valence type), the best equation required only the simple first-order connectivity $^1\chi$ for a good correlation of all derivatives, Eq. (9).

$$\log PC = -21.41/{}^1\chi + (6.31 \pm 0.18) \tag{9}$$

$$n = 49, \quad r = 0.975, \quad s = 0.20$$

The equation is hyperbolic and, of course, does not allow a physicochemical interpretation. But as the authors point out, the equation is sharp enough to allow at least interpolative prediction. One form of prediction is that the contributions of a methyl, chloro, or bromo group to activity will all be equal, and this is borne out by inspection of the data. An interesting aspect of Eq. (9) is that it indicates how such features as chain branching or adjacency of atoms would influence activity inasmuch as these features are reflected in the magnitude of $^1\chi$.

One last word on the Klarmann data is in order. The error in determining the phenol coefficient (*62*) is probably about 10%, so we should not be concerned with obtaining regression coefficients better than $r = 0.95$. There are very few compounds in the set with log P values greater than 5, so that for a gram-positive organism such as *S. aureus* the vast majority of compounds should be of suboptimal log P. It was of interest to use log P values calculated on the basis of the Rekker additivity scheme and try a simple linear correlation: the result (Eq. 10) is quite satisfactory, bearing in mind the 10% error of assay.

$$\log PC = 0.75 \log P - 0.92 \qquad (10)$$

$$n = 49, \qquad r = 0.97$$

3. Nitrophenols

In the case of halophenols just described, pK_a values did not vary significantly and at the pH of the test medium these phenols would exist as neutral molecules.

Introduction of nitro groups into a phenol dramatically increases acidity. Cowles and Klotz (*30*) noticed that the bacteriostatic activity of nitrophenols against *Escherichia coli* (e.g., of 2,5-dinitrophenol, pK_a = 5.1) increases as the pH of the culture medium is decreased. This suggested to them that it was the neutral species that was the "active" form, by which they meant the form that interacts with the receptor.

Within the framework of the Hansch approach to QSAR, Fujita (*50*) analyzed the results of Cowles and Klotz after first correcting the observed inhibitory concentration (C) through pK_a and pH to derive expressions for potency if this were due solely to the neutral molecule or solely to the anion. The left-hand sides of Eqs. (11) and (12) represent potency of the neutral molecule. Equation (11) was derived for congeners at pH 5.5, and Eq. (12) at pH 8.5. The pK_a term is the difference in pK_a between the nitrophenol and unsubstituted phenol, and thus represents the Hammett effect. It is not a measure of dissociation, which is already dealt with by the transformation of the left-hand side.

$$\log(1/C) + (\log K_A + [H^+])/[H^+] = 0.34\pi + 0.70\,pK_a + 1.26 \qquad (11)$$

$$n = 8, \qquad r = 0.985, \qquad s = 0.083$$

$$\log(1/C) + (\log K_A + [H^+])/[H^+] = 0.36\pi + 0.96\,pK_a + 0.89 \qquad (12)$$

$$n = 8, \qquad r = 0.997, \qquad s = 1.213$$

Equations were also derived for pH 6.5 and pH 7.5. Increase in the coefficient of the pK_a term as pH increases was interpreted as denoting increased susceptibility of the receptor to interact with the neutral phenol molecule, perhaps by increasing ionization of a nucleophilic site on the receptor.

Martin (*94*) reanalyzed the data in terms of her model-based equations (*96*), which retain total inhibitory concentration (C) as the potency term but allow for the variable effects of ionization by constructing a very complex nonlinear function for the independent variables. She concluded that the ionic species is about 4000 times less potent than the neutral form and that binding to the receptor is not hydrophobic. The only hydrophobic binding is between the neutral species and a lipophilic nonreceptor.

In all three studies the authors came to the same conclusion that the neutral species was the important one. Only by the technique of Martin could a ratio of potencies of neutral to ionic species be estimated. There is a discrepancy regarding the role of hydrophobic binding; the equations of Fujita suggest a small degree of hydrophobic binding to the receptor, but Martin's "best fit" is to a model in which there is no hydrophobic binding to the receptor. The Fujita equation (13) for pH 5.5 in which π is not included is still of high quality, so Martin's conclusion is probably correct.

$$\log(1/C) + (\log K_A + [H^+])/[H^+] = 0.64\ pK_a + 1.28 \qquad (13)$$

$$n = 8, \quad r = 0.985, \quad s = 0.287$$

What is not immediately clear from the model by Martin is the actual nature of receptor binding. The equations of Fujita do suggest that this may occur by hydrogen bonding between a nucleophilic group on the receptor and the acidic hydrogen of the phenol.

4. Benzyl Alcohols

Hansch and Kerley (*64*) recognized benzyl alcohol as an "outlier" when constructing Eq. (14) for the activity of aliphatic alcohols against *Salmonella typhosa*. Benzyl alcohol is three times as active as Eq. (14) predicts; its inclusion in the equation drops the correlation coefficient to $r = 0.826$.

$$\log(1/C) = 0.82 \log P - 1.30 \qquad (14)$$

$$n = 7, \quad r = 0.934, \quad s = 0.098$$

Hansch and Kerley postulated that the special effect of a benzyl group was mediated through its ability to stabilize a free radical generated by abstraction of a benzylic proton. As evidence, QSAR equations were generated for sets of benzyl alcohols using the radical parameter E_R. As one example, Eq. (15) was generated for activity against three representative gram-negative bacteria.

$$\log(1/C) = (1.56 \pm 1.1)E_R + (0.58 \pm 0.11) \log P + (0.80 \pm 0.28) \quad (15)$$

$$n = 11, \quad r = 0.976, \quad s = 0.164$$

A very good equation using E_R was also generated to correlate the antibacterial activity of chloramphenicols, which are benzyl alcohol derivatives (*66*).

Kieboom (*75*) has criticized the derivation of E_R (*134*) and concluded that no justification exists for its use in the cases of radical reactions. Hence the conclusions by QSAR that benzyl alcohols react via free radicals may be in error.

5. 4-Hydroxybenzoate Esters

Esters of 4-hydroxybenzoic acid (parabens) are widely used as preservatives. They have a broad spectrum of antimicrobial activity, which probably involves damage to the cell membrane. A number of QSAR studies support the view that the cell membrane is the sensitive site.

Hansch and Lien (*65*) derived Eq. (16) for inhibition of *Candida albicans* by compounds **VIII** (X = H, R = methyl to heptyl).

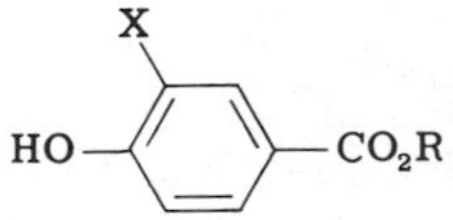

VIII

$$\log(1/C) = (0.70 \pm 0.20) \log P + (0.95 \pm 0.62) \quad (16)$$

$$n = 7, \quad r = 0.971, \quad s = 0.205$$

Hansch *et al.* (*67*) analyzed much of the early literature in terms of the model Eq. (17) for compounds **VIII** against ten gram-positive organisms, two gram-negative organisms, and nine fungi.

$$\log 1/C = a \log P + b \quad (17)$$

Averaged values for a and b indicated that hydroxybenzoates are 30 times as toxic to fungi as to gram-positive cells (b = 1.75 and 0.23); but that gram-positive cells are more sensitive than fungi to changes in hydrophobicity (a = 0.863 and 0.515).

Without doubt, sensitivity to changes in hydrophobicity reflects uptake of parabens into the cell membrane. A sensitive radiotracer technique has been used by Lang and Rye (*89*) to measure uptake of the methyl, ethyl, and propyl esters into *E. coli*. Uptake was studied at an ester concentration in the medium that reduced growth rate by 50%. It was necessary to use 5.1 m*M* methyl, 2.1 m*M* ethyl, or 0.76 m*M* propyl ester. These varying but equieffective doses gave a constant intracellular concentration of $3.5 \pm 0.3 \times 10^{-2}$ *M*/mg dry weight of bacteria.

Alexander *et al.* (*1*) have applied semiempirical molecular orbital (MO) theory (IEHT) to calculate the energy of trial conformations and their corresponding charge distributions for methyl and ethyl parabens. The calculations show a large energy difference between a stable system in which the ester group is coplanar with the ring, and a perpendicular conformation in which the ester group is at 90° to the ring plane. Despite this, they make the thermodynamically improbable suggestion that perpendicular conformations are involved at the receptor, justifying their argument by suggesting that charge on the hydroxyl oxygen (maximized in the perpendicular conformation) may be important for interaction with a positive center in the receptor. Mutual perturbation between drug and receptor certainly can occur, but in this case it seems unlikely and unnecessary. Although MO calculations can be helpful, interpretation of their meaning is fraught with problems.

6. β-Alanine Thioesters

Clifton and Skinner (*25*) have made a QSAR study of the antimicrobial activity of long chain esters of β-alanine. One may surmise that such

$$H_2NCH_2CH_2COSR$$

IX

chemically reactive esters may have a specific (acylating) activity on a particular receptor. However, for the set of nine derivatives (**IX**: R = butyl to hexadecyl, benzyl) there was a consistent "parabolic" relation between activity and chain length for all organisms (*Escherichia coli, Lactobacillus arabinosus, L. casei,* and *Pediococcus cerevisiae*). Also, when an oxygen ester or even long chain amine of equivalent lipophilicity were substituted, identical inhibition resulted. This case study clearly illustrates the value of QSAR in distinguishing specific and nonspecific mechanisms and in highlighting the importance of hydrophobicity to nonspecific (membrane damaging) activity.

III. ANTIBACTERIAL DRUGS

A. Sulfonamides and Sulfones

Many of the membrane-active compounds discussed in Section II are very potent antibacterial agents but lack that essential quality of a modern drug: selectivity. They can therefore only be used topically as disinfectants, as preservatives, or if sufficiently nontoxic as components of antiseptic throat lozenges. The first compounds to be developed with the required selectivity to be useful *in vivo* were the sulfonamides.

1. The Bell and Roblin Theory

Since the discovery of the first sulfonamides in 1935, medicinal chemists have prepared some 5,000 derivatives of sulfanilamide (**X**: R = H), in

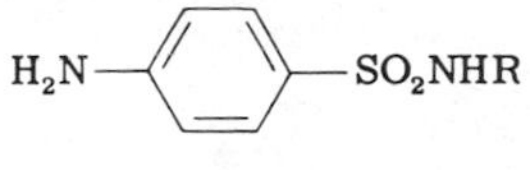

X

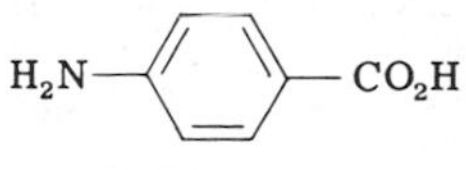

XI

the search for therapeutic advantages. Key biological features of the mode of action of sulfonamides were understood by 1940. Activity *in vivo* is proportional to the concentration in blood and activity in the bacteria results from competition with the microbial growth factor *p*-aminobenzoic acid (PAB) (**XI**). Selectivity is achieved because mammals have no requirement for PAB.

Analog synthesis soon laid the foundations of a structure–activity relationship (SAR). For antagonism of PAB a 4-aminophenyl group is essential. This is preferentially present in the sulfanilamide type of structure, but some other structures are also active. These include 4-aminobenzoyl derivatives and particularly other sulfanilic acid derivatives (**XII**) and sulfones such as the symmetrical analog dapsone (**XIII**), which is especially valuable in the treatment of leprosy. By 1942 it had been found that the

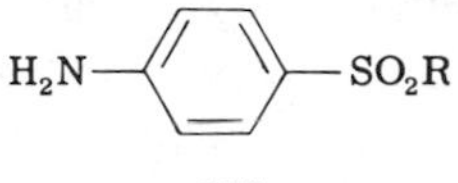

XII

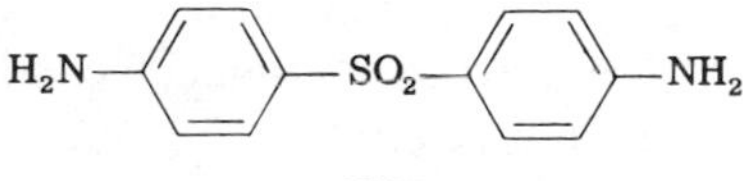

XIII

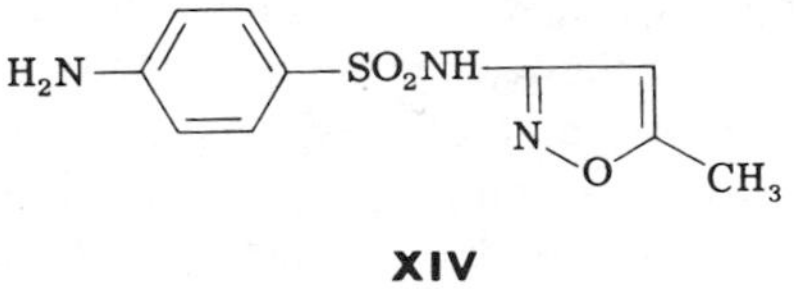

XIV

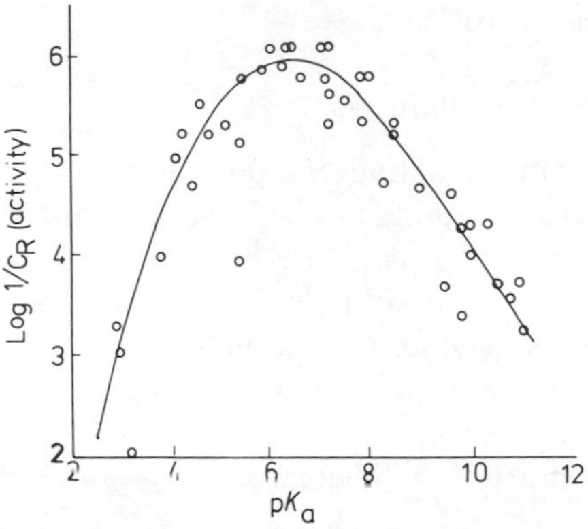

Fig. 1. Effect on bacteriostatic action of variation in the pK_a of a series of sulfonamides. Organism: *E. coli.* The substances on the left are the most highly ionized (as anions) at the pH of the test (pH 7, synthetic medium). From Bell and Roblin (*9*). Reproduced with permission from A. Albert, "Selective Toxicity," 6th ed. Chapman and Hall, London (1979).

most potent sulfonamides were those where R in **X** is a heterocyclic ring. These include sulfamethoxazole (**XIV**), today's market leader. In addition to potency the heterocyclic sulfonamides display a wide variation in pharmacokinetic properties; variations in solubility and duration of action have been made use of in choosing a sulfonamide for a particular clinical application.

In 1942 Bell and Roblin (*9*) published their classic QSAR study of a series of 46 sulfonamides. Activity against *E. coli* at pH 7 was plotted against the pK_a of the sulfonamide, over a range of pK_a values between 3 and 11. A biphasic, almost bilinear curve resulted (Fig. 1). The curve was interpreted as follows: decrease in pK_a over the range from 11 to 7 results in an increasing proportion of ionized sulfonamide; the ion is more active than the neutral species, so activity increases over this range. From pK_a 5 to 3, the sulfonamide is essentially totally ionized and yet activity does not level out but decreases. It decreases because pK_a is now a measure, rather like a Hammett constant, of electron withdrawal by R away from the —SO_2N— group of ionized **X**. The crucial property of the sulfonamide species is not ionization per se, but the charge existing on the oxygen atoms of the —SO_2— group.

The Bell and Roblin study was extremely successful because it provided a rationale for the enhanced potency of heterocyclic sulfonamides that have pK_a values near 7 and also explained the potency of some sulfonamides that cannot ionize at all as acids, such as sulfaguanidine (**XII**: R = —NHC(NH_2)=NH) and dapsone (**XIII**). In these derivatives, a large negative charge can accumulate on the $—SO_2—$ group by resonance delocalization.

2. Contemporary QSAR

The theory of Bell and Roblin was of the utmost importance and has provided a major stimulus to all subsequent investigators. Modifications to the theory were proposed by Cowles (*29*), who considered that only the anion had significant activity but only the neutral form was able to penetrate the cell wall, and by Brueckner (*15*) who differentiated Cowles hypothesis by assuming different intra- and extracellular pH values. In 1968 Seydel reviewed the earlier work and pointed out that there was then no experimental proof for the Bell and Robin theory (*119*).

Convincing proof of any theory concerning events at a molecular level in a biological system, cannot be obtained without the most careful attention to experimental design. Over the past 15 years QSAR has been used as an essential component of many such experiments.

a. Comparison of MIC with Cell-Free Inhibitory Activity. By 1962 the sequential pathway of folate synthesis in bacteria had been established, and sulfonamide shown to be a competitive inhibitor of the incorporation of PAB into dihydropteroic acid, catalyzed by dihydropteroate synthase (Scheme 1).

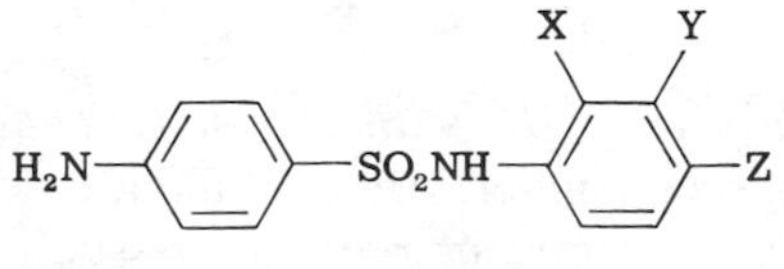

XV

Scheme 1. Reaction inhibited by sulfonamide.

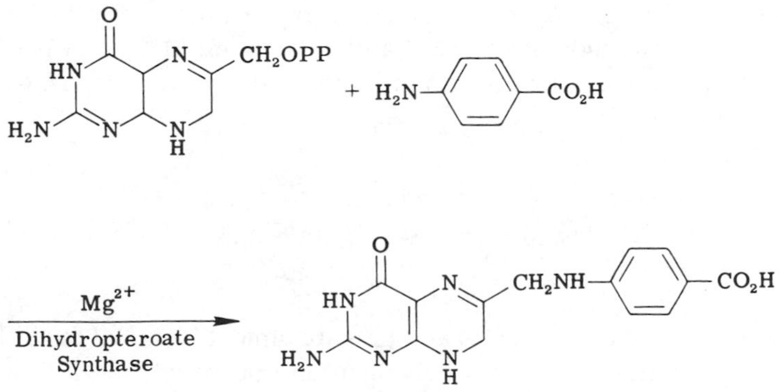

Miller *et al.* (*101*) obtained a cell-free system from *E. coli* and determined the production of dihydropteroic acid under the influence of *N'*-phenyl- (**XV**) and *N'*-pyrid-3-ylsulfonamides (**XVI**).

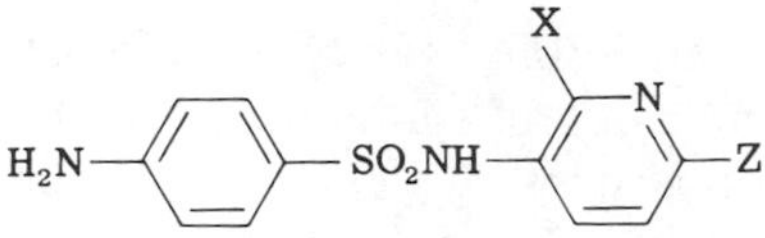

XVI

Combining Series **XV** and **XVI**, Eq. (18) correlates cell-free (enzyme) inhibition with MIC for all except five compounds. The compounds that did not fit this relationship were all less potent as antibacterials than would be expected from Eq. (18). Those compounds were relatively strong acids, having pK_a values such that they are more than 90% ionized at the pH of the test.

$$\log i_{50} = 0.63 \log \text{MIC} + 0.78 \tag{18}$$

$$n = 18, \quad r = 0.951, \quad s = 0.051$$

The equation provides good evidence that permeation of the bacterial cell is not rate limiting, except for the most acidic sulfonamides. This justifies the view of Cowles that ionized sulfonamides do not easily penetrate the cell.

b. Correlations of MIC with Physicochemical Constants. Provided that strongly acidic members are excluded, essentially linear correlations can be found with electronic parameters such as pK_a, σ, or NMR shift in sulfonamides of types **XV** and **XVI** (*52,118*). All such parameters are clearly related, and the best interpretation is that they measure the tendency to provide the more active anion at the enzyme site. Equations (19) and (20), for *E. coli* and *M. smegmatis*, respectively may be compared using compounds of type **XV** and correlating MIC with the NMR shift of NH_2 proton of the corresponding substituted anilines (*120*).

$$\log \text{MIC} = -0.89 \text{ ppm} + 5.65 \tag{19}$$

$$n = 25, \quad r = 0.976$$

$$\log \text{MIC} = -0.84 \text{ ppm} + 5.37 \tag{20}$$

$$n = 25, \quad r = 0.971$$

The regression lines of Eqs. (19) and (20) are almost identical for different bacteria, suggesting a similar mechanism and no problem with penetration. Variation in hydrophobicity has no effect, again consistent with the absence of a penetration problem, and no contribution from any nonspecific (membrane-damaging) effect.

Fujita and Hansch (*51*) attempted to deal with a mixed series of heterocyclic sulfanilamides by correcting the potency term $\log(1/C)$ for degree of dissociation. Relating potency to concentration of the neutral species, Eq. (21) was derived, and relating to the ionic species, Eq. (22) was derived, for activity against *E. coli*.

$$\log(1/C) + (\log K_A + [H^+])/[H^+] = 0.61 pK_a + 0.99 - 0.30\pi^2 - 2.09 \quad (21)$$

$$n = 17, \quad r = 0.975, \quad s = 0.223$$

$$\log(1/C) + (\log K_A + [H^+])/K_A = -0.39 pK_a + 1.01 - 0.31\pi^2 + 0.79 \quad (22)$$

$$n = 17, \quad r = 0.839, \quad s = 0.216$$

For conditions where the corrections are not necessary, that is $pK_a \gg pH$ (compounds un-ionized) or $pK_a \ll pH$ (compounds ionized) these equations are simplified to two straight line plots of activity of un-ionized and ionized molecules against pK_a. The intersection of the two lines corresponds to a $pK_a = 7$, the most favorable for this series, tested at pH 7.2.

Although Fujita and Hansch (*51*) included π and π^2 terms in their "best" equations, (21 and 22), equations in pK_a alone are almost of the same quality ($r = 0.965, 0.764$). It may be that the terms in π appear because the culture medium utilized in this study contained proteins, which were excluded from the later study of Seydel (*120*).

A similar approach to ionization has been followed by Yamazaki *et al.* (*135*) who related optimal pK_a of a series of heterocyclic sulfonamides against *E. coli* to changes in pH of the culture medium. They found that pK_o values at pH 7.4, 7.0, 6.5, and 6.0 were 7.04, 6.82, 6.52, and 6.22, respectively. This work has relevance to the choice of sulfonamide drug for clinical use in that the pK_a should apparently be close to the pH of the body fluid in which maximal activity is desirable.

The Fujita treatment of ionization has been criticized by Martin (*95*) on the grounds that it is too simplistic. In a real situation several pK_a-dependent processes can affect potency, and perhaps both ion and neutral forms can bind to the receptor. Martin analyzed a set of data supplied by Seydel of antibacterial potency measured by microbial kinetics (*52*) for a set of 24 compounds of structure **X** against *E. coli* at pH 8.00. On the basis of her equations, Martin could not decide between two models:

1. Only the ion binds to the receptor, and its effect on the receptor is not a function of its pK_a,
2. Only the neutral form binds to the receptor, and its effect is proportional to its pK_a.

The first model was preferred by analogy to the natural substrate PAB, which is an ionized molecule.

It is not clear whether the model showing activity in both ionic and neutral forms was considered; it is clear from independent study not involving QSAR that not only totally ionized but also totally un-ionized neutral species have activity at the enzyme level. Studies using QSAR methods at the level of bacterial cultures have not taken our understanding much beyond that of Bell and Roblin and still have not provided conclusive proof of molecular mechanism.

c. Correlations in Cell-Free Systems. Brown (*13*), Miller *et al.* (*101*), and Thijssen (*126*) have looked at the influence of sulfonamides on cell-free dihydropteroate synthesis. Miller *et al.* (*101*) derived Eq. (23) for cell-free activity of the Series (**XV**); including five compounds that deviated from Eq. (18) because they were substantially ionized at pH 7.

$$\log I_{50} = 0.43 pK_a - 2.28 \qquad (23)$$

$$n = 14, \quad r = 0.976, \quad s = 0.028$$

On the basis of this linear fit, they argued against the Bell and Roblin theory. However, it must be remembered that the local pH of the enzyme may be rather lower than the pH 7 of the whole-cell culture medium; for compounds of $pK_a = 6–7$ the proportion of ionized to un-ionized compound would change significantly with pK_a in the region of pH = 6. In fact, the lowest pK_a was 5.7, and for this compound there was a significant deviation from Eq. (23), the compound being highly active but less so than predicted on the basis of pK_a, in accord with Bell and Roblin.

Thijssen (*126*) reinvestigated cell-free inhibition and chose to examine a broad range of 18 sulfonamides including seven compounds in the low range of $pK_a = 2.92$ (sulfanilylcyanamide) to $pK_A = 5.7$ (sulfamethoxazole). Three totally un-ionized sulfonamides were also examined, and these also inhibited dihydropteroate synthesis. The biphasic curve between a cell-free inhibitory index, and pK_a (Fig. 2) substantiates the Bell and Roblin theory.

Dihydropteroate synthesis in the presence of sulfathiazole ($pK_a = 7.12$) was measured at various pH values. If only the ionized species is active, altering pH in order to double the percentage ionized should have the same effect as doubling the concentration of sulfonamide at the same pH.

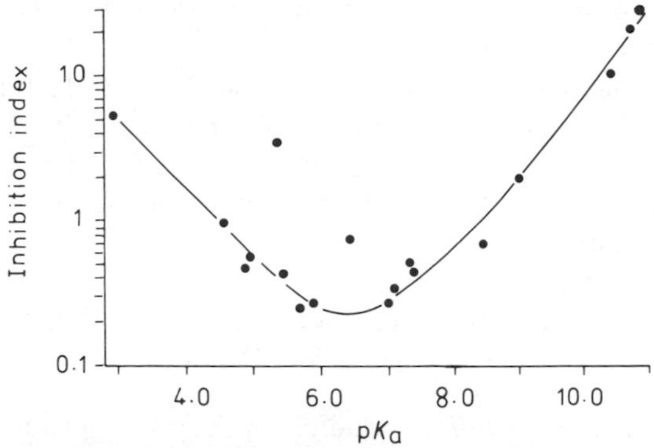

Fig. 2. Plot of the log inhibition index versus pK_a values of the sulfonamides. The inhibition index (I_{50}/S) was determined by plotting the percentage of inhibition of dihydropteroate synthesis versus the logarithm of the inhibitor concentration. Interpolation for 50% gave the relative affinity, expressed as the inhibition index, of the compound. Reproduced with permission from Thijssen (*126*).

In fact, doubling the concentration of sulfonamide gave a much greater enhancement of inhibition, showing that the un-ionized species contributes quite significantly. Comparing inhibitory indices in this paper corrected for the fraction of molecules ionized at pH = 8, one can conclude that the ionic form of any sulfonamide would be at least 20 times as active as the neutral form. Seydel (*121*) has shown that the inhibitory activity of the undissociable sulfone dapsone (**XIII**) in an *E. coli* cell-free system is about 20 times smaller than that of the most active sulfonamide.

Finally, Seydel (*121*) has measured affinities of PAB in the presence of sulfonamides (**XV**) at carefully controlled pH, expressing the affinity of PAB as a function of concentrations of ionized [SA^-] and un-ionized [SAH] fractions. Terms in both [SA^-] and [SAH] are needed for good correlation; comparing coefficients from Eq. (24) suggests a 40-fold difference in affinity between ionized and un-ionized species.

$$K[\text{PAB}] = 6.61[\text{SA}^-] + 0.17[\text{SAH}] - 1.87 \tag{24}$$

$$n = 23, \qquad r = 0.964$$

d. Spectroscopic and Theoretical Studies. Several LCAO–MO calculations have been done for sulfonamides, seeking in particular correlations between charges on oxygens of the —SO_2— group, or primary aromatic amino group, and biological activity (*19,47,83,117*). The validity of such calculations is extremely doubtful because of the gross approximations involved in treating sulfur orbitals. Conformational properties have more recently been studied using EHT and CNDO methods with explicit consideration of sulfur 3d orbitals (*20,111*). No significant correlations have ensued.

Spectroscopic evidence has supported the Bell and Roblin explanation for variation in activity of sulfonamide anions. Rastelli *et al.* (*113*) measured the infrared stretching frequency of the sulfonyl group, and correlated this with a calculated biological activity of the anion, over a wide range of sulfonamides. The stretching frequency of the S—O bond is directly related to bond order and inversely related to the formal negative charge on oxygens. High biological activity of the anion corresponded to low frequency (high polarity) of the S—O bond.

e. Chemical Studies. Studies by Seydel's group (*11,122*) have shown that sulfonamides and various derivatives of PAB will undergo reaction with the dihydropteridine pyrophosphate (see Scheme 1) and are thus incorporated into dihydropteroic acid analogs *in vivo*. However, in the absence of PAB all sulfonamides (and dapsone) studied show the same rate of analog formation despite a large variance in their inhibitory activity. Therefore the rate-determining event in folate inhibition is the competitive binding of the sulfonamide to the enzyme, and not the formation of a dihydropteroic acid analog (*121*). In the case of sulfamethoxazole (**XIV**), the dihydropteroic acid analog formed has been shown (*11*) to be inactive as an antibacterial.

3. Dapsone

Dapsone is the drug of choice for the treatment of leprosy. It is extraordinarily active against the leprosy bacillus *Mycobacterium leprae*, whereas other sulfonamides and sulfones have little effect (*45,90*). It has therefore been suggested that the antimicrobial effect of dapsone on *M. leprae* is qualitatively different from the effect of dapsone, and of related sulfones and sulfonamides, on other mycobacteria.

The QSAR methodology has been used to support and reinforce this suggestion. Colwell *et al.* (*27*) have screened a series of sulfones (**XVII**) including dapsone (**XVII**: R = NH_2) against *Mycobacterium smegmatis* 607 *in vitro*. Objectives of this study were first to see whether *M. smeg-*

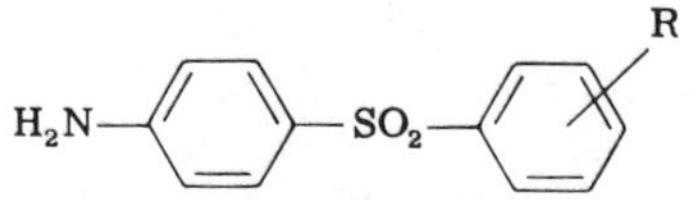

XVII

matis could be used as a model system to evaluate the potential of dapsone analogs against *M. leprae* (an organism that cannot be cultured *in vitro*) and second, to look for similarity or differences in mode of action between dapsone and other sulfones or between sulfones and sulfonamides. Bawden and Tute (*8*) applied QSAR to the results of this study. Parameters examined were σ, the position-dependent field, and resonance components *F* and *R* (*107*), and hydrophobic fragmental constant **f**.

The resulting best equation (25) contains only **R** and **f**; **R** is highly significant and has a high regression coefficient. Though the term in **f** is significant, its coefficient is small, denoting a small sensitivity to changes in hydrophobicity.

$$\log(1/C) = -1.22\mathbf{R} - 0.21\mathbf{f} - 2.22 \tag{25}$$

$$n = 16, \quad r = 0.86, \quad s = 0.31$$

The negative coefficient in *R* denotes that electron release is beneficial. The behavior is entirely analogous to that of sulfonamides, and the equation is thus diagnostic of competitive inhibition of dihydropteroate

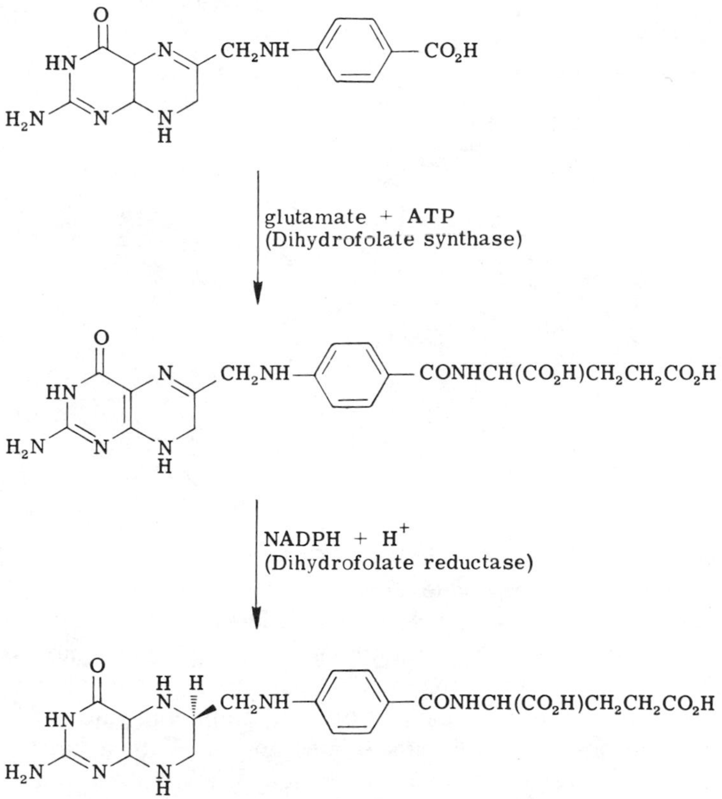

Scheme 2. Final stages in tetrahydrofolic acid biosynthesis.

synthase and charge delocalization from the substituent to the SO_2 group thus enhances activity. Activity of dapsone is high but not exceptional; clearly the action of dapsone against *M. leprae* must be qualitatively different from other sulfones or from sulfonamides.

B. Trimethoprim

After incorporation of PAB into dihydropteroic acid, folate biosynthesis proceeds (Scheme 2) by addition of a glutamic acid unit to give dihydrofolic acid. This is then reduced by NADPH to yield the essential cofactor, tetrahydrofolic acid, a reaction catalyzed by the enzyme dihydrofolate reductase (DHFR). Inhibitors of DHFR have been developed as antibacterials, antimalarials, and antineoplastic agents. A group of antibacterial agents is exemplified by trimethoprim (**XVIII**), a compound that inhibits bacterial DHFR much more effectively than the corresponding mammalian enzyme and thus provides a relatively nontoxic inhibitor of bacteria *in vivo*.

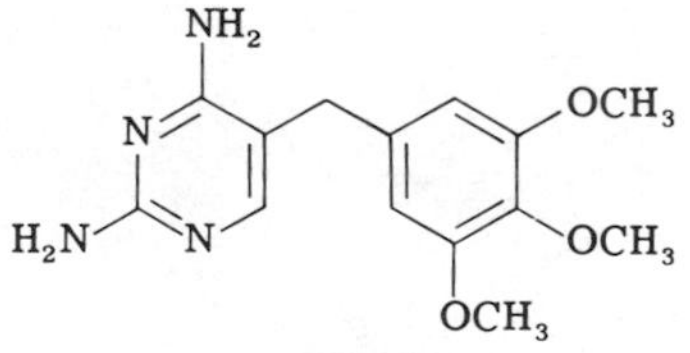

XVIII

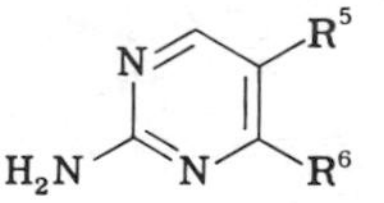

XIX

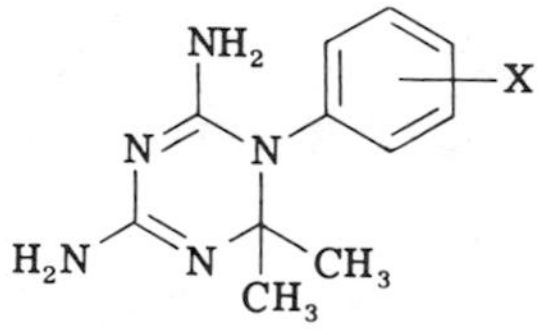

XX

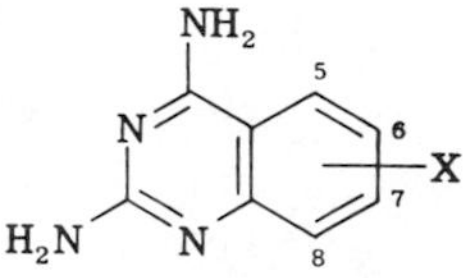

XXI

Many pyrimidines (**XIX**), triazines (**XX**), and quinazolines (**XXI**) have been screened at the enzyme level, and results subjected to QSAR analysis in the search for differential activity between bacterial and mammalian enzymes. Largely from QSAR on quinazolines crude maps have been inferred for the character of "enzymatic space" in the binding region for dihydrofolate. In all correlation equations a hydrophobic parameter for the substituent in position 5 of quinazolines appears with a large positive coefficient, so the region of space into which 5-substituents would project is characterized as hydrophobic. Such a hydrophobic pocket is inferred from the QSAR for both mammalian and bacterial enzymes (*68*). Studies with triazines (**XX**) have provided evidence that this hydrophobic pocket is larger in the bacterial enzyme than in the mammalian enzyme (*37*).

At the enzyme level there is good QSAR evidence that substituents on the benzyl group in close congeners of trimethoprim do not project into a hydrophobic region of the bacterial enzyme. Equation (26) was developed by Hansch *et al.* (*68*) for a set of congeners (**XXII**) tested against DHFR from *E. coli*. Neither π nor molecular refractivity (MR) enter the correlation, indicating neither hydrophobic nor polar contact with the enzyme. Correlation is achieved using an electronic parameter σ_R^+, which represents charge delocalization from substituents to the ortho position of the benzyl group. Resonance interaction as implied by the canonical form **XXIII** can be inferred from the QSAR as being important for high activity (binding) on the bacterial enzyme.

$$\log(1/C) = -(1.13 \pm 0.15)\sigma_R^+ + (5.54 \pm 0.19) \tag{26}$$

$$n = 10, \quad r = 0.986, \quad s = 0.182$$

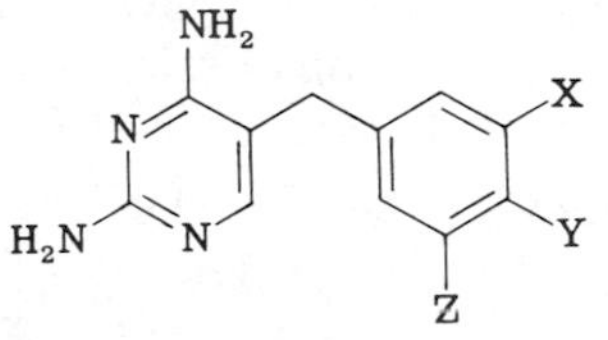

XXII

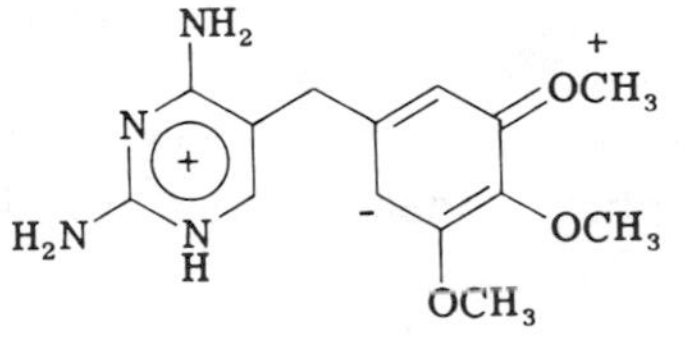

XXIII

This result was particularly exciting when considered with the work of Cayley *et al.* (*21*), who used NMR to study binding of trimethoprim to the *E. coli* enzyme. From observation of a nuclear Overhauser effect they propose that in the bound ligand H-6 on the pyrimidine ring and H-2′ (or H6′) on the benzyl group are very close to one another.

The finding could be interpreted as showing intramolecular charge-transfer stabilization of an active conformer of trimethoprim. In this conformation binding can occur through a polar interaction, which is much more effectively achieved on the bacterial enzyme than on its mammalian counterpart. This particular conformation is quite different from that determined by Koetzle and Williams (*78*) for crystalline trimethoprim. Although it seemed at the time to make mechanistic sense, Eq. (26) is now regarded as misleading. It is an example of the danger of formulating a QSAR from a set of congeners having insufficient variation in the substituents (*36*).

The extraordinary selectivity of trimethoprim results from enhanced activity against the bacterial enzyme in certain 3,4′-di- and 3′,4′,5′-trisubstituted 2,4-diamino-5-benzylpyrimidines (*71*). A 4′-OMe group is not essential for high activity, the 4′-Br analog is equiactive and the 4′-Cl analog more active than trimethoprim. Kompis and Wick (*80*) compared inhibition of *E. coli* DHFR against the Van der Waals radius of the 4′-substituent in the 3′,5′-dimethoxy 4′-H,F,Cl,Br,I,OMe series. The relation between log $1/IC_{50}$ and radius of the 4′-substituent is that of a parabola. A later paper by Kompis *et al.* (*81*) describes trimethoprim analogs with the 4′-OCH_3 group replaced by 4′-CO_2CH_3 and 4′-C(=CH_2)CH_3. The methyl ester inhibits *E. coli* enzyme to the same degree as trimethoprim; the methylstyrene analog is more potent and has a 400,000 times greater selectivity for the bacterial enzyme. These results would not be predicted from Eq. (26) and so demonstrate its unreliability.

A complete understanding of the molecular basis for selectivity of trimethoprim will probably have to await comparison of crystal structures of complexes of trimethoprim with bacterial and mammalian enzymes. The structure of the complex of trimethoprim with an *E. coli* enzyme has been determined by workers at the Wellcome Research Laboratories (5). It is clear from the quality of such studies on methotrexate (**XXIV**) that this could provide the answer and lead to a new generation of selective DHFR inhibitors. Not only crystallographic studies and QSAR, but also computer graphics modeling, have recently been used to study this problem (*91*).

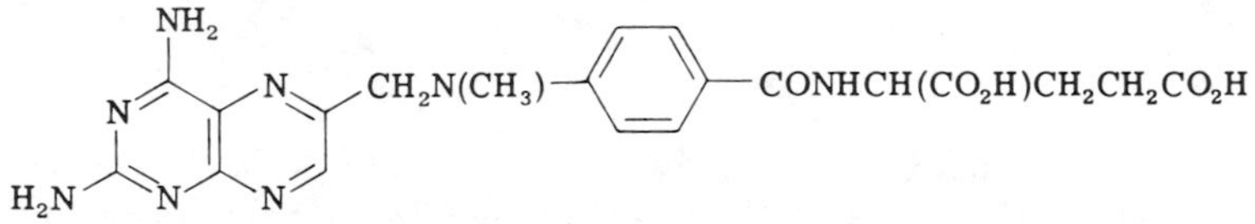

XXIV

Matthews *et al.* (*97,98*) have made an X-ray crystallographic study of the binary methotrexate–*E. coli* enzyme complex and the ternary methotrexate–*L. casei* enzyme–NADPH complex. In both cases methotrexate binds in an open conformation. The pteridine and the aminobenzoyl groups lie with their rings mutually perpendicular in two hydrophobic pockets formed by nonpolar amino acid side chains. Specific H-bond interactions to both 2- and 4-amino groups and an H-bond reinforced charge interaction between the protonated N-1 and an aspartic acid side-chain carboxyl group are in evidence. From their NMR study Cayley *et al.* (*21*) proposed that the pyrimidine ring of diaminopyrimidines (including trimethoprim) binds in the same way as the corresponding part of methotrexate, refuting an earlier suggestion of Hood and Roberts

(*72*)—based on UV spectroscopic studies—that the two rings do not bind in precisely the same location.

Gund *et al.* (*56*) and also Matthews *et al.* (*98*) suggested that the binding of the natural substrate dihydrofolate to DHFR may occur in a somewhat different manner from the binding of methotrexate. The model building experiments of Matthews showed that it was possible to turn the pteridine ring over (through 180°) with respect to the rest of the molecule while still maintaining an excellent fit. Therefore, dihydrofolate may bind with its pteridine ring in this reversed mode, thus presenting the alternate face to the NADPH coenzyme. Confirmation of this alternate binding mode for the natural substrate has now come from two sources; an NMR study (*22*) and crystallographic determination (*48*) of the absolute configuration of tetrahydrofolate prove which face of the molecule accepts the hydrogen transferred from NADPH (see Scheme 2).

Classical Hansch analysis of the antibacterial activity of pyrimidines has been carried out by Coats *et al.* (*26*). The inhibitory activity of 175 pyrimidines (**XXV**) was measured as 50% growth inhibition of *Streptococcus faecium, Lactobacillus casei,* and *Pediococcus cerevisiae*. The set included trimethoprim and seven close congeners but also many bulky 5-substituents with extra aromatic rings, chains, and bridges. Such a large variety of structures forced the extensive use of indicator variables. There

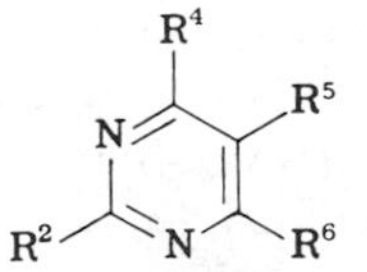

XXV

were minor differences in the equations developed for reversible inhibition of each organism. Equation (27) correlates activity against *L. casei* using hydrophobicity indices and six indicator variables.

$$\log(1/C) = 0.24\pi_5 + 0.46\pi_2 + 1.44I_2 - 1.08I_8 + 1.01I_{10} + 1.48I_{11} + 1.01I_{12} + 1.25I_{13} + 2.86 \quad (27)$$

$$n = 146, \quad r = 0.793, \quad s = 0.668$$

Indicator variable I_2 is for presence of 2-NH_2, I_8 is for bulky groups substituted on the methylene of the 5-aryl methylenedioxy derivatives, I_{10} is for 5-X—Ar where X is —CH_2— or —O— (all trimethoprim congeners included), I_{11} is for 4,6-di-CCl_3, I_{12} for benzimidazole substituents at R^2, and I_{13} for guanidino at R^2.

It transpires that trimethoprim congener activity, and especially trimethoprim itself, is significantly underestimated by Eq. (27). The equation is not very sharp and clearly reflects both the enormous diversity of the considered structures and the lack of sensitivity of a bacterial culture to molecular modification compared with an enzyme assay. Diagnostically it only provides a very crude picture of the receptor, as in Scheme 3.

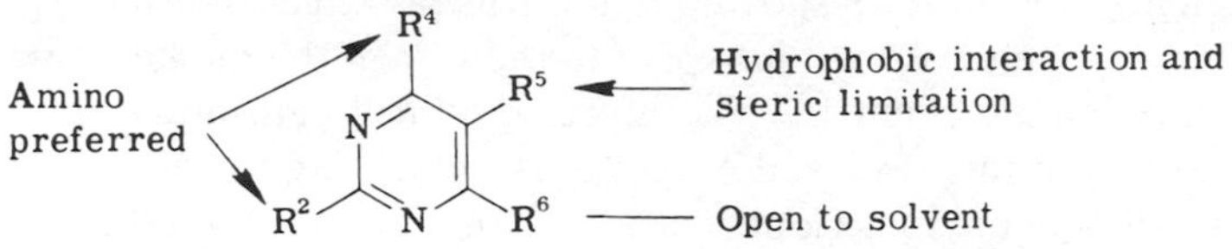

Scheme 3. Reversible inhibition of *L. casei* (*26*).

Although direct information about the receptor is crude, Eq. (27) is helpful in two ways. First, it provides order to a mass of data, allowing one immediately to recognize, for example, that there is something special about the way trimethoprim must act. Second, by comparison with cell-free studies it will enable the assessment of the influence of structure on permeability of the bacterial cell wall and membrane. Unfortunately, very few carefully designed studies at the enzyme level have been published.

A common complication of studying very large sets of compounds, exemplified by the study of Coats *et al.* (*26*), is that the set can include compounds producing the observed effect by more than one mechanism. The action of most of the pyrimidines was reversed by added folic acid, but in some cases the activity was irreversible. Irreversible inhibitors were not included in the development of Eq. (27), and they presumably act in some manner unrelated to folate metabolism. Using these data Smith *et al.* (*124*) applied discriminant analysis to classify the pyrimidines as reversible or irreversible. Applying a random selection, 20% of the data was withheld in order to provide a test of the predictive capability of discriminant functions generated from the remaining 80% of data—the training set.

Discriminant functions were generated for each of the organisms. These show that the presence of a 2-amino group gives reversible inhibition in all organisms, whereas the presence of phenyl or anilino substituents at the 6-position results in classification as irreversible against *L. casei* and *P. cerevisiae* but is not significant in *S. faecium*. Although hydrophobicity is important in determining potency in all systems, it was found insignificant in determining mode of action except for *S. faecium*, where hydrophobicity in the 2-position gives irreversible inhibitors.

Although simple, the discriminant functions were able to provide excellent predictions as tested on the withheld molecules. In the *L. casei* system, for example, the function (28) in three indicator variables correctly predicted 12/13 reversible inhibitors and 16/16 irreversible inhibitors.

$$\text{Discriminant} = 13.39I_2 - 11.70I_6 - 5.70I_8 - 7.28 \qquad (28)$$

In Eq. (28), I_2 is for 2-amino, I_6 is for NHAr or Ar at position 6, and I_8 is for bulky groups on the methylene of certain 5-aryl methylenedioxy derivatives.

C. Triazines

Walsh *et al.* (*130*) measured the antibacterial activity of dihydrotriazine antifolates (**XXVI**) against *S. aureus* and *E. coli* by a standard MIC technique. For regression analysis of the results, hydrophobic, electronic, and steric parameters were explored for a wide variety of substituents R in both meta and para positions of the phenyl ring. Highly significant equa-

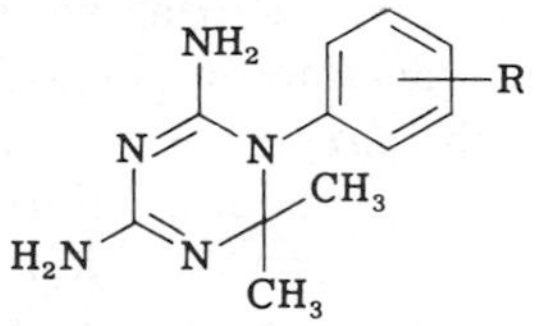

XXVI

tions were generated, showing parabolic dependence on π. The equations were not improved by electronic or steric terms; meta- and para-substituted series could be combined to give Eq. (29) for *S. aureus* and Eq. (30) for *E. coli*.

$$\log(1/C) = (1.05 \pm 0.15)\pi - (0.10 \pm 0.02)\pi^2 + 2.68 \qquad (29)$$

$$n = 52, \quad r = 0.916, \quad s = 0.466, \quad \pi_0 = 5.23$$

$$\log(1/C) = (0.74 \pm 0.16)\pi - (0.07 \pm 0.02)\pi^2 + 2.38 \qquad (30)$$

$$n = 49, \quad r = 0.852, \quad s = 0.468, \quad \pi_0 = 5.15$$

Based on a measured log P for one member of the series, $\log P_0 = 5.8$ for acting against both *E. coli* and *S. aureus*.

Taking only the meta-substituted compounds, Dietrich *et al.* (*37*) reanalyzed the data in terms of the Kubinyi bilinear model, deriving Eq. (31) for *S. aureus* and Eq. (32) for *E. coli*.

$$\log(1/C) = (0.59 \pm 0.05)\pi - (1.52 \pm 0.17)\log(\beta 10^{\pi} + 1) + (2.83 \pm 0.16) \qquad (31)$$

$$n = 23, \quad r = 0.986, \quad s = 0.218, \quad \pi_0 = 5.79, \quad \log\beta = -5.99$$

$$\log(1/C) = (0.51 \pm 0.07)\pi - (1.09 \pm 0.20)\log(\beta 10^{\pi} + 1) + (2.57 \pm 0.23) \quad (32)$$

$n = 22, \quad r = 0.960, \quad s = 0.307, \quad \pi_0 = 5.07, \quad \log \beta = -5.12$

The use of *MR* instead of π in Eqs. (31) and (32) hardly alters the quality, because of covariance between these two parameters in this particular data set. To overcome this problem Wooldridge (*132*) synthesized a few more analogs and was able to use a special highly orthogonal set of 13 meta substituents. He now found π highly significant ($r = 0.917$) but *MR* much less so ($r = 0.671$). Combining all data (meta and para) against *S. aureus*, Wooldridge derived Eq. (33).

$$\log(1/C) = 0.60\pi - 1.89\log(\beta 10^{\pi} + 1) + 2.84 \quad (33)$$

$n = 66, \quad r = 0.963, \quad s = 0.344, \quad \pi_0 = 5.86, \quad \log \beta = -6.20$

Equations (28)–(32) can be compared with an equation of Dietrich *et al.* (*37*) for inhibitory activity of the same triazines against isolated DHFR enzyme from *L. casei*. For strong inhibition in both systems, high hydrophobicity is necessary, but for the enzyme π_0 (4.03) is significantly lower than π_0 for whole bacteria. This may reflect a difference in the enzymes themselves, or the influence of a hydrophobic environment for the enzyme in the bacteria. If the 2,4-diamino heterocyclic system of triazines binds to the enzyme in the same manner as the corresponding system in methotrexate, then the equations suggest that the phenyl ring substituents interact with the same hydrophobic pocket that binds the *p*-aminobenzoyl portion of methotrexate. The X-ray structures of two triazine antifolates of potential use in cancer chemotherapy, have been determined by Camerman and Smith (*18*).

It is clear that these triazines do not offer scope for development as useful antibacterial agents. To achieve useful potency, log *P* would have to be set so high that the compounds would be strongly serum-bound *in vivo*. It was no surprise to find that none of the compounds was active against infections in mice.

D. Isoniazid

When applied to the tuberculostatic activity of isoniazid (**XXVII**: R = H) derivatives, QSAR using physicochemical parameters has provided strong support for a proposed mechanism of action. Though the mode of action of isoniazid (INH) against *Mycobacterium tuberculosis* is not yet firmly established, the "Isonicotinic Acid Hypothesis" (*84*) is very compelling. According to this hypothesis, isoniazid can freely per-

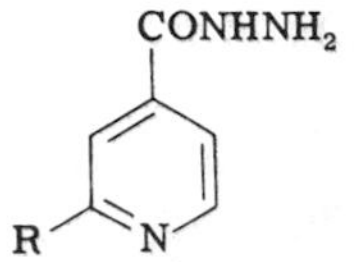

XXVII

meate into the bacterial cell by passive diffusion of the neutral species through the cell wall and membrane. Once inside, a peroxidase enzyme (specific to sensitive mycobacteria) oxidizes the hydrazide group to yield isonicotinic acid (INA), which is completely ionized (pK_a = 4.84) at intracellular pH and cannot therefore diffuse out. Subsequently, the accumulated INA is quaternized and incorporated into an NAD analog, which disturbs the normal metabolism and leads to cell death (Scheme 4).

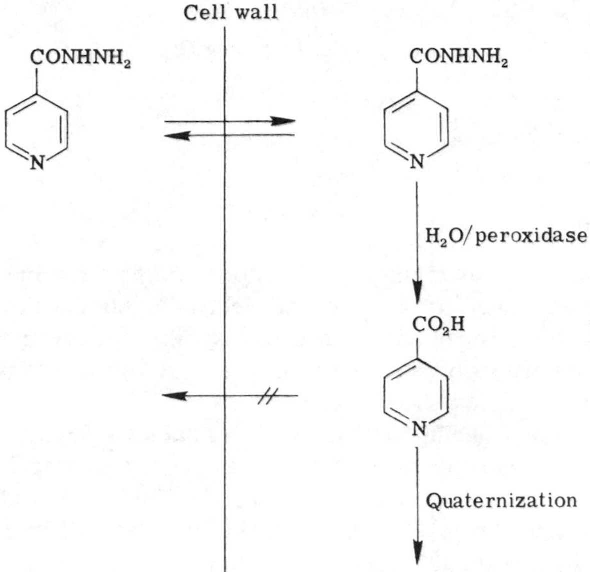

Scheme 4. Essentials of the isonicotinic acid hypothesis.

For derivatives of type **XXVII** the rate (response) determining step in the sequence is likely to be the quaternization reaction. Seydel *et al.* (*123*) have made a QSAR study of these derivatives and found that MIC values against *M. tuberculosis* and quaternization rates with methyl iodide show a similar dependence on steric and electronic effects of the 2-substituent.

Parameterization of steric effects is always problematical in QSAR; there is no generally applicable method or parameter set. Workers in QSAR frequently take the line of using whatever parameters are available for trial correlations, then justify their choice in retrospect, based on the results. Seydel explored π, R_m, Es, and van der Waals volume V_W. For most substituents in set **XXVII**, there is high collinearity between these variables. For some substituents the validity of a total bulk parameter such as π or V_W to represent directional hindrance is very questionable. Clearly, for nonsymmetrical or for conformationally flexible groups (Ph, Ch_2Ph, $CH_2CH{=}CH_2$, CH_2NHAc, for example) one must either make assumptions as to conformation and adjust the parameters accordingly or choose a subset for analysis that omits such problem cases. Using the latter technique, Eq. (34) provides a good correlation of antibacterial activity.

$$\log(1/\text{MIC}) = 0.26\text{p}K_a - 0.06V_W - 1.77 \qquad (34)$$

$$n = 15, \quad r = 0.89, \quad s = 0.45$$

On the same set Eq. (35) provides a good correlation of quaternization rates with methyl iodide:

$$\log k_{\text{rel}} = 0.29\text{p}K_a - 0.02V_W - 1.94 \qquad (35)$$

$$n = 15, \quad r = 0.931, \quad s = 0.32$$

In these equations use of the experimental pK_a is preferable to the theoretical parameter σ as a measure of the electronic influence of the R group on quaternization. The equations are very similar; the lower coefficient in V_W of Eq. (35) probably reflects the smaller size of the attacking electrophile, methyl iodide, in the model reaction.

Moriguchi and Kanada (*103*) have also analyzed Seydel's MIC data. They derived an equation to correlate 19 derivatives using V_W, F, and R as field and resonance components of the electronic effect and a dummy parameter to account for enhanced steric hindrance afforded by certain β-branched 2-substituents. Their equation is no "better" and the interpretation is the same.

Waisser *et al.* (*128*) determined pK_a and quaternization rates (with methyl iodide) for a series of 2-halo-6-alkylpyridines. As there was no correlation between rates of quaternization and pK_a, they concluded that quaternization was influenced mainly by steric approach control.

Isoniazid has been found to inhibit the synthesis of long chain fatty acids, intermediates in the biosynthesis of the mycolic acids that are important mycobacterial cell wall components (*34*). The relationship between the inhibition of mycolic acid synthesis, INA and false NAD production, and the lethal action of INH remains unclear.

E. Quinoxaline 1,4-Dioxides

The antimicrobial agent carbadox (**XXVIII**) has found use in veterinary practice as a growth promotant. Related quinoxaline 1,4-dioxides (**XXIX**) have been tested against *E. coli* and results on 78 derivatives subjected to a QSAR analysis by Dirlam *et al.* (*38*). Using the Free–Wilson method, G values were derived for contributions of 12 different R^1 substituents, 9 different R^2, and 13 different R^3. The analysis, though significant only at the

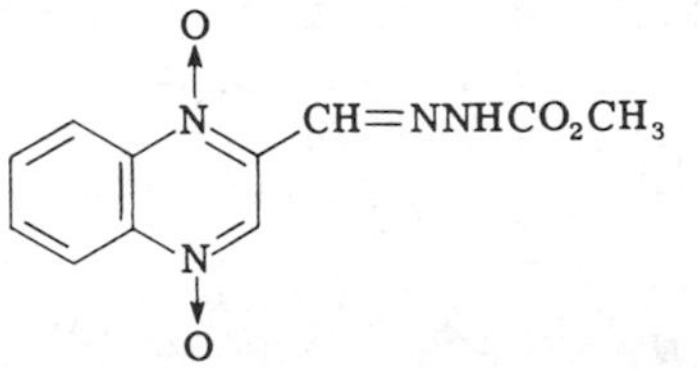

XXVIII

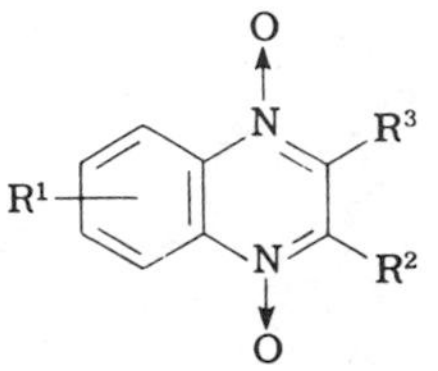

XXIX

5% level, was very useful in predicting a more potent analog that otherwise would not have been made. Although all included compounds having $R^3 = COCH_3$ had only modest activity, the analysis revealed an unexpectedly large G value for this substituent. It had previously been recognized that the substituent $R^2 = CH_2OH$ imparted high activity, so if the additivity assumptions of the Free–Wilson model still held, it was predictable that the derivative with 2-CH_2OH and 3-$COCH_3$ should be very potent. This compound was therefore synthesized as the stable hemiketal **XXX** and possessed not only potent *in vitro* but also exceptional *in vivo* activity—a triumph for QSAR.

XXX

IV. ANTIFUNGAL DRUGS

A. Imidazoles

In 1971 Hansch and Lien (*65*) published their survey of antifungal agents and formulated QSAR correlation for 55 sets of data using electronic and hydrophobic parameters. They suggested that most of these sets acted by causing direct damage to the membrane, a suggestion based on comparison of log P_0 values for similar sets acting as antibacterial, antifungal, or hemolytic agents (Section II,A). The ideal log P for antifungal activity of neutral compounds is in the range of 5–6, and for ionic species is 2–3.

Apart from griseofulvin this survey did not include any of our modern clinically useful antifungal drugs. The last ten years has seen the emergence of several imidazole derivatives, in particular clotrimazole (**XXXI**) miconazole (**XXXII**), and ketoconazole (**XXXIII**). These drugs display a marked broad-spectrum activity against dermatophytes, yeasts (e.g., *Candida albicans*), and gram-positive bacteria.

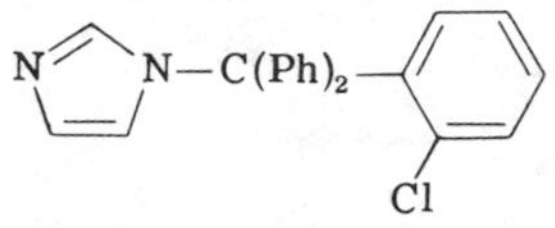

XXXI

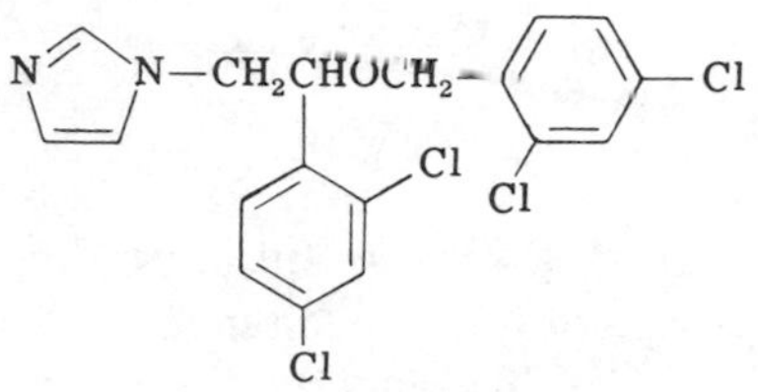

XXXII

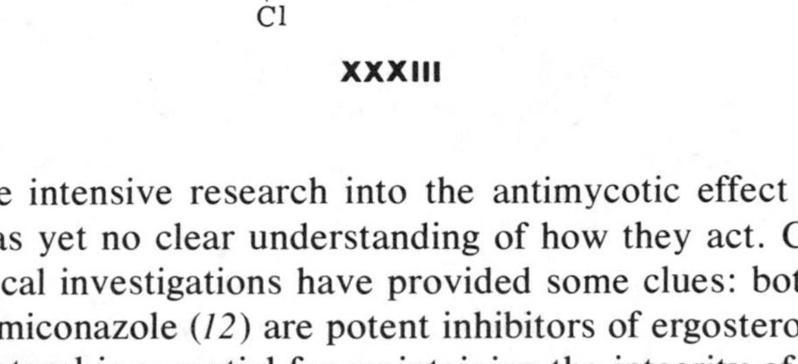

XXXIII

Despite intensive research into the antimycotic effect of imidazoles, there is as yet no clear understanding of how they act. Cytological and biochemical investigations have provided some clues: both clotrimazole (*17*) and miconazole (*12*) are potent inhibitors of ergosterol biosynthesis, and ergosterol is essential for maintaining the integrity of the fungal cell well. Differential effects occur on the behavior of oxidative and peroxidative enzymes of *C. albicans*, treated with miconazole. A fungistatic dose decreases cytochrome *c* oxidase and peroxidase activity and increases catalase activity, but all three enzymatic activities disappear on using a fungicidal dose (*106*). Yamaguchi and Iwata (*133*) contend that a direct physical disruption of the fungal membrane may be responsible on the basis of their research into the effect of fatty acids and sterol composition on the sensitivity of lecithin liposomes to imidazole antifungals.

A great many antifungal imidazoles have been screened, and QSAR techniques have been applied (*129*) but no good correlations have ensued. Buchel *et al.* (*16*) in considering clotrimazole analogs stated that QSAR was difficult because the biological data were poor due to lack of compound solubility in *in vitro* media, low diffusion rates, the compounds being fungistatic rather than fungicidal, and rapid metabolism. Despite these difficulties, a hypothesis—that tritylimidazoles act by giving rise to stabilized carbocations—was tested by applying relevant QSAR parameters. The rate constants for acid hydrolysis and R_m values were determined but were not sufficient to provide a meaningful correlation. It may be shown that steric or conformational features, which are very difficult to quantify for QSAR, are of importance to the activity. An X-ray determination of the structure of miconazole as in a tetramiconazole cobalt nitrate complex (*10*) shows that the three-ring systems lie approximately in three parallel planes. This structure may provide the key to our eventual understanding of some of the molecular features necessary for activity.

B. *N*-Hydroxypyridones

The *N*-hydroxypyridones (**XXXIV**) have been investigated by Dittmar *et al.* (*39,40*). Cicloperox, the ethanolamine salt of the cyclohexyl derivative (**XXXIV**: = C_6H_{11}) is now in clinical trial as an agent for topical use against dermatophytes.

For QSAR, biological response was measured as a reduction in the alopecia formed in guinea pigs after induction of fungal infection by topical application of a suspension of *Microsporum canis,* then local treatment by the compound. In this test the drug is presumably not subject to metabolism and excretion. Steric and electronic variation in the R group was

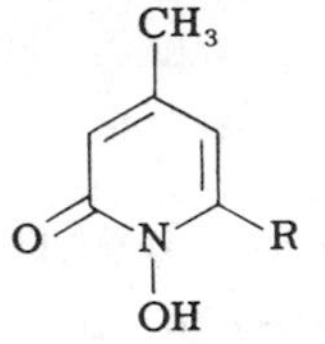

XXXIV

found to be of no consequence. Both free acids and ethanolamine salts were tested and Eq. (36) was developed. The small slope in π is unusual, but then so is the measure of biological activity: *rD* is the reduction in diameter of the alopecia measured 25 days after the infection, the drug being applied once daily from the third to the seventh day. The indicator variable D for presence of the salt is significant. The equation suggests that the rate-determining step is controlled by hydrophobicity and is probably penetration into the stratum corneum; clearly the ethanolamine salts are abut 50% more active than free acids.

$$\log(1/rD) = (0.13 \pm 0.01)\pi + (0.15 \pm 0.02)D + 1.10 \quad (36)$$
$$n = 22, \quad r = 0.983, \quad s = 0.038$$

On the basis of QSAR, the choice of cicloperox for further trial is very sound.

C. Griseofulvin

Griseofulvin (**XXXV**) is used as an oral drug to treat dermatophyte infections. Conventional SAR has shown that activity is critically dependent on the stereochemistry and that the chlorine atom is not necessary. Hansch and Lien (*65*) derived Eq. (37) for analogs **XXXVI**, the biological response being the curling of hyphae of *Botyrtis allii* relative to griseofulvin itself.

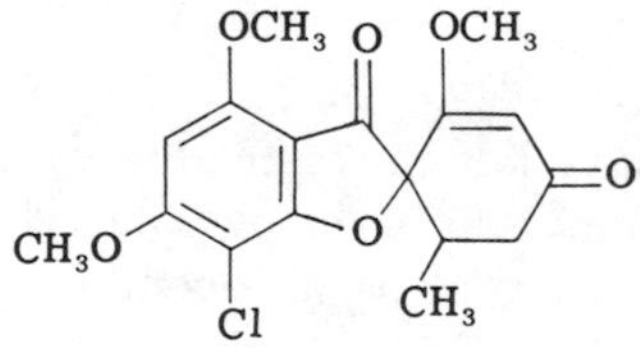

XXXV

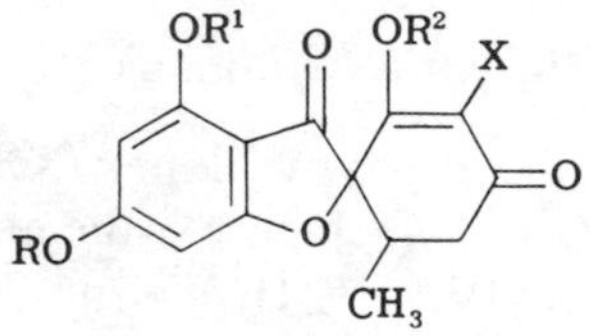

XXXVI

$$\log BR = (0.56 \pm 0.17)\log P + (2.19 \pm 0.77)\sigma_X - (1.32 \pm 0.61) \quad (37)$$
$$n = 22, \quad r = 0.875, \quad s = 0.248$$

The QSAR is not sharp, but the high coefficient in σ_X is interesting and suggests that activity may depend on reaction of the enone system, perhaps adding griseofulvin to a nucleophilic group such as SH in an enzyme involved in fungal metabolism.

D. Phenyl Ethers of Glycerol and Glycol

Phenyl ethers of type (**XXXVII**: X, Y = H, OH; R = 2-, 4-, or 5-alkyl, halogen) have been explored as topical antifungals. Chlorophenesin, 3-*p*-chlorophenoxyl-1,2-propanediol (Mycil), has been used clinically.

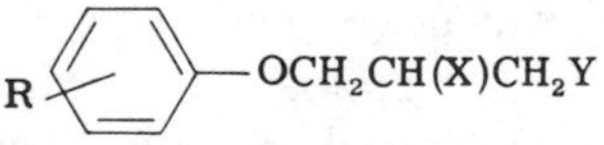

XXXVII

Hansch and Lien (*65*) derived Eq. (38) for inhibition of *Trichophyton mentagrophytes*.

$$\log(1/C) = (0.69 \pm 0.14) \log P + (0.43 \pm 0.51)\sigma_R + (1.21 \pm 0.36) \quad (38)$$

$$n = 26, \quad r = 0.911, \quad s = 0.216$$

Kubinyi and Kehrhahn (*86*) used a modified Free–Wilson method to analyze the same data, obtaining an improved correlation ($r = 0.967$) but using seven variables. The good correlation demonstrated that additivity of group contributions is fulfilled for this set, pointing to the absence of any interaction between adjacent hydroxyls (X, Y = OH, OH) affecting activity. Though both analyses indicate that X, Y = H, H would be more active, a glycerol is necessary clinically if the compound is to be free of any irritant or skin sensitizing properties.

Hall and Kier (*58*) have applied their molecular connectivity method to the data and derived three-variable equations (39) and (40) to describe activity. Both $^4\chi^v$ and $^3\chi$ terms depend heavily on specific branching characteristics and substituent patterns in the molecular skeleton; once decoded in terms of the substructures contributing to variation in these terms, the result suggests that substitution in the para position of the phenyl ring is favorable and that *vic*-dihydroxy substitution is unfavorable.

$$\log(1/C) = (2.44 \pm 0.09)^1\chi - (3.29 \pm 0.09)^3\chi + (2.71 \pm 0.03)^4\chi^v - (1.31 \pm 2.4) \quad (39)$$

$$n = 28, \quad r = 0.957, \quad s = 0.149$$

$$\log(1/C) = (1.30 \pm 0.10)^1\chi - (2.70 \pm 0.08)^3\chi + (2.74 \pm 0.04)^3\chi^v + (0.01 \pm 2.5) \quad (40)$$

$$n = 28, \quad r = 0.955, \quad s = 0.152$$

The three methods applied to this series are complementary to one another and yield information on different aspects of the SAR.

V. ANTIMALARIAL DRUGS

A. 1-Aryl-2-(Alkylamino)ethanols

Over the last 60 years many compounds have been prepared and tested in a still continuing search for drugs to combat malaria. The search has been stimulated because of developing resistance of the malaria parasites to current drugs and resistance of the mosquito to insecticides.

Compounds **XXXVIII** are analogs of the earliest antimalarial drug quinine (**XXXIX**). The aryl moiety has been varied widely, the activity of benzene, naphthalene, and phenanthrene analogs showing that a basic

$ArCH(OH)CH_2NRR'$

XXXVIII

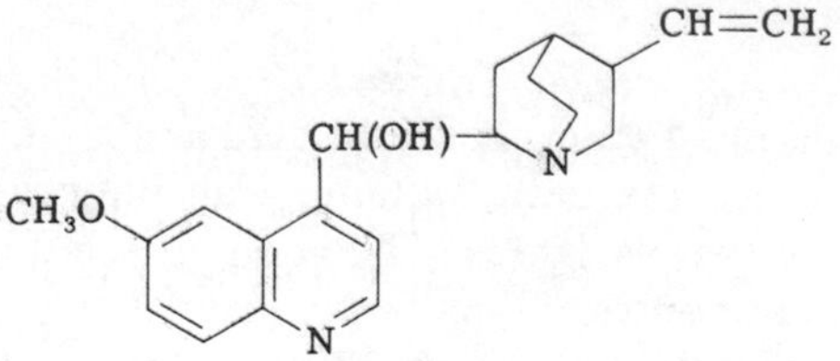

XXXIX

heteroaromatic nucleus is not essential. QSAR techniques (Free–Wilson and Hansch) were applied to 2-phenylquinolines by Craig (*31*) and to phenanthrenes by Craig and Hansch (*32*) to obtain an impressive correlation of *in vivo* data (50% cures in mice) with electronic and hydrophobic parameters. This work was noteworthy in that it showed how, by applying QSAR, the same knowledge concerning SAR could have been obtained by preparing only about half of the compounds.

In a combined study by the Hansch group, Craig, and the Walter Reed Army Institute (*77*), 60 different aryl types were included and a QSAR formulated for no less than 646 antimalarials. In order to include such a varied collection in one QSAR, it was necessary to develop an equation in 14 terms, 9 of which are indicator variables. As with earlier studies, the most important physicochemical determinant of variation in activity was found to be the electron-withdrawing ability of substituents in the aryl moiety; hydrophobic character playing a much less important role.

An interesting feature of the electronic effect is that substituents attached directly to the quinoline ring, or via the 2-phenyl group, have the same electronic effect on activity. When **XL** is compared with the currently most promising antimalarial drug, Mefloquine (**XLI**) it is noted that both have virtually identical observed and predicted activity in the mouse

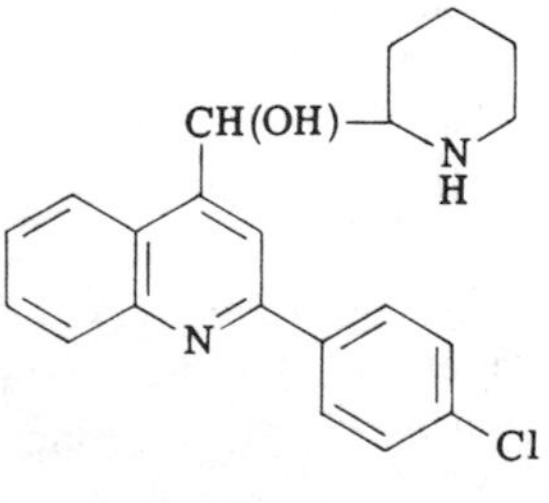

XL

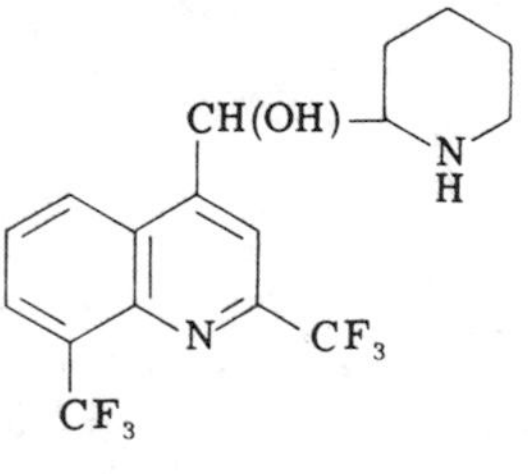

XLI

model and are 250 times more active than quinine. This suggests the importance of the drug acting as an electron acceptor or as a dipole in the drug receptor complexation.

Most forcibly demonstrated in this study is the ability of QSAR to bring some order to a mass of data. Having established this order, tentative predictions can be made for compounds having 1000 times the activity of quinine. The QSAR is not so useful in giving information on mechanism; for although the electronic effects noted are compatible with the suggestion that such antimalarials act by intercalation with plasmodial DNA, there is strong evidence that this is not their mode of action (*35*,*131*).

Ping-Lu Chien *et al.* (*23*) have investigated the effect of varying the aminoalcohol side chain in phenanthrenes of type **XXXVIII** and concluded that the basicity of the nitrogen in the side chain plays an important role in activity. They found also that diastereomers possessed different activity.

The effect of configuration and of conformation of the side chain was investigated by Loew and Sahakian (*93*). The phenanthrene **XLII** and its isomeric 3-piperidyl analog **XLIII** exist as diastereomers due to the presence of two chiral centers. All four optical isomers of **XLII** are highly active antimalarials, whereas only one racemate of **XLIII** is active, and the racemate of a 4-piperidyl analog, having only one chiral center, is inactive. Using PCILO, a study was made of the energies of likely conformations of diastereomers of **XLII** and **XLIII** in cationic forms. The study

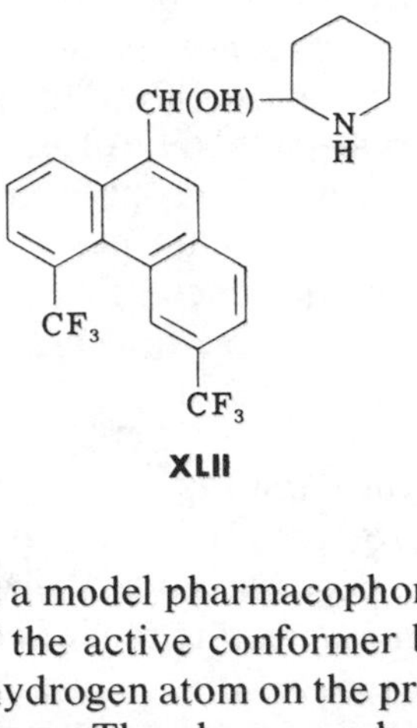

XLII

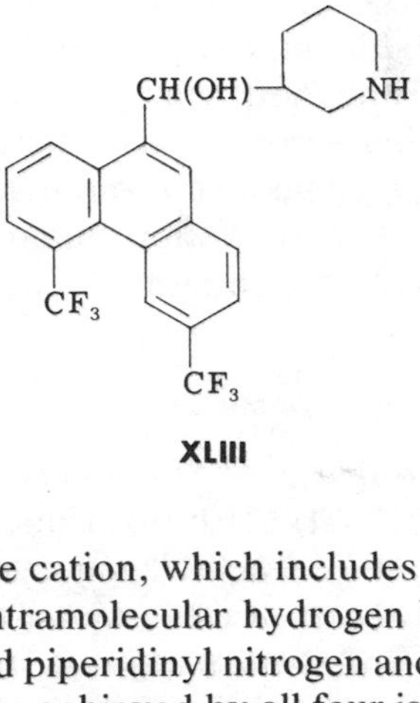

XLIII

proposed a model pharmacophore for the cation, which includes a stabilization of the active conformer by an intramolecular hydrogen bond between a hydrogen atom on the protonated piperidinyl nitrogen and the carbinol oxygen. The pharmacophore can be achieved by all four isomers of **XLII** but by only one, *RS*, of **XLIII**. The *SS* and *RR* isomers of **XLIII** were predicted to be the inactive forms, a prediction open to experimental test.

B. Chloroquine

Useful information has been obtained from application of QSAR to several series of chloroquine (**XLIV**: X = Cl) analogs (**XLIV–XLVI**) by Bass *et al.* (*6*). Parameters considered were hydrophobicities of various seg-

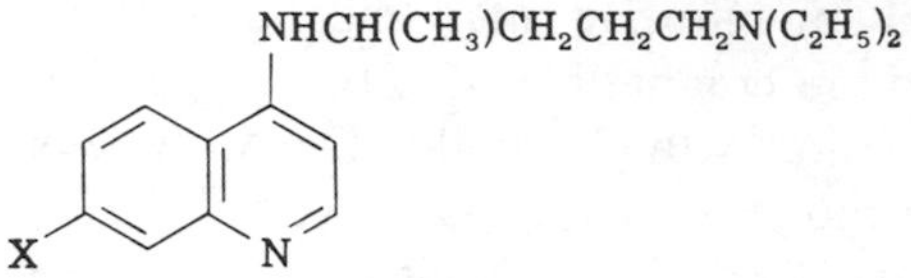

XLIV

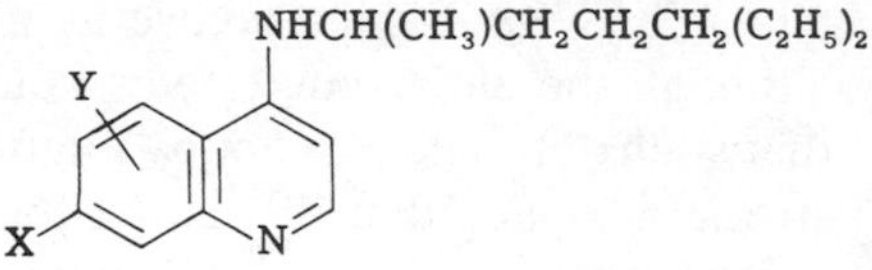

XLV

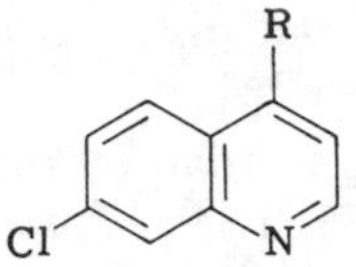

(R = NH-alkyl-NR′ R″)

XLVI

ments, and atom-centered charges calculated by semiempirical MO theory (Huckel and Del Re). The most interesting result came from Series **XLVI**, in which antimalarial activity (against *Plasmodium gallinaceum* in chicks) does not correlate with any single parameter, but when both hydrophobicity and charge on the terminal nitrogen atom are included, a substantial increase in correlation is obtained, suggesting a cooperative effect. The authors' interpretation is that the sizes of the alkyl groups on the terminal nitrogen significantly moderate the ability of the cation to participate in electrostatic binding, perhaps to a DNA phosphate group. This is compatible with an intercalation model, but it would also be compatible with electrostatic binding to any anionic receptor.

C. Arylamidinoureas

Goodford *et al.* (*55*) found that the antimalarial activity of arylamidinoureas (**XLVII**) substituted in meta and/or para positions could be expressed by Eq. (41). The equation was derived by using tabulated values in regression analysis against the oral dose required to reduce parasitemia by half in infected mice.

$$\log(1/C) = 0.28\pi + 0.86\sigma - 0.09 \qquad (41)$$

$$n = 18, \qquad r = 0.68$$

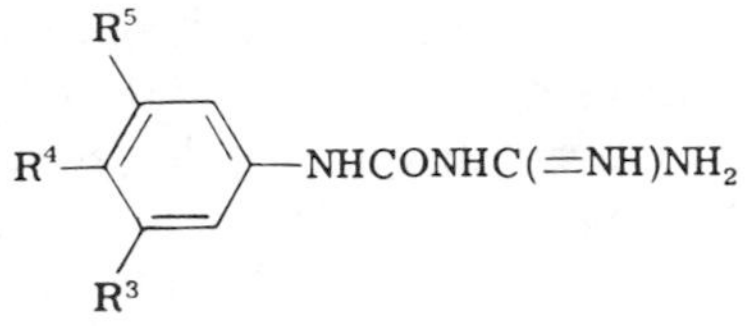

XLVII

The equation gave adequate predictions for new potent compounds despite the low overall correlation coefficient.

The same group (*54*) later examined the possibility that a better correlation would be obtained by the use of measured properties, i.e., partition coefficients, NMR chemical shifts, and pK_a values. Their study showed that the error in using published physicochemical constants could result from intramolecular steric effects. In particular, the 3-chloro-4-nitro derivative showed a large deviation from correlation, traced to the fact that the nitro group is twisted out of the plane of the benzene ring in this molecule. Such derivatives are best avoided in constructing a predictive equation.

D. Quinazolines

Hansch *et al.* (*68*) have analyzed the antimalarial activity of quinazolines (**XLVIII**) against *P. berghei* in mice, and showed that such activity is consistent with *in vitro* antibacterial activity, and no doubt results from inhibition of dihydrofolate reductase of the parasite. Of the sixty com-

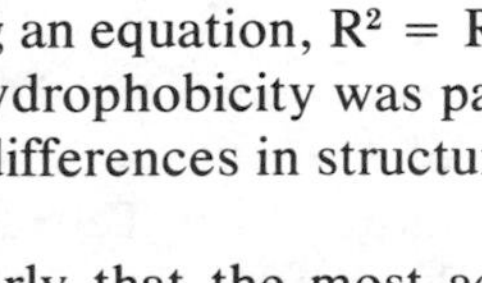

XLVIII

pounds included in deriving an equation, $R^2 = R^4 = NH_2$ for all but three (alkylamino) structures. Hydrophobicity was parameterized by the usual π (sum) and π^2 (sum) and differences in structure at R^6 parameterized by indicator variables.

The analysis shows clearly that the most active congeners have the structural features 6-N(X)CH_2Ar or 6-CH_2NHAr. Furthermore, the magnitude of coefficients shows that the unnatural bridge —N(X)CH_2— gives higher activity (better binding) than the natural —CH_2NH— bridge, as is present in dihydrofolic acid. The simple length of the bridge does not seem important inasmuch as —OCH_2— bridges were less active; the conclusion is that the nitrogen atom of the bridge is the important feature. Hydrophobicity terms allowed the optimum log P to be set at 4.0 for these congeners, a value no doubt associated with *in vivo* distribution processes rather than enzyme binding, and a useful guide for drug design.

VI. Schistosomicidal Drugs

The two most promising drugs in use for the treatment of schistosomiasis are oxamniquine (**XLIX**) and praziquantel (**L**). There are no publications concerning the use of QSAR in development of these agents or analysis of their mode of action, although oxamniquine bears some structural relationship to the earlier schistosomicide hycanthone (**LI**).

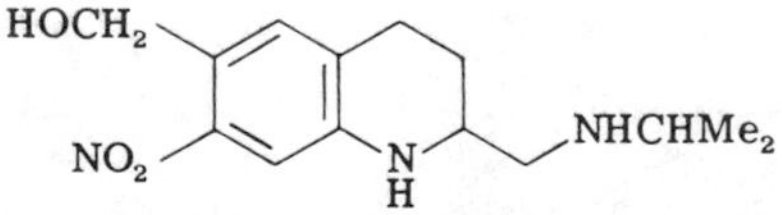

XLIX

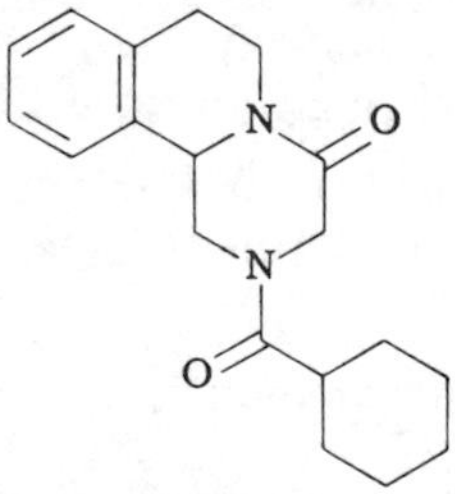

L

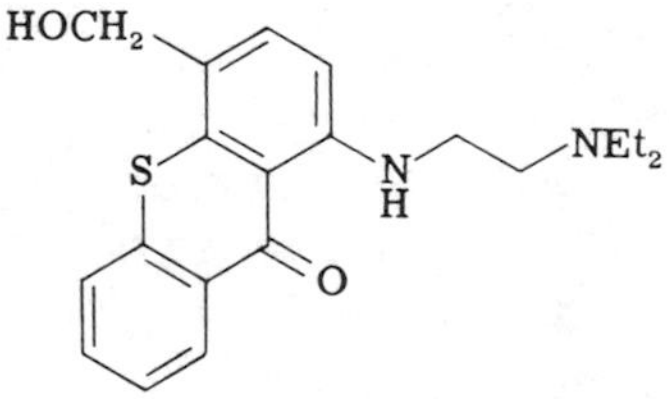

LI

Model building and quantum-mechanical calculations have been applied to an investigation of structure–activity relationships of certain nitro heterocycles, which are active. Thus Robinson *et al.* (*114*) constructed space-filling models of niridazole (**LII**) and of active and inactive analogs. They considered that the ring systems in (**LIII**) should be virtually coplanar. Also, that active analogs should have a 5-nitrothiazolyl or 5-nitrofuryl ring; with a nitrogen substituent linked to C-2 via a rigid side chain, containing either a carbon–carbon double bond or a second nitrogen atom attached directly to C-2. Aldrich and Clagett (*2*) performed

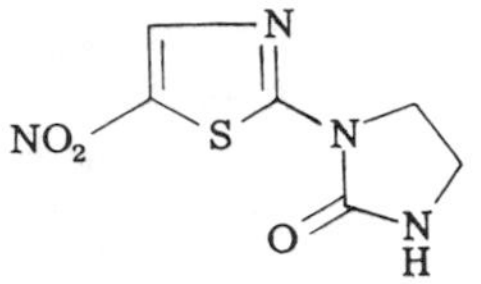

LII

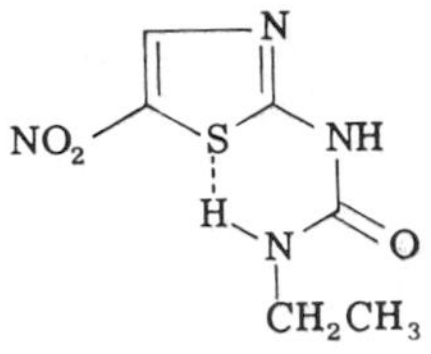

LIII

CNDO/2 calculations on various conformations of **LII** and of its inactive open chain analog (**LIII**). They concluded that **LII** preferred coplanarity of the rings, with the conformation as indicated. By contrast, **LIII** was stabilized in a quite different preferred conformation by an intramolecular hydrogen bond. This caused critical interatomic distances in **LII** and **LIII** to differ greatly and may account for the difference in activity.

Korolkovas and Senapeschi (*82*) applied quantum mechanics in searching for the mechanism of action of hycanthone (**LI**) and its analog, lucanthone (CH_3 replaces CH_2OH). Using minimum energy conformations, electron densities, and HOMO and LEMO energies were calculated by EHT. The parameters were calculated for mono- and dicationic forms. The HOMO and LEMO levels suggest that charge transfer complexation with the guanine–cytosine base pair of DNA is feasible and adds support to the intercalation hypothesis for the mechanism of action. The nitrogen atoms in the chain were calculated to be able to bind to two successive phosphate groups on the same DNA strand, and the LEMO character was found to be more pronounced with the more active drug hycanthone.

The quantum-mechanical studies both on niridazole and on hycanthone and their analogs are of course open to two criticisms; first, the neglect of solvent interaction and second, the assumption that the conformation at the receptor is likely to be the conformation calculated as the minimum. The conclusions must therefore be tentative.

The difficulties of applying classical QSAR to schistosomicides are illustrated by a study of 42 very closely related N^4-(*N*-arylglycyl)-sulfanilamides (**LIV**). Some of these compounds have considerable activity in clearing the mouse of infection with *Schistosoma mansoni*, but most are totally inactive, thus thwarting any application of multiple regression techniques despite the close congenericity involved. The compounds can be considered as two series, 20 compounds with R = $COCF_3$, and 22 compounds with R = $COCH_3$. R′ is a substituted aryl group. When R = $COCF_3$ the best compound has R′ = *o*-chlorophenyl. This compound is weak when R = $COCH_3$. In the series with R =

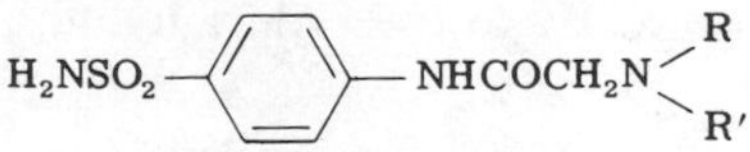

LIV

$COCH_3$, the best compound has R′ = *p*-methoxyphenyl. This compound is inactive in the other series (*73*).

VII. TRICHOMONICIDAL DRUGS

The principal drugs in use for treatment of trichomonal infections are the nitroimidazole derivative metronidazole (**LV**) tinidazole (**LVI**), and nimorazole (**LVII**). These drugs have been developed as particularly effec-

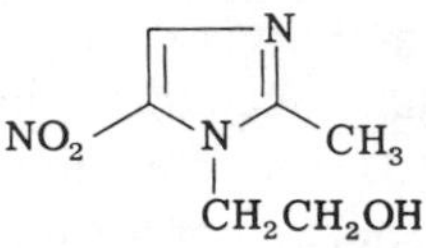

LV

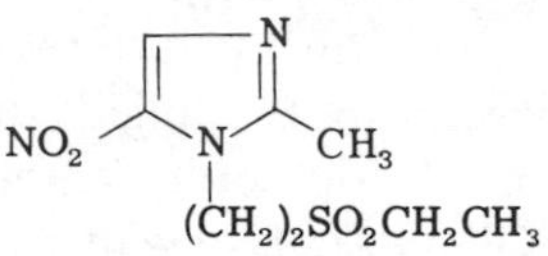

LVI

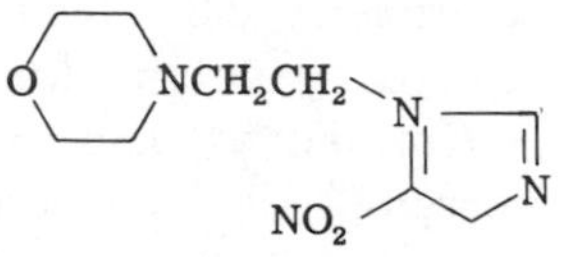

LVII

tive members of a class of antiinfective agents—the nitro heterocycles. Three major groups of nitro heterocycles can be identified: nitrothiazoles, including niridazole, used for treatment of schistosomiasis; nitrofurans used for treatment of bacterial infections of the urinary tract; and nitroimidazoles used for treatment of infections due to anaerobic bacteria and protozoa, especially trichomonads.

All postulated mechanisms of action of the nitro heterocycles involve partial reduction of the system, addition of electrons, or nucleophilic attack. All such properties are reflected in the redox potential of the system and this has frequently been correlated with *in vitro* activity (*70,112*). Kutter *et al.* (*87*) presented evidence that 2-methyleneamino-5-nitrothiazoles (**LVIII**) interfere with microorganisms "by virtue of their reducibility." The redox potential and log *P* parameters together accounted for 90% of the variation in activity *in vitro* against *Trichomonas foetus* (Eq. 42).

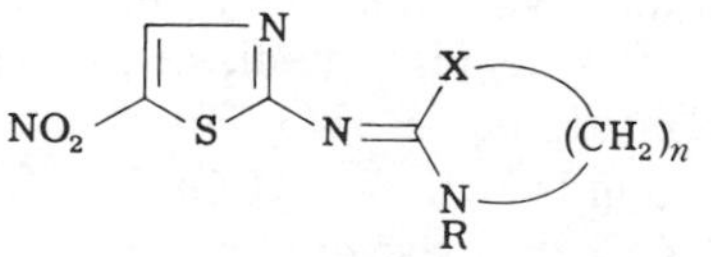

LVIII

$$\log(1/C) = (1.96 \pm 0.77) \log P - (0.54 \pm 0.28)(\log P)^2 + (20.81 \pm 6.37)E_{1/2} + (5.76 \pm 1.68) \quad (42)$$

$$n = 18, \quad r = 0.942, \quad s = 0.229, \quad \log P_0 = 1.83(1.6\text{–}2.4)$$

Chien and Mizuba (*24*) measured *in vitro* activity of metronidazole analogs (**LIX**) against *Trichomonas vaginalis* and derived the correlation equation (43) using a measured log *P* and measured activation free energy for electroreduction ΔG as physicochemical parameters. They concluded that inhibition requires a low ΔG (for reduction) and a high lipophilicity (to aid cell penetration).

$$\log AA = -0.29\Delta G + 0.35 \log P + 4.75 \quad (43)$$

$$n = 9, \quad r = 0.898, \quad s = 0.354$$

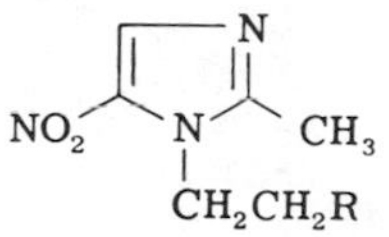

LIX

Miller *et al.* (*102*) measured the lowest oral dose of tinidazole derivatives necessary to completely prevent development of *T. foetus* infection in mice. They found for seven analogs bearing sulfone side chains, a parabolic relation between activity and log *P*, establishing tinidazole itself as having maximum potency in the series.

The mechanism of action of the nitroimidazoles against anaerobic bacteria and against *Trichomonas* has now been elucidated in some detail, largely through the work of Edwards (*44*). Active imidazoles act as an electron sink by accepting electrons from an electron transfer protein (ferredoxin in clostridia), via the nitro group. The redox potential must be less negative than that of the electron transfer protein, and this is a property of the nitro heterocyclic system as a whole. The 4-nitroimidazoles have a more negative redox potential than the 5-nitroimidazoles and are consequently inactive. The nitro group of active imidazole becomes reduced, probably down to the hydroxylamine level, yielding an as yet uncharacterized but certainly very unstable intermediate, which exerts a lethal action on the microbe by binding to DNA.

There are similar features in the antibacterial mechanism of nitrofurans. Their redox potentials are more positive than nitroimidazoles and are not in the range necessary for reduction by anaerobes. But specific nitroreductases are present in aerobic bacteria, and these enzymes will reduce nitrofurans to yield unstable intermediates that then react with DNA, causing strand breakage (*100*).

Inhibition of DNA synthesis by nitro heterocycles has been correlated with half-wave reduction potential (*108*). 4-Nitroimidazole, and various furans and thiazoles lacking the nitro group, showed no inhibition of DNA synthesis.

Overshadowing all nitro heterocycles are their mutagenic properties and carcinogenic potential. Metronidazole and some of its metabolites in humans are mutagens in bacteria when a reductive step is included in the Ames test (*115*). This may be irrelevant to human usage of the drug because mammalian cells are unable to reduce it. Nevertheless, the underlying fear of carcinogenic potential has encouraged the search for safer "nitro surrogates" by replacing the nitro group with groups of similar electron-withdrawing potential. The QSAR studies indicate this to be futile.

VIII. ANTIVIRAL DRUGS

The application of QSAR to antiviral agents has been very disappointing. Given the unique problem of evaluating antiviral agents, it is not surprising that no useful diagnostic or predictive information has accrued from the few published studies. Antiviral chemotherapy poses a unique problem in that the virus is an obligate intracellular parasite, dependent on the integrity of the host cell for its own survival and multiplication. Any compound that damages the host cell can produce an "antiviral" effect. As a consequence the few potentially useful antiviral compounds that are known and that interfere directly and selectively with viral replication (*99*) have a narrow structure–activity relationship, unsuitable for application of QSAR. By contrast, classes of compounds with a wider SAR probably produce their "antiviral" activity by simultaneous interference with both cellular and viral processes, and in such classes it is the absence of a single rate (response) determining step that precludes successful correlations.

Among the first selective inhibitors of intracellular viral replication to be discovered were 2-(α-hydroxybenzyl)benzimidazole and certain derivatives (**LX**). These compounds inhibit poliovirus replication (*109*). O'Sul-

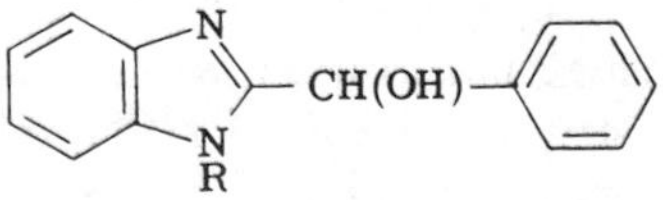

LX

livan *et al.* (*109,110*) noticed a rough parallelism between activity and Hansch π value for the 1-substituent. Activity peaked with R = Ph, but any fit to a parabola was poor. Factors other than lipophilicity operate and have not been defined.

Benzimidazole derivatives have been intensively investigated for antiviral effects. Tamm *et al.* (*125*) reported activity against influenza B virus multiplication for alkyl derivatives (**LXI**), and Hansch (*59*) correlated the activity with a calculated log *P*, to derive Eq. (44).

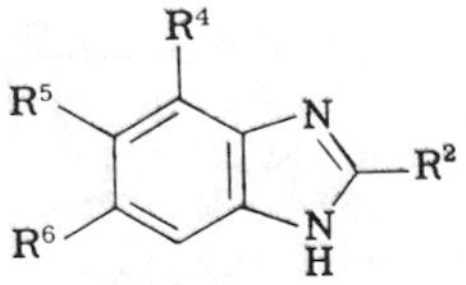

LXI

$$\log(1/C) = (0.58 \pm 0.17) \log P + (1.58 \pm 0.46) \qquad (44)$$

$$n = 15, \quad r = 0.903, \quad s = 0.210$$

Hansch commented that the slope of Eq. (44) was indicative of nonspecific binding to a protein-like receptor and that the intercept was indicative of a weak activity for the benzimidazole functionality. Hall and Kier (*58*) analyzed the same data using their molecular connectivity approach, and examined twenty different chi indices. The "best" onc parameter correlation, that of Eq. (45) predicts that a branched or cyclic alkyl substituent in position 2 would enhance activity relative to a straight chain analog. Unfortunately, only one compound with a branched 2-substituent was included in the data set, and this interesting prediction will probably remain untested.

$$\log(1/C) = (1.40 \pm 0.02)^6\chi + (1.11 \pm 0.29) \qquad (45)$$

$$n = 15, \quad r = 0.950, \quad s = 0.166$$

Bauer and Sadler (*7*) have exploited isatin thiosemicarbazones (**LXII**) a series of compounds with specific activity against vaccinia virus. One derivative, marboran (**LXII**: $R^1 = CH_3$; $R^2 = H$), is quite effective against smallpox in humans. Franke (*49*) applied QSAR to the results of

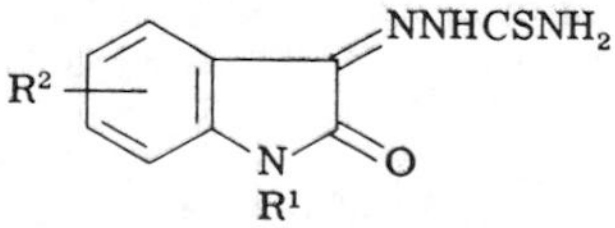

LXII

Bauer and Sadler using standard steric, electronic, and hydrophobic parameters. Using subsets of data, equations were derived with high correlation coefficients but very low statistical significance. Such equations are not reliable.

The unusual sterically hindered amine adamantanamine (**LXIII**) is now marketed as "Symmetrel" and is useful for the prophylaxis of certain types of influenza. It apparently interferes with an early stage in the viral replication cycle, either blocking penetration of virus into the cell or inhibiting removal of its protein coat. This property is shared in varying degree by many other related compounds. Aldrich *et al.* (*3*) have compared

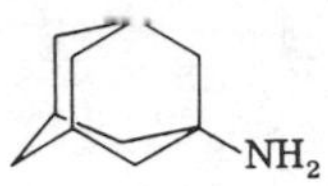

LXIII

the results of activity in mice against influenza A of 87 compounds related to adamantanamine, including *N*- and *C*-alkylated 1-adamantanamines and 1-adamantanemethylamines. No QSAR was attempted. The data should be amenable to discriminate analysis, but because it is clear that no N-substituted derivatives are significantly more active than adamantanamine itself, it is doubtful whether this would prove useful. Dubois *et al.* (*42*) applied the DARC/PELCO treatment to some of the results, providing a rationalization and ordering of the set but no diagnostic information or extrapolative prediction.

The most exciting antiviral agent in prospect at present is ribavirin (**LXIV**). This compound owes its activity to a competitive inhibition of the enzyme inosine monophosphate dehydrogenase, which has an important function only in infected cells. Very close analogs and derivatives have very little or no activity either because they cannot be phosphorylated to the active 5′-phosphate or because they do not achieve the precise fit necessary for competitive inhibition (*41*). Classical QSAR studies have no place in dealing with such restricted specificity.

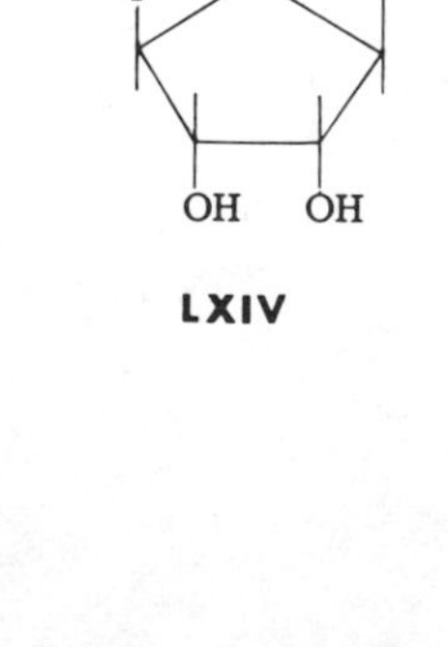

LXIV

IX. OVERVIEW

The application of QSAR methods to the analysis of cell culture or of whole animal data on series of antiinfective agents has frequently provided statistically acceptable correlation equations. The equations generally have proved to be useful only when physicochemical parameters have been employed. They have then provided a framework of reference by which to judge the advisability of synthesis of further analogs, complementing classical medicinal–chemical approaches, and they have frequently given support to theories about the mode of action at the receptor level or insight into the physical properties (ionization state or lipophilicity) required to facilitate drug transport. Most of the successes have come from antibacterial data analysis; there are formidable problems associated with meaningful assay of many other organisms, in particular with viruses and fungi.

In the last five years there has been an admirable trend toward much more careful experimental design of QSAR investigations, in order to avoid statistical pitfalls, and toward obtaining maximum diagnostic and predictive information. Even so, it must be recognized that there is a limit to the information obtainable by the classical regression analysis technique using linear free-energy related or indicator variables. Useful but only crude ideas of electronic, hydrophobic, or steric requirements of the mysterious (usually unidentified) receptor can be obtained. Many more studies at the cell-free, enzyme level (not covered in this chapter) are required to complement and extend studies at the cellular or whole animal level. Much more attention should be given to quantifying the effects of size, shape, and conformation. We can then expect much greater insight into the mode of action of antiinfective agents, and this insight can be used in the design of the novel selective drugs of the future.

REFERENCES

1. A. Albert, "The Acridines." Arnold, London, 1966.
2. H. S. Aldrich and D. C. Clagett, *J. Pharm. Sci.* **65,** 1704 (1976).
3. P. E. Aldrich, E. C. Hermann, W. E. Meier, M. Paulshock, W. W. Pritchard, J. A. Snyder, and J. C. Watts, *J. Med. Chem.*, **14,** 535 (1971).
4. K. S. Alexander, H. Peterson, J. G. Turcotte, and A. N. Paruta, *J. Pharm. Sci.* **65,** 851 (1976).
5. D. J. Baker, C. R. Beddell, J. N. Champness, P. J. Goodford, F. E. A. Norrington, D. R. Smith, and D. K. Stammers, *FEBS Lett.* **126,** 49 (1981).
6. G. E. Bass, D. R. Hudson, J. E. Parker, and W. P. Purcell, *J. Med. Chem.* **14,** 275 (1971).
7. D. J. Bauer and P. W. Sadler, *Br. J. Pharmacol. Chemother.* **15,** 101 (1960).

8. D. Bawden and M. S. Tute, *Eur. J. Med. Chem.—Chim. Ther.* **16,** 299 (1981).
9. P. H. Bell and R. O. Roblin, *J. Am. Chem. Soc.* **64,** 2905 (1942).
10. N. M. Blaton, O. M. Peeters, and C. J. De Ranter, *Acta Crystallogr., Sect. B* **34,** 1854 (1978).
11. L. Bock, G. H. Miller, K. J. Schaper, and J. K. Seydel, *J. Med. Chem.* **17,** 23 (1974).
12. H. van der Bossche, G. Willemsens, W. Cools, W. F. J. Lauwers, and L. Le Jeune, *Chem.-Biol. Interact.* **21,** 59 (1978).
13. G. M. Brown, *J. Biol. Chem.* **237,** 536 (1962).
14. M. R. Brown and E. Tomlinson, *J. Pharm. Sci.* **68,** 146 (1979).
15. A. H. Brueckner, *Yale J. Biol. Med.* **15,** 813 (1943).
16. K. H. Buchel, W. Draber, E. Regel, and M. Plempel, *Arzneim.-Forsch.* **22,** 1260 (1972).
17. H. Buchenauer, *Pestic. Biochem. Physiol.* **8,** 15 (1978).
18. A. Camerman and H. W. Smith, *Biochem. Biophys. Res. Commun.* **83,** 87 (1978).
19. A. Cammarata, *J. Pharm. Sci.* **55,** 1469 (1966).
20. J. F. Cavellier and F. Peradejordi, *Eur. J. Med. Chem.—Chim. Ther.* **16,** 241 (1981).
21. P. J. Cayley, J. P. Albraud, J. Feeney, G. C. K. Roberts, E. A. Piper, and A. S. V. Burgen, *Biochemistry* **18,** 3886 (1979).
22. P. A. Charlton, D. W. Young, B. Birdsall, J. Feeney, and G. C. K. Roberts, *J. C. S. Chem. Commun.* p. 922 (1979).
23. P. L. Chien, D. J. McCaustland, W. H. Burton, and C. C. Cheng, *J. Med. Chem.* **15,** 28 (1972).
24. Y. W. Chien and S. S. Mizuba, *J. Med. Chem.* **21,** 374 (1978).
25. G. Clifton and C. G. Skinner, *J. Med. Chem.* **13,** 575 (1970).
26. E. A. Coats, C. S. Genther, and C. C. Smith, *Eur. J. Med. Chem.—Chim. Ther.* **14,** 261 (1979).
27. W. T. Colwell, G. Chan, V. H. Brown, J. I. De Graw, J. H. Peters, and N. E. Morrison, *J. Med. Chem.* **17,** 142 (1974).
28. H. Commager and J. Judis, *J. Pharm. Sci.* **54,** 1436 (1965).
29. P. B. Cowles, *Yale J. Biol. Med.* **14,** 599 (1942).
30. P. B. Cowles and I. M. Klotz, *J. Bacteriol.* **56,** 277 (1948).
31. P. N. Craig, *J. Med. Chem.* **15,** 144 (1972).
32. P. N. Craig and C. Hansch, *J. Med. Chem.* **16,** 661 (1973).
33. A. Crum-Brown and T. R. Fraser, *Trans. R. Soc. Edinburgh* **25,** 151, 693 (1868).
34. L. A. Davidson and K. Takayama, *Antimicrob. Agents Chemother.* **16,** 104 (1979).
35. M. W. Davidson, B. C. Griggs, D. W. Boykin, and W. D. Wilson, *J. Med. Chem.* **20,** 1117 (1977).
36. S. W. Dietrich, J. M. Blaney, M. A. Reynolds, P. Y. C. Jow, and C. Hansch, *J. Med. Chem.* **23,** 1205 (1980).
37. S. W. Dietrich, R. Nelson Smith, S. Brendler, and C. Hansch, *Arch. Biochem. Biophys.* **194,** 612 (1979).
38. J. P. Dirlam, L. J. Czuba, B. W. Dominy, R. B. James, R. M. Pezzullo, J. E. Presslitz, and W. W. Windisch, *J. Med. Chem.* **22,** 1118 (1979).
39. W. Dittmar and G. Lohaus, *Arzneim.-Forsch.* **23,** 670 (1973).
40. W. Dittmar, E. Druckrey, and H. Urbach, *J. Med. Chem.* **17,** 753 (1974).
41. A. K. Drabikowska, L. Dudycz, and D. Shugar, *J. Med. Chem.* **22,** 653 (1979).
42. J. E. Dubois, D. Laurent, P. Bost, S. Chambaud, and C. Mercier, *Eur. J. Med. Chem.—Chim. Ther.* **11,** 225 (1976).
43. B. Duperray, M. Chastrette, M. C. Makabeh, and H. Pacheco, *Eur. J. Med. Chem.—Chim. Ther.* **11,** 323 (1976).

44. D. I. Edwards, *J. Antimicrob. Chemother.* **5,** 499 (1979).
45. G. A. Ellard, *Lepr. Rev.* **45,** 31 (1974).
46. A. Felmeister, *J. Pharm. Sci.* **61,** 151 (1972).
47. E. C. Foernzler and A. N. Martin, *J. Pharm. Sci.* **56,** 608 (1967).
48. J. C. Fontecilla-Camps, C. E. Bugg, C. Temple, J. D. Rose, J. A. Montgomery, and R. L. Kisliuk, *J. Am. Chem. Soc.* **101,** 114 (1979).
49. R. Franke, *Acta Biol. Med. Ger.* **30,** 467 (1973).
50. T. Fujita, *J. Med. Chem.* **9,** 797 (1966).
51. T. Fujita and C. Hansch, *J. Med. Chem.* **10,** 991 (1967).
52. E. R. Garrett, J. B. Mielck, J. K. Seydel, and H. J. Kessler, *J. Med. Chem.* **12,** 740 (1969).
53. D. Ghosh, *J. Med. Chem.* **9,** 423 (1966).
54. D. Gilbert, P. J. Goodford, and F. E. Norrington, *Br. J. Pharmacol.* **55,** 117 (1975).
55. P. J. Goodford, F. E. Norrington, W. H. G. Richards, and L. P. Walls, *Br. J. Pharmacol.* **48,** 650 (1973).
56. P. Gund, M. Poe, and K. H. Hoogsteen, *Mol. Pharmacol.* **13,** 1111 (1977).
57. L. H. Hall and L. B. Kier, *Eur. J. Med. Chem.—Chim. Ther.* **13,** 89 (1978).
58. L. H. Hall and L. B. Kier, *J. Pharm. Sci.* **67,** 1743 (1978).
59. C. Hansch, *in* "Biological Correlations—The Hansch Approach" (R. F. Gould, ed.), p. 20. Am. Chem. Soc., Washington, D.C., 1972.
60. C. Hansch, *in* "Biological Activity and Chemical Structure" (J. A. Keverling-Buisman, ed.), Pharmacochemistry Library, Vol. II, p. 47. Elsevier, Amsterdam/New York, 1977.
61. C. Hansch and J. M. Clayton, *J. Pharm. Sci.* **62,** 1 (1973).
62. C. Hansch and W. R. Glave, *Mol. Pharmacol.* **7,** 337 (1971).
63. C. Hansch and T. Fujita, *J. Am. Chem. Soc.* **86,** 1616 (1964).
64. C. Hansch and R. Kerley, *J. Med. Chem.* **13,** 957 (1970).
65. C. Hansch and E. J. Lien, *J. Med. Chem.* **14,** 653 (1971).
66. C. Hansch, E. Kutter, and A. Leo, *J. Med. Chem.* **12,** 746 (1969).
67. C. Hansch, J. L. Coubeils, and A. Leo, *Chim. Ther.* **7,** 427 (1972).
68. C. Hansch, J. Y. Fukunaga, P. Y. C. Jow, and J. B. Hynes, *J. Med. Chem.* **20,** 96 (1977).
69. T. Higuchi and S. S. Davis, *J. Pharm. Sci.* **59,** 1376 (1970).
70. K. Hirano, S. Yoshina, K. Okamura, and I. Suzuka, *Bull. Chem. Soc. Jpn.* **40,** 2229 (1967).
71. G. H. Hitchings, (1969). *Postgrad. Med. J., Suppl.* **45,** 7 (1969).
72. K. Hood and G. C. K. Roberts, *Biochem. J.* **171,** 357 (1978).
73. H. Horstmann, S. Schutz, Gonnert, R., and Andrews, S., *Eur. J. Med. Chem.—Chim. Ther.* **13,** 475 (1978).
74. W. B. Hugo, *Int. J. Pharm.* **1,** 127 (1978).
75. A. P. G. Kieboom, *Tetrahedron* **28,** 1325 (1972).
76. L. B. Kier and L. H. Hall, "Molecular Connectivity in Chemistry and Drug Research." Academic Press, New York, 1976.
77. K. H. Kim, C. Hansch, J. Y. Fukunaga, E. E. Steller, P. Y. C. Jow, P. N. Craig, and J. Page, *J. Med. Chem.* **22,** 366 (1979).
78. E. Klarmann, V. A. Shternov, and L. W. Gates, *J. Am. Chem. Soc.* **55,** 2576, 4657 (1933).
79. T. F. Koetzle and G. J. B. Williams, *J. Am. Chem. Soc.* **98,** 2074 (1976).
80. I. Kompis and A. Wick, *Helv. Chim. Acta* **60,** 3025 (1977).
81. I. Kompis, R. Then, E. Boehni, G. Rey-Bellet, G. Zanetti, and M. Montavon, *Eur. J. Med. Chem.—Chim. Ther.* **15,** 17 (1980).

82. A. Korolkovas and A. N. Senapeschi, *Eur. J. Med. Chem.—Chim. Ther.* **13,** 107 (1978).
83. A. Korolkovas and K. Tamashiro, *Rev. Farm. Bioquim. Univ. Sao Paulo* **12,** 37 (1974).
84. E. Kruger-Thiemer, *Ber. Borstel* **3,** 192 (1956).
85. H. Kubinyi, *J. Med. Chem.* **20,** 625 (1977).
86. H. Kubinyi and O. H. H. Kehrhahn, *J. Med. Chem.* **19,** 578 (1976).
87. E. Kutter, H. Machleidt, W. Reuter, R. Sauter, and A. Wildfeuer, *in* "Biological Correlations—The Hansch Approach" (R. F. Gould, ed.), p. 98. Am. Chem. Soc., Washington, D.C., 1972.
88. P. A. Lambert, *Prog. Med. Chem.* **15,** 88 (1978).
89. M. Lang and R. M. Rye, *Microbios* **7,** 199 (1973).
90. L. Levy, *Antimicrob. Agents Chemother.* **14,** 791 (1978).
91. R. Li, C. Hansch, D. Matthews, J. M. Blaney, R. Langridge, T. J. Delcamp, S. S. Susten, and J. H. Freisheim, *Quant. Struct.-Act. Relat.,* **1,** 1 (1982).
92. E. J. Lien, C. Hansch, and S. M. Anderson, *J. Med. Chem.* **11,** 430 (1968).
93. G. H. Loew and R. Sahakian, *J. Med. Chem.* **20,** 103 (1977).
94. Y. C. Martin, *in* "Quantitative Structure-Activity Analysis" (R. Franke and P. Oehme, eds.), p. 351. Akademie-Verlag, Berlin, 1978.
95. Y. C. Martin, *in* "Physical Chemical Properties of Drugs" (S. Yalkowsky and A. Sinkula, eds.), p. 49 Dekker, New York, 1980.
96. Y. C. Martin and J. J. Hackbarth, *J. Med. Chem.* **19,** 1033 (1976).
97. D. A. Matthews, R. A. Alden, J. T. Bolin, S. T. Freer, R. Hamlin, N. Xuong, J. Kraut, M. Poe, M. Williams, and K. Hoogsteen, *Science* **197,** 452 (1977).
98. D. A. Matthews, R. A. Alden, J. T. Bolin, D. J. Filman, S. T. Freer, R. Hamlin, W. G. J. Hoe, R. L. Kisliuk, E. J. Pastore, L. T. Plante, N. Xuong, and J. Kraut, *J. Biol. Chem.* **253,** 6946 (1978).
99. T. H. Maugh, *Science* **192,** 128 (1976).
100. D. R. McCalla, *J. Antimicrob. Chemother.* **3,** 517 (1977).
101. G. H. Miller, P. H. Doukas, and J. K. Seydel, *J. Med. Chem.* **15,** 700 (1972).
102. M. W. Miller, H. L. Howes, R. V. Kasubick, and A. R. English, *J. Med. Chem.* **13,** 849 (1970).
103. I. Moriguchi and Y. Kanada, *Chem. Pharm. Bull.* **25,** 926 (1977).
104. W. J. Murray, L. B. Kier, and L. H. Hall, *J. Med. Chem.* **19,** 573 (1976).
105. H. Nikaido, *Angew. Chem., Int. Ed. Engl.* **18,** 337 (1979).
106. S. de Nollin, H. van Belle, F. Goosens, F. Thore, and M. Borgers, *Antimicrob. Agents Chemother.* **11,** 500 (1977).
107. F. E. Norrington, R. M. Hyde, S. G. Williams, and R. Wooton, *J. Med. Chem.* **18,** 604 (1975).
108. P. L. Olive, *Br. J. Cancer* **40,** 89 (1979).
109. D. G. O'Sullivan, D. Pantic, and A. K. Wallis, *Experientia* **23,** 704 (1967).
110. D. G. O'Sullivan and C. M. Ludlow, *Experientia* **28,** 889 (1972).
111. F. Peradejordi and J. F. Cavellier, *Eur. J. Med. Chem.—Chim. Ther.* **16,** 247 (1981).
112. L. J. Powers and M. P. Mertes, *J. Med. Chem.* **13,** 1102 (1970).
113. A. Rastelli, P. G. De Benedetti, G. G. Battistuzzi, and A. Albasini, *J. Med. Chem.* **18,** 963 (1975).
114. C. H. Robinson, E. Bueding, and J. Fisher, *Mol. Pharmacol.* **6,** 604 (1970).
115. H. S. Rosenkranz and W. T. Speck, *in* "Metronidazole" (S. M. Finegold, ed.), p. 119. Excerpta Med. Found., Amsterdam, 1977.
116. D. Roy, S. Ghosh, and B. C. Guha, *Arch. Biochem. Biophys.* **92,** 366 (1961).
117. R. S. Schnaare and A. N. Martin, *J. Pharm. Sci.* **54,** 1707 (1965).

118. J. K. Seydel, *Mol. Pharmacol.* **2,** 259 (1966).
119. J. K. Seydel, *J. Pharm. Sci.* **57,** 1455 (1968).
120. J. K. Seydel, *J. Med. Chem.* **14,** 724 (1971).
121. J. K. Seydel, M. Richter, and E. Wempe, *Int. J. Lepr.* **48,** 18 (1980).
122. J. K. Seydel and W. Butte, *J. Med. Chem.* **20,** 439 (1977).
123. J. K. Seydel, K. J. Schaper, E. Wempe, and H. P. Cordes, *J. Med. Chem.* **19,** 483 (1976).
124. C. C. Smith, C. S. Genther, and E. A. Coats, *Eur. J. Med. Chem.—Chim Ther.* **14,** 271 (1979).
125. I. Tamm, K. Folkes, C. H. Shunk, D. Heyl, and F. L. Horofall, *J. Exp. Med.* **98,** 245 (1953).
126. H. H. W. Thijssen, *J. Pharm. Pharmacol.* **26,** 228 (1974).
127. E. Tomlinson, M. R. W. Brown, and S. S. Davis, *J. Med. Chem.* **20,** 1277 (1977).
128. K. Waisser, F. Rubacek, R. Karlicek, J. Sora, M. Celadnik, and K. Palat, *Pharmazie* **34,** 197 (1979).
129. K. A. M. Walker, D. R. Hirschfeld, and M. Marx, *J. Med. Chem.* **21,** 1335 (1978).
130. R. J. A. Walsh, K. R. H. Wooldridge, D. Jackson, and J. Gilmour, *Eur. J. Med. Chem.—Chim. Ther.* **12,** 495 (1977).
131. D. C. Warhurst and S. C. Thomas, *Biochem. Pharmacol.* **24,** 2047 (1975).
132. K. R. H. Wooldridge, *Eur. J. Med. Chem.—Chim. Ther.* **15,** 63 (1980).
133. H. Yamaguchi and K. Iwata, *Antimicrob. Agents Chemother.* **15,** 706 (1979).
134. T. Yamamoto and T. Otsu, *Chem. Ind.* (*London*) p. 787 (1967).
135. M. Yamazaki, N. Kakuya, T. Morishita, A. Kanada, and M. Aoki, *Chem. Pharm. Bull.* **18,** 702 (1970).

3

Semisynthetic Antibiotics

YVONNE C. MARTIN AND
ELIZABETH W. FISCHER

I. INTRODUCTION

The QSAR and SAR of semisynthetic antibiotics is different in several respects from that of totally synthetic compounds. The "lead" structure

QUANTITATIVE STRUCTURE–ACTIVITY
RELATIONSHIPS OF DRUGS

ISBN 0-12-695150-0

is typically very complex in both a structural and conformational sense. One consequence of the structural complexity is that much of the analog work is aimed at the definition of the functional groups essential for activity. This analog work is occasionally accompanied by conformational analysis of the products. A second consequence of the structural complexity is that X-ray analysis of the structure is very commonly done, frequently as part of or confirmation of the structure proof of the parent antibiotic. In this chapter conformational analysis of antibiotics will be discussed only if it has been related back to the three-dimensional requirements for activity. Each antibiotic class will be introduced with a stereoview of the generic structure and a brief SAR discussion of the groups that appear to be essential for activity. The QSAR will thus apply to the effect on the essential portion of variation of the nonessential portions of the molecule.

Frequently the details of the molecular mode of action of semisynthetic antibacterials have been studied. Therefore, one may have data on receptor binding and activation, as well as on whole animal and *in vitro* antibacterial activity.

Whole-cell antibacterial activity may be measured by a number of methods that may produce different orderings of potency. The principal methods are two quantitative measures of a few hours duration, growth-kinetic and turbidometric assays, and two semiquantitative assays of 24–48-h duration, dilution or diffusion assays that give minimum inhibitory concentration (MIC) values. In the growth-kinetic assay the growth rate is followed by bacterial cell count in a Coulter counter. It uses a lower concentration of organisms than does the turbidometric assay. Thus one would expect the influence of extraneous factors, such as binding of the drugs to proteins and their metabolism by the bacteria, to increase in the order of growth-kinetic, turbidometric, and MIC assays. Because the clinical effect of antibiotics is typically seen within a few hours, the shorter duration assays would probably be more relevant. A further variable in MIC assays is whether the drug is at uniform concentration throughout the tube or plate, as in various tube- or agar-dilution methods, or whether it is present in a gradient, as in the cup or zone diameter methods. In the former case potency is established by the tube of highest dilution in which no bacterial growth occurs. In the latter case potency is established by the size of the zone of inhibition of bacterial growth as a function of the initial concentration in the well or cup. Hence, in the latter type of assay the relative MIC depends on both the intrinsic potency and the rate of diffusion.

As an example of the complications that may arise in antibacterial testing, two analogs of leucomycin A showed activity equal to it in a twofold agar-dilution method, whereas in the cup diffusion assay their relative potencies were measured as 78% and 57%, respectively (*137*). The correspondence between the short- and long-duration assays is even less, as will be shown in the case of some chloramphenicol analogs. A final complication of the *in vitro* assays is that sometimes the culture medium contains serum albumin to which the analogs bind to differing degrees. The consequences of this addition for QSAR will be illustrated with penicillins.

Because most antibiotics contain ionizable groups, apparent activity usually varies with the pH of the culture medium. This may represent both a complication and an opportunity. The *in vitro* activity of antibiotics is especially suitable for analysis by the use of compartment model-based QSAR equations (*121,123*), because in general the concentration of antibiotic within the bacterial cell has reached steady state well before the relative potency determination is quantified. The evidence for this is in bacterial growth-kinetic studies, which show for erythromycin, for example, that after the addition of antibiotic to a growing culture, the new steady-state growth is obtained within 25 min or less (*68*).

All of the correlations with lipophilicity reported in this chapter are correlations with the equilibrium constant *P*. Because it has been shown that the relationship between the rate and extent of partitioning is not linear, this fact must be kept in mind when the various conclusions are drawn (*53,104,199*).

Usually newly synthesized analogs are tested for activity against several microorganisms. The resulting spectrum of activity is not constant but may differ from analog to analog. An important goal of an analog synthesis program may be to discover a compound with enhanced activity against certain pathogenic targets. In terms of this chapter the reader should be aware that a QSAR may be rather specific for a particular organism or that similar equations may be found for a variety of organisms.

II. INHIBITORS OF BACTERIAL PROTEIN SYNTHESIS

A. Tetracycline Analogs

1. Overview

The tetracyclines are broad spectrum bactericidal antibiotics. Structure **I** in Scheme 1 shows the characteristic structural features: the trio of oxygen atoms at positions 10, 11, and 12; the β-diketone at positions 1, 2, and 3; and the dimethylamino group at position 4. These features are held

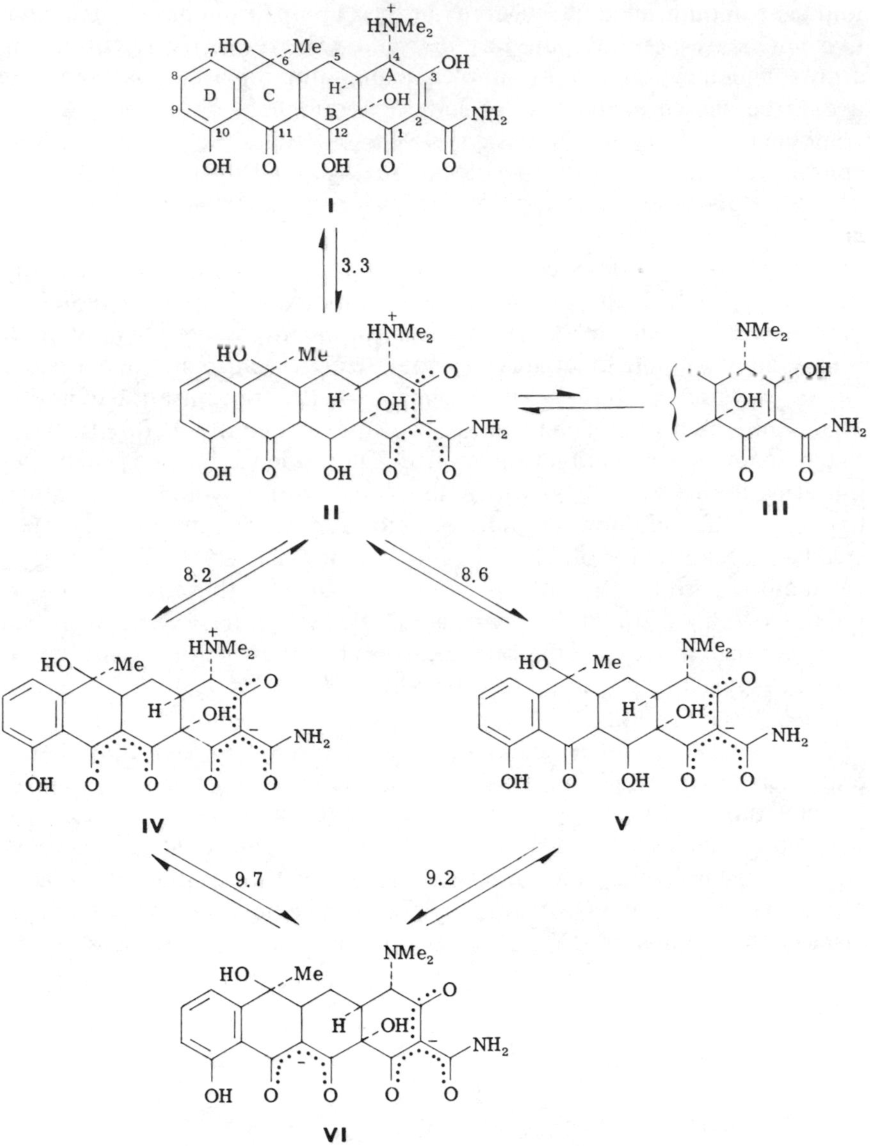

SCHEME 1. Ionization of Tetracycline (*6*).

in the appropriate steric relationship by means of the four fused rings. The extensive structure–activity studies are summarized in many places (*21,22,55,130*). Essentially, no modifications are permitted at positions 1–4 or 10–12, whereas activity is retained with modifications at positions 5–9.

The mode of action of the tetracyclines is thought to be interruption of protein biosynthesis by binding to the bacterial 30 S ribosomal subunit (*55,130*). A role for metal ion-complex formation has been suggested (*4,54,95*).

2. Physical Properties

The combination of functional groups and the ring system of tetracyclines gives rise to a number of subtle equilibria that one must be aware of for careful QSAR work. The most important of these are the structural, solvent, and pH dependence of interactions with protons, interactions with metal ions, and conformational changes. It is likely that in the course of the assessment of antibacterial activity a tetracycline will encounter phases of different pH values, metal ion type and concentration, and polarity. Small changes in these environments could cause subtle changes in the properties of the molecule that are responsible for triggering the observed biological response.

a. Ionization Studies. Scheme 1 shows the ionization scheme for tetracycline. For tetracycline, oxytetracycline (5α-hydroxytetracycline), and 7-chlorotetracycline the following stoichiometric constants have been established: pK_1 is 3.3; pK_2 is 7.8, 7.3, and 7.4, respectively; and pK_3 is 9.6, 9.1, and 9.3, respectively (*4,180*). In 50:50 dimethylformamide:water pK_2 of tetracycline increases to 8.2 and pK_3 to 10.2; similarly those of oxytetracycline increase to 8.0 and 9.8 (*180*). In contrast, in 50:50 methanol:water pK_1 of tetracycline increases to 4.4 and pK_3 decreases to 9.4, while pK_1 and pK_2 of 7-chlorotetracycline increase to 4.3 and 7.6, respectively. In 1:1 dimethyl sulfoxide:water the pK_a values for tetracycline are 4.4, 8.1, and 9.8 (*6*). Finally, in pH partition measurements with 1-octanol the pK_a values of tetracycline are unchanged (*47,188*).

It is important to know the specific pK_a values associated with each site of ionization. Does each stoichiometric pK_a represent only one site of ionization or several? There is general agreement that in water the first proton is lost from the OH group at position 3 (*6,130*). The resulting negative charge can be delocalized as shown in Scheme 1 (**II**). Does the next deprotonation occur from the dimethylammonium group (**V**) or from one of the OH groups in the BCD system (**IV**)? Two published studies were done in 50:50 w:w water:methanol by a combination of potentiometric and NMR titrations (*99,163*). Isochlortetracycline, tetracycline, 4-epitetracycline, and tetracycline methiodide were considered. Both the second and third stoichiometric pK_a values reflect substantial contribution from deprotonation of the OH group of the BCD ring system and deprotonation of the dimethylammonium group. Asleson and Frank used the same technique in 50:50 dimethyl sulfoxide:D_2O to assign the values given in Scheme I for the site constants (*6*). In water and at pH values of biological interest, species **II**, **IV**, and **V** are present. The constants reported in these papers are subject to question because a number of assumptions as to the relative magnitude of various dissociation pathways had to be made. Also, the use of mixed solvents and D_2O probably changed the magnitude of the values. Because of low solubility, no study has been done in pure water, nor have the effects of substituents at the 7 and 9 positions on the site constants been studied. The establishment of site constants useful for QSAR work remains to be accomplished.

Because temperature may dramatically affect pK_a, it is not surprising that Cooke and Gonda observed an effect of temperature and also of concentration on apparent partition coefficients (*48*).

Two groups have investigated the pH partition behavior of the tetracyclines in 1-octanol–water systems and proposed structures of the species in octanol (*47,188*). It was observed that the highest apparent partition coefficient occurs in the range of pH 4–7. The first question is what is present in the octanol? Because thermodynamics (of which partition coefficients are an example) describes only the relative free energy of two states and not their structure, consideration of partition coefficients alone cannot answer the question. However, it is pertinent that both tautomers **II** and **III** of the neutral molecule have been crystallized (*181*). The former was crystallized from hydrated solvent, the latter only when all traces of water were removed. It was also observed that in chloroform solution tetracycline exists as tautomer **III**; additionally, the ultraviolet spectra of octanol and ethanol solutions suggest that in octanol species **III** is predominant (*188*).

Thus the ionization equilibria of tetracyclines are very complex and by no means understood for even a few molecules. From the standpoint of QSAR this means that it will be difficult (1) to parameterize the molecules because both apparent hydrophobicity as well as fraction of each site protonated will depend on the not yet determined site dissociation constants and (2) to interpret existing QSAR, because any electronic effects of an equation may reflect changes in the proportion of the active species available to the receptor as well as changes in the intrinsic strength of the drug–receptor interaction.

b. Metal Ion Binding Studies. Tetracyclines have long been known to have a strong affinity for metal ions (*4,5*). Stability constants have been reported for the interaction of tetracycline 4-epichlortetracycline, 4-epianhydrotetracycline, chlorotetracycline, oxotetracycline, and anhydrotetracycline with such ions as Cu(II), Zn(II), and Ni(II) (*4,11,54*). Conversion of the binding constants to site-specific constants depends on accurate site pK_a values. However, from blocked

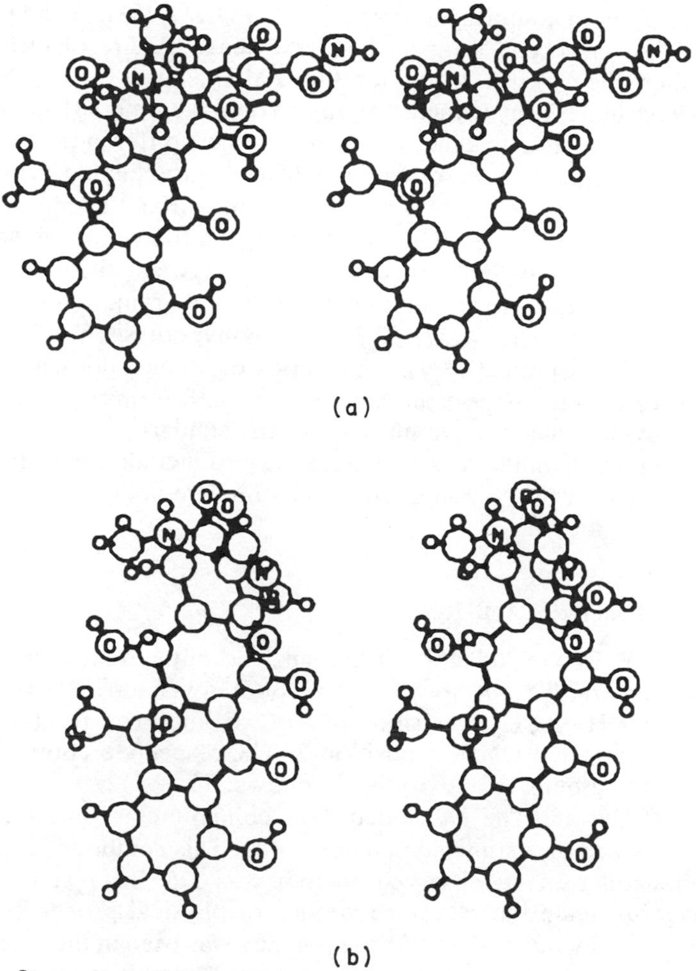

Fig. 1. Stereoviews of the crystal structures of (a) un-ionized and (b) zwitterionic oxytetracycline (structures **III** and **II**, respectively) (*181*).

derivatives Stoel *et al.* have shown that tetracycline binds metals at multiple sites on the A ring (*184*).

c. Conformational Studies. ORD-CD studies have shown that as the 3-OH is deprotonated, the A ring becomes less twisted, and that metal binding induces conformational changes specific to the ions and tetracycline analog involved (*130*). Stezowski and co-workers have reconsidered the effects that variables such as pH and solvent as well as structural variation can have on conformation (*92,95,151–154,181,183*). Although their principal focus has been X-ray analysis, they have used results from solution studies (their own CD and literature PMR) as well (*92,151*).

They have done X-ray crystallography on both tautomers **II** and **III** of tetracycline and oxytetracycline. The two tautomers differ in the conformation of the A ring and the orientation of the carboxamide. The corresponding tautomers of the two analogs do not differ "significantly" in conformation of the A ring. The two species of tetracycline are shown in Fig. 1. They proposed that the equilibrium between the two and the unique conformation of each tautomer are the important determinants of biological activity (*92,150,151,181,182*). This hypothesis has been questioned but not disproved (*139*). This series of studies does not present quantitative data to support the necessity of both forms for activity nor does it provide a quantitative measure of the similarity of the tautomers for different compounds. It seems necessary to include these findings in any new QSAR work; perhaps they will stimulate additional theoretical studies.

3. Antibacterial Activity

Free and Wilson included the QSAR analysis of the relative *in vitro* potency versus *Staphylococcus aureus* of 10 tetracyclines (*63*). The set included either H or CH_3 at position 6; NO_2, Cl, or Br at position 7; and NO_2, NH_2, or CH_3CONH at position 9. The respective contribution of each of these groups to activity is as follows: 75, − 112, − 26, 84, − 16, −218, 213, and 18. The calculated best compound is thus 6-H, 7-Cl, 9-NH_2 for which the estimated potency is 443. This compound is a part of the original data set; its observed potency was 525. Because no attempt was made to relate the relative activities to physical properties in this analysis, potency rather than relative potency was used in the calculation. The equation that was derived explains 91% of the variance in the data.

In 1970–1971 bacterial-growth kinetics were used to assess the relative ability of a series of tetracycline analogs to inhibit the growth of *E. coli*. The QSAR of these results was discussed from different poins of view in three papers. In the first paper, Cammarata *et al.* considered the seven analogs with substituents at only the 7 or 9 position (*43*). The log k values for inhibitory potency for the 7-substituted analogs are positively correlated with σ^2 or E_R values. For the 9-substituted analogs a negative term in the radius of the group is needed in addition to the electronic term. Mager and Barth showed that the two parameters have equal influence on potency in a statistical sense (*111*).

Cammarata and Yau then considered the various 6- and 5-substituted analogs in addition to those above, for a sample size of eleven (*42*). The QSAR was analyzed from several computational viewpoints, all of which can be shown to be equivalent. The best equation is the following:

$$\log k = 0.93\sigma^2 - 0.42r_D + 3.67r_C - 1.99 \quad (1)$$

$$r = 0.93, \quad s = 0.20, \quad n = 11$$

The term r_D is the van der Waals contact distance of the substituent at the 9 position and the term r_C describes the van der Waals contact distance of the OH or H at the 6 position. However, it appears to be an indicator variable that is more positive for the 6-OH compounds. The importance of the electronic effect of substituents is evident from the equations.

Peradejordi *et al.* then added the 5*a*(6)-anhydro, 12*a*-deoxy, and 7-Cl,5*a*(11*a*)-dehydro analogs to those previously considered (*143*). They calculated the physicochemical properties by simple quantum chemical means. Specifically, the oxygen atoms at positions 10, 11, 12 were postulated to be the key to activity. The calculations were done on the molecule as species **II**. The charges were calculated as the sum of the π charges from Hückel calculations plus the σ charges from del Re calculations. Additionally the nucleophilic and electrophilic π superdelocalizability for each atom of interest was calculated from the Hückel results. From these ten predictors, the equation found is the following:

$$\log k = 18.4 + 56.2Q_{O-10} + 48.8Q_{O-11} + 71.3Q_{O-12} + 3.4Q_{C-6} + 16.9E_{O-10} - 1.1E_{O-11} + 18.4E_{O-12} \quad (2)$$

$$r = 0.99, \quad s = 0.167, \quad n = 14$$

The Q terms are the charges on the indicated atoms and the E terms are the electrophilic superdelocalizability, a measure of how easy it is for that atom to delocalize the charge of an approaching electrophile such as a proton or a metal ion. The E_{O-10} and E_{O-11} are significant only at the 10% level; all other terms are more significant. For reference, the charges of O-10, O-11, and O-12 of tetracycline are −0.32, −0.28, and −0.30, respectively. Notice how the charges on these oxygen atoms make them ideally suited for chelation with a metal ion.

Steric terms are not necessary in Eq. (2). This is because in the calculations the lowered activity of the 9-NO_2 and 9-NH_2 analogs is accounted for by considering the proton on O-10 to be hydrogen bonded to the 9-substituent rather than to O-11, **VII** rather than **VIII**. The choice of **VII** was based on literature observations of this hydrogen bond (*130*). The principal calculated difference between forms **VII** and **VIII** is in the charge at atom O-11: for **VII** it is −0.300, whereas for **VIII** it is −0.276. This is translated into a predicted activity of 44 for **VII** whereas that for

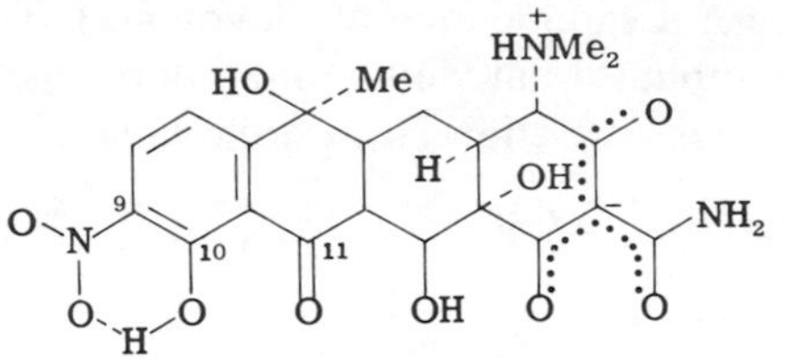

VII

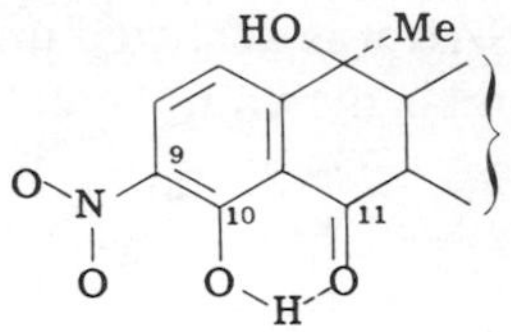

VIII

VIII is predicted to be 635; the experimental activity is 44. In a similar way the calculated activity of the 9–10 hydrogen-bonded form of the 9-NH_2 analog is 24, that of the 10–11 hydrogen-bonded form is 179, and the experimental value is 24.

Although the statistics suggest that this equation is highly statistically significant, later random number simulations suggest that examination of ten possible predictors to find a QSAR with 14 analogs results in an equation with an $R^2 > 0.90$ in 2% of the cases (*194*). This fact, plus the omission of at least three analogs that could have been included suggest that the equation is probably not so statistically secure as might be indicated by the high R^2. In spite of these criticisms and the primitive nature of the quantum chemical calculations, the work as a whole does support the importance of the electrostatic contributions to activity.

In contrast to many other antibiotics, and presumably because of the number of charges on the molecule, tetracycline is transported into sensitive bacteria by an active process that is lost when the bacteria become resistant. One result of this active transport is that the growth rate in the presence of tetracycline may be a hyperbolic rather than a linear function of drug concentration. Only if this is recognized will the inhibitory rate constants be calculated correctly. The same set of compounds studied by Peradejordi *et al.* was reexamined by a turbidometric procedure against a sensitive and a resistant *Escherichia coli* by Miller *et al.* (*128*). There is a good correlation between the inhibitory activity against the sensitive organism and that reported previously, but no correlation between the inhibitory activity against the two strains. These workers also measured octanol (pH 6.6) distribution coefficients, P'. A pH value of 6.6 is a reasonable approximation of the internal pH of a bacterium. They found a linear correlation between log $P'_{6.6}$ and the log of the inhibitory activity with resistant organisms for those analogs for which a hyperbolic fit is needed to determine K_r:

$$\log K_r = 1.98 + 1.74 \log P'_{6.6} \quad (3)$$

$$r = 0.92, \quad s \text{ (not specified)}, \quad n = 11$$

The need for the hyperbolic fit was attributed to the almost equal contribution to potency of the factors: penetration into the cell and binding to the receptor. Those compounds for which a linear fit is possible are modified in such a way that receptor binding is very low. Miller *et al.* (*128*) concluded that resistant bacteria accumulate tetracyclines by a mechanism in which hydrophobicity of the antibiotic is the important characteristic. Including the quantum chemical properties does not improve the correlation. It is possible that the use of the mixed constant P' obscures the separate effects of partition coefficient and basicity (*123*).

The small number of QSAR studies on tetracyclines suggests that the intricacies of the conformational and proton and metal binding kinetics and equilibria have inhibited QSAR investigations. Accordingly, the next stage in the QSAR of tetracyclines could well be an analysis that includes these factors. Such an undertaking may require the use of more sophisticated quantum chemical descriptions of the molecules, the development of new insights into how to handle multiple rates and equilibria in QSAR, and experimental information on the physical properties.

4. Pharmacokinetics and Protein Binding of Tetracyclines

A number of studies have suggested that there is a correlation between hydrophobicity and the serum protein binding of various analogs (*48,76,98,110,149,172–174,175,193,213*). However, in all cases only a few analogs were studied, and usually at least one analog deviated from the apparent relationship. Steric factors may also be involved (*76*). Kellaway and Marriott (*98*) showed a correlation between the number of binding sites of one of the two classes of sites found and the distribution coefficients measured at pH 7.0. They also found a negative parabolic relationship between log P' and the log $(1/K)$ values for both sites and also the number of the first class of binding sites. In all four cases minocycline is an outlier. These studies suggest that hydrophobic binding contributes to the strength of binding to serum proteins but that other factors also make important contributions. Of course, all of these studies may be complicated by the complex ionization equilibria of tetracyclines.

Following earlier preliminary results (*174*), Schach von Wittenau and Delahunt in 1966 published graphs that show that distribution into tissue is also a function of $CHCl_3$ (pH 7.4) log P' values (*173*). They calculated the ratio between the total drug concentration in various tissues (e.g., muscle) and the free or unbound drug concentration in serum. The tissue–serum partition coefficients are a linear function of the log P' values. Hence the tissue depots are lipophilic. In 1979 Toon and Rowland came to the same conclusion from a volume of distribution data calculated

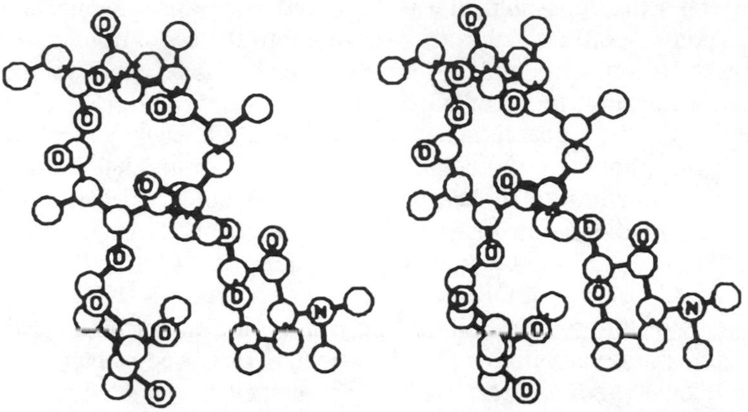

Fig. 2. Stereoview of the crystal structure of erythromycin (*86*).

from pharmacokinetic analysis of seven tetracyclines (*193*). They found no correlation between lipophilicity and the following pharmacokinetic features: overall elimination half-life, renal clearance based on unbound drug, and nonrenal clearance. As was indicated with the QSAR of antibacterial activity, the superimposition of multiple ionization equilibria on the partitioning equilibria could make any property–pharmacokinetic relationship very difficult to untangle (*123*).

B. Erythromycin Analogs

1. Overview

Erythromycin A, (**IX**) is a clinically widely used antibiotic of the macrolide class. Figure 2 shows its conformation as established by X-ray crys-

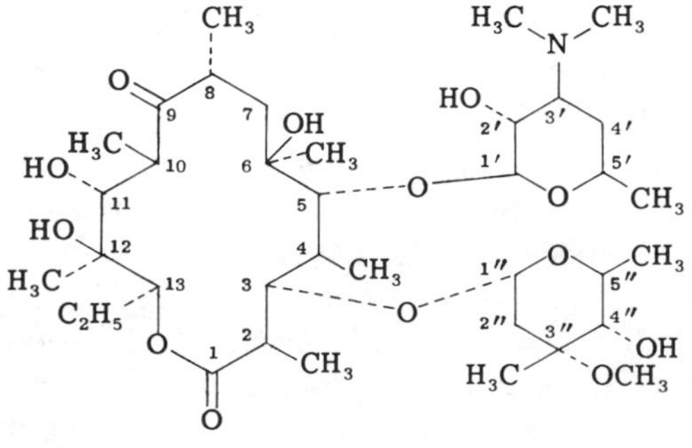

IX

tallography (*86*). It is composed of a 14-membered lactone ring substituted in two positions with sugars, one basic and one neutral. Erythromycin inhibits bacterial growth by inhibition of bacterial protein synthesis by virtue of binding to the bacterial 50 S ribosomal subunits (*208*).

Chemical modification studies have demonstrated that both sugars plus the macrolide ring are essential for ribosomal binding and antibacterial activity (*146*). These biological properties are also abolished by (1) changing the dimethylamino group to the corresponding *N*-oxide, trimethylammonium, or *N*-acetyl analog; (2) esterifying the 2′-hydroxyl group (these esters per se have no activity, but they are hydrolyzed back to the corresponding erythromycin); and (3) certain changes in the macrolide ring, i.e., 8-epierythromycin B, 10,11-anhydroerythromycin A or B, and 11,12-epoxyerythromycin A.

In contrast, the following changes do not substantially change ribosomal binding: (1) esterification of the 4″- or 11-hydroxyl groups; (2) removal of the 12-hydroxyl group to form the naturally occurring erythromycin B; or (3) conversion of the ketone to a hydrazone, substituted or unsubstituted oxime or oxime ester, 11,12-carbonate-6,9-hemiketal, or 9,11-aryl or 9,11-alkyl boronate (*146*).

A close look at the three-dimensional structure of erythromycin shows that the oxygen atoms on the macrolide ring all face one direction from the plane of the ring. Because these appear to be the positions that can be substituted without abolition of ribosomal activity, they must not be involved in receptor binding.

The conformation of erythromycin A and some derivatives has been investigated by NMR (*56,57,129,134,144,145,147*). In general, the macrolide ring is not very flexible (*57*). Substitutions of many types on the macrolide ring do result, however, in subtle conformational changes in the C-6 to C-10 region of the ring but in very little change in the C-1 to C-5 region. For example, in erythromycin A compared to erythromycin B (12-deoxyerythromycin A), the ketone is closer to the C-6 hydroxyl group and hence more strongly hydrogen bonded to it. Thus, although it would be attractive to postulate a series of hydrogen bonds between the macrolide oxygen atoms and the receptor, neither the conformational nor analog studies support such a proposal.

Evidence was also presented to support the possibility that in $CDCl_3/CH_2Cl_2$ solution the desosamine group may move around to the side of the aglycone ring by rotation around the C-5—O bond. This moves the NME_2 group nearer to the 8-Me (*134*). This observation clearly raises the possibility for other rotations of the C-5—O bond under other experimental conditions.

2. Physical Property Measurements

Octanol–water partition coefficient measurements on several molecules showed that changing the 12-substituent from H to OH and the 11-substituent from OH to $OCOCH_3$ or from OCOH to $OCOCH_3$ results in a smaller increase in hydrophobicity than anticipated (*119,120,125*). This observation suggests that there are many intramolecular interactions in the parent molecule. The X-ray structure confirms this in that the following pairs of oxygen atoms are at approximately van der Waals distance: 11–12, 11–9, and 3″–4″ (*86*). An alternative explanation to the irregular π values is (in accordance with the CMR results) that the changed substituent alters the conformation of the ring slightly and as a result the various hydrophobic and hydrophilic groups are in slightly different environments in each analog. The importance of this unpredictability of π values to QSAR analyses is that the log *P* values of other analogs may not be predictable; if it is not possible to calculate log *P* values and if potency depends on log *P*, then the potency of other analogs cannot accurately be predicted.

3. Receptor Binding

All 4″- and 11-esters, 9-oximes, 9-oxime ethers, 9-hydrazones, and *N*-benzyl analogs bind to *E. coli* ribosomes with approximately equal affinity. No significant QSAR has been derived (*119*).

4. 2′-, 4″-, and 11-Esters

One set of 28 analogs consisted of various combinations of OH, OCOH, $OCOCH_3$, and $OCOC_2H_5$ at the 2′, 4″, and 11 positions and either H or OH at the 12 position. The relative potency of the analogs was measured in a turbidometric assay with *S. aureus* as the microorganism. A Free–Wilson analysis of the data resulted in an equation with an R^2 of 0.986, and an s of 0.072 (*117,125*). The coefficients of the group contributions to activity become more negative as the number of carbon atoms increases. Additionally, the coefficient of the group contribution for a given substituent type is always more negative at the 4″ position than the 11 or 2′ position. Because the data fit the Free–Wilson model very well, it was concluded that there is no optimum log *P* or sum of π in this data set, that is, the relationship between potency and log *P* is linear within the range represented by these data.

The same data were also correlated with physicochemical properties (*120*). The result is an equation with negative coefficients of log *P* and indicator variables for esterification at the 4″ or 11 positions and a positive one for erythromycin A compared to B derivatives. In this case R^2 is 0.945 and s is 0.127. Because s is larger than that from the Free–Wilson equation, it was concluded that the physicochemical properties somewhat imperfectly describe the structural changes that the receptor sees.

This data set was reanalyzed by Berntsson who came to the same conclusion after mathematically removing the correlation between log P and $(\log P)^2$ (*12*).

5. 2′-, 4″-, and 11-Esters, 4″-Sulfonate Esters, 4′-Hydroxy Analogs, and Compounds Substituted at the Ketone

The QSAR of the antibacterial activity of a larger set of esters that was synthesized to expand on the previous equation is represented by the following relationship (*119*):

$$\log(1/C) = 1.26 + 1.33 \log P - 0.269 \log P^2 + 0.894\text{Es-4}'' + 0.779\text{Es-11} \quad (4)$$

$$r = 0.965, \quad s = 0.13, \quad n = 32, \quad \log P_0 = 2.47$$

This equation correctly predicted the potency of 33 additional analogs. The prediction may also be expressed as a new equation:

$$\log(1/C) = 1.10 + 1.54 \log P - 0.321 \log P^2 + 0.938\text{Es-4}'' + 0.625\text{Es-11} + 0.189S \quad (5)$$

$$r = 0.963, \quad s = 0.11, \quad n = 65, \quad \log P_0 = 2.39$$

In this equation the indicator variable S suggests that the 4″-sulfonate esters are somewhat more potent than equilipophilic 4″-carboxylate esters. These studies are an example of the correct prediction of potency of new analogs by a QSAR equation.

QSAR analyses were also used to evaluate the possibility that a compound with improved activity against gram-negative bacteria could be found (*119*). The log P_0 varied from 1.97 for activity against the gram-negative *E. coli* to 2.46 for the gram-positive *Haemophilus influenzae* with the gram-negative *Klebsiella pneumonia* and the gram-positive *S. aureus* in between. This similarity in log P_0 values is in contrast to the observation of substantially lower log P_0 values for gram-negative compared to gram-positive organisms reported for other antibacterial compounds by Lien *et al.* (*108*). It points to the limitations in the concept of universal log P_0 values (*198*).

Although the traditional parabolic function rather than a model-based equation was used to fit the data, plots suggest that this is adequate for these data. The evidence for this statement is that the slopes of the low and high log P regions are similar and that there are compounds on both sides of the optimum.

The establishment of these regression equations with an optimum log P and negative steric effects helped us in our decision to terminate the synthesis of further analogs.

Bojarska-Dahlig reported a QSAR analysis of (presumably) the tube-dilution potency versus *Bacillus pumilus* of 16 compounds modified in the macrolide ring (*24*). She reported an equation with a standard deviation of 0.27 and an optimum R_m value equal to that of erythromycin B. The most active compound, the 11,12-carbonate, was omitted from the equation because it was much more potent than expected. (This compound was included in Eq. 2.) The positive deviation from the regression line suggested enhanced receptor binding of the compound.

It is not clear if the similarity in conclusions from Bojarski-Dahlig's study and our own fortuitous or not. It is perhaps so, because we disagree on the relative lipophilicity of the 9-oxime and the cyclic carbonate of erythromycin A and on the relative potency of the cyclic carbonate. Nevertheless, QSAR studies have been successful in highlighting the general influence of lipophilicity on potency of this type of erythromycin analogs.

6. *N*-Benzylerythromycins

The *N*-benzyl analogs, in contrast to those previously discussed, vary in pK_a values. The pK_a values of several analogs were measured by titration (*119,123*). These were then used to calculate the pK_a values of the other analogs. The antibacterial activities had been measured turbidometrically at pH 7.0 for all analogs and also at pH 6.0 and 7.85 for several of them. In order to derive a satisfactory QSAR, it was necessary to consider model-based equations. The one that fit the data best has no term for hydrophobicity (*119,123*).

$$\log \frac{1}{C} = \log \frac{[\mathrm{H}^+]_2/K_a}{\dfrac{[\mathrm{H}^+]_2}{K_a} + a\left(1 + \dfrac{[\mathrm{H}^+]_1}{K_a}\right)} + 0.30\mathrm{Es\ (para)} + 2.37 \qquad (6)$$

$$r = 0.919, \qquad s = 0.186, \qquad n = 38$$

Because of mathematical constraints to get a fit, it was assumed that pH_2, the pH of the internal compartment of the bacteria, was constant at pH 6.0. The fitted value of log a is 1.30. From these results it was concluded that this series behaves as if the bacteria maintain a constant internal pH and that the compounds equilibrate according to their pK_a and to the difference between the internal and external pH values. It was also

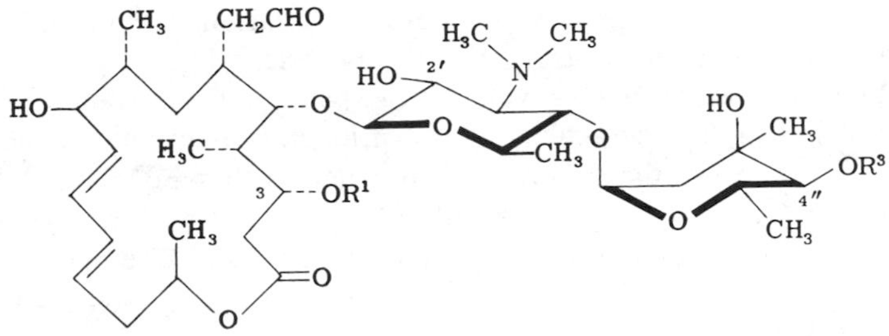

X

concluded that the ionic species is at least as active as, and possibly considerably more active than, the uncharged species and that there is a negative steric effect of substitution at the para position (*119,123*).

C. Leucomycin and Deltamycin Analogs

Leucomycin (**X**) and deltamycin are 16-membered ring macrolides glycosidically attached to a disaccharide. Esterification of the 3 and 4″ hydroxyl groups and various changes in the allylic alcohol do not destroy activity (*137*). Deltamycin differs from leucomycin in that the 9-OH group is oxidized to a ketone and the 12–13 double bond is changed to an epoxide.

The QSAR of the cup (agar diffusion) method versus *Bacillus subtilis* PCI 219 antibacterial activity of a set of eight leucomycin analogs consisting of alkyl esters of the 3 and 4″ positions was reported in 1971 (*119,126*). We found a positive dependence of whole-cell antibacterial activity on π, that is, the optimum log P value is ≥ 2.2, the calculated value of the most lipophilic compound.

Ribosomal binding of a set of leucomycin analogs had been determined by displacement of [^{14}C]erythromycin from *E. coli* ribosomes (*136*). Mager reported that the QSAR of ribosomal binding of alkyl esters of the 3-, 2′-, and 4″-hydroxyl groups is described by the following equation (*112*):

$$\log I_{50} = 9.995 + 0.493\pi + 0.232\pi^2 + 1.64\sigma \qquad (7)$$

$$r = 0.95, \qquad s \text{ (not reported)}, \qquad n = 27$$

This equation corresponds to an optimum π value of approximately zero; π is less than zero in all analogs. The σ term is in reality an indicator variable because it assumes only two values: esterification of the 2′-hydroxyl increases σ by 0.68 and lowers the expected log-binding I_{50} by 1.12. Although 41 analogs were included in the original source of data, only 29 of these were analyzed in the QSAR study.

The original workers observed a good correlation between ribosomal binding and antibacterial activity with the exception of the 2′-esters, which bind to ribosomes less well than expected (*136*). Mager found no significant QSAR for the agar dilution antibacterial activity of the set of derivatives that he studied. Three factors suggest that Eq. (7) may be less reliable than suggested by its r value: (1) omission of approximately one-third of the compounds, (2) special properties of 2′-esters that may distort the variance in I_{50} values, and (3) lack of correspondence with the whole-cell data.

There are seven compounds from the 1971 analysis in Mager's data set. The fact that the 1971 analysis did show a correlation of MIC with log P, whereas the larger data set did not reveal such a correlation, indicates a lack of predictive ability of the original equation and/or reinforces the differences between the potency established by diffusion and dilution methods. In a diffusion assay the leading edge of the antibiotic front contains very small concentrations of antibiotic in the presence of relatively large amounts of bacteria: this is an ideal situation for the bacteria to hydrolyze some of the ester. The authors of the paper that contains the ribosomal binding and agar dilution data state that "some 2′-O-acyl derivatives apparently underwent gradual hydrolysis during antimicrobial assays" (*136*, p. 732). Perhaps the 3 and 4″ positions are also labile under the conditions of the diffusion assay. One must remember that the "A" of a QSAR may change dramatically with a different assay system.

In 1981 Shimauchi *et al.* reported a graphical QSAR of a series of 4″-(*p*-substituted phenylacetyl)deltamycins (*177*). Antimicrobial activity in a broth dilution technique using *S. aureus* and *Mycoplasma gallisepticum* is positively correlated with the chemical shift of the methylene proton of the benzyl group. The chemical shift value is in turn correlated with the Hammett σ_p values. Hence, electron-withdrawing substituents increase antibacterial potency. It would be interesting to know if these compounds are active per se or if they must be hydrolyzed in order to bind to the ribosomes.

D. Lincomycin Analogs

1. Overview

Lincomycin (**XI**) is an antibiotic that is characterized by the presence of sugar and pyrrolidine rings. From structural modification studies we know that the features essential for antibacterial activity appear to be the correct stereochemistry about C-2′ (Fig. 3); an amide (not a thioamide) link; an alkyl substituent at C-4′, which cannot be replaced by one at C-5′;

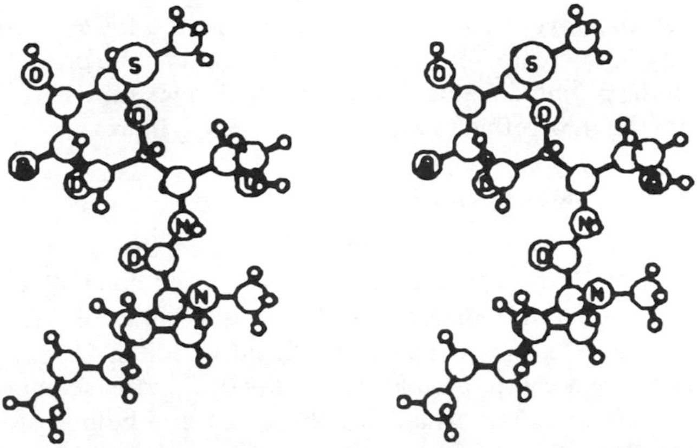

Fig. 3. Stereoview of the structure of lincomycin in the neutral form found by calculation (*44*).

a group C_2H_5 or smaller at N-1′; no changes in the C-2—C-4 portion of the molecule; and the same stereochemistry and not too large a group at C-1 (*115*). The calculated conformation of the free base is shown in Fig. 3.

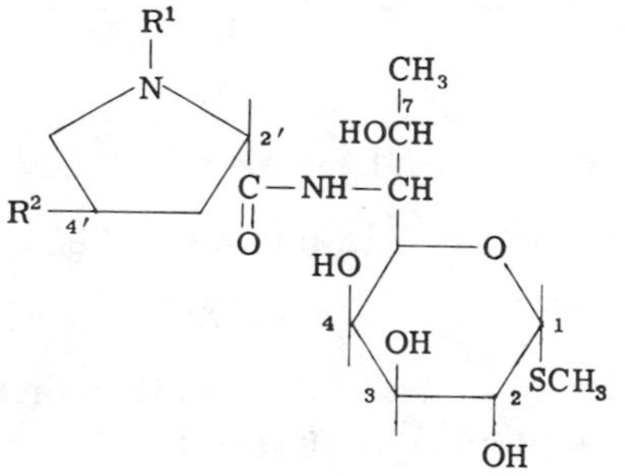

XI

2. Physical Properties

The partition coefficients of several analogs have been reported (*80*). The antibiotic clindamycin differs from lincomycin in that the 7(*R*)-OH has been converted to the 7(*S*)-Cl analog. From three comparisons the average change in log *P* in the transformation from a lincomycin to the corresponding clindamycin is 1.4; this is slightly lower than that expected, 1.7. *Ab initio* quantum chemical calculations on molecular fragments suggest that the structural conversion from lincomycin to clindamycin is accompanied by a conformational change (*178*). In contrast to the experience with erythromycins, alkyl groups increase the log P of lincomycin and clindamycin by a greater than expected amount: the conversion from 3′-propyl to the 3′-butyl analogs increases log P by 0.72, whereas the conversion from the thiomethyl to the thioethyl analog increases log P by 0.8.

3. *In Vitro* Antibacterial Activity

The first QSAR studies were of the effect of modification of the alkyl substituent at N-1′ and C-4′ (*126*). This study used calculated π values. The parabolic equation indicates an optimum π value of ~2.7. The *N*-methyl and *N*-ethyl compounds can be fit into one QSAR equation that also includes an indicator variable attributing 0.23 increase in potency for trans analogs compared to cis and a 0.20 increase in potency for *N*-ethyl compared to *N*-methyl analogs of the same π value. The NH analogs show a linear increase in potency with increasing π values.

These results became more interpretable after the model-based equations for QSAR were developed (*119,123*). All 28 analogs can be fit with one equation having seven variables including an indicator variable for cis versus trans and the pK_a values of NH and *N*-ethyl analogs:

$$\log\frac{1}{C} = \log\frac{1}{1 + P^{0.61} + \dfrac{340(1 + 10^{pK - pH})}{P^{0.61}}} + 0.22D_{tr} + 1.86 \qquad (8)$$

$$pK_a \text{ of NEt analogs} = 8.26$$

$$pK_a \text{ of NH analogs} = 8.86$$

$$r = 0.979, \qquad s = 0.099, \qquad n = 28$$

The standard deviation from this fit is lower than that from any of the parabolic equations. From this work it was concluded that there is hydrophobic bonding between the substituents at the 1′ and 4′ positions and the receptor, that only the neutral form binds to the receptor, and that trans analogs bind more strongly than the corresponding cis analogs. Verification of hydrophobic binding of the substituent at the 4′ position comes from the observation that 4′-depropyl-4′-ethoxylincomycin, in which a methylene has been replaced by its isostere O, is approximately equipotent with the equilipophilic 4′-H analog and not lincomycin (*114*). Harris and Symons have also postulated hydrophobic binding between the 4′-substituent and the ribosome; this was based on comparisons of Dreiding models of 20 substances that interact with *E. coli* ribosomes (*87*).

An early QSAR study of clindamycin analogs that vary in the alkyl substituent at 4′ suggested an optimum π for the 4′-substituent of 2.14 (*126*). This decrease in optimum π value compared to Eq. (8) is consistent with the model-based equation results in which the optimum π decreases with decreasing pK_a of the molecule.

Shipman *et al.* studied the structure–activity relationships of lincomycin analogs with ab initio quantum chemical methods (*44,178*). The results revealed a distinctly different conformational preference for the nonprotonated compared to the protonated species. From consideration of these results and rigid analogs, they concluded that the active species is the nonprotonated one and that the active conformation is that in which there is a hydrogen bond formed between the amide (donor) and pyrrolidine (acceptor) nitrogens (Fig. 3). Lincomycin and clindamycin differ substantially in the preferred conformation about the C-6—C-7 bond. Finally, the calculations showed that the chemically important orbitals, the HOMO, NHOMO, and LUMO are all quite localized on the amide unit, in accordance with the essentiality of the amide for antibacterial activity. These conclusions were based on calculations involving model structures of portions of the molecule only, in spite of the observation that long-range interactions between the carbohydrate and the pyrrolidine ring are sometimes significant.

The two theoretical studies converge in the conclusion that it is the nonprotonated form that binds to the receptor.

4. Whole-Animal Activity

The original QSAR paper included an analysis of the *in vivo* activity of the lincomycin and clindamycin analogs (*126*). The optimum π is not significantly different in the two series in spite of the fact that the change in lipophilicity due to the conversion from 7(*R*)-OH to 7(*S*)-Cl was not included in the calculation of π.

E. Chloramphenicol Analogs

Chloramphenicol (**XII**) is another antibiotic whose mechanism of action is inhibition of protein synthesis by binding to the 50 S bacterial ribosomal subunit. It inhibits protein chain elongation rather than chain initiation. Analog studies have shown that antibacterial activity is lost in all stereois-

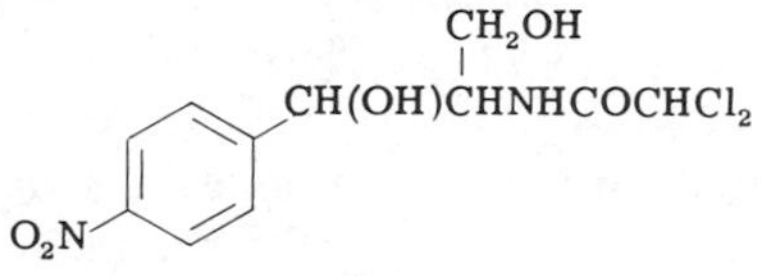

XII

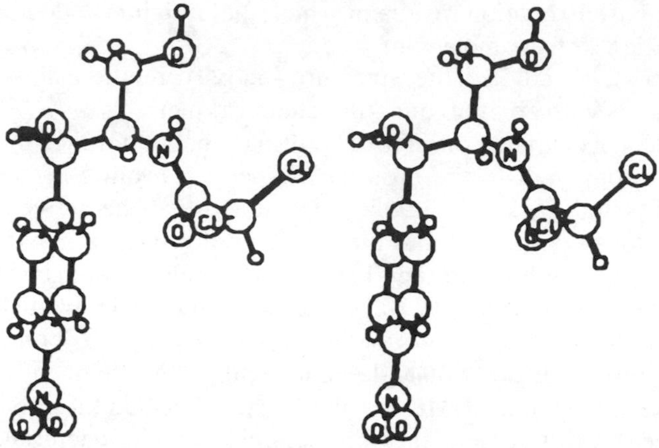

Fig. 4. Stereoview of chloramphenicol in the conformation found by Bustard *et al.* (*40*).

omers (Fig. 4) except the D-threo. However, extensive changes can be made for the *p*-nitrophenyl and dichloromethylene groups (*79*).

Hansch and Fujita's first QSAR paper, published in 1963, reported a correlation of the effect of modification of the 4-NO_2 on antibacterial potency of nine analogs as measured in a tube-dilution assay (*83*). From an equation in which all terms were statistically significant ($R^2 = 0.89$, $s = 0.26$) it was concluded that there is a negative dependence of potency on Hammett σ value and an optimum π of 0.2–0.6 for activity against both gram-positive and gram-negative microorganisms. A better correlation is found when σ_m rather than σ_p is used. The π value used for SO_2CH_3 was higher than that currently used; when the newer value is substituted the statistics do not deteriorate (*122*).

Garrett *et al.* determined relative potencies by microbial kinetics (*69*). Ten analogs were studied, including the 3-NO_2 derivative. A number of equations were reported, but none of these was statistically significant (*41*). The difference between this data set and that analyzed by Hansch and Fujita is not in the physical properties of the analogs studied but rather in the biological properties. There is a much larger spread in the values of potency measured by tube-dilution methods than in those derived from growth kinetics. In the former case the sum of squares of deviation from the mean $\log(1/C)$ is 3.229 ($n = 8$) whereas in the latter case it is 1.38 ($n = 10$). Such clues as to the differences between biological assays may be important to the design of assay procedures that quantitatively measure the parameter relevant for analog selection.

This same data set was analyzed by Cammarata in 1967 according to the hypothesis that dispersion binding governs the drug–receptor interaction (*41*). For this purpose molar polarizability, (P_E) is used as the physical property. (P_E is the same as molar refractivity, *MR*.) Although *MR* had been previously used in qualitative SAR, this is apparently the first time that it was used in QSAR. When potency is used as the dependent variable in this correlation R^2 equals 0.991. This analysis is compromised by the following problems: (1) it was assumed that the OCH_3, NO_2, and SCH_3 groups bind entirely but that the SO_2CH_3 binds only as a sulfonyl and isopropyl binds only as a methyl group; (2) the wrong biological activity was used for the 4-SO_2CH_3 analog; (3) the SCH_3 group was assumed to bind as an anion rather than the neutral substituent; and (4) the 4-NO_2 analog was omitted (its observed potency is outside the 95% confidence interval predicted). Hence, there are four adjustments made to 10 data points. Hansch *et al.* showed that when standard values of *MR* are used R^2 deteriorates to 0.02 (*82*).

Hansch *et al.* reanalyzed these data in 1969 (*82*). Correlations were made with the hydrophobic parameter π and with E_R, which is a measure of the influence of substituents on a radical reaction:

$$\log A = 3.07E_R + 0.23\pi + 0.77 \tag{9}$$

$$r = 0.977, \qquad s = 0.140, \qquad n = 8$$

This equation suggests an optimum π beyond the range of the π values in the data set (> 1.40) and a positive correlation with the ability of the substituent to delocalize a radical. Two compounds were not included in the analysis: the 3-NO_2, for which the log *A* value was 0.58 less then predicted, and the 4-NH_2, for which there was no E_R value available. Inspection of the data did suggest that the 4-NH_2 analog would be quite well predicted. The use of radical constants was not pursued because later these same workers concluded that special constants for radical reactions are not necessary because σ or σ^+ correlates radical reactions reasonably well (*80*). In the case of this set of chloramphenicols, this is not true.

A different equation for the same data was reported in a review but its source could not be verified (*198*). It was claimed that there is an optimum π of 0.4 and positive coefficients for *MR* and the square of the dipole moment. That is, there are four terms for 10 analogs.

Cammarata *et al.* reported still another pair of equations for this set of data (*43*):

$$\log k - \sigma^2 = 0.34\pi - 0.26\pi^2 + 1.26 \tag{10}$$

$$r = 0.92, \qquad s = 0.24, \qquad n = 9$$

and

$$\log k - E_r = 0.22\pi - 0.23\pi^2 + 1.30 \quad (11)$$

$$r = 0.88, \quad s = 0.22, \quad n = 9$$

The left side of the equation was assumed to give the biological potency in excess of that which is a consequence of the interaction implied by σ^2 or E_r. That is, it was assumed that the coefficient of the electronic term is $+1.00$, probably a questionable assumption. Note that the standard deviation from both of these equations is larger than that from Eq. (9). The statistics of the significance of the individual terms in this equation were not explicitly stated; a plus-or-minus value was given but it was not stated whether this is the standard deviation of the coefficient or whether it is the 95% confidence limit.

Chloramphenicol has a number of biochemical activities that appear not to be related to its mode of antibacterial action. Freeman reported a QSAR study of the inhibition of mitochondrial NADH oxidase. In contrast to antibacterial activity, the inhibition of the enzyme does not depend on the configuration of the side chain but is linearly correlated with the hydrophobicity of the substituent at the para position of the phenyl ring (*64*). He found no correlation between physical properties and the inhibition of protein synthesis in bacterial or mitochondrial extracts or in intact bacteria (*65*).

Hansch *et al.* in 1973 reported a new QSAR in bacteria after more analogs had been synthesized and tested in the growth kinetic assay (*84*). For a series of 16 ring-substituted analogs the most important determinant of potency is log *P*:

$$\log k = -0.34(\log P)^2 + 1.13 \log P + 1.08\sigma^2 + 0.02MR + 0.071 \quad (12)$$

$$r = 0.93, \quad s = 0.27, \quad n = 16$$

The optimum log *P* is 1.62, which corresponds to a π of 0.47 if the only modification is in the aromatic ring. The σ and *MR* terms are statistically justified at the 10% level. The values for the radical parameter E_R were apparently not available. Hence, hydrophobicity is the dominant factor, but some sort of electronic property of the molecules is also important in the determination of potency. The QSAR equation was used to predict the potency of the 4-pyridyl analog. It is much less potent than expected. The series is very well designed according to criteria published in 1979 (*127*). The standard deviations of log *P*, σ, and *MR* are large enough and there are no multiple correlations within the physical property data (*122*). The rather high standard deviation from the equation suggests that the typical linear free energy descriptors are inadequate for this series.

Hansch *et al.* also examined the influence on potency of variation of the substituent that replaces the dichloromethyl group on the amide (*84*). The QSAR of this set of 19 compounds reveals no steric effect. Rather, the best equation indicates an optimum log *P* of 0.93 (the log *P* of chloramphenicol is 1.15), a positive correlation with σ^*, and a negative correlation with *MR*:

$$\log k = -0.94(\log P)^2 + 1.76 \log P + 0.62\sigma^* - 0.05MR + 0.50 \quad (13)$$

$$r = 0.925, \quad s = 0.369, \quad n = 19$$

The σ^* correlation is consistent with the amide function being involved in the mechanism of action; the lack of correlation with the Taft steric parameter E_s and the negative dependence of activity on *MR* were not explained. In our evaluation this series is not so well designed (*122*). The standard deviation of log *P* is 0.65, which is low. However, the more serious problem is that two (rather than four) eigenvalues explain 88% of the variance in the correlation matrix of log *P*, σ^*, E_s, and *MR*. Log *P* is correlated with both E_s and *MR*, and its multiple R^2 or fraction of variance explained with the other variables is 0.79; that of *MR* is 0.69. It is possible that the data set is designed in such a way that the subtle interrelationships between potency and physical properties cannot be untangled.

The conformation of chloramphenicol has also received attention. In 1963 Jardetzky proposed that the solution conformation is approximately that shown in Fig. 4. This was based on NMR and Raman spectroscopy (*94*). He also noted a similarity between chloramphenicol and uridine 5′-phosphate. The essentials of these conformational conclusions were confirmed 10 years later in a combined potential energy, NMR, and IR study by Bustard *et al.* (*40*). They found that the conformation is not stabilized by a hydrogen bond and that there are two low-energy conformations that differ only in the positions of the hydroxyl groups. No relationship between these results and biological activity was discussed.

About a year later Holtje and Kier reached similar conformational conclusions from Extended Hückel Theory (EHT) calculations (*90*). Although EHT calculations are quite crude, they can give correct conformational trends within a set of analogs. They also reconsidered the QSAR study (*84*) and used the same biological data. There is no correlation between the antibacterial activity of analogs in which the acylamino side chain has been modified and the charges on the atoms of the corresponding *N*-monomethylamide calculated by the CNDO/2 method. CNDO/2 should give reliable trends in charges. No consideration was given to the possibility that more than one charge may be involved. Furthermore, only 11 of the 20 analogs were considered. Because of limitations of the quantum chemical calculation procedures, no analogs with Br or I in the side chain could be included: the phenyl, benzyl, $CHCNC_6H_5$, and CMe_3 were also omitted. Finally, as can be seen from Fig. 4, there is a possibility of dipole–dipole interactions between the chlorine atoms and the aromatic ring. The use of model compounds that lack the aromatic ring rule out investigation of changes in such an interaction as an underlying basis of the differences in antibacterial potency.

Holtje and Kier also used model interaction calculations to investigate the basis for the differences of activity of analogs substituted in the phenyl ring (*90*). For these interactions CNDO/2 calculations were made on model compounds in which the $CHOHNHCOCHCl_2$ side chain was replaced by CH_3. The charges interacted with a number of amino acid side chains in several relative orientations and distances. The most significant interaction is with indole at a 4.5 Å distance. For 12 of the 14 analogs studied the R^2 is 0.83. Two analogs do not fit the relationship; this was explained by the size of the 4-phenyl analog and possible metabolism of the 4-amino analog. Additionally, four analogs of the original data set were not considered. The large number of possible models considered plus the number of compounds omitted suggests that the apparent relationship may be a statistical artifact (*194*). The comments about the interaction between the aromatic ring and the side chain apply to this set of calculations also. The data studied involve whole-cell antibacterial activity. Because there is little correlation between whole-cell and cell-free potency of analogs (*65*), this study is not receptor mapping as claimed.

Brown *et al.* published a quantum chemical study in 1977 (*37*). There is an apparent error in the structure of chloramphenicol in this paper; it is not clear on what structure the calculations were done. Seven different acyl side chains on the parent molecule were studied by the CNDO/2 method in the conformation shown in Fig. 4. The best single variable correlation with the Hansch *et al.* data has an R^2 of 0.40. They concluded that electrostatic as opposed to frontier orbital indices give the best results and that the electrostatic potential in the vicinity of the carbonyl group may be instrumental in initiating the interaction between the drugs and the target. They also studied six ring-substituted analogs, again in the preferred conformation for chloramphenicol. Two regression equations were highlighted: one with the charge on the variable substituent and one with the charge on the whole phenyl ring. However, a data table suggests that the electric field, generated by the molecule, perpendicular to the benzene ring and at a point 4.5 Å above the center of the ring also correlates with potency. It would be interesting to know if these preliminary results were confirmed in a more detailed study.

A brief conformational study by CNDO/2 methods on $CHCl_2CONHCH_3$ and $CFCl_2CONHCH_3$ suggests that these two compounds have very different conformations (*214*). In the former case a Cl atom eclipses the N atom whereas in the latter case the F atom does. However, CNDO/2 is not the method of choice for conformational calculations.

The ambiguous result of the carefully planned and conducted QSAR studies (*84*) points to the limitations of the linear free-energy method in terms of descriptors of the electronic and conformational properties of molecules (*124*). To date none of the studies using quantum chemical approaches has been complete enough to have solved the QSAR of chloramphenicol. This emphasizes the large amount of effort required to use quantum chemical calculations to go beyond simple QSAR. It is estimated that such studies require at least 10 and probably 100 times the human effort as well as several orders of magnitude more computer time to accomplish (*124*). The QSAR of chloramphenicol analogs may also be made clearer by considering receptor-level potency rather than whole-cell activity.

F. Chloramphenicol, Lincomycin, and Erythromycin: General Models of the Mode of Inhibition of Protein Synthesis by These Compounds

It has long been known that erythromycin, lincomycin, and apparently chloramphenicol compete with each other for a ribosomal binding site (*68,87,200,208*). In 1974 Cheney proposed a model of the mode of interaction of these compounds and substrates with peptidyltransferase (*44*). The basic proposal is that ribosomal binding involves the amide or ester atoms plus the OH on the carbon β to the NH or O. Lincomycin was proposed to bind via other heteroatoms of the sugar and erythromycin via the 11-OH group.

He proposed that since interaction of each participating group with the ribosome is weak, the bound drug should not deviate much from its solution conformation (*44*). The necessary conformation of erythromycin is not one seen experimentally and the available evidence is that the macrolide ring is relatively stiff (*56,57*). Analog studies have shown that two of the atoms proposed to be involved in the ribosomal binding (the oxygens at C-11 and C-12), are not necessary for such binding. Hence, the proposed mode of erythromycin binding can be rejected. The conformation of chloramphenicol proposed as the binding conformation had been shown to be at least 10 kcal higher in energy than the global minimum (*40*).

A year earlier Harris and Symons had published a much more comprehensive analysis of substrates and inhibitors of ribosomal peptidyltransferase in a study using Dreiding models (*87*). It uses chloramphenicol in its X-ray conformation and is more specific in its comparison of phenylalanyl-RNA with lincomycin.

Hahn and Gund reviewed these two models using interactive computer graphics (*79*). This showed that the Cheney model does not predict the inactivity of the L-(+)-erythro isomer of chloramphenicol. They pointed out that the Harris model suggests that chloramphenicol should show preferential antagonism to particular amino acids. Such preferences are not observed. Additionally, the CH_2OH proposed by Harris to be critical for binding is, in fact, not essential (*78*). Hence Hahn and Gund proposed a rather ambiguous receptor map and pleaded for more data. Gund (*77*) later claimed that a transition-state analog that inhibits protein synthesis was designed on the basis of this model, but the report of this inhibitor does not cite the model (*176*).

More recently Bhuta *et al.* pointed out two more deficiencies in the Cheney model: (1) chloramphenicol is principally an inhibitor of the peptide bond acceptor site but the model was of binding to the peptidyl binding site, and (2) the important role of the amide was ignored (*13*). These workers suggested that chloramphenicol is a retro–inverso analog of the aromatic amino acid ester of an aminoacyl-tRNA or puromycin, substrates of the reaction inhibited by chloramphenicol.

G. Aminoglycosides

Aminoglycoside antibiotics are pseudo di- or trisaccharides that contain from four to six amino groups (*157*). They are conformationally flexible and are also characterized by several overlapping pK_a values. The only QSAR study found a positive linear correlation between both the logarithms of the acute LD_{50} and the logarithm of the kidney level with the energy of binding to the polyanion heparin (*103*). Studies involving pH changes confirmed the electrostatic nature of this interaction.

III. INHIBITORS OF NUCLEIC ACID SYNTHESIS

A. Rifamycins and Related Ansamacrolides

1. Overview

The rifamycin antibiotics (**XIII**), exemplified by rifampicin (Fig. 5), are structurally characterized by a naphthalene nucleus bonded on opposite

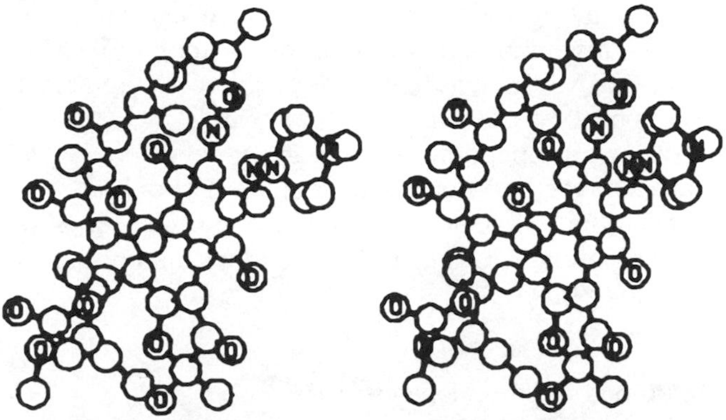

Fig. 5. Stereoview of the crystal structure of rifampicin (*67*).

sides to the ends of an aliphatic (ansa) chain. Modification studies suggest that the naphthohydroquinone and naphthoquinone forms are equally active; acetylation or methylation of the phenolic hydroxyl group in position

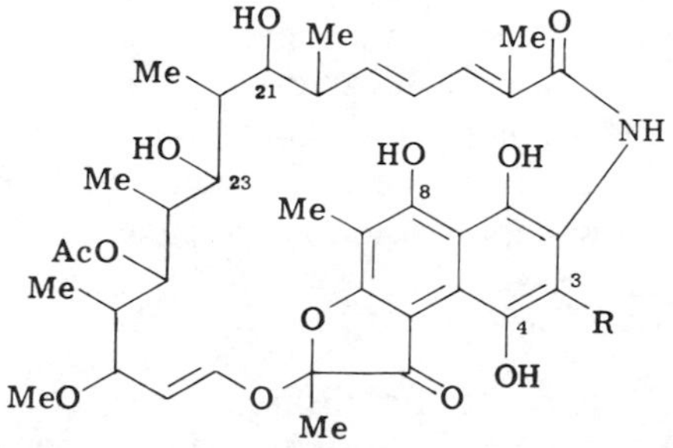

XIII

8 gives an inactive derivative; and opening or reduction or epoxidation of the ansa bridge either abolishes or severely reduces antibacterial activity (*105*). From a comparison of the X-ray and solution conformations of a number of compounds it has been concluded that for activity it is essential to have (1) the aromatic nucleus with oxygen atoms at C-1 and C-8 in either the quinone or the hydroquinone form, (2) the hydroxyls on C-21 and C-23, and (3) a conformation of the ansa bridge (such as shown in Fig. 5) that leads to a required steric relationship between the two hydroxyls and the aromatic nucleus (*38,39*). Most of the QSAR analyses have involved modifications in the substituent at positions 3 and 4 of the aromatic nucleus. It must be noted, however, that there is some evidence that a change of substituent at these positions can result in a change in the conformation of the ansa bridge (*39,52*).

Rifamycins inhibit bacterial growth by virtue of their inhibition of RNA synthesis (*39*). This inhibition is due to direct inhibition of the enzyme DNA-dependent RNA polymerase. The compounds are selective for the bacterial as opposed to the mammalian enzyme.

The rifamycins are lipophilic. Pelizza *et al.* reported R_m values (*141*). The pK_a values of the hydroquinone form are approximately 1.8 for loss of a proton from the C-1–C-8 center and 6.0–8.0 for loss of proton from the side chain piperazine nitrogen (*7*). The more lipophilic analogs lower surface tension (*140*).

2. Inhibition of DNA-dependent RNA Polymerase

Dampier and Whitlock (*52*) studied the inhibition of the *E. coli* enzyme by 18 rifamycin S analogs with substitutions at the 3 position. Both the naphthoquinone and hydroquinone forms are inhibitors in the same concentration range. The dramatic changes in inhibitory potency are a positive linear function of σ_p and not σ_m, van der Waals radius of the attached atom, or conformation of the ansa bridge. The authors concluded that the substituents change the rate of formation of the drug–enzyme complex. They postulate that this complex is a donor–acceptor π complex formed by insertion of a tyrosine from the enzyme into the hole formed between the ansa bridge and the naphthoquinone nucleus.

3. Antibacterial Activity

Following a preliminary study by Barbaro *et al.* (*10*), Pelizza *et al.* reported an extensive QSAR study on rifamycins in 1973 (*141,142*). A total of 76 analogs was studied; this includes 40 oximes of 3-formylrifamycin SV(3-CH=NOR, 4-OH), 16 amides of rifamycin B (3-H, 4-$OCH_2CONR^1R^2$), and 13 iminomethylpiperazines of rifamycin SV (3-CH=N–N⟨piperazine⟩NR, 4-OH). In general the substituents are alkyl or alkyl ether structures; the principal property varied was hydrophobicity. This was assessed by reversed phase thin-layer chromatography extrapolated to the R_f in acetone:water(4:6) solution. They found a correlation between the MIC against *S. aureus Tour* and R_m value:

$$\log(1/C) = 8.02 - 0.18R_m - 0.84R_m^2 \qquad (14)$$

$$r = 0.86, \quad s = 0.39, \quad n = 79, \quad R_{m,0} = -0.11$$

Both terms are statistically significant. There is no correlation between the MIC value against *E. coli* and R_m values.

The correlation is significantly improved if the series is divided into subseries. For *S. aureus Tour* the oximes were fit by Eq. (15):

$$\log(1/C) = 8.12 - 1.56R_{\mathrm{m}} \tag{15}$$

$$r = 0.96, \quad s = 0.26, \quad n = 39, \quad R_{\mathrm{m,0}} < -0.50.$$

The corresponding equation for the iminomethylpiperazines is

$$\log(1/C) = 8.17 - 0.03R_{\mathrm{m}} - 0.45R_{\mathrm{m}}^2 \tag{16}$$

$$r = 0.95, \quad s = 0.08, \quad n = 13, \quad R_{\mathrm{m,0}} = -0.04$$

and that for the amides is

$$\log(1/C) = 7.86 + 0.18R_{\mathrm{m}} - 0.60R_{\mathrm{m}}^2 \tag{17}$$

$$r = 0.89, \quad s = 0.18, \quad n = 16, \quad R_{\mathrm{m,0}} = 0.15$$

Hence, each series is fit reasonably well, each with a slightly different optimum R_{m} value. The curves suggest that consideration of the pK_{a} values of the various series and using model-based equations (*123*) might lead to a better fit of the data in one equation. Similar correlations were reported for the antibacterial activity of the oximes against the other gram-positive organisms *Streptococcus hemolyticus*, *Streptococcus faecalis*, and *Diplococcus pneumoniae*. In every subseries a parabolic function with higher optimum $R_{\mathrm{m,0}}$ fits the data from a resistant *S. aureus Tour*. The potency of seven additional iminomethylpiperazines against *S. aureus Tour* is well predicted by the previous equations (*51*).

Although no general correlation was found between the MIC values against *E. coli* and R_{m} values, equations were found for the individual series. For the oximes the equation is:

$$\log(1/C) = 5.02 - 0.33R_{\mathrm{m}} - 0.68R_{\mathrm{m}}^2 \tag{18}$$

$$r = 0.74, \quad s = 0.18, \quad n = 28, \quad R_{\mathrm{m,0}} = -0.25$$

For the iminomethylpiperazines it is:

$$\log(1/C) = 5.31 - 1.11R_{m} - 1.11R_{m}^2 \tag{19}$$

$$r = 0.79, \quad s = 0.21, \quad n = 11, \quad R_{\mathrm{m,0}} = 0.50$$

For the amides the correlation is not significant.

Quinn *et al.* studied 44 amides and 25 hydrazides of rifamycin B in five bacterial systems (*159*). There is more variation in the electronic properties of the substituents in this series. The log *P* values of the compounds were calculated from that of the parent. The QSAR equations for the amides indicates an optimum log *P* of 3.94, 3.68, and 2.37 for activity against *M. aureus*, *S. faecalis*, and *S. hemolyticus* respectively. The parabolic term is not significant for *B. subtilis:* activity increases linearly with increasing log *P*. In all four cases an indicator variable of 1.0 for *N,N*-disubstituted amides is statistically significant with a positive coefficient. Because of collinearity in the physical properties, it is possible to derive statistically significant equations with a positive linear term in log *P* and a negative linear term in the Taft steric parameter E_s. This equation was discarded when two additional analogs were tested and shown to fit the parabolic log *P* equations but not those linear in log *P* and E_s.

For the series of hydrazides the electronic parameter σ^* is the most important predictor of activity; it has a negative coefficient for all four microorganisms, that is, electron-donating substituents increase activity. However, to quote the authors, "It is difficult to draw any firm conclusions about the hydrazide QSAR. The large amount of collinearity between E_s and log *P*, σ^* and E_s, and log *P* and σ^* seriously obscures the details of the QSAR, (*159*, p. 338)."

Next, Kiritsy *et al.* reported on a series of 14 3-formylrifamycin SV *N*-(4-substituted phenyl)piperazinoacethydrazones (*101*). It was designed by cluster analysis to be suitable for QSAR analyses. Potency against *B. subtilis* and *Mycobacterium phlei* increases linearly with π; the relationship is parabolic for potency against *S. aureus* with an optimum π of 0.52. A positive dependence of potency on *R* and on *MR* are also noted. This leads to a four-variable equation with a sample size of 14. The *R* and *MR* terms are also significant for the correlation with *M. phlei* activity, but in this case the coefficient of the *R* term is negative. No equations were found for potency against *Clostridium perfringens* or *Mycobacterium tuberculosis*.

Lukovits *et al.* (*109*) performed a principal component analysis of just the biological data considered by Quinn *et al.* (*159*). In some cases it is possible to derive an equation with a lower *s* value than that from QSAR if, rather than physical properties, one uses the principal components from the analysis of all biological activity except that used as the dependent variable. Such an equation cannot be used to predict the activity of an unknown molecule because its activity in the other tests would not be known. However, this could be a useful procedure to use to get one estimate of the best (lowest *s*) QSAR equation for a data set.

In 1980 Mager (*113*) reported an unusual QSAR equation for the potency of rifamycin imines and oximes in protecting mice against a lethal bacterial infection:

$$\ln \mathrm{ED}_{50} = 3.64 + 1.50(0.01MV) - 2.57I_\mathrm{D} + 0.06 \tan^{-1}\pi \qquad (20)$$

MV refers to the molar volume and π to the lipophilicity of the substituent beyond the connecting bridge. The indicator variable, I_D, describes the deteriorating effect of iminomethylpiperazines. The only statistic reported is r, which has a value of 0.94. The more traditional parabolic, bilinear, and even polynomial functions in π were reported to be not statistically significant. Evidence that the correlation is not spurious is provided by fairly accurate predictions of the potency of two compounds that were not included in the derivation of the equaton. However, these compounds are forecast by the equation to be more potent than all other analogs, when in fact they were observed to be equal in potency to the most potent in the original set. No explanation of the biological basis for the $\tan^{-1}$ relationship with π was offered.

4. Binding to Serum Proteins

Assandri *et al.* (*7*) studied the binding to serum albumin of six analogs. From temperature-dependence studies they concluded that both hydrophobic and electrostatic interactions are important.

B. Coumerycins

Coumermycin is structurally characterized as a complex coumarin. It apparently inhibits bacterial growth by inhibition of the enzyme DNA gyrase (*50*). Hydrophobicity appears to be an important determinant of MIC values (*157*) and binding to serum proteins (*49*).

IV. INHIBITORS OF CELL WALL BIOSYNTHESIS: β-LACTAM ANTIBIOTICS

A. Overview

The classical β-lactam antibiotics are represented by penicillins (**XIV**) and Δ^3-cephalosporins (**XV**). The structural features essential for antibacterial activity are (1) the β-lactam ring; (2) the fusion of this ring to a second ring to decrease the resonance in the OC—N bond and thereby increase the reactivity of the β-lactam with nucleophiles; (3) the carboxyl group at C-3 of the penicillins and C-4 of the cephalosporins; (4) the acylation of the 6 or 7 amino group; and (5) the chirality of C-3, C-5, and C-6 of the penicillins and C-3, C-6, and C-7 of the cephalosporins, and (5) the 3 double bond in the cephalosporins (*20,75,91,155,156,170,205*). Accordingly, variation is permitted only in the R group in penicillins and in the R and R′ groups in the cephalosporins. Substantial changes in both potency and spectrum are observed with changes in these groups.

A chemical characteristic of the β-lactam antibiotics is their facile reaction with nucleophiles, Y, to cleave the β-lactam ring and form the corresponding penicilloyl (**XVI**) or cephalosporonyl (**XVII**) compound. For example, Y may be a simple hydroxide ion or a nucleophilic group on a protein.

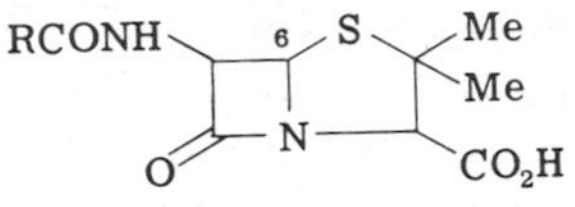

XIV

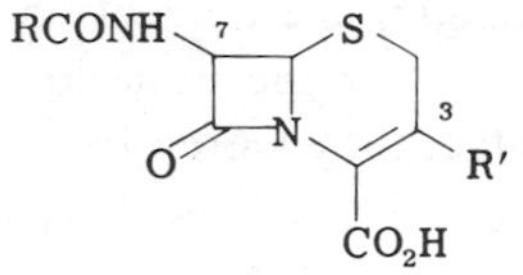

XV

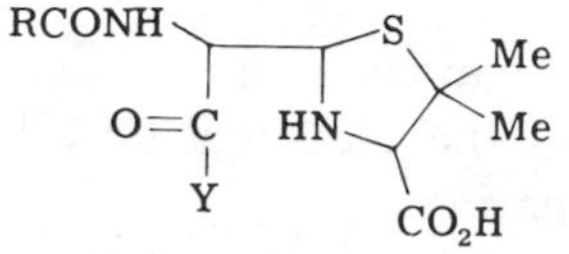

XVI

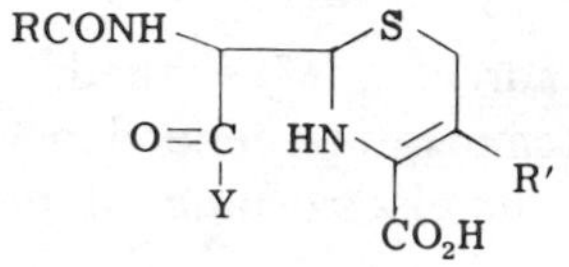

XVII

Penicillins and cephalosporins inhibit bacterial growth by interfering with the formation of the rigid cell wall. They disrupt the cross-linking of strands of peptidoglycan that form insoluble cell wall polymer (*8,204*). The lack of cross-links leads to a weakened cell and ultimately cell lysis or deformation.

Wise and Park (*209*) and Tipper and Strominger (*190*) suggested that the transpeptidase cross-linking enzyme recognizes β-lactams as analogs of either the LAla-D-γ-Glu or DAla-DAla portions of the peptide chains that are involved in the cross-linking reaction. The β-lactam antibiotics acylate and thereby inhibit these transpeptidase enzymes. It is not known whether this acylation is lethal per se or whether it triggers some secondary bactericidal event (*191,192*). Penicillins can also acylate carboxypeptidases (*66,72,74,191,209*). In some species of bacteria this inhibition of carboxypeptidase causes cell death (*66*). However, each strain of bacteria has a spectrum of proteins that are penicilloylated. Physiological roles for all of these proteins have not been determined, nor has the role of acylation of them in cell death been established (*66,72,74,191*). Multiple binding sites may be present in these enzymes. In some of the transpeptidases and carboxypeptidases there is kinetic evidence that suggests that penicillins bind at sites distinct from those at which the peptide substrates bind (*72*). However, for others the isolation of radiolabeled acylated proteins indicates that both the penicillins and peptides acylate the same site (*72,204*).

Bacterial resistance occurs by production of β-lactamases that hydrolyze the β-lactam ring. Sensitive compounds are hydrolyzed by the enzyme whereas resistant compounds are inhibitors of it. Apparently the difference between substrates and inhibitors is in the rate of deacylation of the penicilloyl group from the enzyme (*45*).

There are many similarities between the β-lactamases and the penicillin-sensitive transpeptidases and carboxypeptidases. First, there are homologies in primary and secondary structure (*131,204*). This indicates a common evolutionary origin. Second, major conformational changes occur during the binding of the substrate/inhibitor before any covalent reaction takes place (*46,72,167*). Third, serine is involved in the active site of some of these (*61,204*). Fourth, the same protein may show β-lactamase and transpeptidase or carboxypeptidase activity (*66,72*). The similarities among these enzymes may mean that there is a similarity in their catalytic mechanism.

In 1982 Knox presented a preliminary report of the X-ray crystallographic structure of a penicillin-sensitive enzyme (*102a*). The binding site for penicillin and cephalosporin overlaps that for the DAla-DAla substrate.

In summary, in bacteria there are many penicillin-sensitive enzymes each of which may have a spectrum of enzymatic activities. Any one penicillin can react at different rates with the different enzymes, and a single protein could undergo a spectrum of responses to a closely related series of β-lactams (*72,191*). The effects of the environment and the structure of the β-lactam seem to be important determinants of the ultimate bacterial response (*66,72,73,191,204*).

During 1979–1981 several so-called nonclassical β-lactam antibiotics have been reported (*62,148*). These compounds maintain the β-lactam ring but lack one or another of the other structural features long considered important to activity. Because not much theoretical work has been done on these compounds, they will be included in only a peripheral way in this review.

B. Effects of Modification of the Side Chain

Inasmuch as the side chain of β-lactams is not involved in the covalent bond formation with the target enzymes, it might be anticipated that theoretical structure–activity investigations might be especially applicable to this class of structural analogs. Indeed, Ferres *et al.* have shown a high correlation between the antibacterial spectrum and potency of corresponding members of two series of penicillins, **XIV**, R = X and R = $XCONHCH(C_6H_5)$ (*60*).

1. Measurement of Physical Properties

Bird and Marshall (*17*) measured the octanol–water log *P* values of seven analogs and showed that the method of calculation of log *P* values in use in 1967 was not very reliable for penicillins.

Biagi *et al.* measured the R_m values of many β-lactams by reversed-phase thin layer chromatography (*14,15*). The mobile phase was acetone–water in various proportions and the stationary phase was silicone oil. R_m values were calculated by extrapolation to 0% acetone. The graphs indicate both scatter and nonlinearity. Furthermore, the pH of the aqueous phase is ambiguous. For compounds with ionizable groups in the side chain it is essential to know this pH value (*211*).

Safanda and Sobotka (*165*) also reported measured octanol–pH 7.22 apparent log *P*′ and reversed-phase TLC R_m values. They found good correlations between log *P*′ and R_m values, but the intercept is higher for penicillins that have aliphatic side chains than for those in which the side chain contains an aromatic ring.

The work of Biagi *et al.* was criticized by Bird and Marshall (*19*) and Thijssen (*189*). In the earlier work the R_m values do not change with pH nearly as much as predicted from pH partition theory. Bird and Marshall also determined the pH of such plates and concluded that the silica gel changes the pH of the mobile phase. Hence, they used cellulose coated with octanol as the stationary phase and observed an almost perfect correlation between R_M and log *P*′ at pH values of 3.0, 4.0, and 5.0. The difference in R_M values with pH is very close to theoretical.

Somewhat later Rollo (*164*) measured acid dissociation constants and partition coefficients of 10 penicillins. The acid dissociation constant does not vary with change in structure of the side chain except for very lipophilic compounds, which are probably not soluble enough to be accurately measured. The log *P* values are not remarkable.

Purich *et al.* (*158*) studied the pH dependence of the butanol–water and octanol–water partition coefficients of the ampholyte β-lactams ampicillin, cephalexin, and cephaloglycin. Partitioning is greatest at the highest pH region studied, 7.9. From this it was concluded , in accordance with the measured pK_a values, that at lower pH values the compounds exist in water almost exclusively as zwitterions and not as neutral molecules.

Tsuji *et al.* (*196*) also investigated the pH partition behavior of β-lactams, but they studied only compounds that have no ionizable group in the side chain. They showed a linear correlation with a slope of 1.0 and an intercept of 3.5 of the log *P* of the neutral form compared to that of the ion. Good correlations of their values with previous log *P*, R_m, and HPLC results were also noted.

The hydrophobicity of penicillins has also been studied with reversed-phase high-pressure liquid chromatography (*211*). The stationary phase was silica gel chemically bonded to octadecyl chains; the mobile phase was 0.035 *M* NH_4Cl aqueous methanol adjusted to pH 7.4. Lipophilicity values were calculated from the retention time of the compound compared to that of an unretained sample and extrapolated to *k* values at 0% acetone. There is a high correlation between the log(*k*) values and both octanol–water log *P* values and silicon–water R_m values reported by other workers.

In 1981 Thijssen reported the log *P* values of oxacillin derivatives (*189*). He showed that silica R_m values do not correlate with log *P* values and also that there are nonadditivities in the partition coefficients that are not accounted for by current theories of log *P* calculation.

Finally, Yoshimoto and Watanabe measured log *P* and R_m values of 7-methoxycephalosporin derivatives for use in QSAR analyses (*212*).

2. Binding to Serum Proteins

The studies of binding to serum proteins are important because many of the QSAR studies include analysis of antibacterial activity determined in the presence of serum. The classic paper was published in 1967 by Bird and Marshall (*17*). They studied 79 penicillin analogs and reported a regression equation between calculated octanol–water π values and the log (B/F) value where *B* is the concentration bound and *F* is the concentration free in solution. (Under the conditions of their test B/F is very close to an equilibrium binding constant.) The equation has a positive slope of approximately 0.5. When measured log *P* values are used, the quality of the correlation improves substantially. Hence, they concluded that variation in hydrophobicity is the only important physicochemical change of consequence in the structure–activity relationships of penicillin protein binding. The next year Scholtan published graphs that show a linear correlation between the binding constant to human serum albumin and the log P' value between isobutanol and pH 7.4 buffer for nine analogs (*176*).

Bird and Nayler expanded their studies to include a series of oxacillin derivatives for which no π value had been available earlier (*20*). Better fits of data are obtained when more homogeneous sets of compounds are used. No other physical property improves the quality of the overall regression equation.

Calorimetric determinations of the thermodynamics of serum protein binding of 10 penicillins confirmed that hydrophobic interactions provide the major contribution to the free energy of binding (*106,116*).

Nys and Rekker reanalyzed the protein-binding data on the seven analogs for which log *P* has been measured (*135*). By using the *f* fragmental constant method of log P calculation they were able to calculate log P with a standard deviation of 0.245 compared to the standard deviation of 0.468 using the older method and π values. Hence, although the f method improves the accuracy of the calculation of log P, it is still not perfect. The standard deviations in the correlations of log(B/F) with log P calculated by the π method, the f method, and measured log P are 0.304, 0.201, and 0.106, respectively. Accordingly, as the estimate of log P becomes more precise, the correlation between log(B/F) and log P increases. Thus there is no evidence that structural features other than lipophilicity affect protein binding.

Rekker later expanded these studies (*160*). From an analysis of subsets of compounds he proposed that a stacking interaction of aromatic rings with the serum albumin also contributes to the binding energy. The inclusion of an indicator variable for aromatic compounds decreases the standard deviation from the fit from 0.162 to 0.150.

Adamson and colleagues analyzed the data set of Bird and Marshall by two pattern recognition techniques in which the structure was represented by substructures rather than physical properties (*1*,*2*). In the first, the substructures were generated manually from Wiswesser Line Notation code. In the second, they were generated by the computer from input connection tables. Both studies used stepwise multiple linear regression analysis to derive a function to fit the data. Because these data had been previously shown to correlate with octanol–water log P values, these patterns recognition calculations are in essence calculating log P. Accordingly, they are reduced to an analysis that is a subset of the log P calculation method of Rekker (*161*). For the 79 analogs Bird and Marshall reported an R value of 0.924 and an s of 0.257; the first pattern recognition paper reported values of 0.945 and 0.294, respectively, whereas the second reported 0.976 and 0.225. For the pattern recognition papers 12 and 29 variables, respectively, are included in the equation. The optimist would conclude that the computer is able to generate automatically a set of descriptors of these hydrophobicity–protein binding data. The use of the computer promises to be easier and less biased than hand calculations. The pessimist, however, would point out that the computer-generated fragments require more variables and hence more observations and that they are more difficult to interpret in terms of mechanism or physical chemistry of interaction.

3. Gastrointestinal Absorption

Tsuji *et al.* (*197*) studied the intestinal absorption rate and decomposition rate of seven penicillins. At pH 4.0, where absorption rate and apparent partition coefficients are high, there is a linear correlation between absorption rate and lipophilicity. Data at higher pH values suggests absorption of the ionized form by a lipophilicity insensitive process. Kimura *et al.* (*100*) also showed that there is no correlation between absorption rate and $CHCl_3$–pH 6.5 buffer partition coefficients. Rather, liposome experiments suggest that release of the antibiotics from the membrane is the rate-controlling factor.

4. Antibacterial Activity

The earliest appliction of computerized structure–activity analysis of the antibacterial activity (*S. aureus*) of β-lactam antibiotics was published by Hansch and Steward in 1964 (*85*). They correlated both whole-cell *in vitro* activity and the mouse CD_{50} values. For the mouse CD_{50} values and *in vitro* activity measured in the presence of serum, potency is negatively correlated with the calculated octanol–water π value. The 4-$NHCOCH_3$ was omitted from the CD_{50} correlation because it was observed to be 1.20 log units less potent than predicted. Its *in vitro* potency was not reported. There is no correlation between physicochemical properties and potency measured in the absence of serum. Since the addition of serum decreases potency (by an amount depending on log P), they concluded that the correlations reflect correlations of lipophilicity with protein binding. This was later verified in the direct experiments discussed above.

Shortly thereafter Hansch and Deutsch reported correlation equations for a series of eight penicillin analogs in which the aromatic ring was in direct conjugation with the amide (*81*). There is a negative correlation of the π value with *in vitro* MIC values against *S. aureus* in the presence of serum. The correlation is improved by the inclusion of the Hammett σ value: the ρ is -1.70. The set is too small to be certain of the true interpretation of this apparent electronic effect.

In 1971 Bird and Nayler (*20*) reported correlation equations for three series of penicillins: those for which R is alkyl, ring-substituted α-aminobenzyl, and monosubstituted methylpenicillins. All data is for *in vitro* MIC activity measured in the absence of serum. Four microorganisms were studied: *E. coli*, *Salmonella typhi*, *S. aureus*, and *S. faecalis*. In most cases there are significant correlations with the octanol–water π value and an appropriate electronic parameter. The QSAR relationships are always more homogeneous in the first two sets compared to the heterogeneous $R'CH_2$ analogs. In all cases there is a positive slope for correlation of π with activity against gram-positive microorganisms and a negative one for the correlation of π with activity against gram-negative ones. This result is in accord with the observation by Lien *et al.* (*108*) of a higher optimum log *P* for synthetic antibacterials tested against gram-positive organisms than when the same compounds are tested against gram-negative organisms.

Because the σ^* values of alkyl groups are now considered to be equal to each other (*118*), the reported correlations in the alkyl series may instead reflect steric effects or nonlinear nonparabolic correlations with π.

In the α-aminobenzylpenicillins, activity against *S. typhi* and *S. faecalis* is a negative function of Hammett σ (*20*). This may reflect changes in the pK_a of the NH_2 group and/or the stability of the aminoacyl bond. The three series are not well designed for the investigation of steric effects, but the two equations reported both include a positive coefficient of E_s. That is, more bulky or conformationally restricted groups increase potency. Such results suggest that investigation of conformational correlations of activity may be worthwhile. The observation of an apparent steric effect of substituents on potency is related directly to the experimental observation of conformational responses on binding that differ depending on the nature of the side chain (*46,72*).

The whole animal CD_{50} data set correlated in (*85*) has been a popular one for other workers in the QSAR field. For example, it was shown that the $\log(1/CD_{50})$ values are also correlated with molar attraction constants calculated from regular solution theory (*138*), parachor (*3*), and van der Waals volume (*132*). A high collinearity between van der Waals volume and the molar attraction constants was noted (*132*). Presumably this collinearity extends to π and *MR* also. Finally, Santora and Auyang applied the Fibonacci search technique using log *P* as the search variable to find the most active of the 22 analogs in six steps (*169*).

Biagi and colleagues (*16*) studied the QSAR of penicillins with varying side chains and cephalosporins for which both the side chain and the 3-substituent were varied. Whole-cell antibacterial activity against *S. aureus* and *E. coli* was measured by an agar diffusion zone diameter method. The activity against *Treponema pallidum* was measured by a turbidometric assay in the presence of 1% serum albumin. For the 14 cephalosporins and all 3 microorganisms they reported parabolic equations in reversed phase TLC R_m values. The value of the optimum R_m value is higher for activity against *S. aureus* and *T. pallidum* than that against *E. coli*. For the 11 penicillins studied, a negative correlation of potency against *E. coli* with R_m values was found. No acceptable QSAR equation was found for all 11 analogs using either *S. aureus* or *T. pallidum* activity. However, omission of three analogs (methicillin, cloxacillin, and dicloxacillin) results in parabolic equations with slightly lower optimum R_m values than those calculated from the cephalosporins. The deviations were ascribed to unparameterized electronic, steric, or conformational effects on potency.

Yoshimoto and Watanabe studied the MIC values of a series of 7-

methoxy cephalosporins (**XV**) against *E. coli* (*212*). They found that the optimum π value for the R substituent is − 1.8. All 139 compounds could be included in one equation if they used indicator variables for the R′ substituents.

In 1972 Retsema and Ray demonstrated that hydrophilic compounds compete less well than hydrophobic ones for the whole-cell acylation sites of penicillin G (*162*).

Garzia *et al.* (*70*) demonstrated that QSAR may be used to analyze structure–selectivity as well as structure–activity relationships. Their regression analysis was based on ratios of activities rather than individual activities as such. Considering the same 11 penicillin analogs, they reported that selectivity of the compounds for *S. aureus* as opposed to the two other microorganisms is a positive linear function of the TLC R_m value. The coefficient of the slope is 2.00 of which 1.55 is due to the selectivity for *S. aureus* compared to *E. coli* and 0.45 for that compared to *T. pallidum*. From the value of the standard deviations from the equations, these selectivity relationships are no more precise than the regression equations for all 11 analogs reported previously (*16*).

In 1977 Saikawa *et al.* reported on a series of four penicillin analogs that differed only in the chain length of one substituent in the R group (*166*). The following qualitative correlations were noted with chain length: increased stability against β-lactamases, decreased blood levels, increased binding to serum proteins, increased toxicity, and increased *in vitro* antibacterial activity. Although the *in vitro* antibacterial effect increases fourfold in going from C-1 to C-4, the potency in the whole-animal mouse protection test of *in vivo* efficacy decreases fourfold. In optimizing a structure by QSAR or any other means, one must not forget pharmacokinetic properties.

Ferres *et al.* (*59*) reported that side-chain configuration and not log *P* is the critical determinant of potency in a series of ureidoacylamino penicillin analogs.

Later Sawai and colleagues (*171*) did a direct determination of the bacterial outer-membrane permeability of two penicillins and five cephalosporins. They showed a graphical (apparently parabolic) correlation between chromatographic R_m values and membrane permeability. Except for the most lipophilic compound, cephaloridine, there is a positive linear correlation between permeability and hydrophilicity.

In 1980 Starnes *et al.* showed a linear correlation between the K_i for inhibition of a *B. subtilis* aminopeptidase and rotational flexibility around the bond between the side chain and the β-lactam ring estimated from CPK models (*179*). As in the whole-cell activity, conformationally restricted analogs are more potent.

Finally, Wetzel *et al.* (*207*) reported a very practical application of the

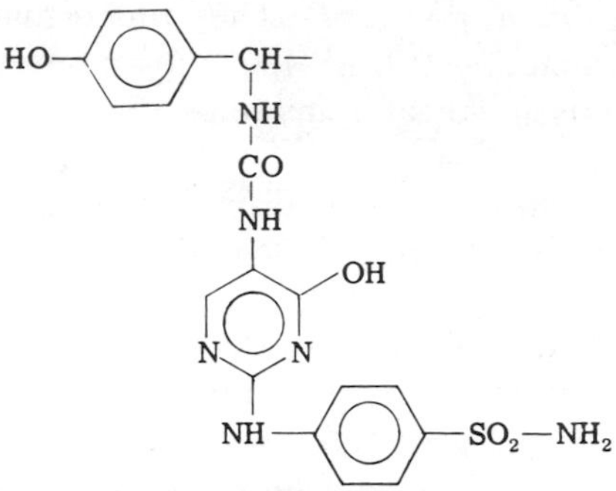

XVIII

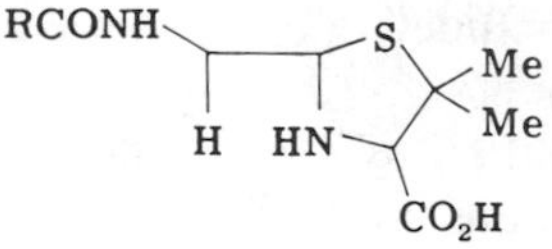

XIX

concepts of QSAR to the development of VX-VC 43, a novel analog of ampicillin, for which the side chain is structure **XVIII**. Early work on the 2-substituent of the pyrimidine ring showed that *in vitro* potency versus the target gram-negative organisms is increased with substituents, such as C_2H_5NH, that have negative Hammett σ values. Concurrently, investigation of a set of para-substituted *N*-benzyl analogs, for which hydrophobic but not electronic properties were varied, showed that increases in hydrophobicity increase potency against *Klebsiella* but decrease it against *E. coli, Pseudomonas,* and *Proteus*. Accordingly, it was decided to halt synthesis in the latter series. The two preliminary series led directly to the decision to synthesize a series of *N*-phenyl analogs with a large and uncorrelated spread of σ and π values. Testing these analogs showed that there is a $+\sigma$ dependence of potency and that analogs with negative π values are more active *in vivo*. This qualitative analysis on 11 analogs led directly to the correct prediction of both good *in vitro* and *in vivo* potency of the optimum compound VX-VC 43.

5. Acid Stability

Penicillins are acid labile: to be clinically useful as oral therapeutic agents they must be stable enough to be absorbed from the gastrointestinal tract. Bird and Nayler (*20*) summarized the early work that suggested that the stability of the compound (in 50% aqueous ethanol at pH 1.3) is increased as the σ^* or σ value of the side chain is increased. That is, withdrawal of electrons from the acylamino group increases the stability of the β-lactam ring.

6. β-Lactamase

Bird and Nayler (*20*) reported that they were unable to find statistically significant equations between the enzymatic K_m or V_{max} values for hydrolysis by β-lactamase and side chain π and σ^* values. This is in accord with the body of evidence that steric or conformational effects are the predominant factor in the penicillin–β-lactamase interaction and that different side chains result in different conformational responses of the enzyme (*46,72,167*).

Samuni and Meyer studied the rotation about the C—N bond to the acyl side chain of three penicillins with the quantum chemical PCILO calculations (*168*). PCILO is probably the quantum chemical method of choice for conformational calculations. The analog that is a good substrate for β-lactamase is conformationally flexible, whereas the two inhibitors are conformationally restricted. Blanpain *et al.* confirmed and extended these observations by a combination of X-ray, NMR, IR, and PCILO methods (*23*). Whereas there are no differences in thiazolidine ring conformation between the substrates and inhibitors, they also found that the side chain is relatively rigid in the inhibitors and flexible in the substrates.

7. Cerebral Toxicity

Weihrauch *et al.* correlated the neurotoxic effects of six penicillins with their isobutanol (pH 7.4) partition coefficients (*206*). Neurotoxicity was assessed by EEG changes in rabbits following drug administration by intravenous infusion at equimolar doses. The r value for the correlation between time after administration at which spike-wave paroxysms were first observed and the partition coefficient (not log P or log P') is 0.928. A graph of log P' versus the log of a neurotoxicity index that includes both time to response and minimal effective dose shows that the four inactive analogs all have butanol buffer log P' values ≤ 0.5, whereas for the four neurotoxic analogs, neurotoxicity increases as a linear function of log P'.

A very similar study was performed by Safanda and Sobotka in rats (*165*). For penicillins with only aliphatic side chains, there is a positive linear correlation between measured log P′ or R_m values and the log($1/C$) to produce epileptogenic EEG discharges 10 min after topical application to the exposed brain. The correlation for the compounds with aromatic groups in the side chain deteriorates to an r value of 0.512; in neither case is the standard deviation specified, but the range in log($1/C$) values in the two series is not drastically different. A plot of the data shows that the aromatic series does indeed have more scatter; however, it provides evidence that the 2,4-dinitrophenyl analog is an outlier and much less potent than expected.

8. Allergic Reaction

Another side effect of penicillins involves the allergic reaction. Bird (*18*) analyzed data on the cross-reaction with benzylpenicilloyl-specific antibodies of 20 penicilloic (**XVI**: X = OH) and penilloic (**XIX**) acids. Regression analysis with the variables log *P*, molar volume, and pK_a showed that only the first two properties are statistically significant. There is a positive correlation with log *P* and a negative one with molar volume. Penilloic acids are approximately one log unit less active than penicilloic acids. Interestingly, just as in the QSAR of serum protein binding of the penicillins, the allergic cross-reactivity of the analogs with carboxyl groups in the side chain fits with that of the other penicillin derivatives when log *P* for the un-ionized form is used. This points out the problem that arises when using apparent log *P′* values in a correlation analysis (*123*). The equations correctly predicted the antibody binding constants of six other benzoyl penicilloic acids. However, methyl- and ethylpenicilloic acids are not well predicted and are hence outside the range of the data set.

C. Variations in the Substituents on the Bicyclic Nucleus

1. Changes in Reactivity of the Amide Bond

Because these antibiotics produce their lethal effect by acylation of susceptible proteins, one would expect that there would be a relationship between antibacterial activity and changes in the intrinsic stability/reactivity of the lactam bond. Investigation of such correlations has been approached mainly with quantum chemical calculations.

The first question posed by these theoretical calculations is this: what is special about the penicillins and cephalosporins that gives them antibacterial activity, whereas ordinary β-lactams and even Δ^2-cephalosporins do

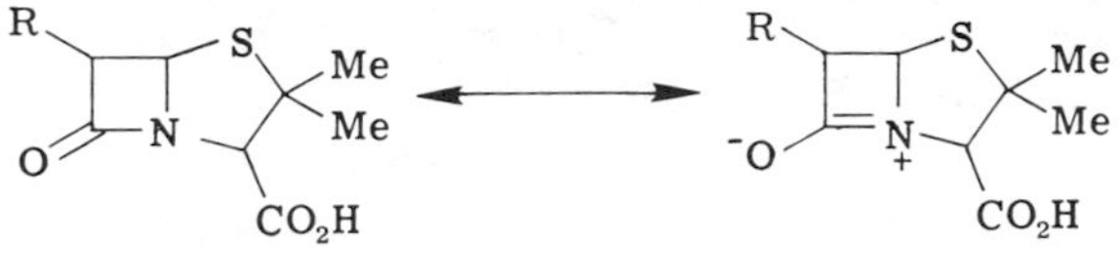

XX

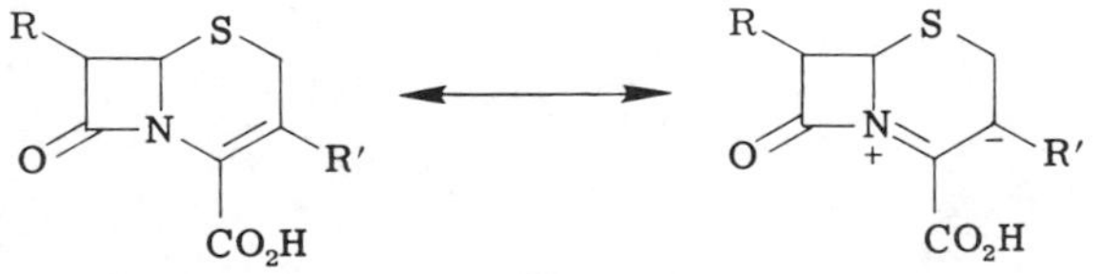

XXI

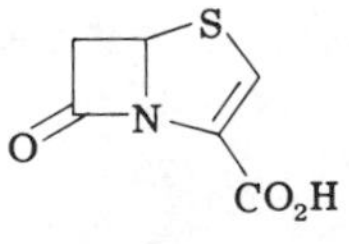

XXII

not have antibacterial activity? As soon as he saw the first X-ray crystal structure, Woodward (*210*) realized that the ring fusion increases the pyramidal character of the nitrogen and hence decreases the OC—N amide resonance (**XX**) and its reactivity. In 1969 Morin *et al.* (*133*) noted that the C=O stretching frequency of penicillin and Δ^3-cephalosporins suggests increased C=O bond character and hence decreased C—N resonance. As a result, the C—N bond should be more labile than that in the Δ^2-cephalosporins for which the C=O character is lower. In 1970 Sweet and Dahl (*186*) reported on X-ray crystallography of examples of these three nuclei. They found that the nitrogen in penicillins is quite pyramidal (0.4 Å above the plane of its attached atoms); in Δ^3-cephalosporins it is 0.24 Å above the plane, but it is nearly planar in the inactive Δ^2 analog. They suggested that besides these geometric considerations the C—N bond in the Δ^3-cephalosporins is further weakened by enamine resonance (**XXI**). Enamine resonance is not possible in the Δ^2-cephalosporins. Early attempts to mimic this increased reactivity by preparation of potential antibiotics with amides other than β-lactams were not successful (*20*). However, in 1978 the Woodward group used such considerations in the decision to prepare penems (**XXII**) shown to have antibacterial activity (*58*).

In 1973 Hermann used EHT and CNDO/2 methods to study the effects of various 3-substituents on the electronic properties of Δ^3-cephalosporins (*88*). Seven analogs were calculated and antibacterial activity was available for four of these. The calculations were done on the β-lactam ring with the attached double bond and the variable 3-substituent. The calculations showed that compounds that are more potent tend to have more reactive β-lactam rings. In other words, electron withdrawing substituents at the 3 position increase antibacterial activity.

Following calibration of the EHT method to handle sulfur properly (*26*), in 1973 Boyd published charge distributions and bond overlap populations for the following nuclei with no 3-substituent or carboxyl group: 3-cephem, 2-cephem, penam, and cepham (the saturated cephalosporin nucleus) (*25*). The results corroborate the previous experimental evidence that acylating activity of the nuclei parallels biological activity.

The next year Topp and Christensen reported CNDO/2 calculations on the complete penicillin and Δ^2- and Δ^3-cephalosporin nuclei (*195*). From comparison of the starting β-lactam to its hydrolysis products, the ring strain is 40 kcal/mol for penicillins and 20 kcal/mol for the cephalosporins. The energy difference between the ground state and the transition state in the acylation reaction was modeled by comparing the total energy of the molecule plus SH^- at infinite distance to that with SH^- 1.82 Å below the susceptible carbonyl. No other geometry changes were included. The Δ^2-cephalosporin is estimated to be 11 kcal less reactive than the Δ^3-cephalosporin. Although penicillin is 17 kcal/mol less reactive than the Δ^3-cephalosporin, the release of its strain energy was expected to be able to overcome this. They found no evidence of the 3′-acetate group leaving during formation of the transition state. Several months later Boyd published electron density maps of 7-amino-3-cephem (*27*).

In 1974 Indelicato *et al.* reported the rate of base catalyzed hydrolysis of the β-lactam ring of penicillins and cephalosporins (*93*). This rate does not change with side-chain structure unless the side chain contains a substituent that participates directly in the chemical reaction. Graphs show a positive relationship between the observed rate and (1) the infrared frequency of the β-lactam carbonyl, (2) the CNDO/2 calculated electron density at the carbonyl carbon atom, and (3) the σ_I value of the R′ substituent of the cephalosporins. Thus electron withdrawing substituents decrease the double bond character and destabilize the amide bond by enhancing enamine resonance. These relationships were pursued by Kawano *et al.* (*97*) who prepared a series of 3-CF_3 analogs of cephalosporins for which the 3-Cl analog was known to be active. For comparison purposes, the 3-CH_3 analog was also prepared. Although a number of active 3-CF_3 compounds were reported, only one set of corresponding 3-CH_3, 3-Cl, and 3-CF_3 analogs was tested. They show the expected trend—the 3-Cl and 3-CF_3 analogs are approximately equipotent.

In 1975 Boyd *et al.* used CNDO/2 calculations to monitor the charge redistribution as a hydroxide ion approaches the carbonyl carbon of 7-amino-3-acetoxymethyl-3-cephem (*32*). As it approaches, the bond to the leaving group is weakened. Although they did not do geometry optimization, they found that the hydroxide attacks from the α face and that the transition state is tetrahedral. This α-face attack has been confirmed experimentally (*71*). Later Boyd further demonstrated the concertedness of the nucleophilic attack on the carbonyl and the departure of the acetate group from 7-amino-3-(acetoxymethyl)-3-cephem (*35*).

In 1977 Boyd reported MINDO/3 calculations on the strain involved in making the nitrogen pyramidal by varying the dihedral angle of the amide (*28*). Only 1–2 kcal/mol and 5–7 kcal/mol are required to twist a flat amide into the dihedral angle of cepham and penam, respectively. These relatively low energies are in accord with the observed antibacterial activity of several monocyclic β-lactams. These calculations also show weakening of the C—N bond and strengthening of the C=O bond as the nitrogen becomes very pyramidal.

More recently Boyd *et al.* used CNDO/2 to study the reaction of a hydroxide ion with 22 cephalosporins that differ in the substituent at the 3 position (*31,33,34*). The transition state energy, TSE, is the difference in energy between the postulated transition state (the compound in its original geometry plus a hydroxide ion group 1.5 Å from the α face) and the reagents at infinite separation. There is a parabolic relationship between the TSE and the average antibacterial MIC measured against five gram-negative microorganisms. The data set consists of two series, those with direct attachments to the 3 position and those in which a variable substituent is present with a CH_2 bridge between it and the ring. Both series are fit by a single regression equation. The parabolic relationship reflects an optimum reactivity; at low TSE values the compounds are not reactive enough to react quickly with the target enzymes, whereas those with high TSE values may react with other nucleophiles before they have a chance to reach the target. These studies could not have been done with linear free energy methods because substituent constants for most of the substituents are not available.

The extension of these theoretical studies to the nonclassical β-lactams would be very interesting. Already the Woodward group has observed that pyramidality of the nitrogen is not the sole requirement for activity (*148*).

Recently Gensmantel *et al.* have reviewed the available data and concluded that compared to ordinary β-lactams, penicillins are only modestly more reactive and that the experimental evidence for inhibition of amide resonance is not convincing (*71*). They also point out that complexing with transition metals causes an approximately 10^8-fold increase in the rate of aminolysis and hydrolysis of penicillins. The metal is coordinated to the carboxyl groups in both penicillins and cephalosporins. In penicillins it is also coordinated to the β-lactam nitrogen and in cephalosporins to the carbonyl oxygen. Clearly, the last word has not been said on the special chemical characteristics of the β-lactam antibiotics.

On a more empirical level, Yoshimoto and Watanabe used a Free-Wilson analysis on a set of cephalosporins (**XV**) in which the R′ was an aromatic heterocycle (*212*). Satisfactory correlations were found for the MIC versus *E. coli* as well as the *in vivo* dose to protect mice against a lethal *E. coli* infection and the area under the time–blood level curve. The side chain in this series was either 2-, 3-, or 4-hydroxypenylglycine. The coefficient of the acetoxy substituent goes from −0.53 in the *in vitro* test to 1.08 in the *in vivo* test. In contrast, the respective values for the α-thioether of pyridine *N*-oxide are −0.78 and 0.43. No correlations of these data with physical properties were reported.

2. Conformational Resemblance between the Antibiotics and the Ground or Transition State of the Substrate of the Enzymatic Reaction

Theoretical studies have also been used to study two conformational properties: (1) the pucker of the fused nonlactam ring and accordingly the orientation of the carboxyl group with respect to the β-lactam and (2) the structure of the transition state in the reaction of the normal peptide substrate with the enzyme.

In 1970 Sweet and Dahl used X-ray structures to show the different steric relationship between the β-lactam and the carboxyl group in penicillin G compared to cephaloridine (*186*). However, shortly thereafter Sweet reviewed the X-ray data that show that the thiazolidine ring of penicillins can assume two conformations: that in which C-2 is out of the

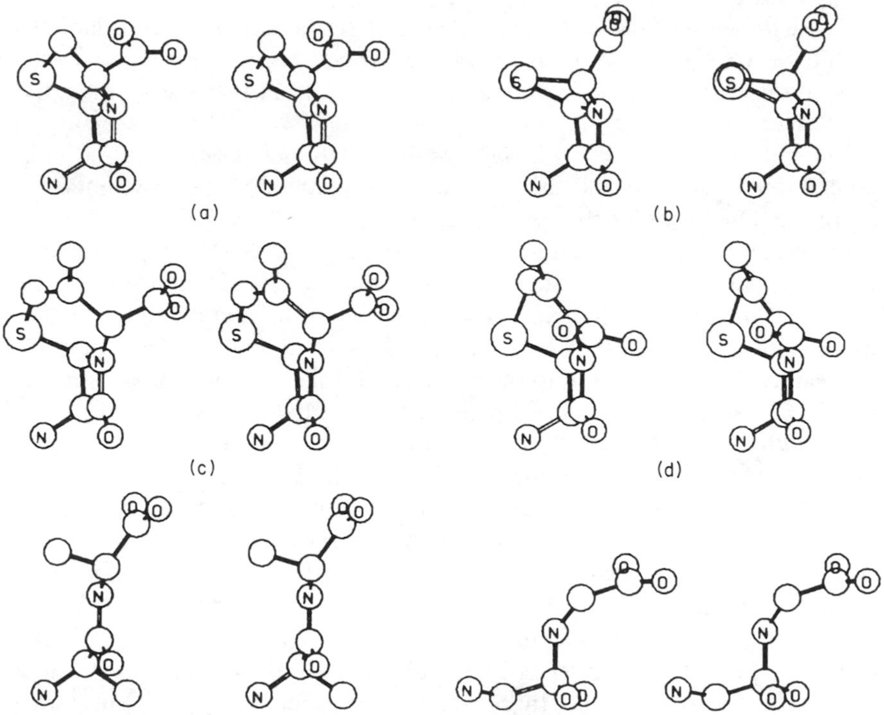

Fig. 6. Stereoviews of the structures of (a) penam in the C-2 conformation, (b) penam in the C-3 conformation, (c) Δ^2-cephem, (d) Δ^3-cephem, (e) DAla-DAla in the ground state conformation that best matches the β-lactams (*30*), and (f) the transition state in the α-face attack of hydroxide on Gly-Gly (*29*).

plane of the other atoms and that in which C-3 is out of the plane (Fig. 6) (*185*). In the former the carboxyl is equatorial and in the latter it is axial. Retsema and Ray demonstrated that the ionized carboxyl is required in order for a molecule to be able to compete with the whole-cell sites for acylation by penicillin G (*162*). From pH studies they concluded that there is an electrostatic bond between the CO_2^- and the binding site. In 1974 Topp and Christensen calculated, with CNDO/2, no conformational barrier and little energy difference for these ring puckers (*195*). Boyd *et al.* reported a similar conclusion in 1976 from EHT calculations (*36*) as did Joshi *et al.* from empirical potential energy calculations (*96*). The latter group showed that clavulinic acid, a β-lactamase inhibitor that is not an antibiotic, has only the C-3 type pucker.

Balsamo *et al.* reviewed the X-ray data on the 12 penicillins (some crystallized as esters) that had been reported up to that time (*9*). They found that penicillins with the C-3 pucker are active against gram-positive organisms only, whereas those with the C-2 pucker are broad spectrum. Although there are still large differences, the C-2 pucker leads to a dihedral angle between the carboxylate and the β-lactam that is more similar to that in cephalosporins and thienamicin, both of which are broad spectrum. Future studies must address the question of the relationship between this conformational correlation with spectrum and the indications in Section IV,B,4 that lipophilicity is the important determinant of this property.

As noted in Section IV,A, in 1965 Tipper and Strominger (*190*) and Wise and Park (*209*) pointed out the resemblance between the penicillin structure and the substrate of the cross-linking reaction. Lee noted in 1971 that the conformational resemblance between penicillin and Gly-DAla-DAla is best when the first peptide bond is distorted from the ground state 180 to 135.7° at an energy cost of an estimated 10 kcal/mol (*107*). In other words, penicillin is an analog of the transition state in the enzymatic reaction. Boyd *et al.* used PCILO to get a corresponding estimate of 8.5 kcal/mol to distort the peptide to a conformation resembling a penicillin and 2.5 kcal/mol to one resembling a cephalosporin (*32*).

Holtje used EHT calculations to investigate methylpenicillin and *N*-acetyl-DAla-DAla (*89*). He proposed resemblances between penicillin and the substrate by comparing the following distances: the carboxyl to both the carbonyl and the nitrogen of the side-chain amide, the β-face methyl group to both the carboxyl group and the carbonyl of the exocyclic amide, and the β-lactam to the exocyclic amide nitrogen atoms. The penicillin was in the C-3 pucker.

From contact distance criteria (*201–203*) Virudachalam and Rao concluded that the β-lactams are more analogous to the DAla-DAla than to the LAla-DGlu segment of the substrate. They also showed that 6-substituents on penicillins and 7-substituents on cephalosporins restrict the conformation of the side chain. Both X-ray crystallography (*102*) and EHT calculations (*89*) show that there is little resemblance between penicillins and *N*-acetyl-α-D-muramic acid, another portion of the substrate in the cross-linking reaction. Virudachalam has done extensive conformational calculations on the repeating unit of the substrate (*203*).

In 1977 Boyd used MINDO/3 to calculate the structure of the compound formed by the nucleophilic attack of glycylglycine by hydroxide (*29*). The conformational similarity with the antibiotics is greatest with attack at the α face. He later extended this with MINDO/3 calculations of Gly-Gly and the α- and β-face transition structures (*30*). Least-squares fitting of the carboxyl carbon, carbonyl carbon, and exocyclic amide nitrogen of various structures and conformations led to the conclusion that the substrate or transition intermediate best fit depends on the ring pucker of the thiazolidine ring as well as on the conformation of the substrate. No clear conclusions could be drawn. It is of course possible that the variety of acylations by penicillins may in fact be a reflection of the fact that penicillins can change conformation to resemble a variety of transition and ground states. Careful combined structure–activity, biochemistry, and theoretical studies may unravel these problems.

V. ANALYSIS OF SEVERAL CASES

As mentioned in the introduction, changing the spectrum of antibacterial activity may be as important a goal of an analogs program as is increasing potency. Takahashi *et al.* performed cluster analysis and nonlinear mapping to the antibacterial data against 27 organisms of 29 antibiotics of various classes (*187*). There were 21 gram-negative and 6 gram-positive bacteria and penicillins, cephalosporins, aminoglycosides, macrolides, tetracyclines, and peptides in the data set. Simply on the basis of the antibacterial $\log(1/C)$ data alone the compounds were classified into groups of similar chemical structure. We also have done such studies within one class of antibiotics but using the MIC value relative to that against *S. aureus*. We found two well-defined clusters, each of which is composed of compounds modified at only certain positions. This is in spite of the fact that there is no obvious pattern when the antibacterial activities are considered one or two at a time.

VI. COMMENTARY ON THE CONTRIBUTION OF QSAR TO THE STUDY OF ANTIBIOTICS

What have been the accomplishments of QSAR of antibiotics? Is it an endeavor worth the effort?

This chapter demonstrates that classic linear free-energy relationship methods have correctly highlighted the relative importance of various physical properties in the determination of potency and side effects of many series of compounds. These simple QSAR methods have established the critical role of hydrophobicity in the following cases: serum protein binding of tetracyclines and penicillins; *in vitro* antibacterial activity of certain series of substituted erythromycins, leucomycins, lincomycins, refamycins, coumermycins, and β-lactams; and *in vivo* antibacterial activity of penicillins. Steric effects added to hydrophobic ones have also been seen. QSAR has quantified straightforward negative steric effects in erythromycin esters and a difference between stereoisomers in lincomycin analogs. A more subtle result is the positive steric effect of substitution in the side chain of β-lactams. Finally, in the pyrimidinylureidopenicillins QSAR showed that potency is primarily determined by electronic effects that are well described by Hammett σ, but π also plays a role in the determination of potency.

Such classic QSAR studies provide valuable summaries of existing structure–activity relationships and may be used to predict the potency of newer analogs proposed for synthesis. More than half of the data presented in this review are of this type, characterized by clear answers from relatively simple methods. The work is not necessarily easy to practice, because for such complex structures an experimental measure of the hydrophobicity of at least some of the analogs may be necessary.

In at least five series (*N*-benzylerythromycins, tetracyclines, chloramphenicol analogs, 3-substituted cephalosporins, and aminoglycosides) classic linear free-energy methodology was not enough to solve the structure–activity problem. In the first four of these cases, however, it did suggest the direction for more detailed studies. For the *N*-benzylerythromycins, compartment model-based equations are sufficient to describe the QSAR. Such methods also slightly improve the QSAR equations of lincomycins. On the other hand, the QSAR of the cephalosporins require quantum chemical descriptors of reactivity.

The QSAR of three classes of molecules (the aminoglycosides, tetracyclines, and chloramphenicols) have been less completely described by theoretical methods. This may be partly because no one has studied them recently. Although it is not a property unique to them, in these three classes of antibiotics variations in substituents result in changes in the conformations of the molecules. It may be that the QSAR will be solved only when theoretical methods to treat QSAR of conformationally flexible molecules have become well established.

The tetracyclines and aminoglycosides also exhibit a further complication that is not found in any of the other series—they contain several groups that may ionize at biological pH values. Structural changes thus affect both the position of atoms in space and which atoms are electrically charged. Because electrostatic interactions are the principal method whereby the receptor recognizes the molecules with which it interacts, such changes in the position of charges in space may mean that the set of molecules no longer appears homologous to the receptor. Predictive QSAR of such series seems to require the use of still-developing receptor mapping and computer graphics techniques. The QSAR comparison of the different β-lactam nuclear analogs may also require such sophisticated methods.

The validity of the QSAR conclusions has been demonstrated by other types of experiments. For example, in the penicillins direct measurements also demonstrate the (1) hydrophobic binding to serum proteins and (2) differences in conformational responses of target enzymes to different analogs. Thus QSAR studies can provide hypotheses that can be checked by other methodologies. The theoretical work on the reactivity of the β-lactam ring has also provided hypotheses that were verified by other types of experiments. The clearest example of this is the experimental demonstration of α-face attack of hydroxide on the penicillins. Other examples of the interplay of the various experimental and theoretical measures of reactivity have also been discussed in this chapter. Although both theoretical and experimental groups were working on the same problems, in many cases workers remained unaware of others' results.

There are also lessons to be learned from the work reported here that challenge the ideas of how certain theoretical methods should be practiced. Fig. 6 contains interesting information for those who would map receptors by superimposing active molecules. The carboxyl group is essential for activity; presumably it acts as a key site of interaction of the molecules with the receptor. Another key atom must be the carbonyl carbon atom of the β-lactam because it is the atom that reacts with the target enzyme. Notice, however, that the relative positions of the carboxyl and the carbonyl of the inactive Δ^2-cephalosporins resembles that in both the ground and transition states of the peptide substrate, whereas for all active antibiotic nuclei the conformational resemblance to the ground and transition states is less. The lesson is that one must not pursue spatial analogies at the expense of the chemistry of the compounds. In the same vein, Fig. 1 reminds us that the same molecule can have a completely different conformation and distribution of charges under different conditions. Any method that neglects such possibilities cannot be correct. Finally, the detailed mode of action studies on the β-lactams should also prompt those who would map receptors from activity or even crude binding studies of analogs to remember that any one compound may have several biochemical targets and that the pattern or reaction with these multiple targets may change even for the same compound.

Acknowledgments. The authors would like to thank D. B. Boyd for furnishing the coordinates for Figs. 6a and f, and B. V. Cheney for furnishing those for Fig. 3. The stereoviews were made using the computer program XRAY written by R. Feldmann of N.I.H. and extensively modified by T. Koschmann of Abbott Laboratories.

REFERENCES

1. G. W. Adamson and J. A. Bush, *Nature (London)* **248,** 406 (1974).
2. G. W. Adamson and D. Bawden, *J. Chem. Inf. Comput. Sci.* **15,** 215 (1975).
3. P. Ahmad, C. A. Fyfe, and A. Mellors, *Biochem. Pharmacol.* **24,** 1103 (1975).
4. A. Albert, *Nature (London)* **172,** 201 (1953).
5. A. Albert and C. W. Rees, *Nature (London)* **177,** 433 (1956).
6. G. L. Asleson and C. W. Frank, *J. Am. Chem. Soc.* **98,** 4745 (1976).
7. A. Assandri, A. Perazzi, and M. Berti, *J. Antibiot.* **30,** 409 (1977).
8. J. Baddilley and E. P. Abraham, *Philos. Trans. R. Soc. London, Ser. B* **289,** 165 (1980).
9. A. Balsamo, P. Domiano, B. Macchia, F. Macchia, and M. Nardelli *Eur. J. Med. Chem.—Chim. Ther.* **15,** 559 (1980).
10. A. M. Barbaro, M. C. Guerra, and G. L. Biagi, *Boll. Soc. Ital. Biol. Sper.* **47,** 556 (1971).
11. L. Z. Benet and J. E. Goyan, *J. Pharm. Sci.* **54,** 983 (1965).
12. P. Berntsson, *Acta Pharm. Suec.* **17,** 199 (1980).
13. P. Bhuta, H. L. Chung, J. Hwang, and J. Zemlicka, *J. Med. Chem.* **23,** 1299 (1980).
14. G. L. Biagi, A. M. Barbaro, M. F. Gamba and M. C. Guerra, *J. Chromatogr.* **41,** 371 (1969).
15. G. L. Biagi, A. M. Barbaro, and M. C. Guerra, *in* "Biological Correlations—The Hansch Approach" (R. F. Gould, ed.), p. 61. Am. Chem. Soc., Washington, D.C., 1972.
16. G. L. Biagi, M. C. Guerra, A. M. Barbaro, and M. F. Gamba, *J. Med. Chem.* **13,** 511 (1970).
17. A. E. Bird and A. C. Marshall, *Biochem. Pharmacol.* **16,** 2275 (1967).
18. A. E. Bird, *J. Pharm. Sci.* **64,** 1671 (1975).
19. A. E. Bird and A. C. Marshall, *J. Chromatogr.* **63,** 313 (1971).
20. A. E. Bird and J. H. C. Nayler, *in* "Drug Design" (E. J. Ariëns, ed.), Medicinal Chemistry, Vol. 11-II, p. 277. Academic Press, New York, 1972.
21. R. K. Blackwood and A. R. English, *Prog. Mol. Subcell. Biol.* **2,** 237 (1970).
22. R. K. Blackwood and A. R. English, *in* "Structure–Activity Relationships among the Semisynthetic Antibiotics" (D. Perlman, ed.), p. 397. Academic Press, New York, 1977.

23. P. C. Blanpain, J. B. Nagy, G. H. Laurent, and F. V. Durant, *J. Med. Chem.* **23,** 1283 (1980).
24. H. Bojarska-Dahlig, *in* "Abh. Akad. Wiss. DDR, Abt. Math., Naturwiss., Tech. 1978" (R. Franke and P. Oehme, eds.), p. 343. Akademie-Verlag, Berlin, 1978.
25. D. B. Boyd, *J. Med. Chem.* **16,** 1195 (1973).
26. D. B. Boyd, *J. Am. Chem. Soc.* **94,** 6513 (1972).
27. D. B. Boyd, *J. Phys. Chem.* **78,** 2604 (1974).
28. D. B. Boyd, *Int. J. Quantum Chem.* **4,** 161 (1977).
29. D. B. Boyd, *Proc. Natl. Acad. Sci. U.S.A.* **74,** 5239 (1977).
30. D. B. Boyd, *J. Med. Chem.* **22,** 533 (1979).
31. D. B. Boyd, *Ann. N.Y. Acad. Sci.* **367,** 531 (1981).
32. D. B. Boyd, R. B. Hermann, D. E. Presti, and M. M. Marsh, *J. Med. Chem.* **18,** 408 (1975).
33. D. B. Boyd, D. K. Herron, W. H. W. Lunn, and W. A. Spitzer, *J. Am. Chem. Soc.* **102,** 1812 (1980).
34. D. B. Boyd and W. H. W. Lunn, *J. Antibiot.* **32,** 855 (1979).
35. D. B. Boyd and W. H. W. Lunn, *J. Med. Chem.* **22,** 778 (1979).
36. D. B. Boyd, C. Yeh, and F. S. Richardson, *J. Am. Chem. Soc.* **98,** 6100 (1976).
37. R. E. Brown, A. M. Simas, and R. E. Bruns, *Int. J. Quantum Chem.* **4,** 357 (1977).
38. M. Brufani, S. Cerrini, W. Fedeli, and A. Vaciago, *J. Mol. Biol.* **87,** 409 (1974).
39. M. Brufani, *Top. Antibiot. Chem.* **1,** 147 (1977).
40. T. M. Bustard, R. S. Egan, and T. J. Perun, *Tetrahedron* **29,** 1961 (1973).
41. A. Cammarata, *J. Med. Chem.* **10,** 525 (1967).
42. A. Cammarata and S. J. Yau, *J. Med. Chem.* **13,** 93 (1970).
43. A. Cammarata, S. J. Yau, J. H. Collett, and A. N. Martin, *Mol. Pharmacol.* **6,** 61 (1970).
44. B. V. Cheney, *J. Med. Chem.* **17,** 590 (1974).
45. N. Citri and M. R. Pollock, *Adv. Enzymol. Relat. Subj. Biochem.* **28,** 237 (1966).
46. N. Citri and N. Zyk, *Biochim. Biophys. Acta* **99,** 427 (1965).
47. J. L. Colaizzi and P. R. Klink, *J. Pharm. Sci.* **58,** 1184 (1969).
48. D. T. Cooke and I. Gonda, *J. Pharm. Pharmacol.* **29,** 190 (1977).
49. C. J. Coulson and V. J. Smith, *J. Pharm. Sci.* **69,** 799 (1980).
50. N. R. Cozzarelli, *Science* **207,** 953 (1980).
51. R. Cricchio, V. Arioli, and G. C. Lancini, *Farmaco, Ed. Sci.* **30,** 605 (1975).
52. M. F. Dampier and H. W. Whitlock, *J. Am. Chem. Soc.* **97,** 6254 (1975).
53. J. C. Dearden and J. Williams, *J. Pharm. Pharmacol.* **30,** 50P (1978).
54. J. T. Doluisio and A. N. Martin, *J. Med. Chem.* **6,** 16 (1963).
55. W. Durckheimer, *Angew. Chem., Int. Ed. Engl.* **14,** 721 (1975).
56. R. S. Egan, T. J. Perun, J. R. Martin, and L. A. Mitscher, *Tetrahedron* **29,** 2525 (1973).
57. R. S. Egan, J. R. Martin, T. J. Perun, and L. A. Mitscher, *J. Am. Chem. Soc.* **97,** 4578 (1975).
58. I. Ernest, J. Gosteli, C. W. Greengrass, W. Holick, D. E. Jackman, H. R. Pfaendler, and R. B. Woodward, *J. Am. Chem. Soc.* **100,** 8214 (1978).
59. H. Ferres, M. J. Basker, D. J. Best, and F. P. Harrington, *J. Antibiot.* **31,** 1013 (1978).
60. H. Ferres, M. J. Basker, and P. J. O'Hanlon, *J. Antibiot.* **27,** 922 (1974).
61. J. Fisher, J. G. Belasco, R. L. Charnas, S. Khosler, and J. R. Knowles, *Philos. Trans. R. Soc. London, Ser. B* **289,** 309 (1980).
62. J. L. Fox, *Chem. Eng. News,* Nov. 5, p. 19 (1979).
63. S. M. Free and J. W. Wilson, *J. Med. Chem.* **7,** 395 (1964).
64. K. B. Freeman, *Can. J. Biochem.* **48,** 469 (1970).
65. K. B. Freeman, *Can. J. Biochem.* **48,** 479 (1970).

66. J. M. Frere, *Biochem. Pharmacol.* **26,** 2203 (1977).
67. M. Gadret, M. Goursolle, J. M. Leger, and J. C. Colleter, *Acta Crystallogr., Sect. B* **31,** 1454 (1975).
68. E. R. Garrett, S. M. Heman-Ackah, and G. L. Perry, *J. Pharm. Sci.* **59,** 1448 (1970).
69. E. R. Garrett, O. K. Wright, G. H. Miller, and K. L. Smith, *J. Med. Chem.* **9,** 203 (1966).
70. A. Garzia, A. Villanti, and G. Tuccini, *J. Pharm. Sci.* **68,** 1081 (1979).
71. N. P. Gensmantel, D. McLellan, J. J. Morris, M. I. Page, P. Proctor, and G. S. Randahawa, *in* "Recent Advances in the Chemistry of beta-Lactam Antibiotics" (G. I. Gregory, ed.), p. 227. Royal Soc. Chem., London, 1981.
72. J. M. Ghuysen, J. M. Frere, M. Leyh-Bouille, H. Perkins, and M. Nieto, *Philos. Trans. R. Soc. London Ser. B* **289,** 285 (1980).
73. J. Ghuysen, *in* "Beta-Lactamases" (J. M. T. Hamilton-Miller and J. T. Smith, eds.), p. 181. Academic Press, New York, 1979.
74. J. Ghuysen, J. Frere, M. Leyh-Bouille, J. Coyette, J. Dusart, and M. Nguyen-Disteche, *Annu. Rev. Biochem.* **48,** 73 (1979).
75. M. Gorman and C. W. Ryan, *in* "Cephalosporins and Penicillins" (E. H. Flynn, ed.), p. 532. Academic Press, New York, 1972.
76. R. G. Green, J. R. Brown, and R. T. Calvert, *J. Pharm. Pharmacol.* **28,** 514 (1976).
77. P. Gund, *Annu. Rep. Med. Chem.* **14,** 299 (1979).
78. F. E. Hahn, *Naturwissenschaften* **67,** 89 (1980).
79. F. E. Hahn and P. Gund, *in* "Drug Receptor Interactions in Antimicrobial Chemotherapy" (J. Drews and F. E. Hahn, eds.), p. 245. Springer-Verlag, New York, 1975.
80. C. Hansch and A. J. Leo, "Substituent Constants for Correlation Analysis in Chemistry and Biology" Wiley, New York, 1979.
81. C. Hansch and E. W. Deutsch, *J. Med. Chem.* **8,** 705 (1965).
82. C. Hansch, E. Kutter, and A. Leo, *J. Med. Chem.* **12,** 746 (1969).
83. C. Hansch, R. M. Muir, T. Fujita, P. P. Maloney, F. Geiger, and M. Streich, *J. Am. Chem. Soc.* **85,** 2817 (1963).
84. C. Hansch, K. Nakamoto, M. Gorin, P. Denisevich, E. R. Garrett, S. M. Heman-Ackah, and C. H. Won, *J. Med. Chem.* **16,** 917 (1973).
85. C. Hansch and A. R. Steward, *J. Med. Chem.* **7,** 691 (1964).
86. D. R. Harris, S. G. McGeachin, and H. H. Mills, *Tetrahedron Lett.* p. 679 (1965).
87. R. J. Harris and R. H. Symons, *Bioorg. Chem.* **2,** 266 (1973).
88. R. B. Hermann, *J. Antibiot.* **26,** 223 (1973).
89. H-D. Holtje, *Arch. Pharm. (Weinheim, Ger.)* **309,** 26 (1976).
90. H-D. Holtje and L. B. Kier, *J. Med. Chem.* **17,** 814 (1974).
91. J. P. Hou and J. W. Poole, *J. Pharm. Sci.* **60,** 503 (1971).
92. L. J. Hughes, J. J. Stezowski, and R. E. Hughes, *J. Am. Chem. Soc.* **101,** 7655 (1979).
93. J. M. Indelicato, T. T. Norvilas, R. R. Pfeiffer, W. J. Wheeler, and W. L. Wilham, *J. Med. Chem.* **17,** 523 (1974).
94. O. Jardetzky, *J. Biol. Chem.* **238,** 2498 (1963).
95. K. H. Jogun and J. J. Stezowski, *J. Am. Chem. Soc.* **98,** 6018 (1976).
96. N. V. Joshi, R. Virudachalam, and V. S. R. Rao, *Curr. Sci.* **47,** 933 (1978).
97. Y. Kawano, T. Watanabe, J. Sakai, H. Watanabe, M. Nagano, T. Nishimura, and T. Miyadera, *Chem. Pharm. Bull.* **28,** 70 (1980).
98. I. W. Kellaway and C. Marriott, *Can. J. Pharm. Sci.* **13,** 90 (1978).
99. U. W. Kesselring and L. Z. Benet, *Anal. Chem.* **41,** 1535 (1969).
100. T. Kimura, M. Yoshikawa, M. Yasuhara, and H. Sezaki, *J. Pharm. Pharmacol.* **32,** 394 (1980).
101. J. A. Kiritsy, D. K. Yung, and D. E. Mahony, *J. Med. Chem.* **21,** 1301 (1978).

102. J. R. Knox and N. S. Murthy, *Acta Crystallogr., Sect. B* **30,** 365 (1974).
102a. J. R. Knox, *Abs. Pap. A.C.S. Mtg.* **184,** MEDI 070 (1982).
103. I. Komiya, K. Umemura, M. Fujita, A. Kamiya, K. Okumura, and R. Hori, *J. Pharm. Dyn.* **3,** 299 (1980).
104. H. Kubinyi, *Arzneim.-Forsch.* **29,** 1067 (1979).
105. G. Lancini and W. Zanichelli, *in* "Structure–Activity Relationships among the Semisynthetic Antibiotics" (D. Perlman, ed.), p. 531. Academic Press, New York, 1977.
106. M. A. Landau, M. N. Markovich, and L. A. Piruzyan, *Biochim. Biophys. Acta* **493,** 1 (1977).
107. B. Lee, *J. Mol. Biol.* **61,** 463 (1971).
108. E. J. Lien, C. Hansch, and S. M. Anderson, *J. Med. Chem.* **11,** 430 (1968).
109. I. Lukovits and A. Lopata, *J. Med. Chem.* **23,** 449 (1980).
110. J. K. H. Ma, H. W. Jun, and L. A. Luzzi, *J. Pharm. Sci.* **62,** 1261 (1973).
111. H. Mager and A. Barth, *Pharmazie* **34,** 557 (1979).
112. P. P. Mager, *Acta Histochem.* **66,** 40 (1980).
113. P. P. Mager, *Pharmazie* **35,** 708 (1980).
114. B. J. Magerlein, *J. Med. Chem.* **10,** 1161 (1967).
115. B. J. Magerlein, *in* "Structure–Activity Relationships among the Semisynthetic Antibiotics" (D. E. Perlman, ed.), p. 601. Academic Press, New York, 1977.
116. M. N. Markovich, E. A. Rudzit, and M. A. Landau, *Antibiotiki (Moscow)* **23,** 654 (1978).
117. Y. C. Martin, "Quantitative Drug Design. A Critical Introduction," p. 329. Dekker, New York, 1978.
118. Y. C. Martin, "Quantitative Drug Design. A Critical Introduction," p. 96. Dekker, New York, 1978.
119. Y. C. Martin, "Quantitative Drug Design. A Critical Introduction," p. 271. Dekker, New York, 1978.
120. Y. C. Martin, "Quantitative Drug Design. A Critical Introduction," p. 215. Dekker, New York, 1978.
121. Y. C. Martin, *in* "Drug Design" (E. J. Ariëns, ed.), Medicinal Chemistry, Vol. 11-VIII p. 1. Academic Press, New York, 1979.
122. Y. C. Martin, unpublished observations (1980).
123. Y. C. Martin, *in* "Physical Chemical Properties of Drugs" (S. H. Yalkowsky, A. A. Sinkula, and S. C. Valvani, eds.), p. 49. Dekker, New York, 1980.
124. Y. C. Martin, *J. Med. Chem.* **24,** 229 (1981).
125. Y. C. Martin, P. H. Jones, T. J. Perun, W. E. Grundy, S. Bell, R. R. Bower, and N. L. Shipkowitz, *J. Med. Chem.* **15,** 635 (1972).
126. Y. C. Martin and K. R. Lynn, *J. Med. Chem.* **14,** 1162 (1971).
127. Y. C. Martin and H. N. Panas, *J. Med. Chem.* **22,** 784 (1979).
128. G. H. Miller, H. L. Smith, W. L. Rock, and S. Hedberg, *J. Pharm. Sci.* **66,** 88 (1977).
129. L. A. Mitscher, B. J. Slater, T. J. Perun, P. H. Jones, and J. R. Martin, *Tetrahedron Lett.* p. 4505 (1969).
130. L. A. Mitscher, "The Chemistry of the Tetracycline Antibiotics." Dekker, New York, 1978.
131. P. C. Moews, J. R. Knox, D. J. Waxman, and J. L. Strominger, *Int. J. Pept. Protein Res.* **17,** 211 (1981).
132. I. Moriguchi and Y. Kanada, *Chem. Pharm. Bull,* **25,** 926 (1977).
133. R. B. Morin, B. G. Jackson, R. A. Mueller, E. R. Lavagnino, W. B. Scanlon, and S. L. Andrews, *J. Am. Chem. Soc.* **91,** 1401 (1969).
134. J. G. Nourse and J. D. Roberts, *J. Am. Chem. Soc.* **97,** 4584 (1975).

135. G. G. Nys and R. F. Rekker, *Eur. J. Med. Chem.—Chim. Ther.* **9,** 361 (1974).
136. S. Omura, A. Nakagawa, H. Sakakibara, O. Okekawa, R. Brandsch, and S. Pestka, *J. Med. Chem.* **20,** 732 (1977).
137. S. Omura, M. Katagiri, I. Umezawa, K. Komiyama, T. Maekawa, K. Sekikawa, A. Matsumae, and T. Hata, *J. Antibiot.* **21,** 532 (1968).
138. J. A. Ostrenga, *J. Med. Chem.* **12,** 349 (1969).
139. G. J. Palenik, M. Mathew, and R. Restivo, *J. Am. Chem. Soc.* **100,** 4458 (1978).
140. G. Pelizza, G. C. Allievi, and G. G. Gallo, *Farmaco, Ed. Sci.* **31,** 31 (1976).
141. G. Pelizza, G. C. Lancini, G. C. Allievi, and G. G. Gallo, *Farmaco, Ed. Sci.* **28,** 298 (1973).
142. G. Pelizza, G. Lancini, G. Allievi, and G. G. Gallo, *in* "Quantitative Structure–Activity Relationships" (M. Tichy, ed.), p. 53. Akadémiai Kiadó, Budapest, 1976.
143. F. Peradejordi, A. N. Martin, and A. Cammarata, *J. Pharm. Sci.* **60,** 576 (1971).
144. T. J. Perun, R. S. Egan, P. H. Jones, J. R. Martin, L. A. Mitscher, and B. J. Slater, *Antimicrob. Agents Chemother.* (*1969*) 116 (1970).
145. T. J. Perun, R. S. Egan, and J. R. Martin, *Tetrahedron Lett.* p. 4501 (1969).
146. T. J. Perun, personal communication (1981).
147. T. J. Perun and R. S. Egan, *Tetrahedron Lett.* p. 387 (1969).
148. H. R. Pfaendler, J. Gosteli, R. B. Woodward, and G. Rihs, *J. Am. Chem. Soc.* **103,** 4526 (1981).
149. P. G. Popov, K. I. Vaptzarova, G. P. Kossekova, and T. K. Nikolov, *Biochem. Pharmacol.* **21,** 2363 (1972).
150. R. Prewo and J. J. Stezowski, *Acta Crystallogr., Sect. A* **34,** 81 (1978).
151. R. Prewo and J. J. Stezowski, *J. Am. Chem. Soc.* **99,** 1117 (1977).
152. R. Prewo and J. J. Stezowski, *J. Am. Chem. Soc.* **101,** 7657 (1979).
153. R. Prewo and J. J. Stezowski, *J. Am. Chem. Soc.* **102,** 7015 (1980).
154. R. Prewo, J. J. Stezowski, and R. Kirchlechner, *J. Am. Chem. Soc.* **102,** 7021 (1980).
155. K. E. Price, *in* "Structure–Activity Relationships among the Semisynthetic Antibiotics" (D. Perlman, ed.), p. 1. Academic Press, New York, 1977.
156. K. E. Price, *in* "Structure–Activity Relationships among the Semisynthetic Antibiotics" (D. Perlman, ed.), p. 61. Academic Press, New York, 1977.
157. K. E. Price, J. C. Godfrey, and H. Kawaguchi, *in* "Structure–Activity Relationships among the Semisynthetic Antibiotics" (D. Perlman, ed.), p. 239. Academic Press, New York, 1977.
158. E. D. Purich, J. L. Colaizzi, and R. I. Poust, *J. Pharm. Sci.* **62,** 545 (1973).
159. F. R. Quinn, J. S. Driscoll, and C. Hansch, *J. Med. Chem.* **18,** 332 (1975).
160. R. F. Rekker, *Farmaco, Ed. Sci.* **34,** 346 (1979).
161. R. F. Rekker, "The Hydrophobic Fragmental Constant." Elsevier, Amsterdam/New York, 1977.
162. J. A. Retsema and V. A. Ray, *Antimicrob. Agents Chemother.* **2,** 173 (1972).
163. N. E. Rigler, S. P. Bag, D. E. Leyden, J. L. Sudmeier, and C. N. Reilley, *Anal. Chem.* **37,** 872 (1965).
164. I. M. Rollo, *Can. J. Physiol. Pharmacol.* **50,** 976 (1972).
165. J. Safanda and P. P. Sobotka, *in* "Quantitative Structure–Activity Relationships" (M. Tichy, ed.), p. 145. Akadémiai Kiadó, Budapest, 1976.
166. I. Saikawa, T. Yasuda, H. Taki, M. Tai, Y. Watanabe, H. Sakai, S. Takano, C. Yoshida, and K. Kasuya, *Yakugaku Zasshi* **97,** 987 (1977).
167. A. Samuni and N. Citri, *Mol. Pharmacol.* **16,** 250 (1979).
168. A. Samuni and A. Y. Meyer, *Mol. Pharmacol.* **14,** 704 (1978).
169. N. J. Santora and K. Auyang, *J. Med. Chem.* **18,** 959 (1975).

170. M. L. Sassiver and A. Lewis, *in* "Structure–Activity Relationships among the Semisynthetic Antibiotics" (D. Perlman, ed.), p. 87. Academic Press, New York, 1977.
171. T. Sawai, K. Matsuba, A. Tamura, and S. Yamagishi, *J. Antibiot.* **32,** 59 (1979).
172. M. Schach von Wittenau, *Proc. Int. Congr. Pharmacol., 4th, Basel, 1969* **4,** 160 (1970).
173. M. Schach von Wittenau and C. S. Delahunt, *J. Pharmacol. Exp. Ther.* **152,** 164 (1966).
174. M. Schach von Wittenau and R. Yeary, *J. Pharmacol. Exp. Ther.* **140,** 258 (1963).
175. W. Scholtan, *Arzneim.-Forsch.* **18,** 505 (1968).
176. F. Seela and V. A. Erdmann, *Biochim. Biophys. Acta* **435,** 105 (1976).
177. Y. Shimauchi, M. Sakamoto, K. Hori, T. Ishikuro, and J. Lien, *J. Antibiot.* **34,** 245 (1981).
178. L. L. Shipman, R. E. Christoffersen, and B. V. Cheney, *J. Med. Chem.* **17,** 583 (1974).
179. W. L. Starnes, E. P. Desmon, and F. J. Behal, *Biochim. Biophys. Acta* **616,** 290 (1980).
180. C. R. Stephens, K. Murai, K. J. Brunings, and R. B. Woodward, *J. Am. Chem. Soc.* **78,** 4155 (1956).
181. J. J. Stezowski, *J. Am. Chem. Soc.* **98,** 6012 (1976).
182. J. J. Stezowski and R. Prewo, personal communication (1980).
183. J. J. Stezowski, R. J. Stojda, and D. R. White, *J. Am. Chem. Soc.* **101,** 2171 (1979).
184. L. J. Stoel, E. C. Newman, G. L. Asleson, and C. W. Frank, *J. Pharm. Sci.* **65,** 1794 (1976).
185. R. M. Sweet, *in* "Cepalosporins and Penicillins" (E. H. Flynn, ed.), p. 280. Academic Press, New York, 1972.
186. R. M. Sweet and L. F. Dahl, *J. Am. Chem. Soc.* **92,** 5489 (1970).
187. Y. Takahashi, Y. Miyashita, H. Abe, S. Sasaki, Y. Yotsui, and M. Sano, *Anal. Chim. Acta* **122,** 241 (1980).
188. H. Terada and T. Inagi, *Chem. Pharm. Bull.* **23,** 1960 (1975).
189. H. H. Thijssen, *Eur. J. Med. Chem.—Chim. Ther.* **16,** 449 (1981).
190. D. J. Tipper and J. L. Strominger, *Proc. Natl. Acad. Sci. U.S.A.* **54,** 1133 (1965).
191. A. Tomaz, *Rev. Infect. Dis.* **1,** 434 (1979).
192. A. Tomaz, K. Kitano, R. Lopez, and C. de Freitas, *in* "Drug Action and Design: Mechanism-Based Enzyme Inhibitors" (T. I. Kalman, ed.), p. 197. Elsevier/North-Holland, New York, 1979.
193. S. Toon and M. Rowland, *J. Pharm. Pharmacol.* **31,** 43P (1979).
194. J. G. Topliss and R. P. Edwards, *in* "Computer Assisted Drug Design" (E. C. Olson and R. E. Christoffersen, eds.), p. 131. Am. Chem. Soc., Washington, D.C., 1979.
195. W. C. Topp and B. G. Christensen, *J. Med. Chem.* **17,** 342 (1974).
196. A. Tsuji, O. Kubo, E. Miyamoto, and T. Yamana, *J. Pharm. Sci.* **66,** 1675 (1977).
197. A. Tsuji, E. Miyamoto, O. Kubo, and T. Yamana, *J. Pharm. Sci.* **68,** 812 (1979).
198. M. S. Tute, *Adv. Drug Res.* **6,** 1 (1971).
199. H. Van der Waterbeemd, S. VanBoeckel, A. Jansen, and K. Gerritsma, *Eur. J. Med. Chem.—Chim. Ther.* **15,** 279 (1980).
200. D. Vazquez, *Biochim. Biophys. Acta* **114,** 277 (1966).
201. R. Virudachalam and V. S. R. Rao, *Int. J. Pept. Protein Res.* **10,** 51 (1977).
202. R. Virudachalam and V. S. Rao, *in* "Biomolecular Structure, Conformation, Function, and Evolution" (R. Srinivasain, N. Yathindia, and E. Subramarian, eds.), Vol. 2, p. 525. Pergamon, Oxford, 1981.
203. R. Virudachalam, *Diss. Abstr. Int. B* **41,** 798 (1980).
204. D. J. Waxman, R. R. Yocum, and J. L. Strominger, *Philos. Trans. R. Soc. London, Ser. B* **289,** 257 (1980).
205. J. Webber and J. L. Ott, *in* "Structure–Activity Relationships among the Semisynthetic Antibiotics" (D. Perlman, ed.), p. 161. Academic Press, New York, 1977.

206. T. R. Weihrauch, H. Koehler, D. Hoeffler, and J. Krieglstein, *Naunyn-Schmiedeberg's Arch. Pharmacol.* **289,** 55 (1975).
207. B. Wetzel, E. Woitun, W. Reuter, R. Maier, U. Lechner, H. Geoth, and R. Werner, *in* "Recent Advances in the Chemistry of beta-Lactam Antibiotics" (G. I. Gregory, ed.), p. 27. Royal Soc. Chem., London, 1981.
208. J. M. Wilhelm, N. L. Oleinick, and J. W. Corcoran, *Antimicrob. Agents Chemother.* (*1967*) p. 236 (1968).
209. E. M. Wise and J. T. Park, *Proc. Natl. Acad. Sci. U.S.A.* **54,** 75 (1965).
210. R. B. Woodward, *in* "The Chemistry of Penicillins" (H. T. Clarke, J. R. Johnson, and R. Robinson, eds.), p. 444. Princeton Univ. Press, Princeton, New Jersey, 1949.
211. T. Yamana, A. Tsuji, E. Miyamoto, and O. Kubo, *J. Pharm. Sci.* **66,** 747 (1977).
212. M. Yoshimoto and H. Watanabe, *Kagaku no Ryoiki Zokan, No. 136,* 151 (1982).
213. H. Zia and J. C. Price, *J. Pharm. Sci.* **65,** 226 (1976).
214. G. Ziebell, G. Bradler, T. Nagel, and M. Scholz, *in* "Abh. Akad. Wiss. DDR, Abt. Math., Naturwiss., Tech. 1978" (R. Franke and P. Oehme, eds.), p. 233. Akademie-Verlag, Berlin, 1978.

4

Antitumor Agents

W. J. Dunn III

I. INTRODUCTION

The first article describing the quantitative structure–activity relationships (QSAR) of antitumor agents was published in 1969 (*75*). Since that time more than 50 reports have appeared presenting in a quantitative manner structure–activity relationships on diverse structure types. Included in these reports are three brief reviews (*43,67,83*). The scope of this chapter is to report in a critical manner the literature of QSAR of anticancer agents. Extremely helpful in this endeavor was the *Chemical Abstracts* series on *Antitumor Agents*.

The approach taken in this chapter is to provide a brief background for the data that serves as the basis of the relationships reviewed here. The discovery and development processes of anticancer agents is necessarily

QUANTITATIVE STRUCTURE–ACTIVITY RELATIONSHIPS OF DRUGS

ISBN 0-12-695150-0

a complex one. Therefore, the derivation and development of QSAR for antitumor agents must be approached with some knowledge of their complexity and the assumptions underlying their development. It is felt by this author that a brief discussion of this process is necessary to provide the ground work for their interpretation.

A. Antitumor Drug Screening

1. The Linear Array

In 1955 the Cancer Chemotherapy National Service Center was formed with the mission to develop chemotherapeutic agents. This was continued in 1965, and in 1972 it became part of the Division of Cancer Treatment of the National Cancer Institute (NCI). As part of this program, potential antitumor agents are procured and submitted to testing (*42*). The flow of development of potential antitumor agents is detailed in a document called the *Linear Array* available on request from the Division of Cancer Treatment. This decision network is briefly diagrammed in Fig. 1.

The objective of stage I of this network is the discovery of lead compounds and the agents selected are from two broad classes: synthetic compounds and natural product extracts. The major portion of the QSAR reported concern synthetic agents, so only the testing strategy of these substances will be dealt with here. On submission of compounds for evaluation they are prescreened in the lymphoid leukemia P-388 tumor of the mouse. If activity can be confirmed, the compound is then tested in leukemia L1210 in the mouse. If the compound has been shown elsewhere to have activity, it is tested directly in the L1210 system. Also, a number of laboratories carry out their own prescreening using a variety of tumors; one of the most common is Sarcoma-180 (S-180) in the mouse.

The advantages and disadvantages of this approach to the search for lead compounds has been reviewed, especially the use of the mouse as a model for the host (*72*), and alternatives have been suggested (*61*).

Once a lead compound has been identified by this process, the problem of optimization of activity as a function of structural change is then faced by the discoverer. It is at this point that the systematic approach of drug design (*63*) can have a great impact. The result of the application of this approach to the problem is a series of compounds on which dose-response data are obtained.

2. The Dose-Response Curve for Antitumor Agents

In the quantification of anticancer drug activity a discussion of the dose-response curve is imperative because the selection of an end point

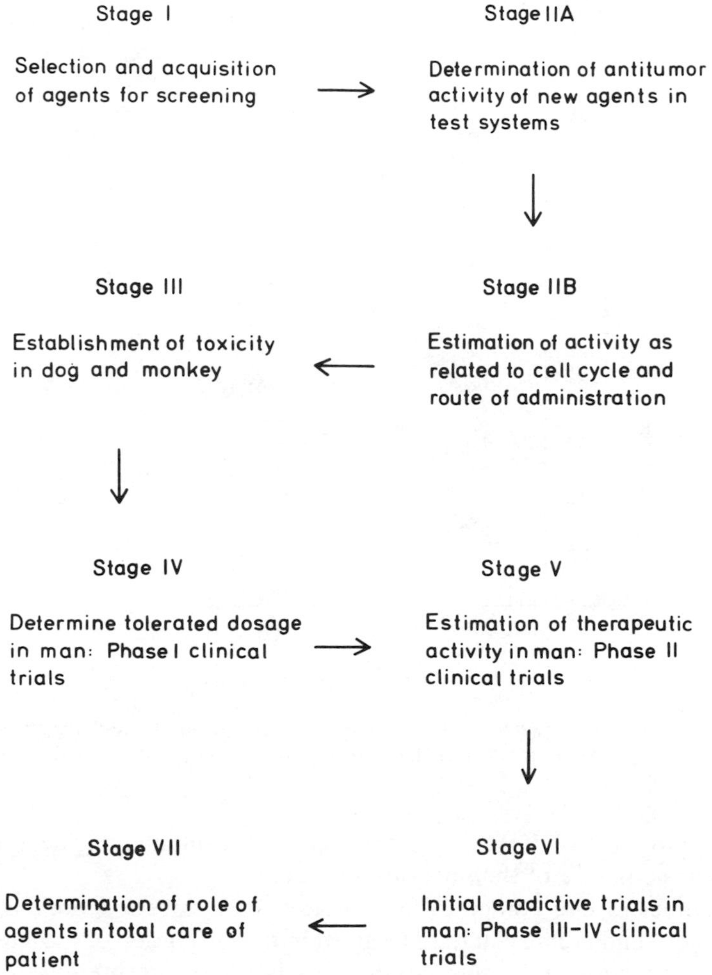

Fig. 1. The Division of Cancer Treatment Program Linear Array (used with permission).

for response can be the most important factor in the derivation of QSAR for a series of compounds. A convincing indication of activity for a compound is demonstration that it can increase the life span of a tumor-bearing animal relative to that of a nontreated tumor-bearing control. The dose-response curve from such an experiment is given in Fig. 2. One aspect of this dose-response curve is significant and that is its biphasic nature. Antitumor agents are characteristically selective cell toxins in that they rely for their effectiveness on some differentiating factor between the tumor cell and the cells of the host. At some dose, therefore, a toxic

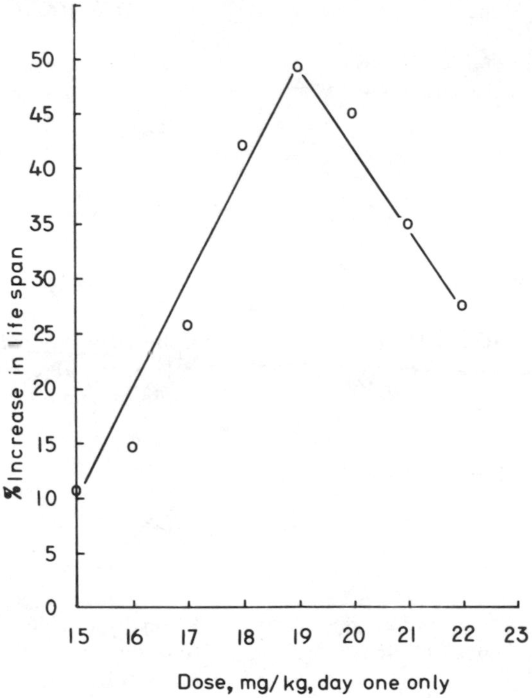

Fig. 2. Dose-response curve for 1-(3-acetamidophenyl)-3,3-dimethyltriazene. Data obtained in author's laboratory against S-180 in the mouse.

response to the host of the test compound will result and this accounts for the biphasic nature of the dose-response curve.

A number of end points are derivable from a dose-response relationship. These end points can then be used in the derivation of QSAR. If the QSAR for a series of active compounds is to be interpreted strictly in terms of the Hansch theory (*63*), in an extrathermodynamic sense, the end point should be selected as the dose (in equimolar terms) required to give a statistically significant increase in life span over that of the control. It is usually considered that a 25% increase in life span is statistically significant. More demanding levels of activity can be used but caution must be taken that all compounds within the series studied achieve this level of activity. One other point should be made in this regard: the dose for this response should be obtained from the portion of the dose-response curve that is in the phase of the curve in which life span is increasing with dose rather than in the toxic phase of the curve. Compounds that cannot give at least a 25% increase in life span are considered inactive.

If an empirical view of QSAR is assumed, then other end points can be used. This is usually reported as the dose that gives maximum increase in life span. The ratio of the optimum dose to that which gives a predetermined increase in life span is the therapeutic index. In this review the former two activity indices predominate.

B. Methods of Data Analysis Applied to Antitumor Structure–Activity Data

1. Regression Methods

Various methods of data analysis have been applied to structure–activity data for the purpose of deriving QSAR. Details of these methods appear elsewhere in this volume. The method selected obviously depends on the objective of the analysis, and because optimization of activity with structural variation is the usual objective, the applications of regression methods are predominant in the literature through the period covered by this review. For the purpose of classification of compounds as active or inactive, discriminant analysis and the linear learning machine have been applied to structure–activity data (*4,27,34,48,49*). Even though these represent a small fraction of the reported QSAR work on antitumor agents, the use of these and more sophisticated classification techniques in the design of antitumor drugs is inevitable.

A recent report by Hodes (*74*) describes a method of data analysis that, though not as quantitative as regression and the various classification methods, can be applied to a large data base of structure–activity data with the resulting selection of structure types with high probabilities of having antitumor activity. As such this is a unique method in that it can potentially generate a lead compound.

A discussion of regresson methods is presented in Chapter 1. The reader is also referred to a 1978 tertiary source (*81*) for a more detailed discussion of the application of linear and nonlinear regression in QSAR.

2. Classification Methods

Classification methods include those methods of discriminant analysis, e.g., the linear learning machine, and pattern recognition methods of which *k*-Nearest Neighbor and SIMCA (*87*) are examples. All methods except SIMCA have been applied to the problem of classifying structures of compounds as active or inactive in anticancer screens (*4,27,34,47,78*).

Using these methods, drugs of known classification whose structures

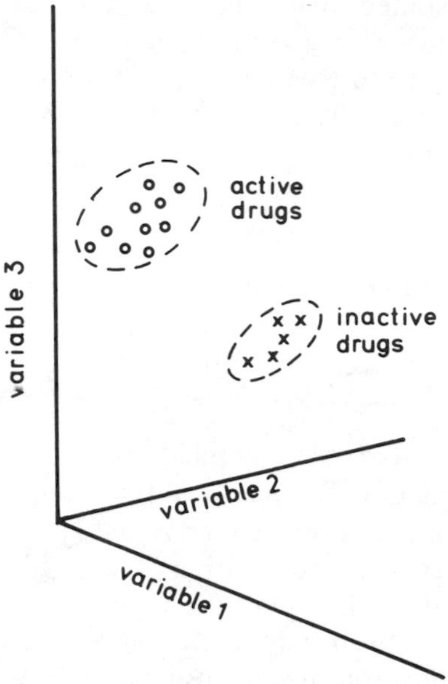

Fig. 3. Symmetric data structure obtained in classification studies.

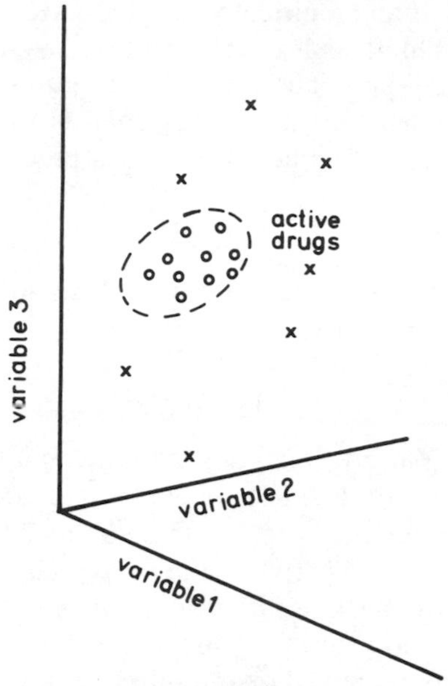

Fig. 4. Asymmetric data structure obtained in classification studies.

are described by various types of descriptors are called the *training set*. These descriptors vary with the presence or absence of molecular fragments, connectivity indices (*77*), or Hammett-like physicochemical constants. A critical assumption made at this point is that the descriptors are assumed to be continuous in a mathematical sense. A coordinate system is constructed with one axis for each descriptor, and the data describing the training set compounds are plotted in this descriptor space. For coordinate systems in three dimensions this can be shown graphically, as in Fig. 3. The ideal result is obtained if the active compounds cluster in one region while the inactive ones cluster in another. This type of data structure has been termed *symmetric data structure* (*49*). The data analytic method applied to the training sets must select the variable(s) that are important for separation of the training sets and then separate the distinct classes. Linear discriminant analysis and the linear learning machine construct a plane separating the classes and then classification is based on which side of the plane a new or untested compound lies.

Another situation is illustrated in Fig. 4. Here the active compounds cluster in one region of descriptor space while the inactives are scattered randomly around the class. This type of data structure has been termed *asymmetric* (*49*) and is probably the rule rather than the exception in classification problems of compounds as active versus inactive.

The origins of these two types of data structure in structure–activity analyses have been discussed (*40*). Clustering as is observed in both cases is due to the presence within a cluster of chemically and pharmacologically similar compounds. Chemical similarity implies that the class members are in some way described to be similar, whereas pharmacological similarity implies that activity within a class is due to a common mechanism. Accepting this, one would expect that cases in which a class of inactive compounds are all inactive by the same mechanism would be extremely rare and that most active versus inactive classification problems would result in an asymmetric data structure; each compound would be inactive by a unique mechanism. Needless to say, discriminant analysis and the linear learning machine will not separate actives from inactives when an asymmetric data structure is observed.

3. Hode's Statistical Heuristic Method for Automated Selection of Lead Structures

At the present time the screening capacity for testing new synthetic compounds is about 15,000 per year. The number of such compounds that are available for primary evaluation is almost limitless. Therefore a method for the preselection of structures for testing with higher or enhanced probabilities for being active would improve the efficiency of the search for new clinically useful compounds. Such a method has been described (*58,74*).

The method is in some ways similar to one used by Cramer *et al.* (*39*) and appears in some ways similar to the Free–Wilson method (*56*). Subtle differences exist and these will be pointed out.

The method begins, as in the previously discussed classification methods, with training sets composed of known active and inactive agents. The training sets are used to derive weights for structural features present, which can in turn be used to derive activity and inactivity scores for a particular compound.

Consider as a particular structural feature, which may be present in a compound, the sequence C—C—N where both single bonds are part of a ring. On the basis of its incidence of occurrence in a 280,000-compound file, a weight can be calculated that will be an estimate of its association with activity. If its incidence of occurrence is p and there are n active compounds in the file containing this feature, then np actives would be expected to have this feature if it is assumed that this feature has nothing to do with the compound being active. From this a weight can be calculated for the feature according to the statistical significance of the difference in its number of occurrences in the active and inactive training sets. This feature was found to be present in 17.7% of the 280,000 compounds. In a trial set of 33 actives, 5.83 are expected to contain this fragment with a standard deviation of 2.19 about the mean. The actual incidence of this feature in the 33 compounds in the trial set is 11 and the number of standard deviations away from the mean is $(11 - 5.83)/2.19$ or 2.36. This has a probability for significance of $P = 0.0183$. For convenience this is converted to $\log(1/P)$. In order to calculate an activity score for a compound, the relationship $\Sigma\,[\log(1/P_i)]$ is used, where i refers to structural features coded. This score is not an activity but a measure of the probability of activity of a compound based on the statistical incidence of its features.

There are obviously some problems encountered with the use of this method. The major problem is that of molecular description and the selection of relevant, nonredundant features. The method is also sensitive to finding chance correlations. Even so, in a trial study of 170 compounds tested against mouse ependymoblastoma, activity scores so calculated were able to distinguish actives from inactives at a significant level statistically.

II. QUANTITATIVE STRUCTURE–ACTIVITY RELATIONSHIPS OF ANTITUMOR COMPOUNDS

Most QSAR reported in the literature are derived from the application of the Hansch Model (*63*) to structure–activity data. Application of this method assumes all compounds in the data set are acting by the same mechanism. Therefore, with additional experimental information regarding the mode of action of some members of the data set, QSAR can be interpreted in terms of this mechanism of action. This makes it possible, in principle, to organize and present the material that follows in terms of what is thought to be the mechanism by which the anticancer agents studied exert their effect.

A. Alkylating Agents

The first compounds discovered to have anticancer activity and the first used clinically to treat neoplastic disease (*40*) were those classified as alkylating agents. These substances are thought to be cytotoxic by general inhibition of DNA synthesis (*84*). Although the precise mode of cytotoxicity that such compounds exert is not known, for the purpose of this work such agents have been subclassified into two groups: (1) nonmetabolically activated alkylating agents and (2) metabolically activated alkylating agents. Not surprisingly, in some cases this classification cannot be made unambiguously. However, this subclassification is made with regard to current thinking, and when a controversy exists it will be pointed out.

1. Nonmetabolically Activated Alkylating Agents

Compounds that exert their cytotoxic effect by being converted to a reactive species, generally electrophilic in nature, via a nonmetabolic pathway are discussed under this category. Mechanisms of activation will not be generalized and are dependent on the organic functional groups in the cytotoxic agent.

The first QSAR reported in the literature on anticancer drugs was derived for the tumor inhibitory 5-aziridino-2,4-dinitrobenzamides of general structure **I**. Activity was determined in the rat against Walker 256, a solid tumor.

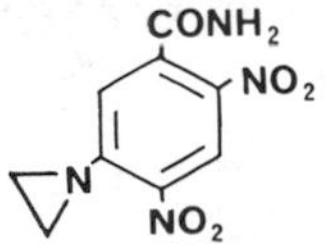

I

$$\log(1/C) = (-0.82 \pm 0.49) \log P - (0.54 \pm 0.38) \quad (1)$$

$$n = 8, \quad r = 0.860, \quad s = 0.320$$

The negative coefficient for the log P term indicates activity to be a decreasing function of lipophilicity. The aziridino group is thought to be converted to a reactive electrophilic center by protonation to the aziridinum intermediate. This process could be sensitive to steric and/or electronic influences but because the site of structural alteration in this series is far removed from the aziridinium group, the structure–activity relationship probably reflects changes in transport properties.

A number of studies have been carried out in the nitrogen mustards. These substances are represented by **II**. Like the aziridines these com-

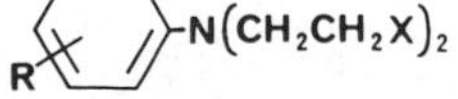

II

pounds undergo an internal nucleophilic displacement of halogen as in Fig. 5. With reactive nucleophiles mustards would be expected to react directly as in reaction (1), whereas poorer nucleophilic centers would require the activated form of the mustard. As can be seen, this mechanism

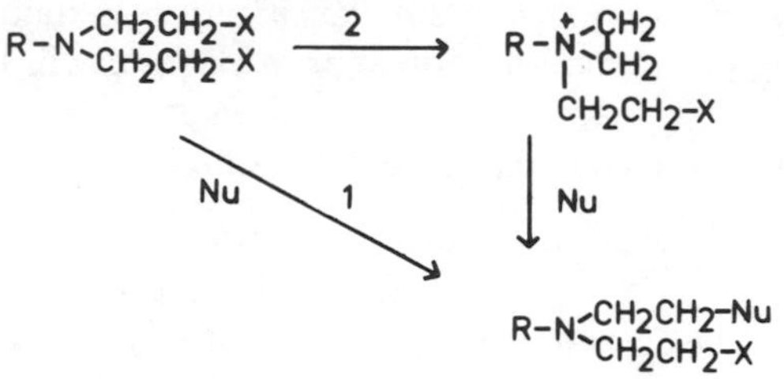

Fig. 5. Activation and reactions of nitrogen mustards.

at a number of points will be susceptible to structural variation and these should lead to rather interesting QSAR.

Lien and Tong (*79*) were the first to explore the QSAR of aromatic nitrogen mustards. Eq. (2) is the relationship reported for these data. Unfortunately no confidence limits were reported. There does appear to be a large electronic effect on activity with electron donating groups enhancing activity.

$$\log(1/C) = -0.26\pi_R - 1.62\sigma_R + 3.66 \tag{2}$$

$$n = 9, \quad r = 0.840, \quad s = 0.450$$

Unfortunately, and this is a general problem with anticancer drug development, toxicity parallels cytotoxicity (*7*). This is shown in Eq. (3). Also it should be noted that the equations were derived using the substituent constants for the un-ionized form of ionizable groups.

$$\log(1/LD_{50}) = -0.27\pi_R - 1.58\sigma_R + 3.48 \tag{3}$$

$$n = 9, \quad r = 0.930, \quad s = 0.270$$

Equation (4) was derived by Hansch *et al.* (*64*) for aniline mustards where activity is against Walker 256 in the rat.

$$\log(1/C) = (-1.19 \pm 0.51)\sigma^- + (0.75 \pm 0.41)I + (-1.00 \pm 0.87)\pi$$
$$-(0.53 \pm 0.55)\pi^2 + (3.84 \pm 0.33) \tag{4}$$

$$n = 14, \quad r = 0.940, \quad s = 0.290, \quad \pi_0 = -0.95, \quad \log P_0 = 1.95$$

the term I is an indicator variable given a value of 1 for X = Br and O when X = Cl, I; σ^- is used to model electronic influences of the R group in structure **II** on the activity term. The point that should be stressed here is that the coefficient for the electronic term is negative. This again emphasizes the enhancement of activity by electron donating groups. It is curious that I and Cl compounds are similar as is indicated by the common value of the indicator variable for these two halogen-containing mustards. Even though this is discussed by the authors no explanation is given although it is consistent with the mechanism proposed in Fig. 5. Iodine and chlorine mustards may be active by the same pathway whereas Br mustards are active via the other. Equation 4 suggests that more hydrophilic groups enhance activity but the lack of statistical significance of the π^2 term makes quantitation of this questionable.

A comparison of the QSAR for activity against two solid tumors can be made by comparing Eqs. (4) and (5). The latter equation was derived for activity against B-16 melanoma in the mouse (*66*).

$$\log(1/C) = (-2.06 \pm 0.48)\sigma - (0.15 \pm 0.12)\pi - (0.13 \pm 0.07)\pi^2 + (4.13 \pm 0.20) \quad (5)$$

$$n = 19, \quad r = 0.940, \quad s = 0.300, \quad \pi_0 = -0.57, \quad \log P_0 = 2.33$$

These equations indicate that for designing chemotherapeutic agents for solid tumors, lipophilicity of $\log P = 2$ should be considered, all other factors being held constant.

Equation 6 was derived by Hansch *et al.* (*64*) for aniline mustards against L1210 in the mouse. Here, I_0 is used as an indicator variable to stress the activity enhancing effort of ortho substitution.

$$\log(1/C) = (-0.31 \pm 0.10)\pi - (0.96 \pm 0.54)\sigma^- + (0.86 \pm 0.37)I_0 + (4.07 \pm 0.21) \quad (6)$$

$$n = 19, \quad r = 0.930, \quad s = 0.310$$

This relationship is qualitatively similar to Eq. (4) even though some differences might be expected because Eq. (4) is derived from solid tumor response data whereas data against L1210, an ascitic tumor, were used to derive Eq. (6).

This similarity in QSAR also extends to those of leukemia P-388 as is seen in Eqs. (7) and (8), respectively.

$$\log(1/C) = (-0.40 \pm 0.08)\pi - (1.00 \pm 0.35)\sigma + (4.59 \pm 0.13) \quad (7)$$

$$n = 19, \quad r = 0.950, \quad s = 0.240$$

$$\log(1/C) = (-0.35 \pm 0.11)\pi - (1.38 \pm 1.00)\sigma + (4.17 \pm 0.20) \quad (8)$$

$$n = 16, \quad r = 0.900, \quad s = 0.320$$

Leukemia P-388 is more sensitive to chemotherapy. These relationships were reported by Hansch *et al.* (*64*), and it was pointed out that the analog of **II** with R = $(CH_2)_3CHO$, X = Cl is 32 times more active than predicted. This is probably due to the fact that it is converted *in vivo* to chlorambucil (**III**). The same compound was used in the derivation of Eq.

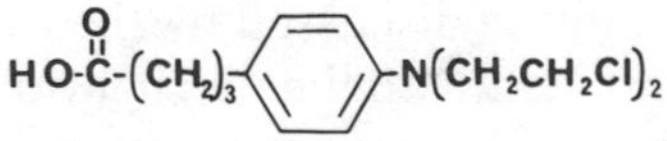

III

(7), however, and is only 3.8 times more active than predicted. No explanation can be extended for this inconsistency even though there are differences in the standard response for activity in the two data sets.

In addition to the halogen leaving groups, sulfonate analogs of the aniline mustards, X = OSO_2-R′, also show significant activity. Data on such anticancer compounds were used to derive Eqs. (9) and (10) (*64*).

$$\log(1/C) = (2.09 \pm 0.63)\mathrm{I}_2 + (4.06 \pm 0.32) \tag{9}$$

$$n = 16, \quad r = 0.880, \quad s = 0.510$$

$$\log(1/C) = (3.03 \pm 0.68)I_2 - (0.94 \pm 0.48)\sigma^- - (0.86 \pm 0.53)I_1 + (4.78 \pm 0.31) \tag{10}$$

$$n = 16, \quad r = 0.960, \quad s = 0.330$$

Here I_2 is an indicator variable given a value of 1 for those compounds containing the R = 4-NO group and I_1 is given a value of 1 for X = tosyl. The activity enhancing effect of the 4-NO group is stressed by the large positive coefficient for I_2. This term accounts for 77% of the variation in activity ($r^2 = 0.77$) for Eq. (9) with only small effects on activity stressed by σ^- and I_1. No effect on activity by lipophilic terms was observed.

In almost every case studied the role of hydrolytic activation is indicated by relationships such as Eq. (11). The indicator variable I_0 is given a value of 1 for ortho-substituted substrates, and I is given a value of 1 for X = Br.

$$\log(\%\ \text{hydrolysis}) = (-1.49 \pm 0.22)\sigma + (0.46 \pm 0.18)I_0 + (0.74 \pm 0.13)\mathrm{I} + (1.19 \pm 0.07) \tag{11}$$

$$n = 43, \quad r = 0.940, \quad s = 0.190$$

Both substitutions apparently enhance hydrolysis considering their regression coefficients. The large negative coefficient for σ mirrors the enhancement to activity expected by electron donation. A poorer correlation was observed with σ^-, indicating the possibility of an inductive mechanism for the electronic effect of the R group.

N-Methylisatin-3-Thiosemicarbazone (**IV**), a compound with known antiviral activity, was used by Ban *et al.* (*23*) as a model for the design of the series of nitrogen mustards. These mustards were then tested against HeLa cells in culture and from the activity data against this model Eq. (12) was derived.

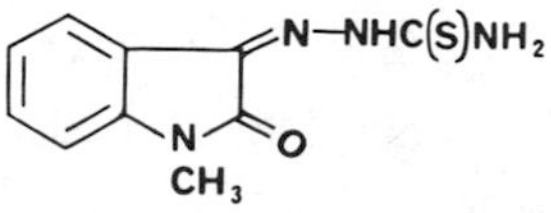

IV

$$\log(1/C) = -0.26(\log P)^2 + 1.16 \log P + 3.15 \quad (12)$$

$$n = 7, \quad r = 0.850, \quad s = 0.180, \quad \log P_0 = 2.19\ (0.57 - 2.69)$$

This is a relationship reflecting a typical parabolic lipophilic effect on activity. It is interesting that three of the nitro-substituted compounds were not fitted to the relationship and that some of the compounds used to derive the equation do not have alkylating potential.

Mitomycin C(**V**) is a naturally occurring antibiotic with antineoplastic activity (*8,55*). The substance does not exhibit high activity and is highly toxic. Using it as a lead compound, a group of Japanese workers (*8*) have systematically designed a series of 39 benzoquinones (**VI**) and evaluated

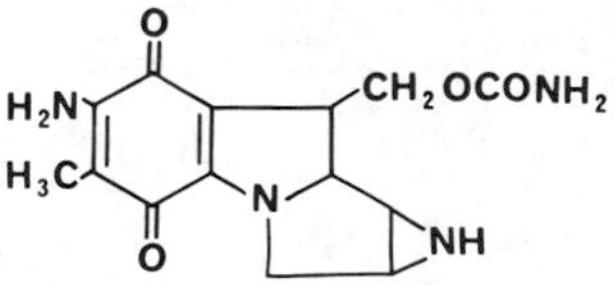

V

them against L1210 in the mouse. It should be pointed out that four different activity indices were obtained from the data. Two types of tests were used: (1) chronic treatment with daily injection for 12 days and (2)

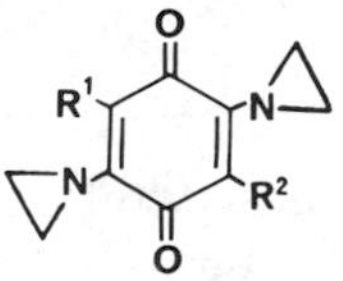

VI

single injection on day one only. From the dose-response data, the minimum effective dose (MED), or the dose giving a 40% increase in life span, and optimal dose (OD), or that dose giving maximal increase in life span, were calculated. These parameters were converted to a standard response of log(1/*C*) where *C* is in *M*/kg.

The relationships between the chronic injection MED are given in Eqs. (13) and (14).

$$\log(1/C) = (-0.45 \pm 0.10) \sum \pi_{1,2} + (6.35 \pm 0.17) \tag{13}$$

$$n = 37, \quad r = 0.850, \quad s = 0.340$$

$$\log(1/C) = (-0.51 \pm 0.10)\pi_2 - (0.34 \pm 0.14)MR_1 - (1.78 \pm 1.12)\mathbf{F} - (0.82 \pm 0.54)\mathbf{R} + (6.09 \pm 0.26) \tag{14}$$

$$n = 37, \quad r = 0.920, \quad s = 0.260$$

Here $\Sigma\, \pi_{1,2}$ is the sum of π values for the substituents R^1 and R^2. Using other combinations of variables for the substituents, Eq. (14) is obtained, which indicates an electronic effect on activity. *MR* was assumed to model steric effects of R^1, which is a reasonable assumption in view of the predominance of alkyl substituents in this position. The dominant role of lipophilicity is certain from Eq. (13) with little gained in terms of reduction in variance in going to the four-variable Eq. (14).

Equations (15) and (16) were derived for the optimal dose-dependent variable.

$$\log(1/C) = (-0.34 \pm 0.09) \sum \pi_{1,2} + (5.75 \pm 0.16) \tag{15}$$

$$n = 37, \quad r = 0.790, \quad s = 0.320$$

$$\log(1/C) = (-0.35 \pm 0.09)\pi_2 - (0.29 \pm 0.13)MR_1 - (2.08 \pm 1.05)\mathbf{F} - (1.16 \pm 0.51)\mathbf{R} + (5.38 \pm 0.25) \tag{16}$$

$$n = 37, \quad r = 0.890, \quad s = 0.250$$

These equations are virtually identical with Eqs. (13) and (14), respectively.

The single dose parameter MED data were used to derive Eqs. (17) and (18). Here again Eq. (17) reflects the strong effect of lipophilicity on activity.

$$\log(1/C) = (-0.38 \pm 0.15) \sum \pi_{1,2} + (5.72 \pm 0.25) \tag{17}$$

$$n = 35, \quad r = 0.670, \quad s = 0.490$$

$$\log(1/C) = (-0.49 \pm 0.09) \sum \pi_{1,2} - (3.95 \pm 1.05)\mathbf{F} - (1.49 \pm 0.49)\mathbf{R} + (5.30 \pm 0.20) \tag{18}$$

$$n = 35, \quad r = 0.910, \quad s = 0.290$$

However, the variance reduction in going from the one-variable equation to the three-variable Eq. (18) is probably real and a strong electronic effect is suggested by the presence of **F** and **R**, the Swain-Lupton substituent constants.

The optimal dose data again are reflective of the minimal effective dose data as is seen in Eqs. (19) and (20), with Eq. (20) being a significant improvement over Eq. (19).

$$\log(1/C) = (-0.34 \pm 0.13) \sum \pi_{1,2} + (5.14 \pm 0.22) \quad (19)$$

$$n = 37, \quad r = 0.680, \quad s = 0.450$$

$$\log(1/C) = (-0.37 \pm 0.07) \sum \pi_{1,2} - (3.25 \pm 0.83)\mathbf{F} - (1.39 \pm 0.43)\mathbf{R} + (4.71 \pm 0.18) \quad (20)$$

$$n = 37, \quad r = 0.910, \quad s = 0.260$$

These equations (13–20) suggested three mytomycin C analogs of greater activity and these were synthesized to test these relationships. The structures of these analogs are given below (**VII**, **VIII**, and **IX**). It can

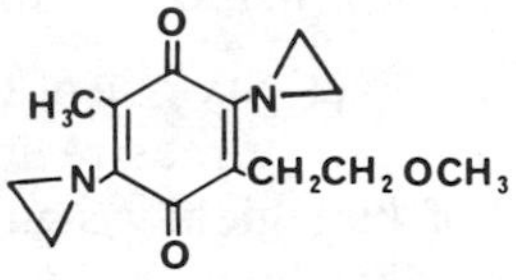

VII

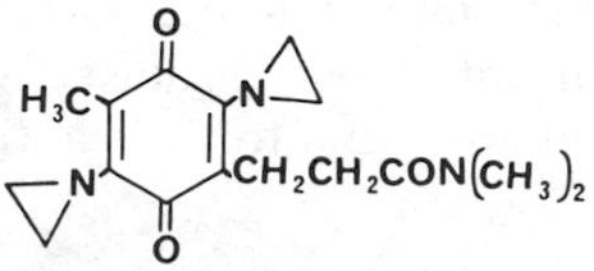

VIII

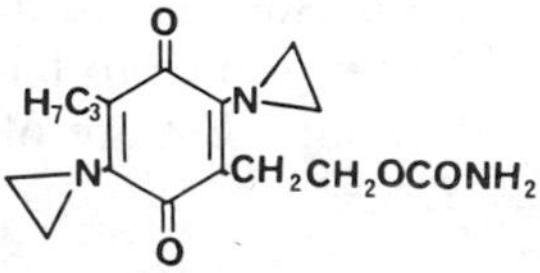

IX

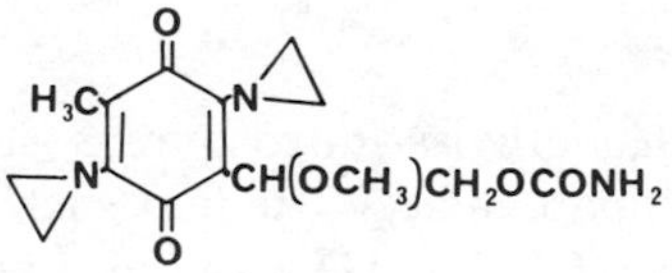

X

be seen that the results were quite good. Another structure (**X**), which resulted from this systematic study, and one of the most active analogs, has been cleared for clinical use in Japan. It is more active and less toxic than mitomycin C. QSAR on similar aziridines have been published in the Russian literature (*26*).

Lien *et al.* (*80*) derived Eqs. (21) and (22) for a series of bis(1-aziridinyl)phosphinyl carbamates (**XI**). Such compounds are thought to be alkylating agents and the effect of their activity against Walker 256 tumor in the rat is shown in Eq. (21).

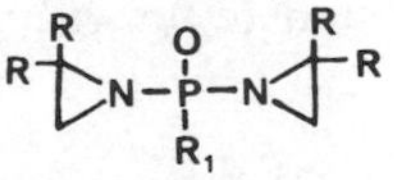

XI

$$\log(1/C) = 2.74\sigma^*_R + 3.34 \tag{21}$$

$$n = 10, \quad r = 0.940, \quad s = 0.260$$

This result is somewhat better than the single variable equation in π (r = 0.71) found by these workers. There is apparently a parallel between activity and toxicity as seen by comparing Eqs. (21) and (22).

$$\log(1/LD_{50}) = 1.73\sigma^*_R + 3.03 \tag{22}$$

$$n = 10, \quad r = 0.770, \quad s = 0.390$$

For their potential anticancer activity one of the more studied classes of organic compounds is the *N*-nitrosoureas related to structure **XII**. Such substances have a variety of biologically significant effects (*9*) and the chemistry relevant to these effects was the subject of a review published in 1979 (*45*). As anticancer agents, those analogs of **XII** with X = halogen and R = alkyl or substituted alkyl are the most important. These compounds have been shown to have significant activity against a variety of transplanted tumors, but are of major interest due to their antileukemia activity (*29,82*).

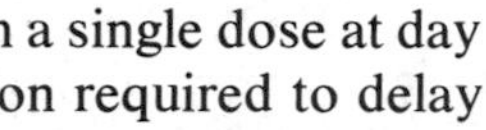

XII

Most QSAR for 2-haloethyl-*N*-nitrosoureas suggest that activity is strongly dependent on lipophilicity. The first such result (Eq. 23) was reported by Hansch *et al.* (*70,71*). Here activity was determined against Lewis lung carcinoma from a single dose at day one of infection. The term C is the molar concentration required to delay tumor growth 4 days.

$$\log(1/C) = (-0.08 \pm 0.05)(\log P)^2 + (0.14 \pm 0.15)\log P + (1.23 \pm 0.26) \tag{23}$$

$$n = 13, \quad r = 0.760, \quad s = 0.280$$

The marginally significant log P term can be dropped and the log $P_0 = 0$ results. Because of the diversity of structure in the series, however, it is doubtful that effects other than lipophilicity can be modeled. The importance of this parameter, though, cannot be overstressed and later studies

(*69,71*) have pointed this out by comparing relationships for activity with those of toxicity. Equations (24) and (25) are examples derived for analogs of **XII**.

$$\log(1/C) = (-0.17 \pm 0.04)\log P - (0.66 \pm 0.18)I_1 + (0.38 \pm 0.21)I_2 - (0.26 \pm 0.14)I_3 + (1.76 \pm 0.11) \quad (24)$$

$$n = 95, \quad r = 0.790, \quad s = 0.260$$

The term C is the molar concentration required to give a 10^3-fold decrease in L1210 cells in the mouse. The indicator variable I_1 is used to distinguish those compounds with substituents on R ($I_1 = 1$); I_2 is given a value of 1 for those congeners of **XII** that contain oxidizable sulfur groups, e.g., —S—, whereas $I_3 = 1$ indicates X = F. This equation indicates that an optimum in log P is not reached but that lipophilic compounds are to be less active than those that are hydrophilic. Comparing this with Eq. (25),

$$\log(1/C) = (-0.04 \pm 0.01)(\log P)^2 - (0.62 \pm 0.15)I_1 + (1.04 \pm 0.06) \quad (25)$$

$$n = 96, \quad r = 0.830, \quad s = 0.220, \quad \log P_o = 0$$

where C is the molar LD_{10}, the optimum log $P_o = 0$ is well established. This suggests that a separation of active and toxic responses may be possible and it is proposed in this work that R = disaccharide be introduced to achieve a more hydrophilic and less toxic drug. More hydrophilic analogs of **XII** are less toxic to bone marrow and as cytotoxic (*55*).

In addition, toxic responses other than those of general toxicity as measured by LD_{10} are of interest to those involved in the design of antitumor agents. One response that has been shown to be significant to monitor is mutagenicity. This can be modeled by the effect of the cytotoxic agents on various strains of *Salmonella* (*3*). For one series of (*o*-phenylenediamine)platinum dichlorides (**XIII**), some of which are clinically

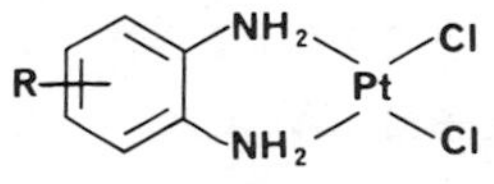

XIII

significant as antitumor agents, QSAR have been derived. In such a study, Eq. (26) resulted (*69*).

$$\log(1/C) = (2.23 \pm 0.32)\sigma^- + (5.78 \pm 0.18) \quad (26)$$

$$n = 13, \quad r = 0.980, \quad s = 0.260$$

Here C is the molar concentration required to produce 30 mutations/10^8 bacteria. The process is clearly controlled by electronic erffects having those compounds containing R groups that are electron withdrawing as the most active. This was shown to be an additive electronic effect and lipophilicity was not found to be a significant physicochemical property of the mutagens.

2. Metabolically Activated Compounds

There are classes of anticancer compounds that are thought to require activation by a metabolizing enzyme of the host as the tumor. Typical of such compounds are the dialkyltriazenes of which 5-(3,3-dimethyl-1-triazeno)imidazole-4-carboxamide (DTIC) (**XIV**: $R^1 = R^2 = CH_3$) and 1-aryl-3,3-dimethyltriazenes (**XVI**) are examples.

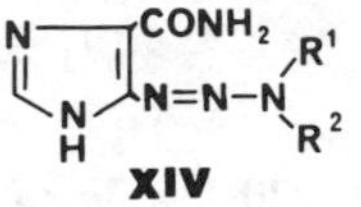

XIV

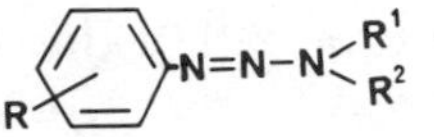

XV

Evidence points to a role of cytochrome P-450 in the activation of the triazenes, and the triazenes' mode of action is thought to involve the steps shown in Fig. 6 (*59,73*). Metabolically activated compounds usually lead to the generation of an electrophilic species with the potential for forming covalent linkages with key nucleophilic centers in the cell. In Fig. 6 this is the methyl cation or its precursor, the methyldiazo cation. In most cases the key reaction leading to cytotoxicity can only be postulated, inasmuch as the reactivity of the intermediate is high and its specificity not great. As a result the QSAR for such drugs are complex and usually multivariable.

Derivatives of **XIV** with structural variation at the 3 position of the triazene moiety were the first of the triazenes to be studied using quantitative methods (*5,51,560*). Equation (27),

$$\log(1/C) = (-0.28 \pm 0.19)(\log P)^2 + (0.59 \pm 0.24) \log P + (3.45 \pm 0.18) \quad (27)$$

$$n = 10, \quad r = 0.930, \quad s = 0.150, \quad \log P_0 = 1.10$$

which was derived by these workers, shows a parabolic dependence on log P. This probably reflects the role of transport prior to metabolic activation.

The analog of **XIV** with $R^1 = R^2 = CH_2CH_2Cl$ was not used to derive Eq. (27) because it is 4.3 times more active than predicted. From its structure it is obvious that it functions as an alkylating agent that would not require metabolic activation.

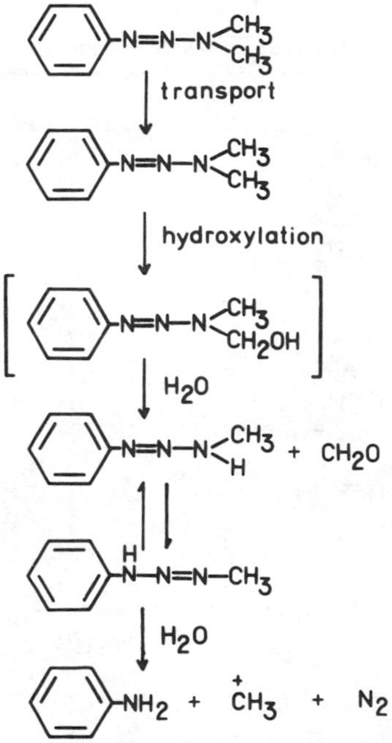

Fig. 6. Activation and reaction of dimethyltriazenes.

The imidazole group at the 1 position of the triazene function in **XIV** can be replaced by the phenyl group with no loss in activity. The result is general structure **XV**. Several of such triazene series have been studied extensively from the QSAR standpoint. The first QSAR work on these compounds was published by Dunn *et al.* (*33*).

For the 13 compounds that were active in the series studied, structure and activity were related by Eq. (28). Activity was determined against *S*-180 in the mouse.

$$\log(1/C) = (-0.69 \pm 0.09)\sigma + (3.41 \pm 0.03) \quad (28)$$

$$n = 13, \quad r = 0.920, \quad s = 0.090$$

The role of electronic effects in determining activity is clearly stated in this relationship (*28*). No other single variable equation was significant, and the parabolic relationship in log *P* explained only 22% of the variance in activity.

A study of the relationship between structure and toxicity (LD_{50}) resulted in Eq. (29), which even though significant, shows considerable scatter in the toxicity term. Toxicity is parallel to activity and a separation of the two parameters appears unlikely.

TABLE I
Activity Data Used to Derive Eq. (29) for **XV** Analogs, $R^1 = CH_3$

Structure	R	R^2	Log(1/C^a)
XVa	4-$NHCOCH_3$	CH_3	4.04
XVb	4-$NHCONH_2$	CH_3	3.97
XVc	3-$CONH_2$, 6-OCH_3	CH_3	3.95
XVd	4-$NHCONH_2$	CH_2CH_3	3.87
XVe	4-NHCOH	CH_3	3.85
XVf	H	CH_3	3.85
XVg	3-$CONH_2$	CH_3	3.80
XVh	4-CH_3	CH_3	3.76
XVi	4-$NHCONH_2$	$CH_2CH{=}CH_2$	3.77
XVj	4-SO_2NH, 2-pyrimidyl	CH_3	3.74
XVk	2-CO_2H	n-C_3H_7	3.74
XVl	4-$CONH_2$	CH_2CH_3	3.66
XVm	2-COOH	CH_3	3.64
XVn	2,6-F_2	CH_3	3.63
XVo	4-SO_2NH_2	CH_3	3.60
XVp	4-$(CH_2)_3CONHNH_2$	CH_3	3.60
XVq	H	H	3.60
XVr	m-$COCH_3$	CH_3	3.58
XVs	4-$(CH_2)_3CO_2C_2H_5$	CH_3	3.54
XVt	4-$CONH_2$	CH_3	3.51
XVu	4-$CONH_2$	n-C_4H_9	3.47
XVv	2-COOH	n-C_8H_{17}	3.47
XVw	2-$CONH_2$, 4-CN	CH_3	3.46
XVx	3-Pyridyl nucleus	CH_3	3.46
XVy	2-$CONH_2$	$CH_2CH{=}CH_2$	3.43
XVz	3-CO_2CH_3	CH_3	3.42
XVaa	3-CH_3	CH_3	3.40
XVbb	4-$CONH_2$	$CH_2CH{=}CH_2$	3.38
XVcc	2-$CONH_2$, 4-SO_2NH_2	CH_3	3.32
XVdd	2-$CONH_2$	CH_3	3.31
XVee	2-NO_2	CH_3	3.28
XVff	2-$CONH_2$, 4-$CONH_2$	CH_3	3.27
XVgg	3-$CONH_2$, 5-$CONH_2$	CH_3	3.27
XVhh	2-$CONH_2$, 4-NO_2	CH_3	3.26
XVii	2-Cl	CH_3	3.26
XVjj	2-$CONH_2$	n-C_3H_7	3.26
XVkk	2-$CONHCH_3$	CH_3	3.25
XVll	2-$CONHCH_2CONH_2$	CH_3	3.25
XVmm	2-$CONHCH_2CN$	CH_3	3.22
XVnn	4-COOH	CH_3	3.22
XVoo	4-CO_2CH_3	CH_3	3.20
XVpp	4-$CONH_2$	i-C_3H_7	3.17
XVqq	2-COOH	n-C_4H_9	3.15
XVrr	2-CO_2H, 4-Cl	n-C_8H_{17}	3.14
XVss	2-$CONH_2$, 4,6-Cl_2	CH_3	3.14

(*continued*)

TABLE I *(continued)*

Structure	R	R^2	Log(1/C^a)
XVtt	2-CO_2CH_3	i-C_4H_9	3.12
XVuu	2-$CONH_2$	n-C_4H_9	3.10
XVvv	2-$CONH_2$, 4-NO_2	n-C_4H_9	3.08
XVww	2-$CONH_2$	CH_2CH_2OH	3.07
XVxx	2-$CONHNHCOCH_3$	CH_3	3.05
XVyy	4-OCH_3	COC_6H_5	3.05
XVzz	3-$CONH_2$, 2,5-Cl_2	CH_3	3.04
XVaaa	H	$CH_2C_6H_5$	3.03
XVbbb	4-$(CH_2)_2CO_2C_2H_5$	n-C_4H_9	3.02
XVccc	4-$CO_2C_2H_5$	CH_2CH_3	3.01
XVddd	2-$CONHNH_2$	Cyclohexyl	2.99
XVeee	2-$CONHCH_2CH_3$	CH_3	2.92
XVfff	4-$CONH_2$	s-C_4H_9	2.90
XVggg	4-$CONH_2$	n-C_8H_{17}	2.84
XVhhh	4-$CO_2C_2H_5$	i-C_4H_9	2.80
XViii	4-CH_3	$COCH_3$	2.78
XVjjj	3,5-$(CN)_2$	CH_3	2.63
XVkkk	4-CN	$CH_2C_6H_4$-OCH_3	2.72
XVlll	2-$CONHNHCOCH_2CN$	CH_3	2.63

[a] C: Concentration in M/kg required to give a 40% increase in life span. Tumor model was L1210 in the mouse.

$$\log(1/C) = (-0.33 \pm 0.10)\sigma + (2.84 \pm 0.04) \quad (29)$$

$$n = 14, \quad r = 0.690, \quad s = 0.110$$

It should be pointed out that the series of compounds in this work was designed using the cluster analysis approach of Forsythe *et al.* (*54*). Using the clusters published by these workers, 14 compounds were designed from the 10-level based on the physicochemical variables π^2, π, σ, MR, and MW. The advantages of the use of this method are that the resulting series will contain little, if any, convariance in the physicochemical properties and that it will span variable space extracting the optimum in structure–activity information.

From the point of view of drug development, a number of compounds from the **XV** series were requested from NCI for further testing in L1210 in the mouse. Of these the R = 3-$NHCOCH_3$ (**XVI**) and R = 4-CH=CHCOOH (**XVII**) analogs were shown to have reproducible and significant activity and were considered for advanced testing.

In a similar study of the R^1 = CH_3 analogs of **XV** ihn Table I, Hansch *et al.* (*65*) derived Eq. (30).

$$\log(1/C) = (0.10 \pm 0.08) \log P - (0.04 \pm 0.02)(\log P)^2 - (0.31 \pm 0.11)\sigma^+ - (0.18 \pm 0.08)MR_{2,6} + (0.39 \pm 0.18)E_s + (4.12 \pm 0.27) \quad (30)$$

$$n = 61, \quad r = 0.840, \quad s = 0.190, \quad \log P_o = 1.18$$

Three of the compounds were deleted from the analysis. This equation was interpreted as follows. The σ^+ term with the negative coefficient indicates that electron release through resonance increases activity, whereas the negative coefficient for $MR_{2,6}$ shows that large groups in the ortho position decrease activity. The role of the E_s term, the Taft steric parameter for R^1 and R^2, was not discussed, although it was pointed out that the optimum log P_o of 1.18 agrees well with that for the triazenes of structure **XIV** in Eq. (27).

A test of the predictability of Eq. (30) can be made. Recently data have become available on the activity of the three compounds below (**XVI**, **XVII**, and **XVIII**). These substances were synthesized in this

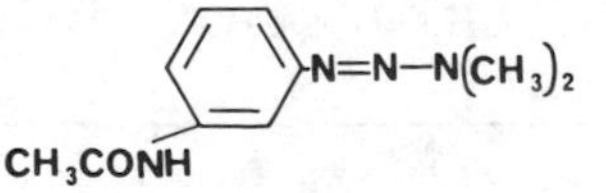

XVI

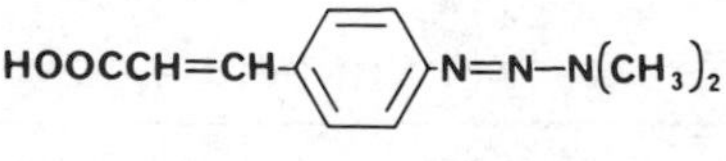

XVII

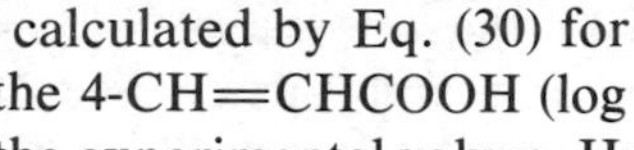

XVIII

author's laboratory and submitted to NCI for testing against L1210 in the mouse, and their activities can be estimated from Eq. (30).

The activities of 3.57 calculated by Eq. (30) for the 3-$NHCOCH_3$ (log P = 1.61) and 3.28 for the 4-CH=CHCOOH (log P = 2.41) analogs are in good agreement with the experimental values. However, the high activity of 3.34 estimated for the inactive 4-C_6H_5 compound (**XVIII**) log P = 4.37) is surprising, especially because its lipophilicity is much greater than log P_o = 1.18.

An explanation can be given if the data in Table I are examined. Only four compounds have log $P > 4.00$ and all owe their lipophilicity to large alkyl groups at the 3 position of the triazene function. Such groups also have large and negative E_s values. This term in Eq. (30) is heavily weighted, and this tends to balance the positive contribution to activity from the log P term for those four compounds. Therefore, the E_s term acts as a dummy variable to bring the estimated activities of these lipophilic compounds into line. Equation (30) appears not to be valid for compounds with very lipophilic groups in the aryl portion of the molecule and overpredicts their activity. This overfitting that sometimes results with the use of regression analysis can be detected by proper validation methods (*85*).

In an attempt to classify analogs of **XV** with $R^1 = CH_3$, $R^2 = CH_2C_6H_4X$ as active or inactive against Sarcoma-180 in the mouse, Dunn and Greenberg (*47*) were able to derive a discriminant function that would separate active from inactive triazenes at the rate of 85% (11/13). The major variable separating actives from inactives appeared to be σ for R, and the lipophilicity of this substituent was also significant. Within the series of triazenes reported, there was little or no variation in toxicity, so a structure–toxicity study could not be done.

B. Enzyme Directed Agents

1. Dihydrofolate Reductase Inhibitors

The development of anticancer drugs based on differences in the biochemical pharmacology of normal and tumor cells is one of the most powerful approaches to the rational design of anticancer agents. This approach has been used to some extent but it is becoming more important as more differences between normal and tumor cells are detected. This is due in part to the ability of the biochemist to isolate and purify key enzymes and to describe at the molecular level the function of these enzymes. This, coupled with the X-ray crystallographer's use of computer graphics to display macromolecules (i.e., enzymes) in a manner useful to those in drug design make this an important method for discovering new and more effective anticancer agents (*67*).

Differences in the biochemistry of normal and cancer cells have been explored extensively, and in instances where differences in enzyme function between the two types of cells can be exploited, the method has shown promise. Data that illustrate species differences in enzyme specificity for trimethoprim are given in Table II.

TABLE II
Differential Sensitivity to Inhibition of Dihydrofolate Reductase by Trimethoprim

Enzyme source	I_{50} (*M*)
Escherichia coli	0.5×10^{-5}
Tapeworm	560×10^{-5}
Frog liver	$20,000 \times 10^{-5}$
Human liver	$30,000 \times 10^{-5}$

An early proponent of this method was Baker (*22*) who carried out extensive syntheses of potentially selective inhibitors of dihydrofolate reductase (tetrahydrofolate dehydrogenase) isolated from L1210 of the mouse and Walker 256 of the rat. Since Baker's untimely death in 1971, Hansch and co-workers, recognizing the significance of this approach, have extended this work by applying regression methods to his data in an attempt to quantify species and tissue differences in this enzyme (*57*).

Using data on compounds of type **XIX** with I_{50} values for rat liver dihy-

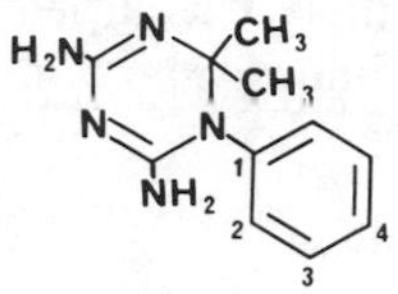

XIX

drofolate reductase and L1210 dihydrofolate reductase from the mouse, Eqs. (31) and (32), respectively, were derived (*67*).

$$\log(1/C) = (0.80 \pm 0.13)\pi_3 - (0.19 \pm 0.04)\pi_3^2 + (1.01 \pm 0.62)\sigma_3 + (6.16 \pm 0.22) \tag{31}$$

$$n = 18, \quad r = 0.964, \quad s = 0.190, \quad \pi_{30} = 2.13\ (1.8\text{–}12.5)$$

$$\log(1/C) = (0.93 \pm 0.39)\pi_3 - (0.23 \pm 0.16)\pi_3^2 + (1.28 \pm 2.00)\sigma_3 + (5.59 \pm 0.59) \tag{32}$$

$$n = 9, \quad r = 0.944, \quad s = 0.410, \quad \pi_{30} = 1.99\ (1.3\text{–}4.8)$$

These relationships serve to define optimum lipophilicites for substitution in the 3 position of **XIX** and suggest strong dependencies on the electronic effects of 3-substituents.

A much more extensive QSAR (Eq. 33) has been obtained by Dietrich *et al.* (*44*) for congeners of structure **XIX**.

$$\log(1/C) = 0.68\pi_3 - 0.12\pi_3^2 + 0.23MR_4 + 0.02MR_4^2 + 0.24I_1 - 2.53I_2 - 1.99I_3 + 0.88I_4 + 0.69I_5 + 0.70I_6 + 6.49 \tag{33}$$

$$n = 244, \quad r = 0.923, \quad s = 0.377, \quad \pi_{30} = 2.9\ (2.6\text{–}3.3)$$

This equation is based on inhibition of both dihydrofolate reductase from L1210 from the mouse and Walker 256 in the rat. The indicator variable I is used to differentiate the enzyme sources, with $I_1 = 1$ for the Walker 256 enzyme. Both 3- and 4-substituted analogs were used to derive the relationships. The other indicator variables are as follows: I_2 indicates substi-

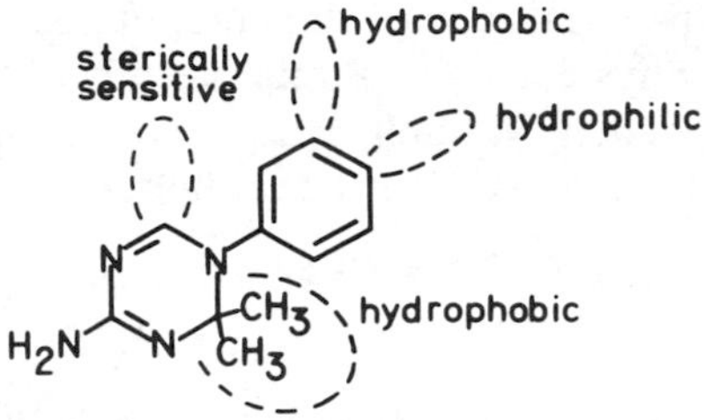

Fig. 7. Regions of the dihydrofolate reductase active site defined by QSAR. (Reprinted by permission of the publisher form QSAR of comparative inhibition of mammalian and bacterial dihydrofolate reductase by triazines, by S. Dietrich, C. Hansch, and R. N. Smith, *in* "Chemistry and Biology of Pteridines" (R. L. Kisliuk and G. M. Brown, eds.), Vol. 4, p. 425. Elsevier/North-Holland, New York, 1979. Copyright 1979.)

tution in the 2 position of the pyrimidine group, I_3 indicates the presence of a carboxyl group in the molecule, I_4 indicates hetroatom bridges or an ethylene bridge from the pyrimidine to the phenyl group, I_5 is a combination of I_1 and I_2, and I_6 is 1 for 6-SO_3Ar.

From these equations the approximation of the binding site for the enzyme can be given as shown in Fig. 7. In addition to the nature of the enzyme active site as implied by Eq. (33), the region of limited hydrophilic character can be spanned by appropriate bridging groups to a region containing a group capable of nucleophilic displacement of the SO_3Ar. This is indicated by the coefficient of 0.88 for I_4. This may be considered a quantitative expression of Baker's "bulk tolerance" concept (*22*).

2. Respiration Inhibitors

In a similar attempt to design biochemical selectivity into a series of potential inhibitors of cellular respiration, Coats *et al.* (*36,37*) have synthesized and evaluated copper(II) chelates of structure **XX**. To obtain a

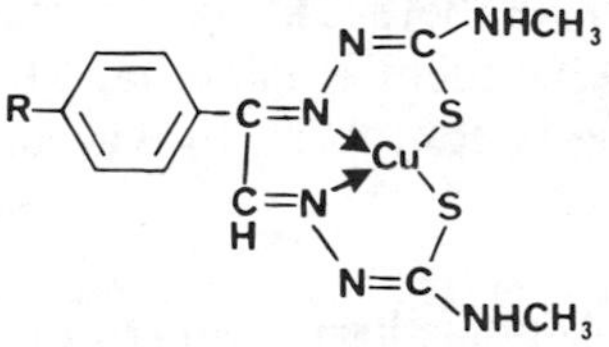

XX

dependent variable for their QSAR study, molar I_{50} values for inhibition of respiration were obtained for each compound against Ehrlich ascites cells and liver slices in culture. The difference in these two parameters was assumed to be the specificity of the compounds for the ascites tumor and to be related to physicochemical expressions of the structures of the substrates. This dependent variable was related to the physicochemical properties of the phenyl substituent according to Eq. (34).

$$\log(1/C_{\text{ascites}}) - \log(1/C_{\text{liver}}) = (0.54 \pm 0.36)\pi - (1.03 \pm 0.81)\sigma_p + (2.52 \pm 0.31) \quad (34)$$

$$n = 8, \quad r = 0.920, \quad s = 0.300$$

This relationship quantifies the differential in response to the two systems due to the lipophilic and electronic character of the substituents on the phenyl group. Using a more extensive series of **XX** analogs, these workers (*37*) were able to obtain Eq. (35), which suggests an optimum in π.

$$\log(1/C_{\text{ascites}} - \log(1/C_{\text{liver}}) = (-0.26 \pm 0.24)\pi - (0.10 \pm 0.02)\pi^2 + (0.65 \pm 0.44)\sigma_p^+ + (2.27 \pm 0.27) \quad (35)$$

$$n = 11, \quad r = 0.810, \quad s = 0.370, \quad \pi_0 = -1.31\ (-1.92 \text{ to } -0.24)$$

In addition to copper(II) chelates, Coats and Shah (*36*) have explored the QSAR of 4-hydroxyquinoline-3-carboxylic acids (**XXI**) as inhibitors of cellular respiration. This result is Eq. (36).

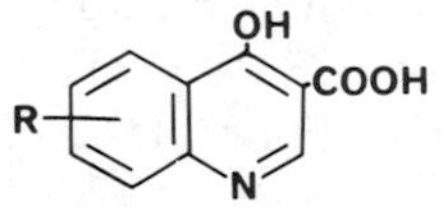

XXI

$$\log(1/C) = (0.45 \pm 0.29)MR + (2.68 \pm 0.47) \quad (36)$$

$$n = 14, \quad r = 0.700, \quad s = 0.550$$

The only significant variable detected by the regression analysis is *MR*. This suggests that the substituent R is perhaps binding in a region of the enzyme in which binding is controlled by van der Waals interactions or dispersion forces.

3. Ribonucleoside-Diphosphate Reductase

A number of α-*N*-formylheteroaromatic thiosemicarbazones such as **XXII** and **XXIII** are known to inhibit DNA synthesis (*2*) in L1210 cells in mice. The point of inhibition in the DNA synthesis sequence by these compounds is inhibition of the enzyme ribonucleoside-diphosphate reductase. There are two sources of the enzyme used for inhibition studies: (1)

rat Novikoff tumor and (2) H.Ep-2 tumor of human origin. Dunn and Hodnett (*48*) have obtained QSAR for inhibition of the enzyme obtained from these two sources by analogs of **XXII** and **XXIII.**

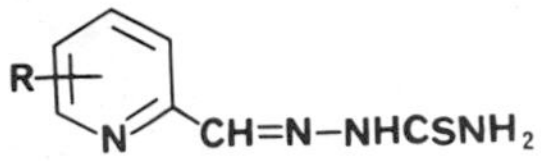

XXII

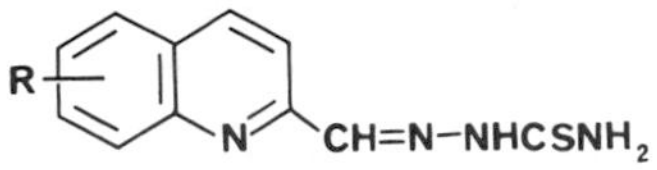

XXIII

For 50% inhibition of the reductase from H.Ep-2 tumor from human sources by **XXII** analogs, Eq. (37) was obtained. Here *C* is in moles per liter and F is the Swain–Lupton field effect constant. All terms are significant at the 99% level of confidence.

$$\log(1/C) = -0.81 \sum \mathbf{F}_{3,5} + 0.29 \sum \pi_{3,5} - 0.24MR_5 + 6.30 \quad (37)$$

$$n = 28, \quad r = 0.880, \quad s = 0.330$$

Against tumor of human origin analogs of **XXII** gave Eq. (38) and against rat Novikoff tumor a similar set of **XXII** analogs gave Eq. (39).

$$\log(1/C) = 6.70 - 1.81MR_5 \quad (38)$$

$$n = 13, \quad r = 0.800, \quad s = 0.370$$

$$\log(1/C) = 7.67 - 0.44MR_5^2 \quad (39)$$

$$n = 12, \quad r = 0.930, \quad s = 0.350$$

In all cases interpretation of the equations in mechanistic terms is difficult. The inverse dependence of inhibition with *MR* could be interpreted to reflect a steric interface by the ring substituents to binding. This is the authors' interpretation.

Another interesting outcome of comparing Eqs. (38) and (39) is the similarity in response of the enzymes from the two sources to changes in structure. The active sites of the two enzymes are very similar, implying that the rat Novikoff tumor enzyme is a good model for anticancer drug design studies.

C. DNA Binding Agents

1. Acridines

In the design and synthesis of acridines as potential anticancer agents, the work of Cain and co-workers at the Cancer Chemotherapy Research Laboratory in Auckland, New Zealand, represents some of the most thorough and exhaustive in the field. Cain (*31*) was one of the first to recognize the role of relative lipophilicity in the design of anticancer agents. From his laboratory has come an extensive series of reports describing the synthesis and anticancer activity of 9-anilinoacridines **(XXIV)** (*10–21,30–32,41*).

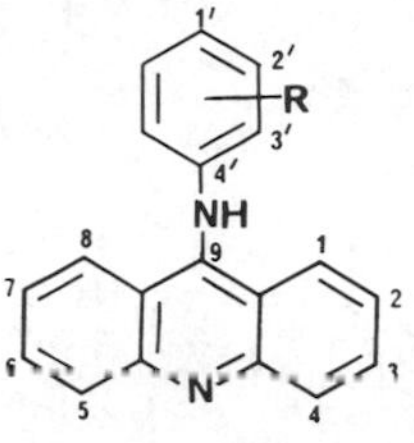

XXIV

The acridines bind strongly to DNA and it is known that the 9-anilinoacridines bind to DNA with the anilino group positioning itself in the minor groove. The cytotoxic effect of these substances is thought to be the result of this intercalation.

In all, over 700 acridines have been synthesized and evaluated for antileukemic activity and toxicity. In a 1982 report by Atwell *et al.* (*10*) the QSAR for these compounds were presented. In this QSAR study, activities were derived from various dose-response parameters. Also, to model lipophilicity, R_m, an experimental parameter obtained from the R_f value of a compound on thin layer chromatography was used. For the acridines this parameter has been shown to be highly correlated with isobutyl–water partition coefficients. Because the acridines are generally basic with a wide range of pK_a values, this parameter was determined at pH 1. This assures that effects due to variation in pK_a, such as degree of ionization, need not be considered in the derivation of their QSAR. This assumes activity is due to the ionic form of the acridine.

The acridines are most effective against leukemia L1210, and the measure of *in vivo* antitumor activity used in this study is the dose required to give a standard response of 40% increase in life span in mice. This parameter is considered by these workers to be a measure of drug selectivity. The relationship between drug potency and physicochemical properties is given in Eq. (40).

$$\begin{aligned}\log(1/C) = {} & (-0.14 \pm 0.03)\pi - (0.01 \pm 0.006)\pi^2 - (1.08 \pm 0.09)\sigma \\ & - (0.32 \pm 0.16)MR_2 + (1.04 \pm 0.13)MR_3 \\ & - (0.25 \pm 0.05)MR_3^2 - (0.77 \pm 0.13)I_{3,6} - (1.68 \pm 0.21)E_{sR^{3'}} \\ & + (0.78 \pm 0.13)I_{NO_2} + (0.70 \pm 0.32)I_{DAT} + (0.50 \pm 0.18)I_{BS} \\ & - (1.25 \pm 0.37)R_{BS} + (3.73 \pm 0.07) \qquad (40)\end{aligned}$$

$$n = 509, \quad r = 0.878, \quad s = 0.323, \quad \log P_o = -0.6$$

The range in the dependent variable in molar terms is 3300, and with 13 variables in the equation there are 39 compounds for each variable. A fit to a bilinear model gave a steeper negative slope of the π terms with the statistical parameters $r = 0.893$ and $s = 0.305$. This slightly better correlation is probably not significant. Therefore, this is no improvement over the parabolic relationship.

Because the π term refers to π constants for all substituents on the acridine system, it was shown that $\log P_0$ for the set is -0.6, which is in agreement with most other results of QSAR for antileukemia drugs. Considering this, the lipophilic terms suggest a dependence on distribution.

An explanation of the dependence of activity on electronic properties of the substituents is not clear. It is known that DNA binding is enhanced by electron release. Also the acridines are deactivated by a mechanism that involves initially attack by a thiol group on the C-9 position of acridine. This eventually results in displacement of the side chain. This is enhanced by electron releasing groups on the acridine system, conferring greater stability to thiol attack. Thus the electronic term may reflect a resultant of a combination of effects.

The MR and E_s terms were interpreted to reflect steric effects, and the optimum in MR_3 is consistent with this. The negative coefficient for E_s indicates a cooperative effect on activity, as E_s constants are less than zero. Such effects are rare but could in this case be due to substituents forcing the side chain into a conformation more favorable for intercalation. Another steric term, $I_{3,6}$, indicates 3,6-disubstitution; its negative coefficient indicates a detrimental effect of substitution at these positions on activity.

The remaining terms are all indicator variables of ambiguous interpretation in terms of discrete interactions or effects. The I_{NO_2} term is given a value of 1 for those compounds with a 3-NO_2 group. This group at the 3 position gives enhanced activity and also toxicity.

In an effort to derive a structure–toxicity relationship for the acridines, Eq. (41) resulted.

$$\begin{aligned}\log(1/C) = {} & (-0.07 + 0.02) \sum \pi - (0.76 + 0.09) \sum \sigma \\ & - (0.56 + 0.48)MR_1 - (0.24 + 0.13)MR_2 \\ & - (0.59 + 0.12)MR_3 - (0.12 + 0.04)MR_3^2 - (0.09 \pm 0.16)E_{s3'} \\ & - (0.61 \pm 0.11)E_{s3'}^2 - (0.51 \pm 0.14)I_{3,6} + (0.43 \pm 0.12)I_{NO_2} \\ & - (1.13 \pm 0.33)I_{BS} + (0.50 \pm 0.13)I_{NH_2} + (3.57 \pm 0.12) \qquad (41)\end{aligned}$$

$$n = 643, \qquad r = 0.771, \qquad s = 0.362$$

The dependent variable is the molar LD_{10} with toxicity varying over a 700-fold range in molar terms. The relationship is almost identical with Eq. (40) except for a slightly poorer statistical fit. This similarity again indicates that the potency and toxicity may not be separable.

A result of this work by Cain and his research group is the analog of **XXIV**, *m*-AMSA (R = 1′-$NHSO_2CH_3$, 3′-OCH_3), which has been cleared for clinical trials and shows promising results.

2. Anthracyclines

The anthracyclines (**XXV**) represent one of the more potent and promising new leads to anticancer agents (*38*). An analog of **XXV**, adriamycin (R = $COCH_2OH$; R^1 = NH_2), has been shown to be very effective against various experimental tumors. One of the difficulties with the therapeutic use of the anthracyclines, however, is their extreme cardiac toxicity, which appears to be cumulative. In an attempt to use QSAR to separate these two responses and minimize the undesirable toxic effects, Fink *et al.* (*53*) derived what they called quantitative structure–selectivity relationships (QSSR). From activity data against B-16 melanoma in the mouse for 23 analogs of **XXV**, Eq. (42) was derived. Here *C* is the molar concentration giving a 25% increase in life span in the test group.

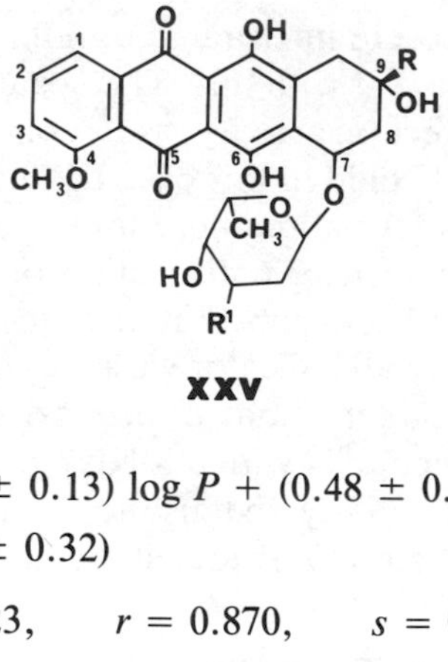

XXV

$$\log(1/C) = (-0.41 \pm 0.13) \log P + (0.48 \pm 0.35)I_0\ (0.81 \pm 0.38)I_1 + (6.57 \pm 0.32) \qquad (42)$$

$$n = 23, \quad r = 0.870, \quad s = 0.290$$

The indicator variable I_0 refers to the presence of the 4-OH substituent and I_1 implies the presence of a very lipophilic hydrazone substituent in position 9.

Cumulative cardiotoxicity is modeled by Eq. (43), which includes the same variables as Eq. (43) with the exception of I_2, which indicates the three analogs with R^1 = tertiary amine.

$$\log(1/C) = (-0.30 \pm 0.11) \log P + (1.01 \pm 0.25)I_0 + (0.69 \pm 0.33)I_1 + (0.74 \pm 0.34)I_2 + (4.82 \pm 0.22) \qquad (43)$$

$$n = 21, \quad r = 0.930, \quad s = 0.180$$

From these relationships the effect of lipophilicity on both activities is almost equivalent and from the series of compounds examined it appears that the separation of antitumor activity and cardiac toxicity may not be feasible. The authors suggest a reasonable alternative: to explore more hydrophilic analogs in an effort to find an optimum in lipophilicity, if possible. This has been done with other types of anticancer agents, and the use of QSAR in this way could lead to more useful and effective anthracyclines.

Kessel (*76*) has shown that various pharmacological effects of the three anthracyclines below (**XXVI**, **XXVII**, and **XXVIII**) are a function of lipophilicity as modeled by log *P* in the 1-octanol–water system.

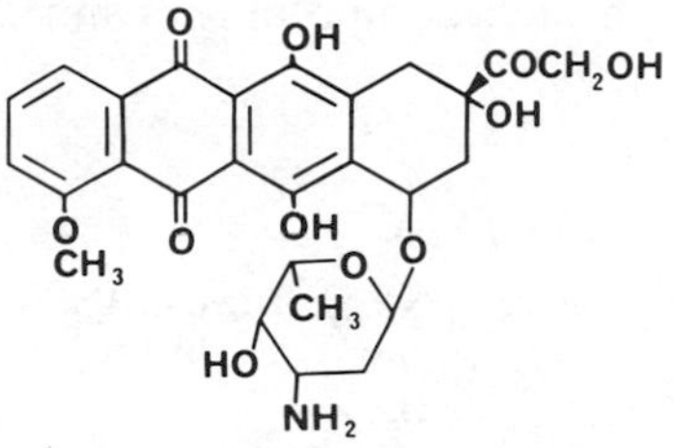

XXVI

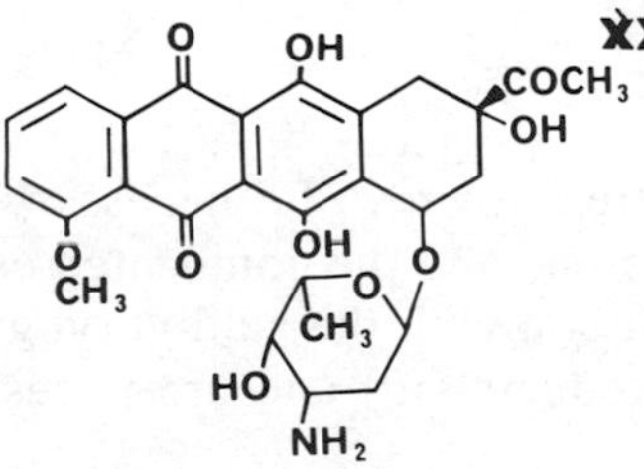

XXVII

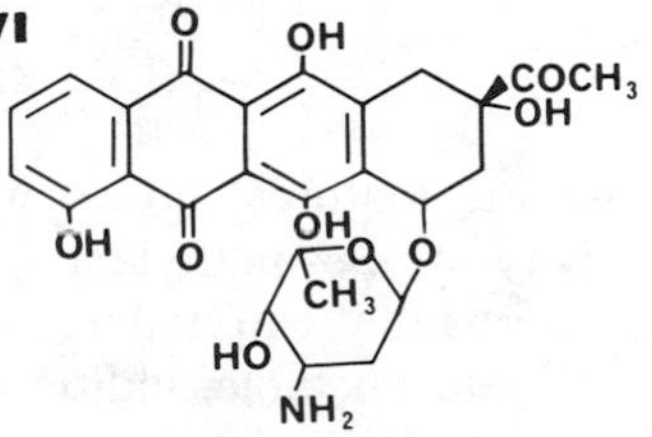

XXVIII

These results are given in Table III. In this case the activity is cytotoxicity to L1210 cells in culture, and ID_{50} is the dose inhibiting growth of cultured cells by 50%. It can readily be seen from the data that activity increases

TABLE III
Structure–Activity Data for Anthracyclines

Compounds	Log *P*	ID_{50} (mg/ml)
XXVII	−1.00	15.00
XXVIII	−0.66	7.50
XXIX	0.16	3.00

with log P, and it is reported (*76*) that the rate of uptake and amount of accumulation of the drugs in the tumor cells also are directly related to log P.

D. Miscellaneous Antitumor Agents

1. Sesquiterpene Lactones

Using plants as sources of potential anticancer agents Eakin *et al.* (*50*) have isolated a number of structurally complex and cytotoxic sesquiterpene lactones. An example of such compounds is elephantonin (**XXIX**). The mode of action of such compounds is not thoroughly understood.

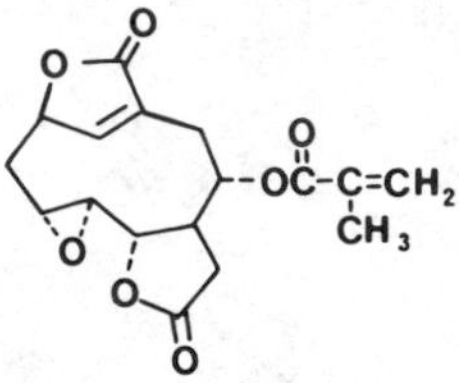

XXIX

Some structural features, however, are known to be necessary for optimum activity. The α-methylene-γ-lactone and the conjugated ester side chain are groups that can undergo addition with the sulfhydryl groups of cysteine to yield unstable addition products (*50*) and are necessary for high activity.

If such groups are present in the molecule, then variations in activity within a series of sesquiterpene lactones can be shown to be a function of differential transport (*50*). For lactones containing only the α-methylene-γ-lactone function, activity depends on the octanol–water log P according to Eq. (44) where C is the micromolar concentration giving a 50% inhibition of KB cell growth in culture.

$$\log(1/C) = 0.58 \log P + 4.56 \tag{44}$$

$$n = 9, \quad r = 0.870, \quad s = 0.220$$

For compounds containing only the α, β-unsaturated ester side chain, activity was similarly a function of partitioning, as shown in Eq. (43). The parameters in both equations are similarly defined. Comparing Eqs. (44) and (45), the differences in slope terms might suggest differences in transport mechanisms because the intercepts are identical for all practical purposes.

$$\log(1/C) = 1.02 \log P + 4.54 \quad (45)$$

$$n = 12, \quad r = 0.810, \quad s = 0.410$$

If both functions required for activity in the sesquiterpene lactone class are present, no significant relationship between activity and lipophilicity was observed for five compounds, possibly indicating a dual mechanism of action.

2. Inhibitors of Mitotic Cell Division

In some recent studies with the *Vinca* alkaloids, Donigian *et al.* (*46*) have shown that these compounds exert their cytotoxic effect by inhibiting cell division. This cytotoxic activity is due to the alkaloid interacting with the microtubulin protein tubulin, forming a drug–protein complex. This disrupts the mitotic spindle apparatus and leads to cellular malfunction and cell death.

Vindoline (**XXX**) is an example of such an alkaloid. By obtaining drug–tubulin binding constants (K_d) for a series of *Vinca* alkaloids and using measured and calculated log P values, Donigian *et al.* (*46*) derived Eq. (46).

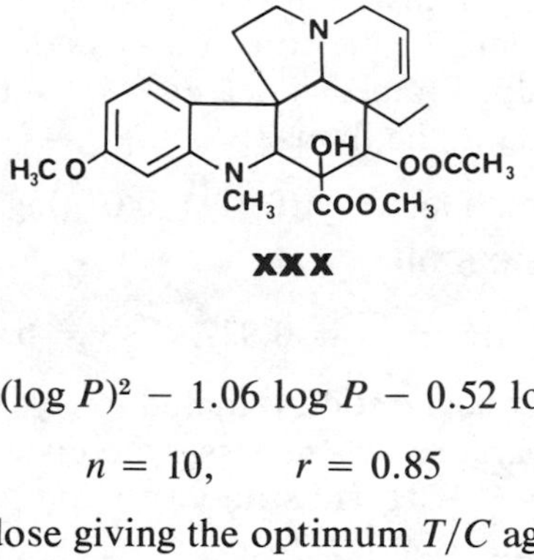

XXX

$$\log C = 0.22(\log P)^2 - 1.06 \log P - 0.52 \log K_d + 5.37 \quad (46)$$

$$n = 10, \quad r = 0.85$$

In this case C is the dose giving the optimum T/C against P-388 leukemia in the mouse. This relationship reflects an optimum in activity with log P because the activity is not expressed in the usual reciprocal manner. The optimum log P is approximately 2.40, somewhat higher in general than that found for alkylating agents and other anticancer drugs.

Equation (47) shows the relationship between toxicity and these parameters. Here again C is the LD_{50} in μmol/kg.

$$\log C = 0.13(\log P)^2 - 0.52 \log P - 0.48 \log K_a + 4.65 \quad (47)$$

$$n = 10, \quad r = 0.84$$

The difference between Eqs. (46) and (47) is the intercept term, indicating that there is some selectivity in the mode of action of these alkaloids.

One of the most potent inhibitors of mitotic cell division is colchicine (**XXXI**: R = $COCH_3$, R^1 = OCH_3). Colchicine itself is a naturally occur-

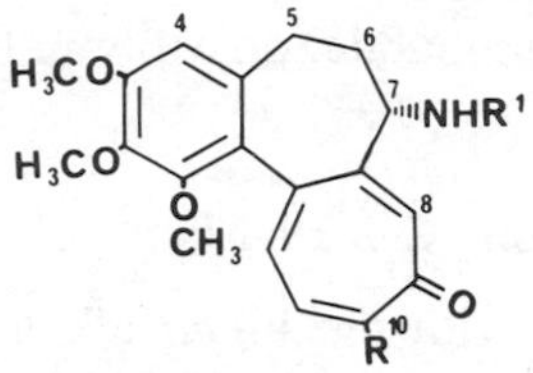

XXXI

ring compound and was known in ancient times to have anticancer properties. This activity is thought to be due to its ability to bind to a cysteine residue in the tubulin polypeptide (*24,25*), thus preventing cell division.

Even though there has been some clinical interest in the use of colchicine its extreme toxicity has limited its use in treatment of human cancer. Such use has also been hindered by the more favorably acting *Vinca* alkaloids.

Attempts have been made to study the QSAR of colchicine and its analogs in an effort to separate activity and toxicity. Beisler and Quinn (*24*) have obtained data from NCI files on 16 analogs that were sufficiently active for a QSAR study. From this set Eq. (48) was derived for activity against P-388 leukemia in the mouse.

$$\log(1/C) = (0.67 \pm 0.28) \log P - (0.19 \pm 0.07)(\log P)^2 + (1.77 \pm 0.59)I + (4.13 \pm 0.620) \quad (48)$$

$$n = 16, \quad r = 0.927, \quad s = 0.499$$

Here C is the molar concentration required to give a 40% increase in life span. The indicator variable was necessary to distinguish the activity enhancing effect of R = $COCH_3$ substitution. From this relationship $\log P_0$ is estimated to be about 1.30.

On the basis of this relationship twelve compounds were designed, synthesized, and tested. Of the twelve compounds nine were active, and Eq. (49) which resulted is an indication of its very good predictability.

$$\log(1/C) = (0.58 \pm 0.28) \log P - (0.20 \pm 0.08)(\log P)^2 + (1.72 \pm 0.51)I + (4.22 \pm 0.56) \quad (49)$$

$$n = 25, \quad r = 0.883, \quad s = 0.546, \quad \log P_0 = 1.45$$

The log $P_0 = 1.45$ estimated agrees well with that obtained by Eq. (48).

Toxicity studies on this same series of compounds led to Eq. (50) in which C is the molar LD_{50}.

$$\log(1/C) = (0.40 \pm 0.29) \log P - (0.14 \pm 0.08)(\log P)^2 + (1.24 \pm 0.52)I + (3.65 \pm 0.57) \quad (50)$$

$$n = 26, \quad r = 0.790, \quad s = 0.564$$

Unfortunately, this relationship suggests a strong intercorrelation between activity and toxicity. Because the analogs studied here were all 7- and 10-substituted derivatives of structure **XXXI**, it was decided to abandon variation in these two positions in search of more active agents. Variation in position 4 has been undertaken and at the time of this writing promising results are indicated for substitution here.

3. Radiosensitizing Agents

Attempts to develop agents that can selectively sensitize cancer cells to the effects of ionizing radiation represent a novel approach to cancer therapy (*1*,*6*). This approach to cancer treatment is not chemotherapy but instead an indirect use of drugs to obtain a selective cytotoxic effect by ionizing radiation.

As a general model for studying the radiosensitizing effects of such compounds, hypoxic (oxygen deficient) bacterial cells in culture are used. In the testing of potential radiosensitizing agents, hypoxic cells are treated with a given concentration of the test compound for a given time period, usually 2 h (*1*), then a dose of ionizing radiation is given. The enhancing effect (increased lethality) of the radiation is determined as the ratio of the slopes of the accumulated dose versus the surviving fraction of cells from the treated and control groups. This enhancement ratio (CER_1) is usually reported as $C_{1.4}$ or $C_{1.6}$.

Compounds that have been shown to be radiosensitizing are generally nitro aromatics and nitro heterocyclics. In a study of the QSAR for such compounds Adams *et al.* (*1*) derived Eq. (51), where C is in mol/dm^3, giving a 1.4 enhancement of cell (Chinese hamster) kill by ionizing radiation and E/V is the one-electron reduction potential of the test compounds.

$$\log(1/C) = (7.01 \pm 0.64)E/V + (6.48 \pm 0.26) \quad (51)$$

$$n = 42, \quad r = 0.860, \quad s = 0.280$$

This dependence on reduction potential is not unexpected. The fact that activity was not dependent on the 1-octanol–water log P is unexpected since one might expect selective transport or uptake to be important. Log P varied within the series of 42 compounds from -1.30 to 2.38 and there was almost a 10,000-fold range in the activities, so if this were the case it would have been detected.

In a similar study limited to the effects of nitroimidazoles (**XXXII** and **XXXIII**) on hypoxic bacterial cells, Anderson and Patel (*6*) derived Eq. (52).

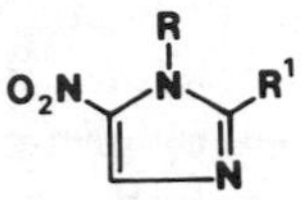

XXXII

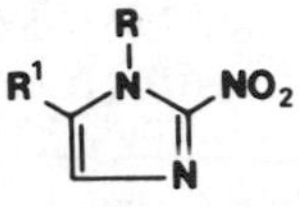

XXXIII

$$\log(1/C) = (9.32 \pm 1.06)E/V + (0.25 \pm 0.05) \log P + (6.71 \pm 0.41) \tag{52}$$

$$n = 9, \quad r = 0.970, \quad s = 0.160$$

Here C is the molar concentration giving an enhancement of cell (*Escherichia coli*) kill of 1.7. Likewise against *Streptococcus lactis* the same radiosensitizing effects of the set of heterocycles were related to physicochemical properties by Eq. (53). Higher order terms in log P were not statistically significant.

$$\log(1/C) = (9.53 \pm 2.47)E/V + (1.49 \pm 0.12) \log P + (6.74 \pm 0.97) \tag{53}$$

$$n = 9, \quad r = 0.910, \quad s = 0.360$$

It is obvious that for this set of heterocycles transport apears to be significant. These authors do state that in preliminary experiments sensitizing efficiency can be obtained from compounds having high lipophilicity.

III. CONCLUSION

One of the most significant applications of QSAR in antitumor drug design has come from the work of Cain and co-workers (*10–21,30–32,41*). Cain (*10*) was one of the first to realize the importance of systematic variation in structure within a series of compounds in an effort to optimize activity. This systematic approach has been outlined (*10*), and it is suggested that log P_0 be obtained from an homologous series of a lead early on in the optimization process. Once this log P_0 (which is presumed to reflect optimum transport properties) has been obtained, it can then be considered in the problem of optimizing activity with respect to other physicochemical parameters (*68*).

Using this approach the compound *m*-AMSA (**XXIV**: R = 1′-$NHSO_2CH_3$, 3′-OCH_3) was designed, which has now proceeded to the final stages in the Linear Array (Fig. 1).

This same effect of structural variation on lipophilicity (and transport) has been stressed by Hansch (*67*) who has shown that log P_0 can be expected to be quite different for different tumor types. For example, his work shows that a log P_0 of about 0 is found for *N*-nitrosoureas against ascitic tumors (*69*) such as L1210, whereas solid tumors such as Walker 256 respond to more lipophilic drugs with a log P_0 of about 2 (*70*). Numerous cases of this phenomenon, which is not generally obvious if QSAR methods are not applied to the data, have been reported.

Another approach to lead optimization, which is somewhat more straight forward then the method used by Cain, is the use of cluster analysis (*54*). This method is most efficient if the lead compound is to be altered by introduction of standard substituents such as Cl, NO_2, F, and CH_3 into a lead. As has been shown in this writer's laboratory (*33*), this method can lead to optimum activity within a series in a very efficient manner. Using this approach a series of 14 analogs of the triazene **XV** were synthesized and tested against S-180 in the mouse with the result that 13 were active. Two of the compounds designed from the clusters advanced to Stage IIB in the Linear Array. As much information was obtained from this study of 14 compounds as was obtained from a study of a set of 64 similar triazenes (*62,65*).

The use of QSAR methods in the design of mitomycin analogs (**X**) produced one that led to a clinically useful drug (*23*). Another result of the use of QSAR was the design study of colchicine (**XXXI**: R = $COCH_3$, R^1 = OCH_3) analogs in which it was concluded that variation in the 7 and 10 positions should be abandoned and variation in the 4 position undertaken (*24,25*). Although this may have been eventually concluded without QSAR, the conclusion was reached after synthesis of only a small number of colchicine analogs and was the direct result of structure–activity and structure–toxicity studies of the same compounds.

It is encouraging that QSAR methods are being applied to other aspects of cancer therapy such as the search for effective enhancers of radiation therapy (*1,6*). At present this is a little explored area of cancer therapy and only a small number of such reports have appeared. Further work applying QSAR to the design of more effective radiation enhancing agents may prove profitable.

REFERENCES

1. G. E. Adams, E. D. Clarke, I. R. Flockhart, R. S. Jacobs, D. S. Sehmi, I. J. Stratford, P. Wardman, M. E. Watts, J. Parrick, R. G. Wallace, and C. E. Smithen, *Int. J. Radiat. Biol.* **35,** 133 (1979).
2. K. C. Agrawal, E. C. Moore, M. S. Zedeck, and A. C. Sartorelli, *Biochemistry* **9,** 4492 (1970).
3. B. N. Ames, J. McCann, and I. Yamasaki, *Mutat. Res.* **31,** 347 (1976).
4. J. Amirmoazzami, E. M. Hodnett, and G. Prakash, *J. Med. Chem.* **21,** 11 (1978).
5. Y. U. Amrein, B. H. Venger, C. Hansch, and G. J. Hathaway, *J. Med Chem.* **22,** 473 (1979).
6. R. F. Anderson and K. B. Patel, *Br. J. Cancer* **39,** 705 (1979).
7. A. W. Andrews, A. Leo, A. Panthananickal, C. Hansch, J. Theiss, and M. Shimkin, *J. Med. Chem.* **24,** 859 (1981).
8. M. Arakawa, M. Yoshimoto, H. Miyazawa, K. Shinkai, and H. Nakao, *J. Med. Chem.* **22,** 491 (1979).
9. M. C. Archer, K. K. Park, and J. S. Wishnok, *Chem.-Biol. Interact.* **29,** 139 (1980).
10. G. J. Atwell, W. A. Denny, B. F. Cain, C. Hansch, A. Panthananickal, and A. Leo, *J. Med. Chem.* **25,** 276 (1982).
11. G. J. Atwell, B. F. Cain, and W. A. Denny, *J. Med. Chem.* **18,** 1110 (1975).
12. G. J. Atwell, B. F. Cain, and W. A. Denny, *J. Med. Chem.* **19,** 772 (1976).
13. G. J. Atwell and B. F. Cain, *J. Med. Chem.* **19,** 1124 (1976).
14. G. J. Atwell and B. F. Cain, *J. Med. Chem.* **19,** 1409 (1976).
15. G. J. Atwell, B. F. Cain, and W. A. Denny, *J. Med. Chem.* **20,** 987 (1977).
16. G. J. Atwell, B. F. Cain, and W. A. Denny, *J. Med. Chem.* **20,** 1128 (1977).
17. G. J. Atwell, B. F. Cain, and W. A. Denny, *J. Med. Chem.* **20,** 1242 (1977).
18. G. J. Atwell, B. F. Cain, and W. A. Denny, *J. Med. Chem.* **21,** (1978).
19. G. J. Atwell, B. C. Baguley, B. F. Cain, and W. A. Denny, *J. Med. Chem.* **22,** 134 (1979).
20. B. C. Baguley, B. F. Cain, and W. R. Wilson, *Mol. Pharmacol.* **12,** 1027 (1976).
21. B. C. Baguley, B. F. Cain, and W. A. Denny, *J. Med. Chem.* **21,** 658 (1978).
22. B. R. Baker, "Design of Active-Site-Directed Irreversible Enzyme Inhibitors." Wiley, New York, 1967.
23. J. Ban, D. Maysinger, M. Medic-Saric, M. Movrin, and E. J. Lien, *Eur. J. Med. Chem.—Chim. Ther.* **13,** 515 (1978).
24. J. A. Beisler and F. R. Quinn, *J. Med. Chem.* **24,** 251 (1981).
25. J. A. Beisler, Z. Neiman, and F. R. Quinn, *J. Med. Chem.* **24,** 636 (1981).
26. V. V. Belogorodskii, B. A. Ivin, V. A. Filov, B. O. Kraiz, L. L. Malyugina, R. I. Pol'kina, and Y. N. Kozlovskii, (1978) *Khim. Farm. Zh.* **12,** 67 (1978); Engl. transl. p., 481. Plenum, New York, 1979.
27. C. F. Bender and B. R. Kowalski, *J. Am. Chem. Soc.* **96,** 916 (1974).
28. T. Blair and G. A. Webb, *Eur. J. Med. Chem.—Chim. Ther.* **16,** 157 (1981).
29. B. J. Bowden, G. P. Wheeler, J. A. Grimsley, and H. H. Lloyd, *Cancer Res.* **34,** 194 (1974).
30. B. F. Cain and W. A. Denny, *J. Med. Chem.* **20,** 515 (1977).
31. B. F. Cain, *Cancer Chemother. Rep. Part 1* **59,** 679 (1975).
32. B. F. Cain and W. A. Denny, *J. Med. Chem.* **21,** 430 (1978).
33. S. S. Callejas, W. J. Dunn, III, and M. J. Greenberg, *J. Med. Chem.* **19,** 1299 (1976).
34. K. C. Chu, R. J. Feldman, M. B. Shapiro, G. F. Hazard, and R. I. Geran, *J. Med. Chem.* **18,** 539 (1975).

35. E. A. Coats, S. R. Milstein, G. Holbein, J. McDonald, R. Reed, and H. G. Petering, *J. Med. Chem.* **19,** 131 (1976).
36. E. A. Coats and K. J. Shah, *J. Med. Chem.* **20,** 1001 (1977).
37. E. A. Coats, S. R. Milstein, M. A. Pleiss, and J. A. Roesener, *J. Med. Chem.* **21,** 804 (1978).
38. M. Cory, G. L. Tong, W. W. Lee, D. W. Henry, and G. Zbinden, *J. Med. Chem.* **21,** 731 (1978).
39. R. D. Cramer, III, G. Redl, and C. E. Berkhoff, *in* "Quantitative Drug Design," Chemical Society Reviews, p. 273. Chem. Soc., London, 1974.
40. W. Damesher, L. S. Goodman, M. M. Wintrable, M. J. Goodman, A. Gilman, and N. McLennan, *J. Am. Med. Assoc.* **132,** 126 (1946).
41. W. A. Denny and L. R. Ferguson, *J. Med. Chem.* **22,** 251 (1979).
42. V. T. DeVita and L. M. Kershner, *Am. Pharm.* **NS20**(4), 16 (1980).
43. S. Dietrich, C. Hansch, and R. N. Smith, *in* "Chemistry and Biology of Pteridines" (R. L. Kisliuk and G. M. Brown, eds.), Vol. 4, p. 425. Elsevier/North-Holland, New York, 1979.
44. S. Dietrich, C. Hansch, and J. Y. Fukanaga, *J. Med. Chem.* **24,** 544 (1981).
45. G. A. Digenis and C. H. Issidorides, *Bioorg. Chem.* **8,** 97 (1979).
46. D. W. Donigian, R. J. Owellen, C. A. Hartke, and F. O. Hains, *Biochem. Pharmacol.* **26,** 1213 (1977).
47. W. J. Dunn, III and M. J. Greenberg, *J. Pharm. Sci.* **66,** 1416 (1977).
48. W. J. Dunn, III and E. M. Hodnett, *Eur. J. Med. Chem.—Chim. Ther.* **12,** 113 (1977).
49. W. J. Dunn, III and S. Wold, *J. Med. Chem.* **23,** 595 (1980).
50. M. A. Eakin, S. M. Kupchan, and A. M. Thoma, *J. Med. Chem.* **14,** 1147 (1971).
51. R. Engle, C. Hansch, R. N. Smith, and H. B. Wood, *Cancer Chemother. Rep., Part 1* **56,** 443 (1972).
52. M. Eto, Y. Shuto, E. Taniguchi, and K. Maekawa, *Agric. Biol. Chem.* **43,** 861 (1979).
53. S. I. Fink, C. Hansch, A. Leo, M. Jamakawa, and F. Quinn, *Farmaco, Ed. Sci.* **35,** 965 (1980).
54. A. B. Forsythe, C. Hansch, and S. Unger, *J. Med. Chem.* **16,** 1227 (1973).
55. P. Fox, J. M. Heal, and P. S. Schein, *Biochem. Pharmacol.* **28,** 1301 (1979).
56. S. M. Free and J. W. Wilson, *J. Med. Chem.* **7,** 395 (1964).
57. J. Y. Fukunaga, C. Hansch, and E. E. Steller, *J. Med. Chem.* **19,** 605 (1976).
58. R. I. Geran, L. Hodes, G. F. Hazard, and S. Richman, *J. Med. Chem.* **20,** 469 (1976).
59. A. Gescher, J. A. Hickman, R. J. Simmonds, M. F. G. Stevens, and K. Vaughn, *Tetrahedron Lett.* p. 5041 (1978).
60. T. Giraldi, G. Sava, L. Lassiani, and C. Misis, *Cancer Treat. Rep.* **63,** 93 (1979).
61. A. Goldin and M. K. Wolpert-Defilippes, *Bull. Cancer* **66,** 61 (1979).
62. N. Greenberg, C. Hansch, G. J. Hathaway, and F. R. Quinn, *J. Med. Chem.* **21,** 574 (1978).
63. C. Hansch, *Acc. Chem. Res.* **2,** 232 (1969).
64. C. Hansch, A. Panthanaickal, A. Leo, and F. Quinn, *J. Med. Chem.* **21,** 16 (1978).
65. C. Hansch, G. J. Hathaway, K. H. Kim, S. R. Milstein, C. R. Schmidt, N. R. Smith, and F. R. Quinn, *J. Med. Chem.* **21,** 563 (1978).
66. C. Hansch, A. Leo, and A. Panthananickal, *J. Med. Chem.* **22,** 1267 (1979).
67. C. Hansch, *Farmaco, Ed. Sci.* **34,** 89 (1979).
68. C. Hansch, *Farmaco, Ed. Sci.* **34,** 729 (1979).
69. C. Hansch, B. H. Venger, and A. Panthananickal, *J. Med. Chem.* **23,** 459 (1980).
70. C. Hansch, J. A. Montgomery, and J. G. Mayo, *J. Med. Chem.* **17,** 477 (1974).

71. C. Hansch, A. Leo, C. Schmidt, P. Y. C. Jow, and J. A. Montgomery, *J. Med. Chem.* **23,** 1095 (1980).
72. H. B. Hewitt, *Adv. Cancer Res.* **27,** 149 (1978).
73. J. A. Hickman, *Biochemie* **6,** 997 (1978).
74. L. Hodes, *in* "Computer Assisted Drug Design" (R. Christoffersen and E. C. Olson, eds.), ACS Symposium Series, No. 112, p. 582. Am. Chem. Soc., Washington, D.C., 1979.
75. A. H. Kahn and W. C. J. Ross, *Chem.-Biol. Interact.* **1,** 27 (1969–1970).
76. D. Kessel, *Biochem. Pharmacol.* **28,** 3028 (1979).
77. L. B. Kier and L. Hall, "Molecular Connectivity in Chemistry and Drug Research." Academic Press, New York, 1976.
78. K. Komatsu and I. Moriguchi, *Chem. Pharm. Bull.* **25,** 2800 (1977).
79. E. J. Lien and G. L. Tong, *Cancer Chemother. Rep., Part 1* **57,** 251 (1973).
80. E. J. Lien, K. Mayer, P. H. Wang, and G. L. Tong, *Acta Pharm. Jugosl.* **29,** 181 (1979).
81. Y. C. Martin, "Quantitative Drug Design. A Critical Introduction." Dekker, New York, 1978.
82. J. A. Montgomery, *Cancer Treat. Rep.* **60,** 651 (1978).
83. S. Ram and A. K. Saxena, *Prog. Drug Res.* **23,** 199 (1979).
84. W. C. J. Ross, "Biological Alkylating Agents." Butterworth, London, 1962.
85. R. D. Snee, *Technometrics* **19,** 415 (1977).
86. D. J. Straus, R. P. Warrell, and C. W. Young, *Cancer Treat. Rep.* **64,** 1157 (1980).
87. S. Wold, *Pattern Recognition* **8,** 127 (1976).

5

Cardiovascular Agents

STEFAN H. UNGER

QUANTITATIVE STRUCTURE–ACTIVITY
RELATIONSHIPS OF DRUGS

ISBN 0-12-695150-0

I. INTRODUCTION

A surprising amount of literature has been uncovered for this review of cardiovascular QSAR studies. However we have tried to keep tables and figures to a minimum. Appropriate references have been given and coverage of nonquantitative studies has been kept to a minimum. Equations relating only one independent to one dependent variable have not usually been given, but the statistics have been noted, and the sign of the correlation indicates the direction of the correlation.

The variety of methods of reporting statistical information is due to the idiosyncratic nature of the literature itself. The information available has been given. The convention of using D for distribution coefficients ([octanol]/[aqueous]) and P for partition ([free base, neutral or acid in octanol]/[free base, neutral or acid in aqueous]) has been observed. Finally, $pX = \log(1/X)$ has been used for expressing biological activities.

One of the major difficulties of studies on cardiovascular (CV) effects is the pharmacodynamic nature of the CV system. Aside from the usual difficulties in transferring *in vitro* data to *in vivo* systems, the CV system has a host of compensatory mechanisms for maintaining homeostasis. Although the CV area of medicinal chemistry benefits in many cases, from direct measurement of the desired therapeutic effect (as opposed to the CNS area, for example), the parameters are not always independent or straightforward. For these reasons, it is easy to criticize many of the studies reported herein. It is hoped that this review will help to motivate workers to increase their level of interest in this challenging area of drug design.

II. ANTIANGINAL AGENTS

A. β-Blockers

1. Activity and Selectivity

In 1948 Ahlquist (*1*) first proposed the classification of adrenergic receptors into two subtypes, α and β. Sensitivity of the α-receptor to catecholamines in both isolated tissues and intact animal preparations is epinephrine > norepiniphrine ≫ isoproterenol. On the other hand, the β-receptor shows isoproterenol > epinephrine ≫ norepinephrine. Further subdivision of receptors has been proposed, as shown in Scheme I. More recent technology has shown that tissues can possess combinations of β-receptor subtypes (*42*). For example, the lung has been shown to

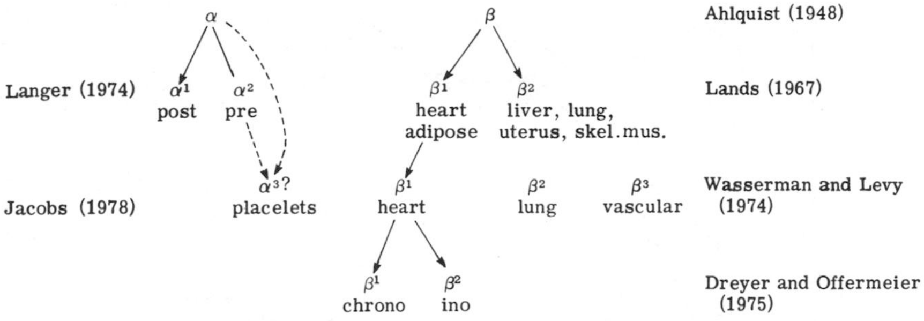

SCHEME I

have $\beta_1/\beta_2 = 0.3$ (*21*); the population of β-receptors has been related to both thyroid state and temperature (*28,129*). Minneman and Molinoff (*166*) have reviewed the latest technology and have proposed an extensive set of criteria for the *in vitro* classification of β-adrenergic subtypes.

Stimulation of the α-receptor in various tissues generally leads to excitatory responses (constriction of skin and splanchnic arterioles, intestinal and bladder sphincters, reduction of intestinal motility, and inhibition of insulin release), whereas stimulation of β-receptors generally leads to inhibitory responses, except in the heart (increase in chrono- and inotropism, dilation of arterioles of skeletal muscles, relaxation of bronchial smooth muscles, and increase in glycogenolysis and lipolysis). See Section II,A,1,a for a discussion of the biochemical mechanism of action involving cAMP.

β-Adrenergic blocking agents were developed as agents that might protect the heart from sympathetic drive (formerly "sympathetic denervation") and therefore prevent further ischemia in patients already compromised by angina pectoris (*35*). The direct result of β_1-blockade is bradycardia, reduced atrio-ventricular conduction, and reduced cardiac output. However, because β-blockers are mostly lipophilic amines, there are a number of side effects that might be due to the membrane properties of these agents (see Section II,A,2). Clinically, β-blockers have found wide use in a number of diverse indications, not all of which depend on direct β-adrenergic blockade: angina pectoris, arrhythmias, hypertension, Fallot's tetralogy, hypertrophic obstructive cardiomopathy, hyperkinetic heart syndrome, myocardial infarction, thyrotoxicosis, pheochromocytoma, Parkinsonism, migraine, tremor, anxiety states, schizophrenia, glaucoma, and narcotic or alcohol withdrawal (*71,76–78*). Numerous excellent reviews have been published (*2–5,13,32,70,83,157,163,177,180,254,266*), including one on the design of β-blocking drugs (*23*).

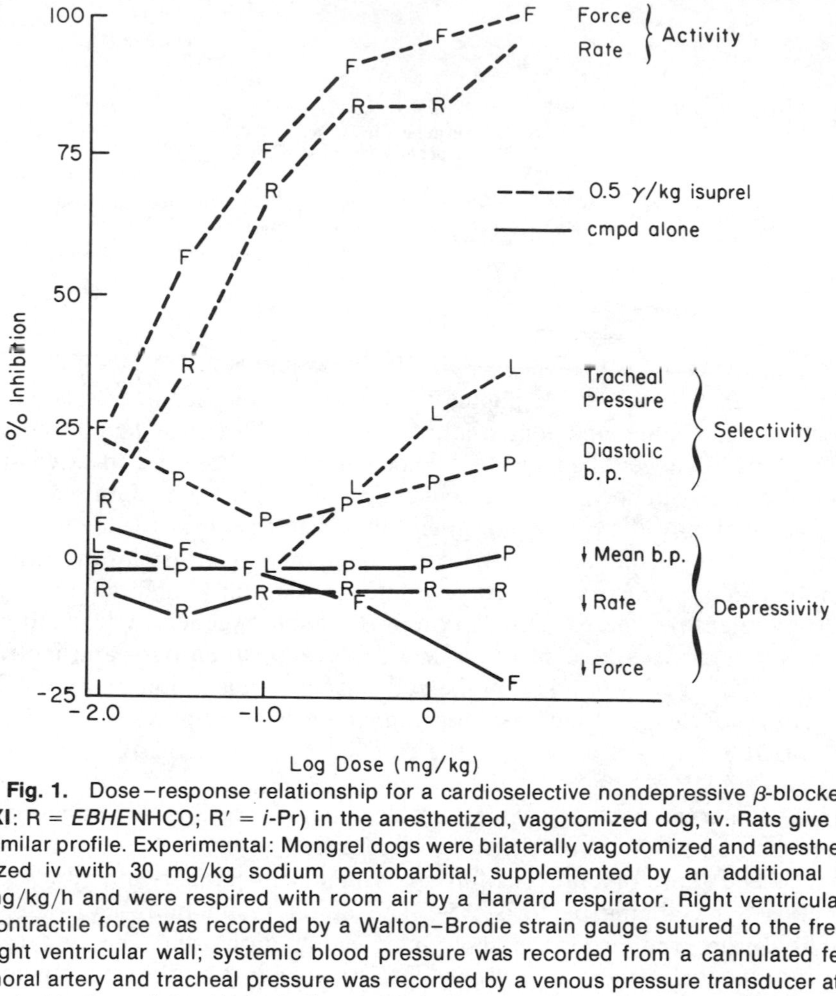

Fig. 1. Dose–response relationship for a cardioselective nondepressive β-blocker (**XI**: R = *EBHE*NHCO; R′ = *i*-Pr) in the anesthetized, vagotomized dog, iv. Rats give a similar profile. Experimental: Mongrel dogs were bilaterally vagotomized and anesthetized iv with 30 mg/kg sodium pentobarbital, supplemented by an additional 5 mg/kg/h and were respired with room air by a Harvard respirator. Right ventricular contractile force was recorded by a Walton–Brodie strain gauge sutured to the free right ventricular wall; systemic blood pressure was recorded from a cannulated femoral artery and tracheal pressure was recorded by a venous pressure transducer attached to the endotracheal tube by a cannula. Data were recorded on a Beckman Type R Dynograph or a Grass Model 7 Polygraph. Drug administration was bolus (iv) into a cannulated femoral vein. Dose levels of 0.09 μg/kg and 0.5 μg/kg of (±)-isoproterenol sulfate dihydrate were administered during the control period and at 10 and 20 min following each dose of β-blocker. A dose of histamine (0.5–2.5 μg/kg), which produced a standard 10–20 mm H_2O increase in tracheal pressure, was administered 30–40 sec following each 0.09 μm/kg dose of isoproterenol. Four to six doses of β-blocker in the range 0.01–3.16 mg/kg were administered with 45 min intervals between doses. One β-blocker was studied per dog. Dose levels were expressed in terms of base. Parameters were calculated from cumulative doses and were fit by unweighted least squares through the logit transformed responses. Molar doses were used.

Rats were anesthetized with pentobarbital, the jugular vein was cannulated for iv drug administration and the carotid artery was cannulated for blood pressure and

The design criteria for β-blockers are therefore: activity (chrono- and/or inotropism), selectivity (heart over lung, vasculature, and other tissues and also pure blocking activity over partial agonist activity, "intrinsic sympathomimetic activity" [i.s.a.]) and cardiodepressivity (membrane side effects). One of the major difficulties in the design of β-blockers is the nature of the pharmacological data. Exclusive use of *in vitro* receptor studies neglects the pharmacodynamic nature of this class of agents. However, because of the dynamic nature of the CV system, it is not clear if independence of measurement is always achieved. Blockage of chrono- and inotropic effects are significantly correlated in a series of alkylcarbamoyl-substituted thiazole β-blockers ($r = 0.898$) (*247*). Inotropism and blood pressure may be related because peak pulse pressure is related to force of contraction. A further difficulty, at least with larger experimental animals, is that of obtaining reproducible results or results on a sufficiently large number of animals because of the extensive surgery, cost, and animal-to-animal variation (e.g., sympathomimetic tone). A final difficulty is the lack of concensus as to the desired profile for these agents because agents with virtually every combination of activity, selectivity, i.s.a., and depressivity have been studied in the clinic (*254,266*). Nonetheless, propranolol is still the dominant agent of choice (*2*). The profile of a potent, cardioselective, nondepressive β-blocker designed by QSAR is shown in Fig. 1.

a. Adenylate Cyclase. Rosen *et al.* (*91,92,194*) have studied the relationship between stimulation or inhibition of frog erythrocyte adeny-

---

heart rate. The animal was placed in a body plethysmograph and ventilated with room air using a Harvard rodent respirator. Transthoracic pressure, tidal volume, and air flow were processed by a computer that provided on-line computation of dynamic compliance and airway resistance. A dose of methacholine (3–6 μg/kg, iv) was selected, which produced a standard decrease in dynamic compliance. Isoproterenol (0.5 μg/kg, iv) was given 30 sec prior to methacholine. This established control levels for heart rate and pulmonary protection. Drug was administered followed by 10 min waiting period, a challenge of isoproterenol and methacholine (30 sec apart), and a 5 min recovery. Each animal received four increasing iv doses of drug. Data reduction was similar to that in the dog experiment. Three to four rats were used per compound.

The following parameters can be defined: activity, $pED_{50} = \log(1/ED_{50})$, dose causing 50% block of isoproterenol induced chronotropic or inotropic (right ventricular) response; depressivity, $-pED_{-20} = \log ED_{-20}$, dose causing 20% drop in rate, force, or mean blood pressure; and vascular effect, $-pED_{20} = \log ED_{20}$, dose causing 20% decrease in isoproterenol induced hypotension (diastolic), or lung effect, dose causing 20% block of isoproterenol protection against histamine (dog) or methacholine (rat) increases in pulmonary overpressure (dog) or decreases in dynamic compliance (rat). All parameters are defined so that a more positive number is more desirable.

late cyclase and β-adrenergic tissue preparations by various compounds, finding qualitative SAR. Frog erythrocyte adenylate cyclase exhibits β_2-receptor responses, however.

Bilezikian *et al.* (*33*) studied binding and inhibition of over 40 β-blockers to turkey erythrocyte adenylate cyclase. This excellent collection of data has not been subjected to QSAR.

For a diverse set of 18 β-blockers related to **I**, significant correlation (r = 0.954) between *in vitro* dog heart and *in vitro* guinea pig heart adenylate cyclase has been found (*10*).

Unger (*247,248*) has described the correlation of inhibition of guinea pig

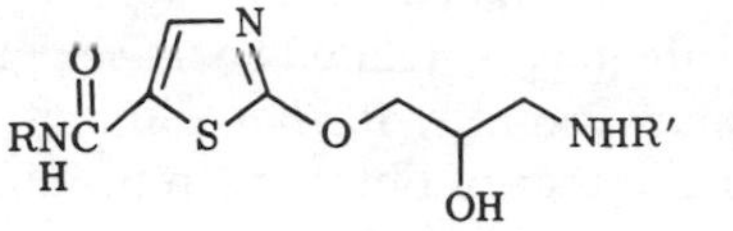

I

lung and heart adenylate cyclase by a series of compounds (**I**: R = aliphatic, including bulky and/or unsaturated; R′ = *i*Pr, *t*Bu).*

$$-pID_{50}^{\text{lung}} = -4.5 + 0.4(\text{C} @ 5) + 0.9(\text{C} @ 8) - 0.5(\text{H} @ 8) + 0.1C_{\text{min}}^{\text{face}} - 0.5D_{\text{cycle}} \quad (1)$$

$$n = 19, \quad s = 0.14, \quad r = 0.924$$

$$pID_{50}^{\text{heart}} = 4.9 + 0.4[(\text{C} \geq 6) \geq 3] + 0.2(\text{C} @ 7) - 0.1C_{\text{max}}^{\text{face}} - 0.2D_{=\equiv} - 0.5D_{i\text{-Pr}} + 0.6D_{i\text{-Pr}}D_{\text{cycle}} \quad (2)$$

$$n = 19, \quad s = 0.14, \quad r = 0.947$$

Note that lipophilicity is not important in Eqs. (1) and (2) but that detailed topographical features are. [See Unger *et al.* (*247,248*) and below for a complete discussion and explanation of variables.] Lung activity is di-

* The numbering scheme and parameter definition is illustrated for 2-Me-hexyl as follows:

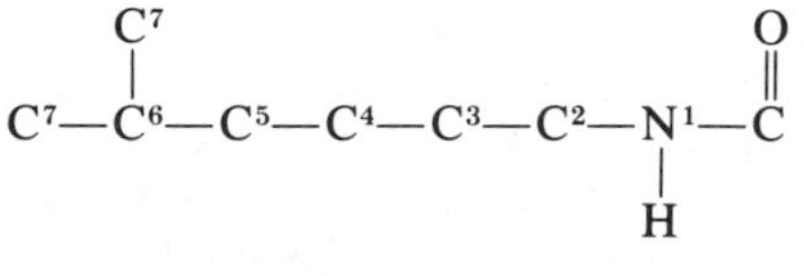

The following types of descriptors are typical of those derived:

(C @ 5) #C at fifth position (= 1)
(H @ 8) #H at eighth position (= 0)
(C @ 8) #C at eighth position (= 0)
(C @ ≥ 7) #C at seventh and higher position (= 2)
[(C ≥ 6) ≥ 3] are #C at sixth and higher positions greater than or equal to 3? (= 1, i.e., yes).

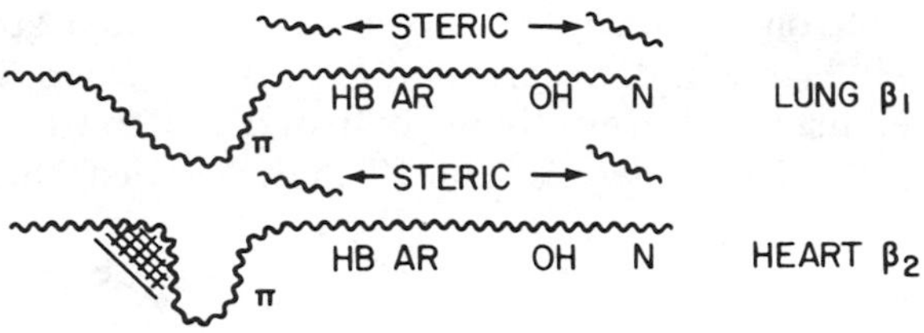

Fig. 2. Model of the lipophilic exoreceptor for β-blockers (**I**).

minished by bulk along the face of the bulk alkyl R, especially by positions 5 and 8 down the alkyl chain from the NH (**II**). Heart activity is

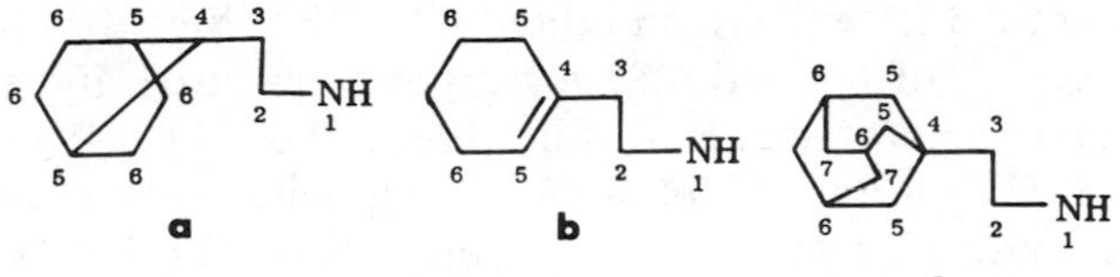

a **b** **c**

II

mainly increased by bulk at the end of the chain (position 6 and higher), but the side chain is preferably cyclic, saturated and R′ = *i*-Pr. These descriptions agree with correlations of *in vivo* data (*vide infra*) (*247,248*). β_1/β_2-selectivity for **I** can be understood from Eqs. (1) and (2) on a molecular basis as arising from slight differences in conformation of the β-adrenergic site. This is illustrated in Fig. 2.

b. Tissue Studies. For a series of compounds (**III**), (*69*) selecti-

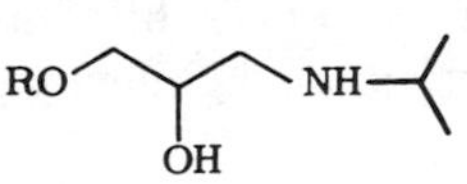

III **a.** R = 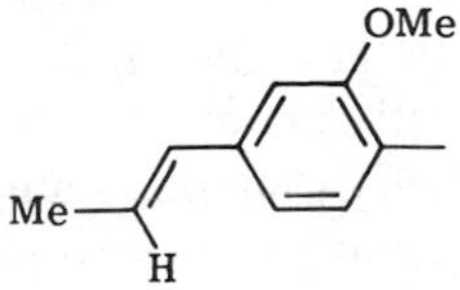

b. R = 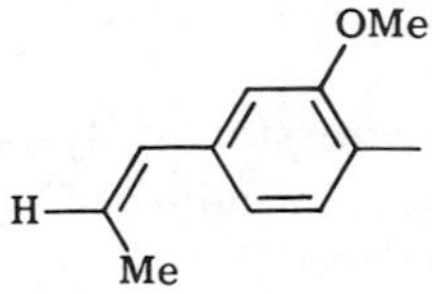

vity of heart rate on isolated rat atria over (β_2) rat fundus strip was found to depend very highly on the steric nature of the R group. For example, **IIIa** possessed high cardioselectivity compared to **IIIb** ($\beta_1/\beta_2 = 25$ compared to 0.1). Similar studies (*206*) on **IV** show identical cardiac:vascular

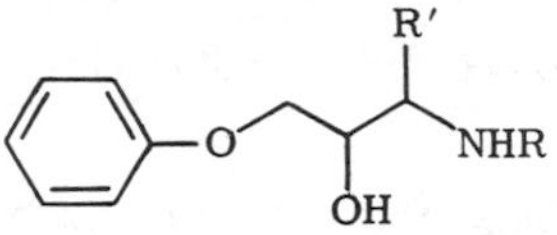

IV

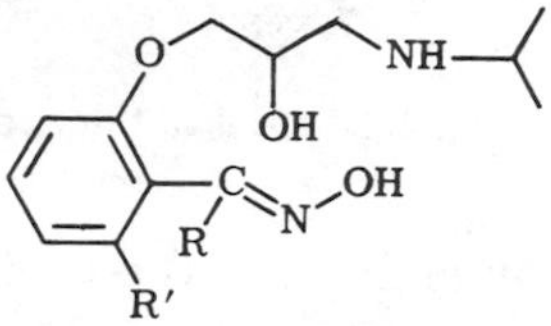

V

selectivities of 0.3 for erythro and threo (**IV**: R′ = Me; R = *i*-Pr) but differing pA_2 values of 6.3 and 6.82 for erythro on heart and vascular receptors versus 5.66 and 6.20 for threo. For **IV** (R′ = Me; R = CH_2CH_2-3,5-$(OMe)_2$-Ph), $\beta_1/\beta_2 > 40$, or a greater selectivity than that found for practolol ($\beta_1/\beta_2 = 22$). No correlation with log D (pH = 7.4, 0.02*M* PO_4) was found for the series of eight compounds.

Vascular selectivity of series **V** was reported (*25,272*) to be positively related to the steric overlap of R′ and R based on molecular models ($n = 18$, $r = 0.903$, $s = 0.226$). This result led to the ketone (**V**: R = Ph)—the oxime could not be formed—which was highly selective. Further methodological details were not published.

A parabolic curve was found to explain variations in myocardial selectivity (tachycardia versus vasodilation) as a function of lipophilicity (both calculated and $CHCl_3$–H_2O) for a series of trimepranol analogs (**VI**) (*278*).

Failure to obtain a QSAR in a series of acetophenone oxime ethers (**VII**) using π, π^2, σ, **F**, E_s, and parachor was reported (*136*). *In vitro* pA_2 values for isoproterenol stimulated guinea pig right atrial strips or trachea were used.

Zaagsma and Nauta (*276,277*) studied the QSAR of series **VIII**, where Ar is substituted benzene, naphthalene, or tetrahydronaphthalene. All compounds were ortho-substituted with respect to the alkanolamine side chains. Isoproterenol stimulated guinea pig right atrium or tracheal strips were used for potency estimation; antagonism of ouabain-induced arrhythmias and inotropic and chronotropic effects were determined on the right atrium. Local anesthetic effects were measured on isolated partially demylinated frog sciatic nerve. See Section II,A,2 for a discussion of the depressant effects.

Stepwise multiple regression analysis using log D (pH 7.4, PO_4), $pK_{a(m)}$ (mean values), π', E_s, R′ and σ_R^{ortho}. No cross correlations were found except between log D and π:

$$pA_2^{\text{atrium}} = 0.57E_s - 0.61 + 5.80 \tag{3}$$

$$n = 7, \quad r = 0.977, \quad s = 0.159$$

$$pA_2^{\text{trachea}} = 0.75E_s - 2.96\text{p}K_{a(m)} + 33.09 \tag{4}$$

$$n = 7, \quad r = 0.999, \quad s = 0.33$$

The importance of steric properties of the R′ group for both trachea and atria was noted by the authors. Addition of $\text{p}K_{a(m)}$ to Eq. (4) was significant, although its exact role was not discussed. These results can be compared with **V** if one assumes that only one alkanolamine side chain interacts with the receptor and the other is merely a complicated ortho substituent.

A series (**VIII**: R′ = H) with greater variation in the aryl moiety had earlier failed to give a QSAR for β-blocking activity but did show simple correlation with lipophilicity for antiarrhythmic and local anesthetic activities (see Section II,A,2,a) (*276*).

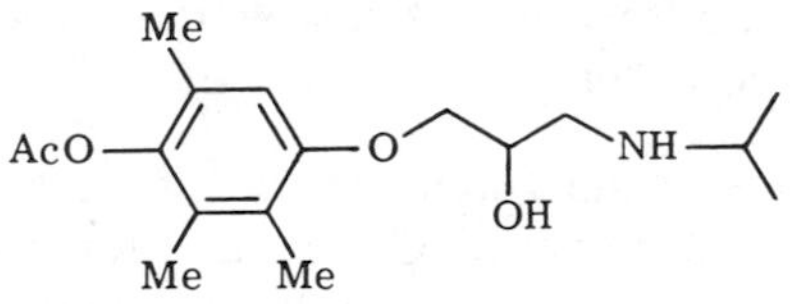

VI

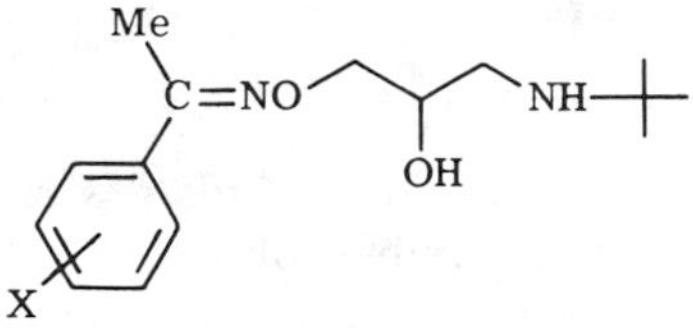

VII

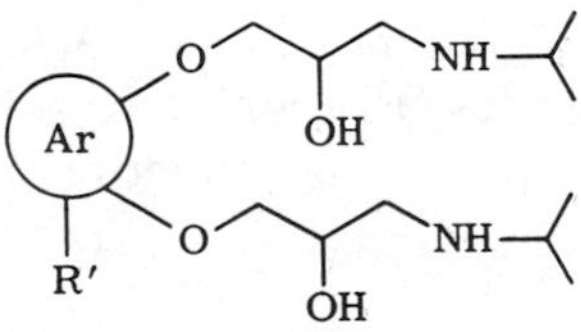

VIII

A discriminant analysis of phenylalkylamines has been reported (*132*) in which 138 compounds have been classified into four groups: antagonists (29 compounds), partial agonists with mainly blocking action (51 compounds), partial agonists with mainly stimulating action (19 compounds), and pure agonists (39 compounds). A large number (>50) of local and global electronic, lipophilic, steric, and special parameters were examined. Separation of the four classes was obtained with a model that employed 15 parameters. Reclassification, however, gave only 46% correct and 4% incorrect classification with poor discrimination between antagonists and partial agonists and with mainly blocking action contributing to the larger error. The following conclusions were drawn.

1. Prediction of blocking activity requires sufficient hydrophobicity and size of the meta or para ring substituents.
2. Effect of electronic substitution on the ring is not clear but seems not to be critical.
3. Other structure modifications are of secondary importance.
4. Electronic-withdrawing substituents on the ring and hydrophobicity and size of amine substituent influence β-mimetic activity.

There are insufficient details to comment further.

Trieff *et al.* (*243*) failed to obtain a relationship between *in vitro* rate of oxidation by *N*-bromosuccinimide (NBS) and the pA_2 values of seven β-blockers. The pA_2 values were the means of eight different tissues. A significant negative correlation was reported for the four nonselective compounds ($r = -0.987$), namely, USUV 65-24, pronethalol, propranolol, and H35-25. NBS oxidation was used because the authors felt that it was appropriate to study quantitatively a chemical reaction that all of the β-adrenergic antagonists might undergo and that might be related to the biological activity (*243*). The justification for this choice was the Belleau model, which, however, is no longer considered valid (Section V,C).

c. In Vivo Models. Clarkson (*48*) and Davies (*52,53*) have summarized a number of QSAR studies on Imperial Chemical Industries (I.C.I.) β-blockers. Qualitative discussions of QSAR results for other analogs can be found (*212,213*).

Cardiac β-adrenergic blocking potency (isoprenaline tachycardia in anesthetized cat, dose in μg/kg infused over 30 min providing 50% block) was correlated for three series (**IX**), where X = CONH (acylamino) (*51*), NHCO (amido) (*210*), or NHCONH (ureido) (*211*).

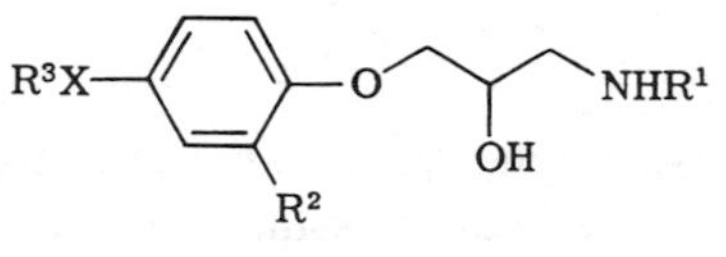

IX

Acylamino

$$\log A = 2.21 - 0.80\pi + 0.13\pi^2 - 1.16\sigma_{m_1} - 0.28\sigma_{m_2} - 0.30\delta_{R^1} + 0.30\delta_{R^3} \quad (5a)$$

$n = 150?$, $s = 0.141$, mean experimental error $= \pm 0.12$

$$\log A = 2.20 - 0.81\pi + 0.13\pi^2 - 1.17\delta_{R^1}\sigma_m - (1 - \delta_{R^1})[0.64\sigma_m + 0.22E_S] - 0.26\delta_{R^1} + 0.33\delta_{R^3} \quad (5b)$$

$n = 25,\quad s = 0.19,\quad r = 0.960,\quad$ mean experimental error $= \pm 12$

$n = 23,\quad s = 0.14,\quad r = 0.980$

Amido

$$\log A = 2.89 - 0.76\pi + 0.07\pi^2 - 0.53\sigma_m - 0.34\delta_{R^1} + 0.30\delta_{R^3} \quad (6)$$

$n = 17$ (27 experimental points), $\quad s = 0.19,\quad r = 0.947$

Ureido

$$\log A = 1.75 - 0.81\pi + 0.13\pi^2 - 1.17\delta_{R^1}\sigma_m - (1 - \delta_{R^1})[0.64\sigma_m + 0.22E_s] - 0.26\delta_{R^1} + 0.45\delta_{R^3} \quad (7a)$$

$n = 12$

In Eqs. (5) through (7a), $A = ED_{50} \times 100/MW$; σ_{m_1} and σ_{m_2} are meta electronic effects of ortho R^2; π is for the total molecule and is referred to practolol. For Eq. (5a), if R^1 = *t*-Bu, then $\sigma_{m_2} = 0$ and $\delta_{R_a} = 1$; if R^1 = *i*-Pr, then $\sigma_{m_1} = 0$ and $\delta_{R^1} = 0$; if R^3 = Me or Et, then $\delta_{R^3} = 0$; and if $R^3 \geq$ *n*-Pr, then $\delta_{R^3} = 1$. For Eqs. (5b) and (6), if R^1 = *i*-Pr or *t*-Bu, then δ_{R^3} = 0 or 1, respectively. For Eq. (7), if R^1 = Me, then δ_{R^3} = 0 or 1 otherwise. The uneven reporting of statistical parameters was in the original references (*48,52,53*). The number of points in Eq. (5a) is not clear. Equation (7) was not obtained by an independent stepwise multiple regression, but rather the terms in the brackets were copied from Eq. (5b). The curve fitting as reported is idiosyncratic and the choice of indicator variables does not appear straightforward, nor is their use or derivation clearly explained.

Nonetheless, the results of the I.C.I. QSAR modeling are shown in Fig. 3. Increased lipophilicity increases activity, according to the authors (despite the parabolic dependence on π). The ortho position is relatively sterically free and electron-withdrawing substituents in this position increase activity due to an electronic effect on the amidic NH. There is a "steric narrows" for R^3 at a distance of 4–5 atoms from the para position of the aryl (compare Fig. 2). Finally, *t*-Bu is consistently more active than *i*-Pr in this series as R^1 substituent.

A modified Free–Wilson–Hansch correlation of 56 of the I.C.I. ureido analogs (*211*) has appeared (*36*). The Free–Wilson analysis $r = 0.935$ was used to help decide which Hansch-type parameters to examine in order to explain the activity of these compounds. The final equations contained five terms, Eq. (7b), but overall correlation was low.

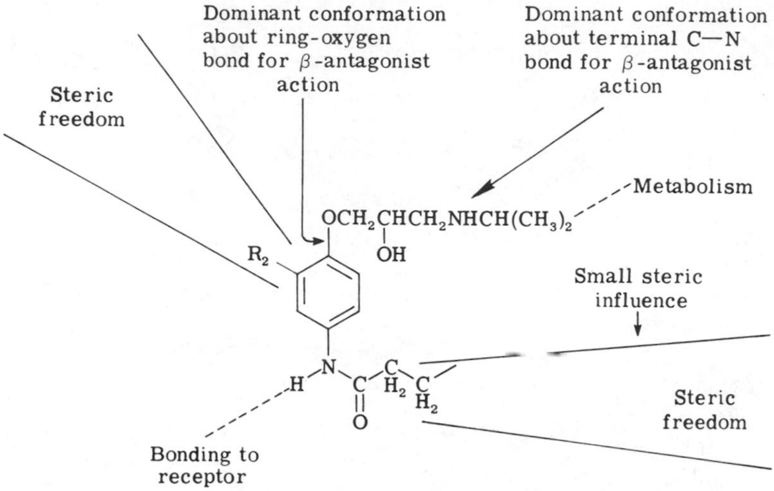

Fig. 3. I.C.I. Model for β-blockers. Reproduced by permission (*52*).

$$pC = -0.94 + 0.52I_1 + 0.81\sigma + 0.58 \sum \pi - 0.06\left(\sum \pi\right)^2 - 0.76I_2 \quad (7b)$$

$$n = 56, \qquad r = 0.838, \qquad s = 0.265$$

Omission of four outliers raised the correlation slightly; $n = 52$, $r = 0.886$, $s = 0.230$. $I_1 = 1$ if R^1 = *t*-Bu (**IX**) and $I_1 = 0$ otherwise; $I_2 = 1$ if $R^1 = CHMeCH_2OPh$ and $I_2 = 0$ otherwise.

Intrinsic sympathomimetic activity was found by the I.C.I. group for most analogs at some level. I.s.a. was measured in rat depleted of catecholamines by syrosingopine by noting the increase in heart rate when 2.5 mg/kg of compound was given iv. No QSAR were reported; however, a tentative correlation between population of specific conformers about 1,2-carbon–carbon bond and i.s.a. emerged from a preliminary molecular orbital study on a series of ortho substituted phenoxypropanolamines (*48*).

Cardiac versus pulmonary selectivity was thought to be due to differences in distribution. Intrinsic blocking activity (i.b.a.) was defined as the β-blocking activity (i.e., binding to receptor) corrected for distribution: i.b.a. = $\log A - B\pi + C\pi^2$ where B and C were taken from regressions such as Eq. (5). Plotting i.b.a. versus $\log P$, one finds a family of curves representing isopotent binding to cardiac receptors. It was noted that protection from histamine induced bronchospasm in the guinea pig (the only measure available for pulmonary effects) showed that compounds on the i.b.a.–$\log P$ plot were also grouped by efficacy in bronchospasm protection. From this long series of extrapolations and assumptions, the authors concluded that selectivity was due to distributional effects. Support was found in the data of Somerville and Coleman (I.C.I.) (*215*). (see also Jack [*115*], but his conclusions are doubtful.) Practolol is selective in tissue, but it becomes nonselective in their membrane (vesicle) fragments. It was noted that purification might have disrupted the receptor. This observation concerning lack of selectivity for practolol in vesicle fragments has not been confirmed in at least two other laboratories. Burges and Blackburn (*39*) found about tenfold selectivity in rat heart and lung. Alvarez (*9*) studied guinea pig heart and lung adenylate cyclase, finding a similar cardiac selectivity for practolol and nonselectivity for propranolol. As shown above, selectivity can be explained by subtle differences in receptor conformation (Fig. 2).

Vascular β-receptor selectivity *in vivo* was measured in the cat as the pattern of blood pressure effects over time. Diastolic pressure reversal of +30 mm Hg for acylamino compounds was shown to be related to lipophilicity, suggesting pharmacokinetic causes. Basil *et al.* (*25*) obtained similar results on series **X**.

$$\log v/c = -0.46 + 1.30\pi - 0.23\pi^2 \qquad (8)$$

$$n = 12, \quad r = 0.900, \quad s = 0.118, \quad \pi_0 = 2.82$$

where v is the vascular 1/2 blocking concentration, c is the cardiac 1/2 blocking concentration (anesthetized cats with isoproterenol challenge), and $\pi = \Sigma\ (\pi_{R^1} + \pi_{R^2})$. The individual activities were correlated with

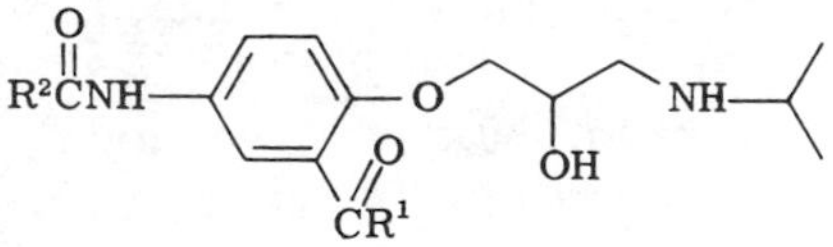

X

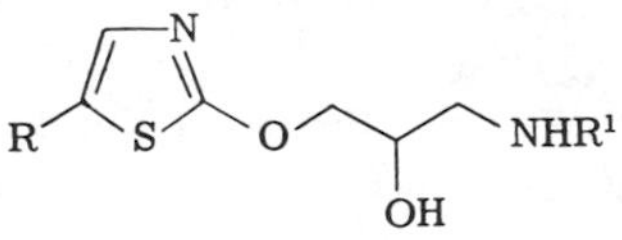

XI

steric terms at low correlation levels because of biological variation, especially for the vascular data. A larger sample of compounds would probably be needed to detect subtle steric properties; the compounds studied were not sufficiently diverse (log alkyl, *i*-Pr, *i*-Bu, CH_2Ph, and Ph). Antiarrhythmic properties (reverting dose for ouabain inducd arrhythmias) were also correlated (see Section II,A,2,a).

$$\log(MW/c) = 2.75 + 0.85\pi - 0.13\pi^2 + 0.50E_s \qquad (9)$$

$$n = 14, \quad r = 0.874, \quad s = 0.193, \quad \pi_0 = 3.19$$

$$\log(MW/v) = 2.90 + 0.70E_s \tag{10}$$

$$n = 12, \quad r = 0.637, \quad s = 0.215$$

Tazolol (**XI**: R = H, R′ = *i*-Pr) is a selective myocardial β-stimulant with mild β-blocking activity (*64,147,195,217,218*). A molecular orbital (MO) study on tazolol has appeared (*151*). Addition of an alkylcarbamoyl, alkylcarbonylamino, alkylcarbamate, or alkylureido side chain gives myocardial selective β-blockers (**XI**: R = R″NHCO, R″COHN, R″OCOHN;R′ = *t*-Bu or *i*-Pr; R″ = alkyl) (*31*).

The QSAR optimization that commenced after one analog (**XI**: R = *i*-HpNHCO; R′ = *t*-Bu) had been selected for development is described below. The result of this QSAR optimization program was the discovery of a highly novel side chain (*247,248*). One of the novel features of this work was the development (*47,219,267*) of a dog preparation that allowed the simultaneous determination of activity, selectivity (both blood pressure and pulmonary), and depressivity in a single animal. Data were also collected in rats (*267*) to confirm the dog data and to allow a more precise measurement of pulmonary function in a rat whole body plethysmograph. (See Fig. 1 for experimental details.)

One side chain with an interesting profile was the cyclohexylethylcarbamoyl moiety, which had a better profile than close analogs such as cyclohexylmethyl or cyclohexylpropylcarbamoyl (e.g., for R′ = *t*-Bu, pED_{50}^{force} = 5.46, 619, and 6.16; $-pED_{-20}^{force}$ = −5.22, −5.02, and −5.50; $-pED_{20}^{po}$ = *nd*, ≫− 5.08 and not vascular selective, as the alkyl bridge between the cyclohexyl and carbamoyl lengthened). Combining knowledge of this profile with a preliminary short-bulky-moderately lipophilic hypothesis derived from correlation of adenylate cyclase data, Eqs. (1) and (2) (see also Fig. 2) give rise to the endobicyclo[3.1.0]hexylethyl (*EBHE*) side chain. This side chain proved to be quite exceptional. Not only was the *EBHE*carbamoyl compound extremely active in the dog

TABLE I
Comparisons of Analogs of **XI** in Dog Model with Standards, Relative to Propranolol[a]

Analog	pED_{50}^{force}	$-pED_{50}^{force}$	$-pED_{20}^{po}$
XI: R = iHpNHCO; R′ = *t*-Bu	0.5	0.5	255
XI: R = EBHENHCO; R′ = *i*-Pr	2.3	≃3	362
Propranolol	(1.0)	(1.0)	(1.0)
Practolol	0.2	>4	173
Acebutolol	0.3	2	179

[a] Parameters are defined in Fig. 1.

model (pED_{50}^{force} = 7.01, $-pED_{20}^{force}$ = −5.02, and $-pED_{20}^{po}$ = −5.35), but it was equiactive in the rat model whereas all other analogs were totally uncorrelated between the two species. It also possessed a very high pA_2 = 8.32 (*47*). This observation suggested that the *EBHE* interacted strongly with an exoreceptor near the β_1-receptor and that this feature was common to both dog and rat heart. The improved selectivity of *EB HE*NHCO is clear from the rat model, and there was no lung effect showing at the highest dose tested (10 mg/kg). Rate and vascular effects were likewise satisfactory in the rat. The compounds (**XI**: R = *EB HE*NHCO, R′ = *i*-Pr) compare very well with standards (Table I). The hypothesis seemed proved, but this compound was actually more active than anticipated.

Up to the time this analog was produced, *in vivo* QSAR were limited to simple plots of activity versus log k', and two very preliminary QSAR models for activity and selectivity were used. Because of the enormous difference between the cyclohexylethyl and bicyclohexylethyl side chain, it was apparent that subtle steric effects were responsible for differences in biological profile, in confirmation of Eqs. (1) and (2). At the time, Verloop's (*260*) steric parameters were not available and other common steric parameters such as E_s and *MR* were of little use (*251*). The concept of Newman's six number (*251*) was then considered as a topological parameter. The atoms in the alkyl chain were numbered, as shown in **II**. Various descriptors could then be developed, such as what is the number of carbons at the 8 position (C @ 8) and is the number of carbons at the 6 and higher positions equal to 3 [(C ≥ 6) = 3]? Further progress could not be made in QSAR until it was assumed that the *EBHE* group was nearly ideal. All other alkyl side chains were then parameterized according to their similarity to it. To do this without sophisticated computer graphics and conformational energy calculations, now more readily available, Dreiding models of all 40 side chains were constructed and put into allowed conformations that would also fit into the putative cleft defined by the *EBHE* group. An objective protocol was followed and no parameters were changed once they had been determined. Fig. 4 shows how these parameters were defined. The number of carbons on the face of the cleft (C-5 to C-6 to C-7 area) that could either maximally or minimally contact the cleft were determined. Some side chains (e.g., those with alkynyl groups) would only fit into the cleft in a down conformation *D*↓ . Certain side chains, especially those of highly active analogs, all appeared to have a point of unsaturation in the 4 position (D¨ @ 4) (for *EBHE* this was the cyclopropyl moiety and for others it was a double or triple bond). We also included fractional lipophilicity *f* values (*139*). Using this extended set of parameters, highly precise QSAR that provided intuitive satisfaction

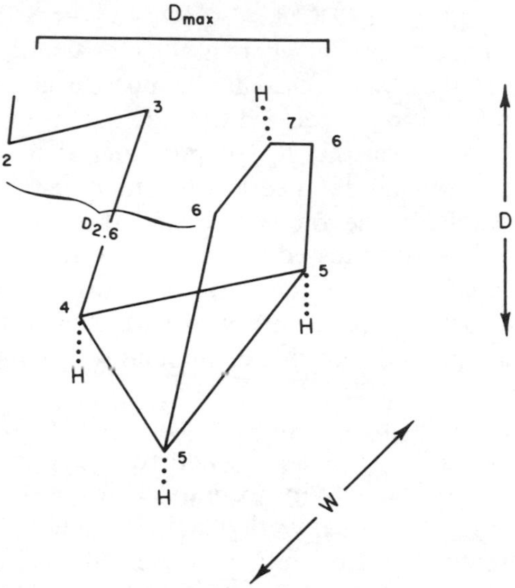

Fig. 4. EBHE Group showing numbering scheme and dimension parameters.

could be derived, shown in Eqs. (11) through (14). For the dog (iv) model we obtained:

$$\mathrm{p}ED_{50}^{\mathrm{force}} = 5.8 + 0.4\,(D^{\cdot\cdot}\ @\ 4) - 0.4\mathrm{D}\downarrow + 0.3\left(\sum f_{\geq 5}\right)$$

$$+0.2[(\mathrm{C} \geq 6) = 3] - 0.1\,(\mathrm{H}\ @\ 4) - 0.1(f_{8,9}) - 0.4DW \quad (11)$$

$$n = 40, \quad s = 0.12, \quad r = 0.918$$

$$-\mathrm{p}ED_{20}^{\mathrm{po}} = -5.0 + 1.1\,(\mathrm{C}\ @\ 8) + 0.2\,(\mathrm{H}\ @\ 5)$$
$$-0.8 \log k' - 0.3[(\mathrm{H}\ @\ 4) = 1] \quad (12)$$

$$n = 14, \quad s = 0.14, \quad r = 0.908$$

The rat (iv) model data is correlated by:

$$\mathrm{p}ED_{50}^{\mathrm{rate}} = 3.3 + 0.7\,(C_{\mathrm{max}}^{\mathrm{face}}) + 0.5D_{==} \quad (13)$$

$$n = 11, \quad s = 0.31, \quad r = 0.927$$

$$-\mathrm{p}ED_{20}^{\mathrm{c}} = -5.4 + 0.7f_5 + 1.1\,(D^{\cdot\cdot}\ @\ 4) \quad (14)$$

$$n = 8, \quad s = 0.08, \quad r = 0.987$$

Equations (11) and (13) for activity are interpreted as having positive contributions from unsaturation at the 4 position and lipophilicity at the 5 to 7 positions. Negative effects are due to down conformation, too many hydrogens at the 4 position (i.e., not unsaturated) or a large cross-sectional area. QSAR for activity in the rat confirms the importance of lipophilic interactions on the face and unsaturation in the chain.

Equations (12) and (14) show that lack of effect in the lung is correlated with relatively less lipophilic substituents containing bulk at the 5 and 8 positions. QSAR for the rat confirms the importance of bulk at the 5 position and unsaturation at the 4 position.

These QSAR results substantially confirm the receptor model described above [Eqs. (1) and (2) and Fig. 2] with the possible modification that the base or far wall of the β_2-cleft should be filled in slightly in order to account for the importance of substitution at the 5 position in diminishing lung activity. The π binding site refers to the importance of unsaturation at the 4 position and may be a site of dispersion or metal binding.

The tailoring of steric effects can be seen in a comparison of the isolipophilic endo- and exobicyclo[3.1.0]hexylethyl moieties. In dog there is a 7.6-fold difference in activity, whereas depressivity differs by an insignificant 1.3-fold, as might be expected. In adenylate cyclase, endo is 2.1-fold more active in heart, but exo is 5-fold less active in lung. A compact group interacts with heart, whereas an extended group interferes with lung binding. Again, this involves substitution at the 5 position; the cyclopropyl is also out of position for the putative π-dispersion binding. In rat, endo is twice as active as exo.

Finally, the *EBHE* can be transferred to some other aromatic nuclei or other polar bridge groups while maintaining or improving the profile (*247*). For example, the α-CH_2 can be replaced by NH, forming a ureido moiety, and the thiazole can be replaced by phenyl. The resulting compound shows $pED_{50}^{force} = 7.11$, $-pED_{50}^{force} > -5.0$, and $-pED_{20}^{po} = -6.06$. Subtle geometric changes due to differences in size and bond lengths may be responsible for some of the differences in profile. However, the high activity shows the uniqueness of this side chain.

Compound **XI** (R = *EBHE*NHCO; R′ = *i*-Pr) has undergone clinical evaluation and has been found to be active, selective, and nondepressive at 200 mg/day in human, but it possesses i.s.a (RS-51288) (*47*).

d. Other Properties. The affinity constants K_s of eight β-blockers for microsomal cytochrome *P*-450 causing type I spectral shifts were correlated (*153*) ($r = 0.98$) with octanol–water distribution coefficients at pH = 7.4, whereas the extent of binding (%*P*-450 binding with β-blocker) was not correlated ($r = 0.07$). For example, the hydrophilic oxprenolol (log $D = 0.10$) and methypranol (log $D = 0.45$) bind to a greater extent (25% and 26.8%, respectively) than the more lipophilic propranolol (19%) with log $D = 0.93$.

Absorption, distribution, metabolism, and excretion of β-blockers are correlated with lipophilicity (*2,157,266*).

e. Physical Properties: Lipophilicity. Vermeij (*261*) has studied the role of lipophilicity on the distribution properties of β-blockers. Tissue storage of propranolol (a lipophilic drug) is 15 times higher in brain than plasma, while it is only 3 times higher for metoprolol (a moderately lipophilic drug) and is equal in concentration for practolol (a hydrophilic drug). Uptake of β-blockers by red cells and plasma binding were also determined by lipophilicity (*11*). The concentration of chloride was found to influence D of propranolol, due presumably to ion pairing (*154,252,275*); however, compare Kulkarni *et al.* (*127*). Vermeij reports $P = 970$ (log $P = 2.99$) for propranolol, assuming only un-ionized drug can be partitioned between both phases (*261*). Our direct shake–flask measurements show log $P = 3.44$ with $pK_a = 0.34$ (*247*), in agreement with other direct literature determinations of log $P = 3.09$–3.56 with $pK_a = 9.32$–9.60 (*179*). The assumption that only un-ionized drugs partition is not correct (*252*).

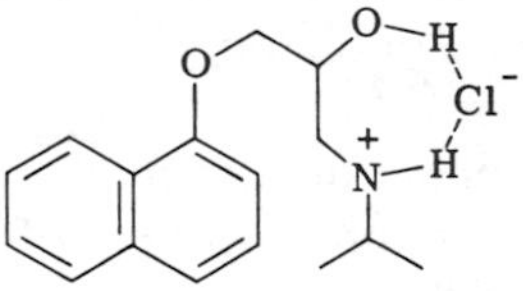

XII

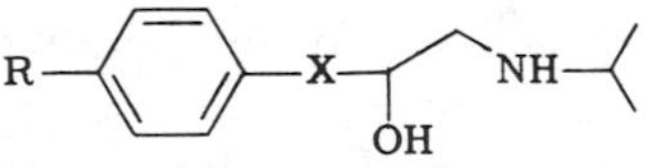

XIII

	R	X
a.	CH_2CH_2OMe	OCH_2
b.	$NHSO_2Me$	–
c.	$CH_2C(=O)NH_2$	OCH_2

Van Zwieten and Timmermans (*229,255*) found a correlation between degree of penetration into cerebrospinal fluid and log D for metoprolol (**XIIIa**) (log $D = 0.35$), sotalol (**XIIIb**) (log $D = -1.553$), and atenolol (**XIIIc**) (log $D = -1.921$) but no correlation with degree of penetration and acute hypotensive effects. These compounds probably do not act as hypotensive agents at central β-adrenergic receptors. For example, (+)-isomers are active hypotensive agents when centrally administered in some animal models; these are devoid of direct adrenergic effects and antihypertensive activity in humans. Most β-blockers, hydrophilic or lipophilic, show effective hypotensive effects *in vivo*.

f. Conclusions. QSAR studies on β-blockers are one of the most fruitful areas of research, although there has been no attempt to derive a unifying picture of the β-receptor. This perhaps may come out of the work at I.C.I. and Syntex, but would require a larger number of more diverse structures to be run in a single pharmacological model.

2. Depressivity and Nonspecific Effects

a. Cardiodepressant and Antiarrhythmic Effects. A study by Levy (*141*) was one of the first to try to link the negative inotropic (cardiodepressant) effect of β-blockers to their nonspecific membrane effects and thus to physicochemical properties. No simple quantitative correlation between lipophilicity ($CHCl_3$–H_2O) and/or pK_a was found by Levy to explain either specific β-blocking activity or nonspecific depression of myocardial contraction on isolated rabbit atria. However, the more lipophilic propranolol and pronethalol were stronger local anesthetics (rabbit cornea) than the hydrophilic sotalol or INPEA: (+)-propranolol (a very weak β-blocker) was equipotent with its racemate as a local anesthetic. There was no general correlation between β-blocking activity and nonspecific effects (*258*). Local anesthetic activity is frequently used to assess cardiodepressant activity (*266*) (see Section IV), so the discrepancy is not clear. Levy also reported (*140*) a correlation between surface tension effects of β-blockers and their negative inotropism. This study was extended by Attwood and Agarwal (*14*).

Levy's work has been criticized on two accounts. Hellenbrecht *et al.* (*103*) have found a good correlation between negative inotropism with a more accurate set of octanol–H_2O partition coefficients (*vide infra*) and Fitzgerald (*71*) has questioned the supposed link between negative inotropism and nonspecific membrane activity from a clinical standpoint. For example, quoting Sowton's results (*29*) on a study of eight patients given 20–25 mg of (+)-propranolol within two days of a myocardial infarction, Fitzgerald notes that no significant changes were observed in heart rate, tension time, or cardiac output. In anesthetized dogs a study by Barrett (*22,24*) showed that (±)-propranolol was more cardiodepressant of rate, contractile force, ejection rate, and tension time index than the (+)-isomer, which gave insignificant effects. The conclusion was that the cardiodepressant effects of propranolol were due to its β-blocking effects and not to its membrane stabilizing activity (MSA). Similarly, Graca and van Zweiten (*85*) found that β-blockers had no effect on guinea pig atrial transmembrane $^{45}Ca^{2+}$ flux, whereas quinidine and lidocaine did. They questioned the use of the term "quinidine-like" to describe cardiodepressant action of β-blockers.

There are several general explanations for this discrepancy: *in vitro* versus *in vivo* comparisons may be invalid in this case because of the complicated hemodynamics, or the severely compromised human heart, or the highly prepared canine heart are not accurate models for their more normal cousins. Furthermore, the high doses needed to observe nonspecific effects *in vivo* may cause other offsetting changes in the system.

Despite these cautions there is a considerable body of QSAR data on various models used to assess negative inotropism.

The number of 1-anilino-8-naphthalene sulfonate (ANS) binding sites in human erythrocyte ghosts was found (*270*) to be increased by the presence of β-blockers. ANS is thought to measure the changes in lipid composition near the polar head groups. β-Blockers also stabilized these erythrocyte ghosts against hypotonic hemolysis. Optical isomers behaved identically. Such effects are expected of membrane-active local anesthetic agents (*161,196,204,214*). Furthermore, the authors note that the percentage of increase in ANS binding sites is correlated both with relative cardiodepression ($n = 8$; $r = 0.927$) and with distribution coefficients ($r = 0.883$). A slight refinement was noted in that alkyl substitution at the aromatic moiety has a somewhat greater effect than an isolipophilic substitution at the aliphatic amine.

Akiyama and Igisu (*8*) obtained similar results with propranolol, pindolol, and practolol in a study of the fluorescence polarization of 1,6-diphenylhexatriene (DPH) labeled human erythrocyte ghosts. Nondepressive practolol and pindolol had no effect, whereas propranolol induced a statistically significant 11% drop. Similarly, Lee (*137*) observed that both chloropromazine and propranolol reduced the gel to liquid–crystalline phase transition temperature in dipalmitoylphosphatidylcholine (DPPC) and dipalmitoylphosphatidylethanolamine (DPPE). This effect was offset by myristic acid because of a reduction in surface charge. However, practolol even at very high concentrations had no effect. We have obtained similar results using differential scanning calorimetry (DSC) in DPPC liposomes for propranolol, practolol, and several Syntex β-blockers.

Hellenbrecht *et al.* (*102*) have directly correlated negative inotropism (conduction velocity in frog heart muscle strips) with octanol–H_2O distribution coefficients ($n = 9$, $r = 0.985$), surface activity ($r = 0.941$) and calculated lipophilicities ($r = 0.932$). The β-blockers were alprenolol, propranolol, KL-255, Kö-592, oxprenolol, INPEA, pindolol, sotalol, and practolol. The authors have also (*269*) observed inhibition of [^{3}H]serotonin uptake in human platelets that followed nearly the same order as in the former series. Because of these correlations, the authors proposed that the nonspecific membrane effects of all β-blockers could be predicted simply from their partition coefficients. Conformational changes in the membrane were thought to be the underlying mechanism of action for the nonspecific membrane effects of β-blockers.

Hellenbrecht and co-workers (*103,104,107*) further tested this hypothesis in a series of Boehringer β-blockers by finding a correlation between octanol–H_2O distribution coefficients and three nonspecific effects, as above: 50% decrease in conduction velocity in isolated frog heart; fourfold elevation of the threshold for electrically induced ventricular fibrillation in anesthetized atropinized guinea cat pretreated with propranolol. In the case of guinea pig arrhythmias, some evidence for increased effects of N-alkylation over ring alkylation was noted (*104*), in agreement with Mylecharane and Raper (*174*) who studied who studied 2-nitrilophenoxypropanolamines in rabbits. Rauls and Baker (*187*), on the other hand, found no difference in position of substitution.

Partition coefficients were determined in octanol–phosphate buffer; some difficulties were reported with the more hydrophilic compounds. A correction was used for the distribution coefficient $P/D = 1 + 10^{(\mathrm{p}K_a - \mathrm{pH})}$; this correction is probably not valid because of ion pairing (*14,252*). In fact, Hellenbrecht reports calculated and observed D did not agree for four hydrophilic compounds, which would be less likely to ion-pair partition than the other analogs.

For depression of conduction velocity in frog heart,

$$\mathrm{p}IC_{50} = 3.07 + 0.33 \log D - 0.88 \log D^2 \tag{15}$$

$n = 20, \quad s = 0.137, \quad r = 0.967, \quad \log D_0 = 2.09\ (1.11–6.25)$

The square term was not statistically significant for a subset of 12 Boehringer compounds (*103*) when 60-min incubations were used, but was significant, as above, for 10-min incubations ($n = 11$, $s = 0.068$, $r = 0.989$, and $\log D_0 = 1.73$). Optimum lipophilicity has been shown to depend upon time parameters (*58*). For another modification—data collected after a second stimulus—$s = 0.076$, $r = 0.988$, and $\log D_0 = 1.04$. The shift in $\log D_0$ under different conditions points up the danger of placing too much emphasis on the particular pharmacological model in cardiovascular studies.

Depression of ventricular contractility in a prepared cat pretreated with propranolol (to block β-receptors and reduce β-tone):

$$\mathrm{p}IC_{50} = 4.99 + 0.30 \log D - 0.13 \log D^2 \tag{16}$$

$n = 15, \quad s = 0.115, \quad r = 0.981, \quad \log D_0 = 1.21\ (0.75–2.19)$

This compares with a subset of 12 Boehringer compounds (63) $n = 12$, $s = 0.10$, $r = 0.984$, and $\log D_o = 1.72$. The study has been extended to include atenolol (*106*).

Protection against ventricular fibrillation in anesthetized guinea pigs:

$$pIC_{400} = 5.31 + 0.22 \log D - 0.14 \log D^2 \qquad (17)$$

$$n = 12, \quad s = 0.201, \quad r = 0.925, \quad \log D_o = 0.83\ (0.22\text{–}5.08)$$

Similar quadratic correlations ($r = 0.976\text{–}0.988$) were given for $\log D_{calc}$ with $\log D_o = 0.91\text{–}3.23$ for the three different activities.

Hellenbrecht and Gortner (*105*) have shown that low doses of β-stimulants (−)-isoprenaline and (+)-salbutamol depress fibrillation threshold; however, higher doses returned threshold to initial values. Epinephrine-induced arrhythmias have been used by Molinengo (*169*) as a model for antiarrhythmic drugs. Ouabain-induced arrhythmias, on the other hand, have been shown to respond neither simply to the β-adrenergic nor local anesthetic properties of β-blockers (*133*).

Hellenbrecht *et al.* (*103*) concluded: "(1) Nonspecific cardiodepression increases parabolically with increasing hydrophobicity . . . characteristic for the given pharmacological system. (2) Nonspecific cardiodepression is solely dependent on the sum of the hydrophobic substituents of the drug molecule, irrespective of the site of the substituents (aromatic ring system and/or amino group). (3) Nonspecific cardiodepressant activity of a β-adrenoceptor blocking drug in a given pharmacological system can be predicted by determination or by calculation of the hydrophobic property of the drug molecule [p. 234]." These claims seem overly optimistic in view of the contradictory clinical evidence.

Davis (*57*) has confirmed many of the above laboratory observations: β-blocking activity (rabbit, isolated ileum) is unrelated to local anesthetic activity ($r = 0.770$, guinea pig intradermal weal; $r = 0.752$, rat phrenic nerve–neuromuscular junction) or to quinidine-like activity ($r = 0.758$, reduction of maximal drive rate in guinea pig). The nonspecific effects were all cross-correlated with $r > 0.98$, when log of relative activity was used. More lipophilic propranolol, pronethalol, and INPEA could penetrate nerve and myelin sheaths, whereas hydrophilic sotalol and MJ 1998 (sotalol with a methyl α to NHMe) could not; nonspecific effects also occurred at 100-fold higher concentrations than β-blocking effects.

Wooldridge *et al.* (*25,272*) obtained Eq. (18) for the reduction in ouabain-induced arrhythmia in conscious dogs for series **X**.

$$\log(MW/RD) = -0.989 + 1.84 \sum \pi - 0.27 \sum \pi^2 \qquad (18)$$

$$n = 11, \quad r = 0.953, \quad s = 0.108, \quad \sum \pi_o = 3.37$$

Addition of a steric term gave no improvement. *MW* is molecular weight and *RD* is reverting dose in mg/day.

Zaagsma and Nauta (*276,277*) correlated local anesthetic activity, LA, (desheathed sciatic nerve of frog) with antiarrhythmic effects, AA, (ouabain-induced arrhythmias in guinea pig right atrial muscle) for a series of compounds (**VIII**). For a diverse set of aryl groups (phenyl, naphthyl, and biphenyl; R′ = H) with different positions of side-chain substitution (*277*), correlation of AA versus LA gave $n = 10$, $r = 0.858$, and $s = 0.460$. The ortho diethers possessed enhanced AA activities compared to other positions of substitution, and there was better correlation ($n = 8$, $r = 0.952$, and $s = 0.284$) when these two compounds were omitted. The QSAR are shown in Eqs. (19) and (20), where $pK_{a(m)}$ is the mean pK_a. Because of the unusual nature of the ortho diethers, a second study (*276*)—devoted to this type of aryl substitution—was undertaken, using **XV** (R′ = H, low alkyl). Results are shown in Eqs. (21) and (22), (values in parentheses are *t* tests). β-Blocking activity for these compounds is discussed in Section II,A,1.

$$\text{LA} = -1.23(\log P)^2 + 4.89\text{p}K_{a(m)} - 42.3 \tag{19}$$

$$n = 8, \quad r = 0.918, \quad s = 0.231$$

$$\text{AA} = -2.33(\log P)^2 + 8.89\text{p}K_{a(m)} - 76.8 \tag{20}$$

$$n = 8, \quad r = 0.955, \quad s = 0.300$$

$$\text{LA} = 1.11\pi - 0.39\pi^2 + 1.27 \tag{21}$$

$$n = 7, \quad r = 0.970, \quad s = 0.91$$

$$\text{AA} = 2.13\pi - 0.84\pi^2 + 3.64 \tag{22}$$

$$n = 7, \quad r = 0.924, \quad s = 0.249$$

Hermannsen (*108*) compared the β-blocking local anesthetic properties of propranolol, INPEA, and Ph QA 33 (**XIV**) with the ouabain-induced arrhythmias in guinea pig, finding that the antiarrhythmic effect of β-

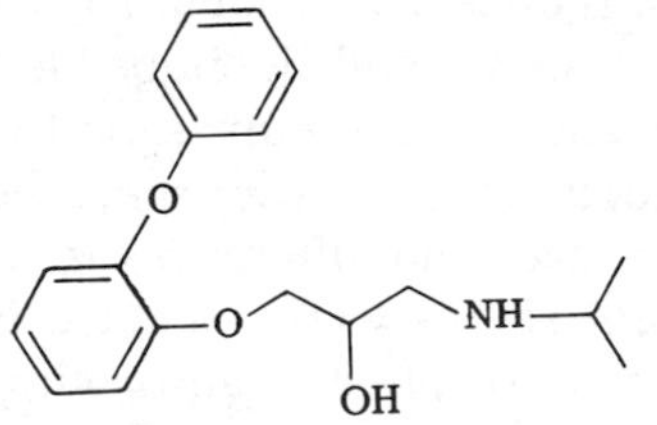

XIV

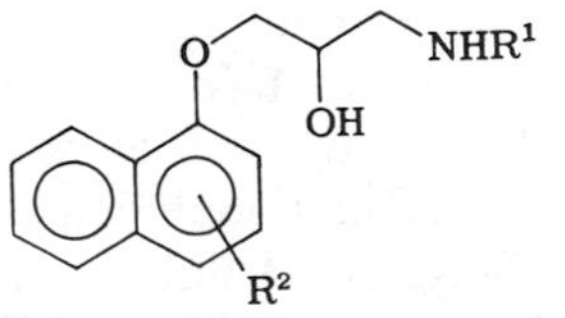

XV

blockers is correlated with local the anesthetic effect (guinea pig cornea), rather than specific β-blocking effect (isolated guinea pig atrium contraction rate). Too few compounds were examined for an adequate quantitative test.

Hellenbrecht and Muller (*101*) also studied the nonspecific effects of β-blockers as inhibitors of serum cholinesterase. Nayler (*175*) has found that both pronethalol and propranolol inhibit—whereas epinephrine and norepinephrine potentiate—lipid facilitated transport of calcium from Ringers buffer into chloroform. Thus the behavior of these β-blockers parallels that of quinidine. Tyramine had no effect on Ca^{2+} transport, even at very high concentrations (0.5 mg/ml). The reported finding that epinephrine and norepinephrine, drugs, which both precipitate cardiac arrhythmias, interact with these extracted lipids to potentiate their calcium transporting activity lends support to the hypothesis that the antiarrhythmic properties of the β-adrenergic antagonists and quinidine involve their interaction with cellular lipids. In general, the presented results are in agreement with the suggestion put forward by Woolley (*273*) (1963) that cellular lipids may provide the receptor site whereby certain drugs and hormones react with cells to effect a particular response (*175*). There are certainly nonadrenergic binding sites on myocardial membranes. On the other hand, the negative inotropic receptor has been identified by Honig and Reddy (*112*) as the protein tropomyosin complex (Ca^{2+} tropomyosin, and actomyosin). Rauls and Baker (*187*) reasoned that because there is evidence linking antiarrhythmic activity of β-blockers to membrane stabilizing (extracellular) events and the negative inotropic activity to depletion of Ca^{2+} stores in the cardiac sarcoplasmic reticulum (intracellular), it might be possible to design antiarrhythmic β-blockers with no negative inotropic component. The extracellular binding of β-blockers was thought to occur with the lipophilic aromatic moiety embedded into the lipophilic region of the bilayer of the cell membrane. The aliphatic nitrogen (which is protonated by physiological pH) interacts with a polar group, possibly displacing Ca^{2+}. Therefore, substitution of polar substituents on the aliphatic nitrogen might reduce transport across the cell membrane and reduce negative inotropic effects, whereas the lipophilic aromatic portion could still be embedded in the lipid bilayer, producing the desired enhanced therapeutic ratio for antiarrhythmic activity. Two series of compounds (**XV**) were prepared, R^1 = *i*-Pr constant or R^2 = H constant. There were no differences in the slope of activity versus lipophilicity. Different slopes were expected in the R series because of the difference between absorption or absorption versus penetration of the β-blockers. There are two comments on this study: the correlations are not of a particularly high order, suggesting that either other factors are involved or the incorrect dependency on lipophilicity was investigated. For example, use of log *D* instead of log *P* might improve results (*202*). Second, partitioning to the surface is a bulk property of the drug; if this step is the rate determining step, then identical dependencies on bulk lipophilicity would be expected. The authors have neither proved nor disproved their hypothesis; further analysis is required (*126,158*).

Unger (*247,248*) has studied the cardiodepressant effects of **I** in dog, finding the bulk (not lipophilicity) of R to determine lack of depressivity. The original idea for a "bulky" R group was that the larger group should sit on or fit into the membrane much less efficiently than an isolipophilic open-chain compound (*247*). Although this statement is correct (*196,204*), the expected effect based on analogy to anesthetics is the opposite of the one found; the compound should be more depressive. For example, Jain *et al.* (*116*) found that a series of adamantane derivatives perturbed phase transitions in artificial lipid membranes in an order that was not related to lipophilicity, size, or polarity alone. The explanation of the discrepancy seems to lie in the evidence cited in Section IV,A and therefore have different effects on depressivity (*116*). To confirm the physicochemical effect of bulky R groups, we have measured the phase transition temperature by DSC as a function of drug concentration in artificial DPPC liposomes for propranolol, practolol, and several Syntex β-blockers. In still preliminary work we have found that the Syntex β-blockers (**I**) are intermediate between the depressive propranolol and nondepressive practolol. Propranolol causes a steep dose-responsive melting of the liposome, whereas practolol has no effect up to very high concentrations. Although isolipophilic with propranolol, RS-51288 is less depressive of melting

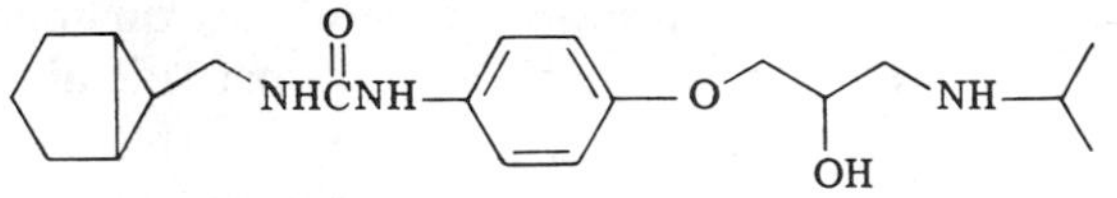

XVI

point. At very low concentrations there is some evidence for slight *freezing*, although this must be confirmed. Further RS-51288 is devoid of local anesthetic activity in a rat phrenic nerve diaphragm preparation except in very high doses (*47*). The phenylureido analog of RS-51288 plateaus out at about 4 mol % and is considerably less depressive that RS-51288 or propranolol at higher concentrations (**XVI**).

Although rate and force inhibition are highly correlated ($n = 62$, $s = 0.16$, $r = 0.898$) in dog, rate inhibition in rat and force in dog are also correlated (*247*), which helps to confirm that depressivity is a nonspecific species-independent effect.

The following QSAR was derived for the dog, iv data:

$$-\text{p}ED_{-20}^{\text{force}} = -4.4 - 1.4W + 0.4DW + 0.4D_{i\text{-Pr}} \quad (23)$$

$$n = 34, \quad s = 0.31, \quad r = 0.783$$

Each term is significant at the 95% confidence limits; W is the width of the R group, D is the depth. $D_{i\text{-Pr}} = 1$ if R′ = *i*-Pr but $D_{i\text{-Pr}} = 0$ otherwise. The dimensions are determined relative to endo[3.1.0]bicyclohexylethyl, which was found to be nearly ideal. The Eq. (23) can be interpreted as follows: DW is the cross-sectional area, which is corrected by W; therefore, R groups with large cross-sectional area, but small width (i.e., large depth) are less depressive of force, as are *N*-*i*-Pr series.

The corresponding equation for rat iv data is:

$$-\text{p}ED_{-20}^{\text{rate}} = 5.9 + 0.6\,(\text{C @ } 6) - 5.8D_{2,6} - 3.6W - 2.5 \log k' \quad (24)$$

$$n = 8, \quad s = 0.24, \quad r = 0.940$$

The term C @ 6 is the number of carbons six atoms away from the carbamoyl nitrogen (nitrogen is counted as 1), $D_{2,6}$ is the distance between the second and sixth atoms and log k' is from HPLC using C-18 Corasil and 35v% CH_3CN in pH 7.0 buffer. Equation (24) is interpreted as showing the importance of bulky but not lipophilic substituents with small width and length ($D_{2,6}$). Although all terms are significant and there is low cross-correlation of terms, less weight can be given to this equation because of the low number of data points.

The example shows that *in vivo* cardiodepressivity is probably dependent in a more complex manner on steric properties of the drugs (at least within a well-defined series) than simple dependency on lipophilicity. This is rationalized by reference to the different microscopic binding modes of anesthetics in artificial membranes, which suggests that simple models of membrane effects of β-blockers are probably oversimplified and that more work needs to be done.

b. Methods. A discriminant analysis (*30*) of 44 antiarrhythmic and 14 nonantiarrhythmic β-blockers found 88% correct reclassification using the hydrophobicity and molecular refraction of the para substituent. Twenty-one cardiodepressive and fourteen nondepressive β-blockers were correctly reclassified to 98% with the following characteristics: electron-donating substituents in meta positions and hydrophilic ring substituents in general, and hydrophilic substituents on the aliphatic nitrogen. This pattern leads to noncardiodepressive β-blockers. Few details were given in the paper.

c. Conclusions. A considerable body of evidence links pharmacological models of cardiodepressant and antiarrhythmic effects with physicochemical properties, but the relationship to the clinical picture is less clear, at least in the case of propranolol (*29,71*).

B. Ca^{2+} Antagonists

A diverse class of agents antagonize slow transmembrane Ca^{2+} flux and the intracellular Ca^{2+} flux of cardiac excitation–contraction coupling. The result is negative inotropism and smooth muscle relaxation, which is translated into hypotension.

Analogs of verapamil (**XVII**) were studied by Mannhold *et al.* (*155*). No

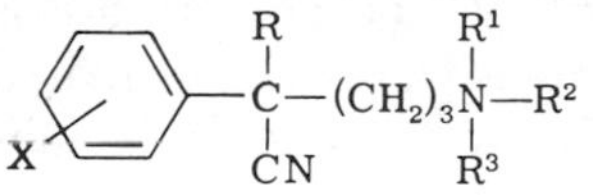

XVII

correlation was found between $\log(1/ED_{50})$ and observed $\log D$ (PO_4 buffer), where ED_{50} is for a cat papillary muscle preparation (isotonic contraction). For a subgroup of compounds (**XVII**: X = varying; R = *i*-Pr; R^1 = Me; R^2 = CH_2CH_2Ph-3,4[$OMe]_2$) MV, E_S, σ, μ, and π were examined, of which σ gives the best correlation ($r = 0.791$). Next, all multiple combinations with σ were determined (incorrect procedure) using Eq. (25). Parameters were standardized by mean and standard deviation.

$$pED_{50} = 0.96\sigma + 0.63MV \tag{25}$$

$$n = 7, \quad s = 0.064, \quad r = 0.994, \quad p < 0.0005$$

A second subset [**XVII**: X = 3,4$(OMe)_2$; R = varying; R = Me; R^2 = CH_2CH_2Ph-3,4-$(OMe)_2$; R^3 = −] of only four compounds gave a better ($r = 0.924$) correlation with $-\pi$ than with $-E_S$ ($r = 0.063$), the only two parameters investigated. Note that π is a literature value, despite the determination of $\log D$.

A second study on nifedipine analogs (**XVIII**) was reported (*190*). Nifedapine is a specific inhibitor of the slow membrane channel, in contrast to verapamil, which also inhibits the fast Na^+ inward current. A similar cat papillary muscle preparation was used. R_M values were determined on paraffin impregnated silica gel plates using 50% MeOH–H_2O as the mobile phase; π, E_S, V_W (van der Waals), L, and B_1–B_4 (Verloop), MR, σ, **F**, and **R** were examined. No significant correlation was obtained with either π, R_M, σ, **F**, or **R** for 14 analogs. However, a significant correlation for

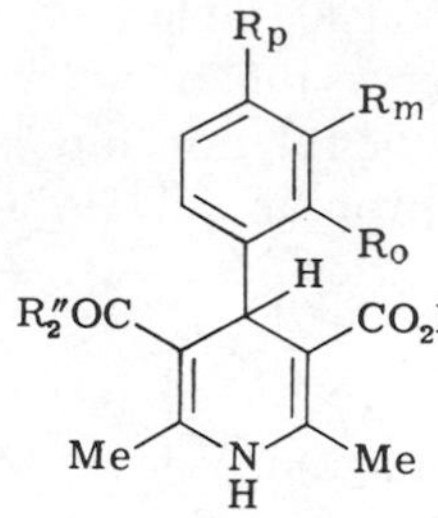

XVIII

eight ortho analogs with $-E_s$ could be obtained ($n = 8$, $r = 0.87$, $s = 0.14$, $p < 0.001$). For five ester analogs (**XVIII**: $R_m = NO_2$; $R_o = R_p = H$), good correlations were obtained with R_m ($r = 0.96$), $-\pi$ ($r = 0.97$), E_s ($r = 0.90$) or V_w ($r = 0.94$) (V and R_m are intercorrelated $r = 0.89$). More hydrophilic derivatives were more active, as were ortho ring substituted analogs. The authors felt that ester substitution influenced potency and not efficacy (receptor fit).

III. ANTIHYPERTENSIVES

Hypertension—a physiological state in which the diastolic blood pressure is ≥90 mm Hg—occurs in over 40 million Americans and is characterized by a complex and not well understood etiology. For example, all of the following agents have been used to treat some form of hypertension: central α-agonists, peripheral α-antagonists, adrenergic neuron blockers, β-blockers, direct vasodilators, ganglionic blocking agents, monoamine oxidase inhibitors, diuretics, and angiotension II converting enzyme inhibitors. Frequently a stepped-care regimen has been used in which diuretics are tried first, and then other agents are substituted or added, although β-blockers have been suggested as the initial agent of choice (*79*). Generally, treatment of severe hypertension (diastolic pressure > 125 mm Hg) is considered a medically urgent necessity; however, although treatment of mild to moderate hypertension has been shown to reduce mortality and incidence of stroke in large scale studies, not all cases are detected or treated (*17,60,95,253,264*).

Several current reviews on qualitative structure activity relations of antihypertensive agents have appeared (*41,160*).

A. *In Vitro* Enzyme Studies

Despite the large number of mechanisms involved in the regulation of blood pressure, only a few QSAR studies that deal with the enzymatic level of action have appeared.

Inhibition of bovine arterial cyclic AMP phosphodiesterase by a series of papaverine analogs (**XIX**) could be correlated by Eq. (26) (*138*):

$$pIC_{50} = 1.03 \sum \pi - 0.16 \sum \pi^2 + 2.62 \quad (26)$$

$$n = 15, \quad s = 0.25, \quad r = 0.82 \quad \sum \pi_o = 3.5$$

The IC_{50} for spasmolytic effect on isolated rat aorta was significantly correlated with the enzyme inhibition ($n = 14$; $r = 0.94$), implying that the pharmacological effect would be correlated with lipophilicity.

Kutter and Hansch (*130*) obtained Eq. (27) for inhibition of rat liver MAO and Eq. (28) for human liver MAO for a series of compounds (**XX**).

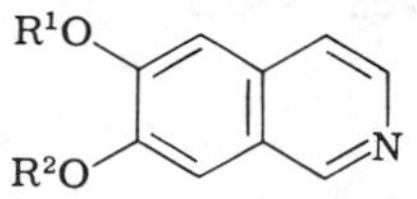

XIX

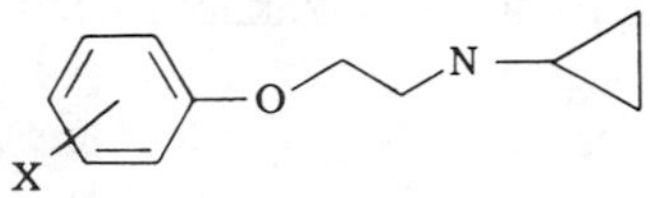

XX

In eq. (27), the π term is not significant but becomes significant if three poorly fit derivatives are omitted ($n = 15$, $r = 0.976$, $s = 0.203$).

$$pIC_{50} = 0.70E_s + 1.64\sigma + 0.198\pi + 4.15 \quad (27)$$

$$n = 18, \quad r = 0.945, \quad s = 0.330$$

For Eq. (28), the σ and π terms are not significant, but the simple equation is not presented by the authors. This equation gives $+E_s$ ($n = 9$, $r = 0.809$, $s = 0.729$).

$$pIC_{50} = 1.03E_s + 1.09\sigma + 0.40\pi + 4.54 \quad (28)$$

$$n = 9, \quad r = 0.955, \quad s = 0.435$$

Fujita (*80*) correlated eleven different types of inhibitors for *in vitro* and *in vivo* activity with similar results using σ, π, and E_s in addition to an indicator variable for certain series. Correlations were in the range $r = 0.84–0.996$. The most significant finding of this study was the high frequency of dependence on steric constants E_s. Smaller substituents gave better inhibition. Electron deficient aromatic rings also consistently enhanced activity.

B. Diuretics

QSAR has been useful in the design of a potent, high ceiling K^+-sparing diuretic muzolimine (**XXIa**), which is currently in Phase III clinical trials (*113*). A simplified Topliss tree optimization search showed that the $+\pi/+\sigma$ branch led to the 3,4-Cl_2 analog. A very rough correlation of

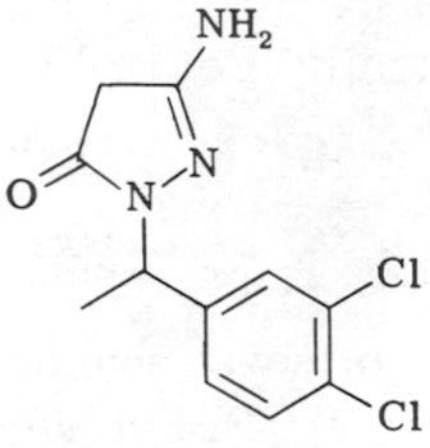

XXIa

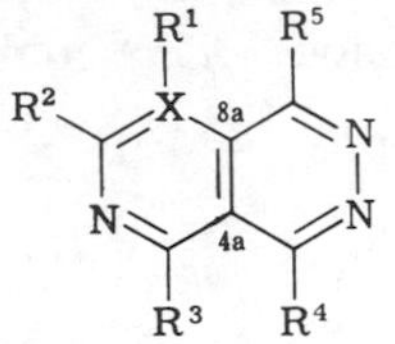

XXIb

sodium excretion in the dog following 3 mg/kg p.o. of test drug versus R_M (dioxane–H_2O) was also reported ($n = 24$, $r = 0.63$).

A series of diuretic azanaphthalene derivatives (**XXIb**) has been studied by Free–Wilson and Extended Hückel calculations (*167*). Urine volume (log V), amount of Na^+ and K^+ (log $U_{Na}V$ and log U_KV), and log(U_{Na}/U_K) at a dose of 30 mg/kg in rats were used as dependent variables. Free–Wilson analysis on 37 analogs (**XXIb**: $R^1 = X = N$) (i.e., pyrimido[4,5-*d*]-pyridazines) gave significant results for log V and log(U_{Na}/U_K) ($r = 0.987$, $s = 0.057$, and $r = 0.979$, $s = 0.045$, respectively). The best substituents were R^2 = phenyl, R^3 = H and $R^{4,5}$ = 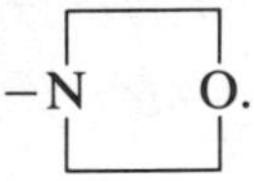.

A similar analysis on 46 (**XXXIb**: X = C-ring (i.e., pyrido[3,4-*d*]-pyridazine derivatives gave significant results for log V, log($U_{Na}V$) and log(U_{Na}/U_K). The best substituents were log V: R^1 = Me, R^2 = phenyl, R^3 = H, $R^4 = R^5$ = 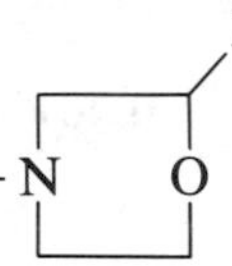 with X = H, Me; log($U_{Na}V$); R^1 = H, R^2 = Et, R^3 = H, $R^4 = R^5$ = 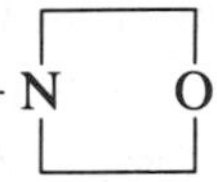; and log(U_{NA}/U_K): R^1 = Me, R^2 = Et, R^3 = H, $R^4 = R^5$ = 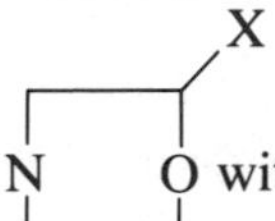 with X = H, Me. Many of these had been synthesized and, in fact, were quite active. A selection of eleven representative azanaphthalene skeletons was chosen for extended Hückel calculations. The correlations are given in Eqs. (29–31):

$$\log V = 0.62N^*_{4a} - 5.01M_{4a,8a} + 4.98 \quad (29)$$

$$n = 11, \quad r = 0.891, \quad s = 0.093$$

$$\log(U_{\mathrm{Na}}V) = 0.52N^*_{4a} - 6.13M_{4a,8a} + 6.16 \tag{30}$$
$$n = 11, \quad r = 0.836, \quad s = 0.120$$
$$\log(U_{\mathrm{K}}V) = 0.53N^*_{4} + 0.36N^*_{4a} - 0.22 \tag{31}$$
$$n = 10, \quad r = 0.835, \quad s = 0.095$$

Terms N^*_{4a} and N^*_4 are the sum of atomic populations of HOMO and NHOMO in the π system at positions 4 or 4a. Term $M_{4a,8a}$ is the atomic bond population between position 4a and 8a. In Eq. (31), if the pyrido[2,3-*d*]pyrimidine (**XXII**) was present, N^*_4 became insignificant and

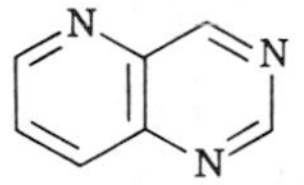

XXII

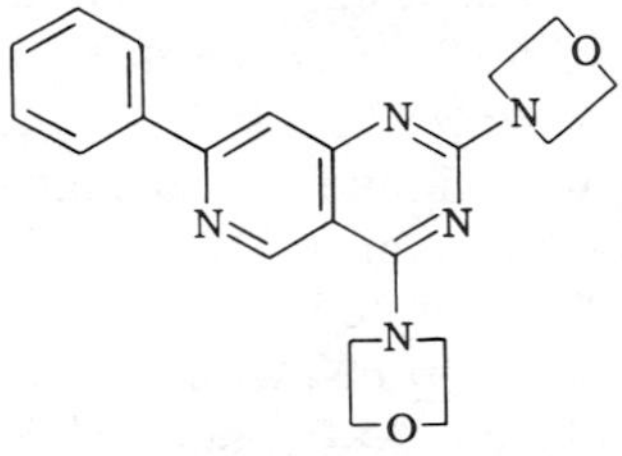

XXIII

so this analog was omitted. Based on these equations, **XXIII** was synthesized and the relatively potent diuretic activity of $V = 2.03$ was determined ($U_{\mathrm{Na}}V = 1.62$) at 10 mg/kg and $U_{\mathrm{K}}V = 1.57$ at 20 mg/kg. Thus **XXIII** was slightly less active than expected. Including **XXIII** in Eqs. (29) through (31) gave slightly poorer correlations ($r = 0.87$, 0.78, and 0.82 respectively).

Singh and Gupta (*209*) subjected the same data to Pariser–Parr–Pople calculations, with similar results indicating the importance of the π electrons at the ring junction. The statistics were somewhat poorer, however, and only the $\log(U_{\mathrm{K}}V)$ Eq. (6) was significant ($n = 10$, $r = 0.818$, $s = 0.117$).

Satzinger (*200*) has discussed the importance of lipophilicity in a series of etozolin diuretics.

Miller *et al.* (*165*) have discussed pK_a effects and Maren (*156*) investigated the qualitative correlation between pK_a and ether–water partition coefficients of sulfonamides acting as (diuretic) carbonic anhydrase inhibitors.

An equation (32) has been reported for inhibition of carbonic anhydrase by sulfonamides (**XXIV**) (*142*):

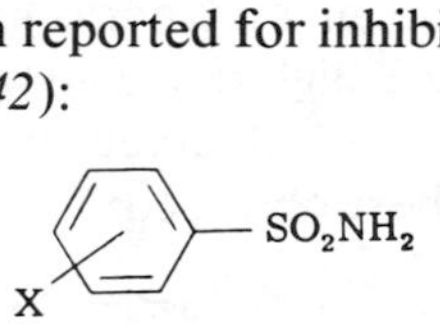

XXIV

$$pK_I = 0.26 \log P + 0.89\sigma + 5.31 \quad (32)$$

$$n = 19, \quad r = 0.923, \quad s = 0.247$$

The most complete study of sulfonamide carbonic anhydrase inhibitors is that of Kakeya *et al.* (*120–123*). Qualitative plots of the various electronic properties (Hammet σ, pK_a, chemical shift of the SO_2NH_2 protons, and S=O valence-force constants in IR) and the aqueous solubility versus the pK_I at both 0.2 and 15°C showed the importance of electron-withdrawing and desolubilizing substituents. Next, the diuretic and natriuretic activities and duration of action in rats were determined. Diuresis and natriuresis were highly correlated ($r = 0.999$), showing correlation of Y = 0.908 and 0.907 between diuresis and natriuresis versus pK_a. Correlations of r = 0.822 and 0.811 for $\Sigma\sigma$ were also obtained. Similar correlations were found for chemical shift ($r = 0.91–0.93$) and S=O valence force constant, $r = 0.90–0.91$. Some compounds were outliers, particularly disubstituted compounds.

Comparing *in vitro* pK_I with *in vivo* diuresis or natriuresis showed reasonable correlation. At 0.2 or 15°C, $r = 0.80–0.81$.

Chloroform partition coefficients and bovine serum albumin association constants at pH = 7.4 were also determined and showed qualitative correlation with duration of action.

The best QSAR are shown in Eqs. (33) and (34), for 15°C:

Ortho

$$\mathrm{p}K_I = 1.23\sigma^* + 0.98E_s - 0.08 \quad (33)$$

$$n = 3$$

Meta and para

$$\mathrm{p}K_I = 0.38\pi - 0.74\Delta \mathrm{p}K_a + 0.52 \quad (34)$$

$$n = 16, \quad r = 0.938, \quad s = 0.216$$

Compounds of the 1,3,4-thiadiazole-5-sulfonamide class that were omitted from Eq. (34) were reasonably well predicted. The independent variables are referenced to benzenesulfonamide; pK_a was determined at 20°C. Similar correlations were obtained at 0.2°C. For diuretic and natriuretic activity, the dose causing a tripling in excretion volume or [Na^+] was reported. Because of the high correlation between these two activities ($r = 0.999$), only pC^+_{Na} was subjected to QSAR. The following Eqs. (35) through (37) were the best obtained:

$$\mathrm{p}C_{Na^+} = -0.14\pi^2 - 0.26\pi - 0.67\Delta \mathrm{p}K_a + 0.34 \quad (35)$$

$$n = 16, \quad r = 0.965, \quad s = 0.089, \quad \pi_o = -0.92$$

$$pC_{Na^+} = -0.15\pi^2 - 0.09\pi + 1.50\Delta ppm + 0.28 \quad (36)$$
$$N = 16 \quad r = 0.939, \quad s = 0.116, \quad \pi_0 = -0.299$$
$$pC_{Na^+} = -0.22\pi^2 - 0.20\pi + 0.70pK_I + 0.05 \quad (37)$$
$$n = 16, \quad r = 0.878, \quad s = 0.163, \quad \pi_0 = -0.446$$

Equation (37) gave somewhat better predictions for omitted compounds; however, this equation contains experimentally determined pK_I values on the compounds in hand. Equations failed for ortho substituted compounds, but predicted 1,3,4-thiadiazole-5-sulfonamide analogs reasonably well. Therefore, electron-withdrawing substituents having π equal to about -0.3 give the most active analogs.

C. Peripheral Vasodilators

The qualitative SAR of peripheral vasodilators have been reviewed by Francis (*73*).

Heilman *et al.* (*100*) failed to obtain a QSAR for the antihypertensive activity of **XXV** in spontaneously hypertensive rats (SHR) using π, σ, or E_s. However, LD_{50} appeared to be correlated negatively with lipophilicity for **XXV** (R′ = H, Me, Ac, and $COCF_3$) but no equations were given.

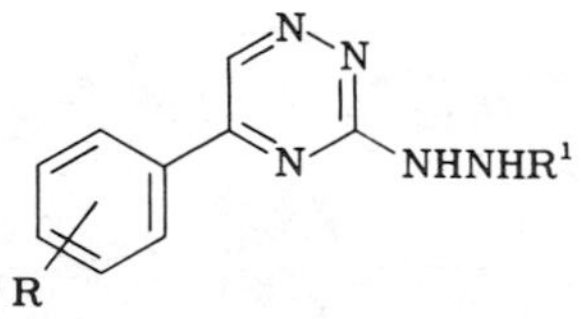

XXV

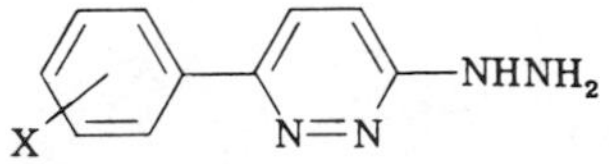

XXVI

Leclerc *et al.* (*135*) obtained the parabolic Eq. (38) for the hypotensive effect of **XXVI** 30 min after iv dosing to anesthetized rats. Addition of σ, E_s, or *MR* was not significant.

$$pED_{20} = 5.30 + 0.28\pi - 0.24\pi^2 \quad (38)$$
$$n = 12, \quad r = 0.91, \quad s = 0.14$$

The peripheral vasodilating activity of **XXVII** is reportedly (*201*) correlated by Eq. (39),

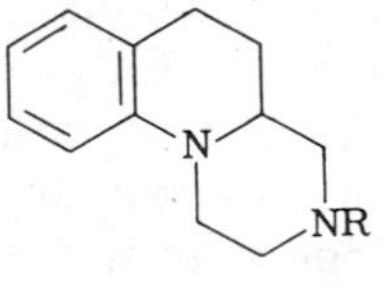

XXVII

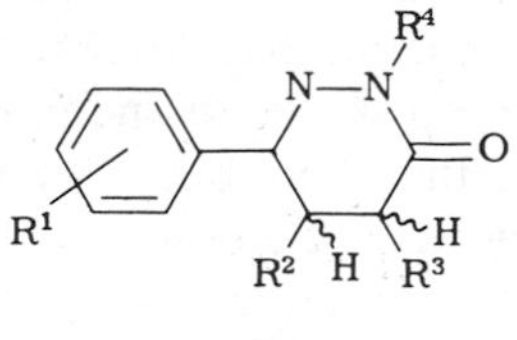

XVIII

$$pC = 4.77 \log P - 0.96 \log P^2 - 5.72 \tag{39}$$

$$n = 10, \quad r = 0.989, \quad s = 0.047, \quad (\log P)_o = 2.47$$

A series of 32 hypotensive pyridazinones (**XXVIII**) of unspecified mechanism of action were correlated by the Free–Wilson method with $r = 0.986$ using either rank order or mean arterial blood pressures (MABP) of normotensive rats four hours post 100 mg/kg p.o. (*128*). The best compounds are (rank order) $R^1 = 4 - CN$, $R^2 = Me$, $R^3 = R^4 = H$, and (MABP) $R^1 = 4\text{-OMe—Ph}$, $R^2 = H$, $R^3 = Me$, and $R^4 = CH_2CH_2Ph$; rank order results are preferred and R^3 and R^4 parameters are statistically insignificant.

Benzothiadiazine (**XXIX**) antihypertensive activity is related to inhibition of Ca^{2+} induced vasoconstriction in the rat aorta. (*271*). A QSAR using extended Hückel MO parameters has been obtained (Eq. 40) in which $S'_{(n)}N$ is the approximate (frontier) nucleophilic superdelocalizability on atom n, $S'_{(n)}E$ is the electrophilic counterpart. $E^{[A]}$ is the electric field created at point [A] by a set of charges, $F^{[A]}$ is the intermolecular Coulombic interaction energy for the molecule and point [A], and $\pi'_{n,n}$ is the frontier self-atom polarizability of atom n and $q(R^1)^{\pi}$ is the summed net regional charge over all atoms in the R^1 group of **XXIX**.

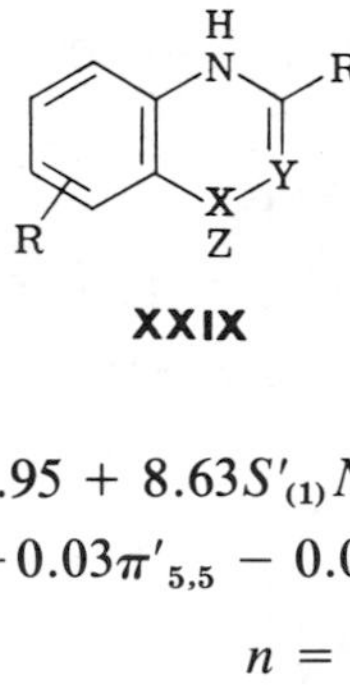

XXIX

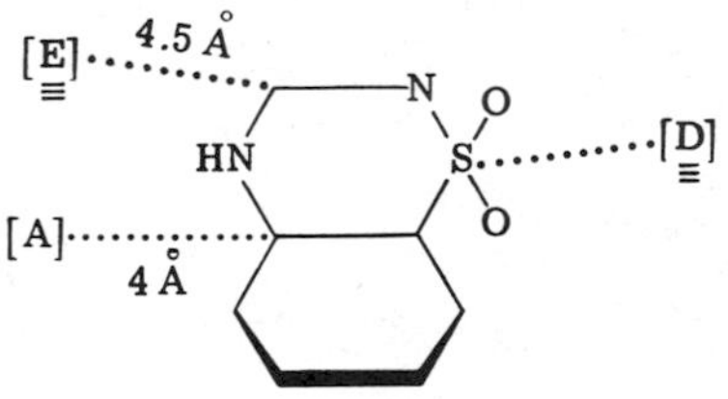

XXX

$$pA_2 = 1.95 + 8.63S'_{(1)}N - 135.09S'_{(4)}E + 78.14E^{[D]} + 54.52S'_{(3)}N$$
$$-0.03\pi'_{5,5} - 0.03\pi'_{1a,1a} + 61.60F^{[E]} + 1.49q(R^1)^{\pi} \tag{40}$$

$$n = 24, \quad r = 0.997, \quad s = 0.12$$

The references should be consulted for further definition of these terms. The most interesting feature of this study is the attempt to calculate interactions with a putative receptor, shown in **XXX**. The distance between [A] and [E] is 3.5 Å, the diameter of a singly hydrated Ca^{2+} (3.7 Å), and is thought to be the likely binding site, with [D] being an accessory binding site. With the molecule bound, an electron transfer occurs to the receptor and reduces the binding at [A], while increasing slightly that to [D] and

[E]. The drug then disengages the receptor. Although this is an interesting model, the data are probably overfit from a statistical viewpoint.

Höltje (*111*) obtained a good correlation ($r = 0.907$, $n = 17$) for these data using the putative interaction with an arginine side-chain receptor at a distance of 4 Å. Asparagine and tryptophan gave insignificant correlations when treated similarly ($r \simeq 0.4$).

A classical QSAR has also been formulated for **XXXI**, (Eq. 41) (*239*):

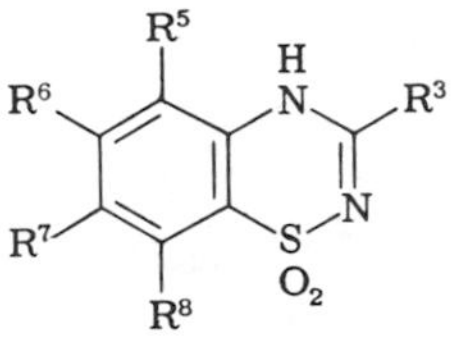

XXXI

$$A^* = 0.42 + 1.28\pi_{R^{6,7}} + 0.72\pi_{R^3} - 0.19\pi^2_{R^3} \quad (41)$$

$$n = 33, \quad r = 0.91, \quad s = 0.35, \quad (\pi_{R^3})_o = 1.95$$

The values are based on experimental observations (*241*); $A^* = \log[2 \times MW/ED_{50}] + \log(K_a + H/H)$ where ED_{50} has been determined for norepinephrine-induced contractile response of the isolated rat aortic ring; A^* and pA_2 are highly correlated ($n = 33$, $r = 0.95$, $s = 0.38$). Therefore, the classical QSAR differes from the MO based correlation in assigning the main substituent effect to the lipophilic rather than electronic substituent effect. In addition, *in vivo* data (DOCA rat) could be correlated as shown in Eq. (42) where $A' = \log(1000/MED)$.

$$A' = 1.23 + 0.43\pi_{R^{6,7}} + 1.42\pi_{R^3} - 0.81\pi^2_{R^3} \quad (42)$$

$$n = 14, \quad r = 0.85, \quad s = 0.25, \quad (\pi R_3)_o = 0.88$$

Position specific effects can be illustrated by comparing two analogs (**XXXIV**: R^3 = Me; $R^5 = R^8$ = H, $R^6 = CF_3$; R^7 = Cl, with **XXXIV**: R^3 = cHx; R^{5-8} = H) whose lipophilicities are similar ($\log P = 2.24$ versus 2.20) but whose activities differ considerably ($A^* = 3.13$ versus 1.15). Finally, Eq. (41) predicted the activities of withheld compounds to within the required accuracy.

A Free–Wilson analysis has also been reported for these data (*238*) with $r = 0.996$. The maximum value of A^* was then predicted as 5.44 for **XXXI** (R^3 = Δ^3-cyclopentenyl; R^5 = Br; $R^{6,7} = CF_3$; R^8 = Cl), in short, highly electron deficient phenyl rings.

The data have also been treated by the DARC–PELCO topological method with $n = 15$, $r = 0.996$, and $s = 0.1$ (*12*).

D. Peripheral α-Antagonists

Hansch and Lien (*97*) studied the antagonism of adrenaline and noradrenaline hypertensive effects in spinal rate by **XXXII** (*87,88*). These

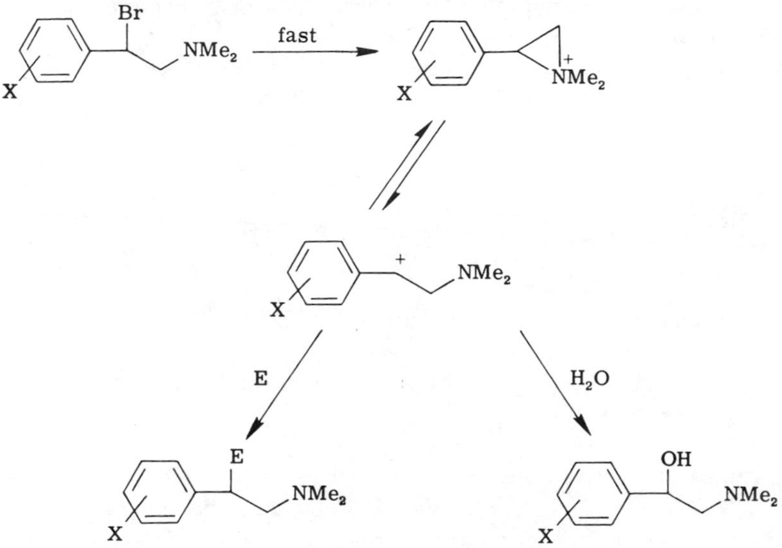

SCHEME II

agents are thought to alkylate the α-receptor according to Scheme II. For 22 compounds (**XXXII**: R = R′ = Me) versus adrenaline (Eq. 43) or noradrenaline (Eq. 44), simple correlations with π and σ were obtained.

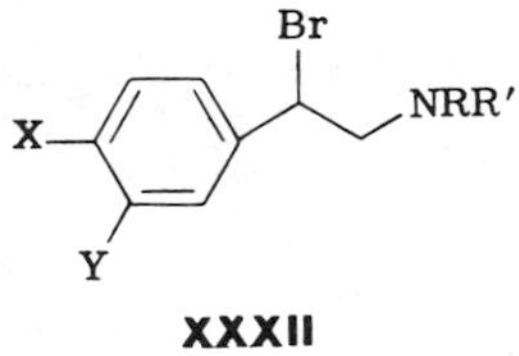

XXXII

$$pC^{ad} = 1.22\pi - 1.59\sigma + 7.89 \tag{43}$$

$$n = 22, \quad r = 0.918, \quad s = 0.238$$

$$pC^{nad} = 1.26\pi - 1.62\sigma + 7.85 \tag{44}$$

$$n = 22, \quad r = 0.911, \quad s = 0.257$$

For ten analogs (**XXXII**: X = Y = H) studied in the cat, Eqs. (45) through (47) were obtained, while Eq. (22) was obtained for nine compounds (**XXXII**: X = Y = H) studied in the mouse.

$$pC^{ad} = 1.11E_s^c + 3.57\sigma^* - 4.43n_H + 11.91 \quad (45)$$

$$n = 10, \quad r = 0.99, \quad s = 0.235$$

$$pC^{nad} = 1.12E_s^c + 3.84\sigma^* - 4.49n_H + 11.86 \quad (46)$$

$$n = 10, \quad r = 0.950, \quad s = 0.452$$

$$pC^{ad} = 0.28E_s^c + 2.70\sigma^* - 3.03n_H + 8.95 \quad (47)$$

$$n = 9, \quad r = 0.924, \quad s = 0.378$$

Finally, Eqs. (48–49) were obtained for eleven compounds of the same series in the rat:

$$pC^{ad} = 0.90E_s^c + 0.83\sigma^* - 3.08n_H + 9.86 \quad (48)$$

$$n = 11, \quad r = 0.927, \quad s = 0.547$$

$$pC^{nad} = 0.81E_s^c + 0.72\sigma^* - 2.95n_H + 9.64 \quad (49)$$

$$n = 11, \quad r = 0.952, \quad s = 0.420$$

For Eqs. (45) through (49), n_H is the number of hydrogens on the amine nitrogen. Rates of solvolysis of **XXXII** (X = Y = H) at 31°C in acetone–water by Chapman and Triggle (*45*) could be correlated as shown in Eq. (50).

$$\log k = 1.10E_s^c + 4.47^* - 1.85 \quad (50)$$

$$n = 6, \quad r = 0.998, \quad s = 0.031$$

Large inductive withdrawing groups on the nitrogen increase solvolysis, but small inductive withdrawing groups propitiate α-blocking activity. The authors (*97*) took this discrepancy to indicate that the biological activity might be driven by an S_N2 mechanism. If the mechanism were S_N1, then one would expect a $-E_s^c$ in Eqs. (45) through (49). Large groups increase solvolysis, reducing the effective concentration of the intermediate for interaction with the enzyme (*193*). Unfortunately, the selection of substituents was not good because σ^* and E_s^c were covariant. The authors also provided a spurious argument attempting to relate the magnitude of the regression coefficient associated with E_s^c to the species, mouse, rat, or cat.

Cammarata (*40*) reinvestigated the correlation of **XXXV**, obtaining Eq. (51), in which there is no lipophilic or electronic effect assigned to para substituents. Further, the van der Waals radii $r_{v,p}$ are accidently correlated to π_p and σ_{p^+} ($n = 6$; $r = 0.983$, $s = 0.073$) (*250*) prompting Unger and Hansch (*250*) to reexamine the original problem from the point of view of factorization of substituent effects by position. In this study $r_{v,m}$,

$r_{v,p}$, π, π_m, π_p, σ, σ_m, σ_p, $\mathbf{S}_m$, $\mathbf{S}_p$, $\mathbf{P}_m$, and $\mathbf{P}_p$ were investigated; **S** and **P** are inductive-field and resonance constants from Unger's thesis (*249*). Because Eq. (53) shows that σ^+ is perfectly explained by its factors **S** and **P**, Eq. (54) was selected as the best equation.

$$pC^{ad} = -0.91\sigma_m + 0.75\pi_m + 1.67r_{v,p} + 5.77 \qquad (51)$$

$$n = 22, \quad r = 0.961, \quad s = 0.168$$

$$PC^{ad} = 0.86\pi + 0.47\mathbf{S}_m - 0.36\mathbf{S}_p + -0.92\mathbf{P}_p + 0.62r_{v,p} + 7.08 \qquad (52)$$

$$n = 22, \quad r = 0.967, \quad s = 0.167$$

$$\sigma^+ = 0.77\mathbf{P}_p + 0.26\mathbf{S}_p + 0.20\mathbf{P}_m + 0.47\mathbf{S}_m + 0.01 \qquad (53)$$

$$n = 22, \quad r = 0.098, \quad s = 0.02$$

$$pC^{ad} = 0.82\pi - 1.02\sigma^+ + 0.62r_{v,p} + 7.06 \qquad (54)$$

$$n = 22, \quad r = 0.964, \quad s = 0.164$$

The absence of $\mathbf{P}_m$ in Eq. (52) was attributed to the small amount of contributed variance and small number of compounds. The importance of σ^+ argues against the ethyleneiminium ion as an important species in the rate determining step (Scheme II).

Unger and Hansch (*250*) gave five criteria for help in selection of a best regression equation.

1. Wide choice of independent variables. Those selected must not be multicolinear.
2. Variables chosen must be statistically significant in the regression.
3. Parsimony. The simplest model is to be preferred, all else being equal.
4. Number of terms in the model must be supported by the number of compounds. [Note: Topliss and Costello (*240*)—updated by Topliss and Edwards (*242*)—refer to variables examined and not variables included. However, see Unger and Hansch (*250*) for a discussion.]
5. Qualitative model must make physicochemical and biomedicinal sense.

E. Central α-Agonists

Clonidine (**XXXIII**: X = 2, 6-Cl_2) was originally developed as an analog of the α-adrenergic naphthazoline (**XXXIV**) for use as a nasal decongestant. However, it was found to possess potent central antihypertensive action via stimulation of α-receptors in the medulla. This central α-stim-

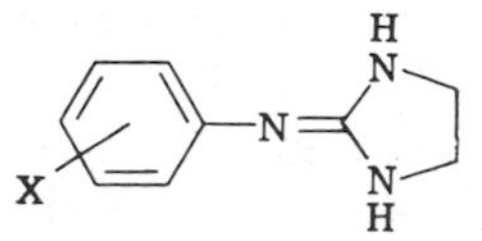

XXXIII

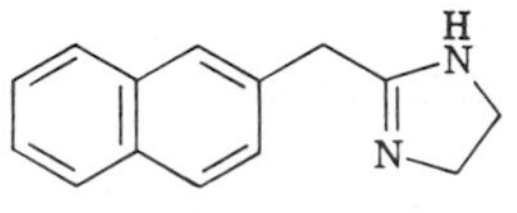

XXXIV

ulation causes a reduction in peripheral sympathomimetic tone and an increase in the vagal reflex. Initially upon dosing, however, clonidine induces a transient peripheral pressor effect due to stimulation of peripheral α-receptors in the vasculature (*110,237,256,257*).

The relationship between centrally and peripherally mediated action has been quantitatively related via the distribution coefficient (*109,265*). Because penetration into the CNS is related to the distribution coefficient, and because the hypotensive effect is due to central α-stimulation, Hoefke *et al.* (*109,265*) fit Eq. (55) for five analogs where

$$\ln \text{(rel. bradycardia in vag. rats)} = 0.224(1 - e^{0.645X}) \tag{55}$$

and X is ln(D × rel. hypertensive effect in spinal rats). Increasing CNS activity therefore occurs with increasing lipophilicity and peripheral activity. It was assumed that there were no differences in the receptors *per se*. One analog (**XXXIII**: X = 2,6-Et_2) was omitted. Because $D = 0.06$ for this analog, versus $D = 3.0$ for clonidine (pH = 7.4), the importance of other factors aside from distribution [which should have been accounted for in Eq. (55)] was assumed.

A similar relationship between central and peripheral effects has been found by Timmermans and van Zwieten (*230–232*) for a larger set of derivatives (Eq. 56):

$$\text{p}C_{30} = 0.63 \log D + 0.84\text{p}C_{100} - 0.30 \tag{56}$$

$$n = 13, \quad r = 0.912, \quad s = 0.501$$

The term pC_{30} is the central hypotensive effect causing a 30% drop in blood pressure as determined in anesthesized normotensive rats (iv); pC_{100} is the dose causing a doubling in arterial pressure in the pithed rat (iv), and is a measure of the peripheral effects. In this equation log D was found to improve the correlation significantly. The authors point out the importance of accounting for lipophilic effects in determining the mode of action of drugs by standard pharmacologic means, a point frequently overlooked.

The central hypotensive effect pC_{30} was directly related to the bradycardia in anesthesized normotensive rats, pC_{25} ($n = 26$, $r = 0.96$, $s = 0.248$) (*233*).

These authors next determined log D and pK_a for 28 analogs (*231,234*). Log P was calculated using $P = D[1 + 10^{(pK-pH)}]$. Satisfactory correlation with $\Sigma\pi$ ($n = 28$, $r = 0.972$, $s = 0.177$F) and with Σf ($n = 28$, $r = 0.859$, $s = 0.255$) were obtained. Brain concentrations in ether anesthesized rats were determined by VPC analysis after iv dosing. The ED_{30} dose was used and the time was taken as that giving peak effect. For example, the hydrophilic 2,6-F_2 analog was dosed at 600 μg/kg at 30 min, whereas the lipophilic 2,6-Cl_2, 4-Br was dosed at 60μg/kg with peak effects at $\leq$5 min. Equation (57) was obtained:

$$\log(C_{\text{brain}}/C_{\text{iv}}) = -0.13 \log D^2 + 0.57 \log D - 0.94 \qquad (57)$$

$$n = 14, \qquad r = 0.987, \qquad s = 0.139, \qquad \log D_o = 2.16$$

Thus clonidine log $D = 0.62$ is suboptimal, whereas 2,4,6-Br_3 is close to ideal for brain penetration, log $D = 2.24$. Although the parabolic fit is statistically significant, many more lipophilic analogs are needed better to define the shape of the optimum reaching curve. However, this is an interesting study.

The bradycardia of **XXXIII** has been qualitatively related to lipophilicity (*162*).

Struyker Boudier *et al.* (*220*) attempted a QSAR study of α-agonists using isolated rabbit intestine and intrahypothalmic injection in rats as a measure of central activity. Chloroform–buffer distribution coefficients were determined; however, the only correlation that could be obtained was that between pD_2 and +pK_a ($n = 11$, $r = 0.837$, $s = 0.242$). Too few analogs of the eleven imidazolines showed central hypotensive effects to allow correlation analysis. However, on the basis of qualitative SAR, the authors concluded that peripheral and central α-receptors differed.

A QSAR has been reported by Rouot *et al.* (*198,199*) in which pD_2 is the −log concentration causing 50% of maximal response in arterial blood pressure in pithed rats and has been corrected for protonation (assumes protonated species is active). Equation (58) shows the importance of steric effects in the ortho position, meta is mainly, but not entirely, steric, and para is not important for this hypotensive activity.

$$pD_2^* = -1.93E_{S2,6} - 0.77E_{S2,6}^2 - 1.19E_{S2} - 0.70E_{S3} - 0.38\mathbf{F} + 6.17 \qquad (58)$$

$$n = 22, \qquad r = 0.93, \qquad s = 0.29$$

Four compounds were synthesized to test this equation and good agreement was obtained between experimental and calculated for the three nontoxic derivatives. No correlation of hypotensive effects (iv or icv dosing) could be obtained; however, there were too few compounds showing a hypotensive effect to allow a full examination of this point.

Local anesthetic activity (rabbit cornea) was correlated by log D ($n = 11$, $r = 0.78$, $s = 0.30$). [See also Kobinger and Pichler (*125*).]

Timmermans and van Zwieten (*235*) have done the most extensive investigation using 27 derivatives (**XXXIII**) in anesthetized normotensive rats, i.v. dosing. A large number of independent variables were examined: seven Hammett-type electronic parameters, eight molecular orbital indices, log D, π and parachor, E_s, and MR. The best equation obtained by stepwise regression was Eq. (59):

$$\begin{aligned} pED^*_{30} = {} & -0.00032\left(\sum \text{par}\right)^2 + 0.11\left(\sum \text{par}\right) - 0.70pK^o_a \\ & + 5.33\ \text{HOMO(P)} + 6.75\ \text{EE(P)} + 2.49 \qquad (59) \\ & n = 27, \quad r = 0.952, \quad s = 0.341 \end{aligned}$$

ED^*_{30} is the dose of drug, corrected for protonation, causing a 30% decrease in mean arterial blood pressure; Σ par is the total substituent parachor (a measure of size), pK^o_a is taken relative to the unsubstituted compound in H_2O; HOMO(P) is the highest occupied molecular orbital of protonated species, EE(P) is the difference HOMO − LEMO for protonated species. The ΔpK_a term is the single most important term and was attributed mainly to effects on lipophilicity. All compounds were predicted to within two standard deviations. This result has been questioned by Topliss and Edwards (*242*) on the basis of statistical significance because of the large ratio of examined variables to observations. The frequency of chance correlations is about 45% for the ratio employed in this study.

Because of the difficulty in using *in vivo* data, the authors next obtained Eq. (60) by calculating the ED_{30} (C) from Eq. (57) in order to give a measure of the brain concentration and to remove distribution effects. This equation (60) predicts activity well, except for meta substitution.

$$\begin{aligned} pED_{30}\ (\text{C}) = {} & -0.401\left(\sum E_s\right)^2 - 1.77 \sum E_s + 1.90 \sum \mathbf{R} \\ & + 5.13\ \text{HOMO(P)} + 6.77\ \text{EE(P)} + 8.03 \qquad (60) \\ & n = 27, \quad r = 0.941, \quad s = 0.326 \end{aligned}$$

Omitting the two meta compounds gives $r = 0.965$, $s = 0.262$. An alternate equation substitutes $-\Sigma\ \mathbf{F}$ for $\Sigma\ \mathbf{R}$ and q_{C-8}(P) for HOMO(P) and $r = 0.935$, $s = 0.340$. The steric effect at different positions was examined, but no improvement over Eq. (60) could be obtained (meta compounds omitted). However, ortho substituents appeared more important with one side dominating (the side with the larger substituent). These results compare reasonably well with those of Rouot *et al.* (*198,199*) (Eq. 58) for peripheral effects.

The QSAR results were used to formulate a working hypothesis for centrally acting α-agonists: the receptor accepts electrons for the donor-protonated drug, the positive NH^+ of the imidazoline binding to a negative receptor site. An electron-deficient phenyl is required (no conjugation between phenyl and imidazoline is preferred), one side of the phenyl dominates the steric requirements.

It is not clear that the interplay between electronic factors has been clarified by these studies, especially in light of remarks (*240,242*) concerning the ratio of variables examined to compounds. However, the general approach taken by these authors is both innovative and useful.

Following Pullman *et al.* (*49,185*) and Wermuth *et al.* (*268*), Hoefke (*110*) has proposed that clonidine can assume a conformation that mimics two critical distances of noradrenaline with the phenyl and imidazoline rings perpendicular. The distance from the center of the phenyl to the distant NH^+ is 5.0–5.1 Å, while the distance from the bridge nitrogen to this distant NH^+ is 1.28–1.36 Å. These distances compare favorably with 5.1–5.2 Å and 1.2–1.4 Å, respectively, for noradrenaline.

The crystal structure of phenmetrazine, an α-agonist, has been taken as evidence confirming this pharmacophoric pattern (*168*).

CNDO/2 calculation (*164,236*) showed that the imidazoline and phenyl may not be perpendicular, and an allene-like structure between the two rings is proposed. The pK_a values could be calculated successfully from this model and it was concluded that the protonated form of clonidine activates the α-receptor. However, UV photoelectron spectra and CNDO/*s* calculations (*59*) show that the phenyl and imidazoline are found to be perpendicular. CNDO/*s* does not correctly calculate energy levels for n_N and σ orbitals but does calculate π orbitals, according to these authors. Further studies showed that there was no correlation between the first ionization energies and hypotensive effects. Therefore, these results contradict Timmermans' results on the importance of steric effects and the protonated form of clonidine.

A considerable amount of work has gone into the study of clonidine and its analogs, and the results have generally been quite fruitful. Unfortunately, there has been much redundancy in the preparation of similar analogs and determination of their physicochemical parameters by different laboratories. Although many more lipophilic compounds should have been examined to better define the optimum and descending portions of the curve, Timmermans' investigations involving Eq. (57) are classical and, it is hoped, will motivate other workers toward more thorough investigations using QSAR.

F. Angiotension II Analogs

Hsieh *et al.* (*114*) presented some semiquantitative arguments concerning the effect of lipophilicity (calculated) and size of substituents in angiotensin II analogs [Asp-Arg-Val-Tyr-Ile-His-Pro-Y (**XXXV**)] on pressor activity in nephrectomized, pentolinium-treated male rats. Increasing lipophilicity of Y led to increasing pressor activity, as long as Y was linear aliphatic. Branching led to reduced activity, aromatic substitution of phenyl (Y = Phe) led to increased activity over that expected from lipophilicity alone. Less bulky aromatic substituents were more active. Families of curves were obtained using the covalent radii of ring substituents. Electron-donating substituents were uniformly more active than isolipophilic electron-withdrawing substituents. In conclusion, the 8 position of **XXXV** seems to respond to aromatic system changes, mainly via electronic, but also through lipophilic and steric effects. Potent inhibitors are therefore found in the class of bulky nonaromatic hydrophilic substituents (e.g., serine or threonine) or with conformationally constrained aromatic rings (e.g., indane).

G. Methods

Discriminant analysis of 15 α-agonist and 18 α-antagonist phenalkylamines were separated by the fractional lipophilicity (Rekker) of the amino substituent with 83% correct reclassification. Hydrophilic (or small) substituents on nitrogen led to α-agonist activity; no systematic effect of aromatic or methine substitution was found (*30*).

Adaptive least squares (ALS) was devised (*172*) for discrimination of ordered classes, as opposed to linear discriminant analysis (LDA) for independent classes. The method was applied to **XXXVI** for three or-

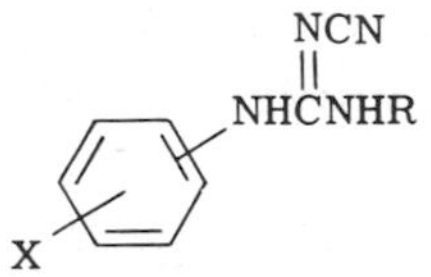

XXXVI

dered/hypotensive classes: poor (32 compounds), moderate (25 compounds), and high (19 compounds). SHR rats with p.o. dosing were used. An unspecified number of variables was examined and those whose weight times standard deviation was greater than 0.1 were selected for inclusion in Eq. (61).

$$L = 0.12N_c - 0.02(N_c)^2 - 1.71V_H + 1.80I_1 + 1.72I_2 - 1.99I_3 + 1.44I_4 + 0.30I_5 + 0.13I_6 - 2.34 \quad (61)$$

$$N = 76, \quad n_{mis}, = 17\%(1), \quad R_s = 0.832, \quad p < 0.001$$

N_c is the number of carbons in R (use of $\Delta N_c = N_c - 5$ to remove colinearity did not change the results); V_H is a measure of hydrophilicity (*171*); I_1 and $I_2 = 1$ for 3-pyridyl- and 4-pyridylguanidines, respectively. $I_3 = 1$ if 6-substituted pyridyl; $I_4 = 1$ if R has ≤ 3 C atoms in the longest chain and one tertiary carbon. $I_5 = 1$ if R has ≤ 1 ring attached to the α carbon of R and $I_6 = 1$ if *i*-Pr is present in the terminal position of R. In Eq. (61), n is the number of compounds, n_{mis} is the number misclassified as a percent with the number in parentheses being the number misclassified into the next class but one. R_s is the Spearman (nonparametric) rank correlation coefficient.

For LDA using the same variables $N = 76$, $n_{mis} = 21\%$ and $R_s = 0.790$ ($p < 0.001$). Nonelementary discriminant analysis (*6*) gave $n_{mis} = 34\%$ (0) with $R_s = 0.694$.

The k-nearest neighbor (kNN; k = 1) method gave $n_{mis} = 28\%$ with $R_s = 0.747$. If 15 to 16 compounds were randomly left out, revalidation averages were 25% for ALS versus 28% for LDA, with $R_s = 0.794$–0.888 and 0.649–0.803, respectively. Therefore, ALS seems worthy of further investigation.

H. Conclusions

The application of QSAR techniques to antihypertensives has been a successful enterprise. The high ceiling K^+-sparing diuretic muzolimine (**XXIa**) (currently in Phase III clinical trials) was designed with the help of QSAR. A number of successful predictions have been made, including an excellent series of studies of clonidine (**XXXIII**: X = 2,6-Cl_2) and related analogs. Antihypertensive data of various types have been the vehicle for several authors to illustrate various methods and critiques.

IV. ANTIARRHYTHMICS

Cardiac arrhythmias arise from disturbances in electrical impulse formation and/or propagation in various cardiac tissues and are therefore ultimately caused by imbalance in ionic fluxes, especially Na^+, K^+, and Ca^{2+}. Because membranes and their permeability to ions regulate these fluxes, membrane-active drugs (e.g., local anesthetics such as procaine) or the membrane-active side effects of drugs (e.g., quinine) have been exploited as antiarrhythmic agents. Thus we have procainamide, quinidine, and propranolol [at high concentrations (*196*)] acting as antiarrhythmic agents. Specific enzymes and modulators regulate the binding and transport of Ca^{2+} [calmodulin and (Ca^{2+}/Mg^{2+})-ATPase] as well as Na^+ and K^+ (Na^+/K^+)-ATPase. However, because ATPase is a membrane bound enzyme, nonspecific agents may act indirectly via changes in membrane fluidity that induce conformational changes in the enzyme, or otherwise deactivate the enzyme (*89,245*). This situation can be contrasted with that of the β-blockers or ouabain, which interact directly with stereospecific receptors at low concentrations. Such interaction is thought to be the mode of antiarrhythmic activity of these compounds in the clinic (*71,76–78*), however, this is a point of controversy (*148*). The reader is referred to an excellent 1974 review by Vaughan Williams (*259*) and two 1976 reviews by Morgan and Mathison (*159,170*) for a thorough discussion of antiarrhythmic drugs, arrhythmias, and their electrophysiological genesis. Courtney (*50*) discusses simple linear QSAR of local anesthetics in terms of the various components of ionic flux, finding size and lipophilicity to be important. Lipophilicity determines closed channel blocking potency. Frequency dependent Na^+ channel blocking is greater for more hydrophilic drugs, whereas smaller drugs show faster escape rates for closed channel block. Molecular weight is the measure of size. Different fixed doses of the drugs were used, making further QSAR work meaningless. Lipophilicities were calculated by the PROPHET system with only fair ($r = 0.87$, $n = 5$) agreement with experimental oleyl alcohol partition coefficients.

A. Nonspecific Effects

Seeman (*204*), Roth (*197*), and Nuhn *et al.* (*176*) have extensively reviewed the membrane action of anesthetics, tranquilizers, and neuroleptics and provide a good general background on membrane effects. Hansch and Glave (*98*) present a general survey of the QSAR approach to nonspecific membrane effects. Büchi and Perlia (*38*) have reviewed the design of local anesthetics. In this section we will review some of the more relevant literature on nonspecific effects not previously covered in detail.

The accumulation of 16 various drugs by isolated guinea pig atria was correlated with log P and binding to atrial homogenate for either resting or 2-Hz stimulated atrial muscles, Eqs. (62) and (63) (*150*).

$$\log(T/M)(0\ \text{Hz}) = 0.25 \log P + 0.46 \log(B/F) + 0.73 \qquad (62)$$

$$n = 16, \quad r = 0.978, \quad s = 0.254$$

$$\log(T/M)(2\ \text{Hz}) = 0.28 \log P + 0.45 \log(B/F) + 0.79 \qquad (63)$$

$$n = 16, \quad r = 0.979, \quad s = 0.267$$

T/M is the equilibrium tissue to medium ratio, corrected for the extracellular space of the muscle, and B/F is the % bound/% free in atrial homogenates. Addition of $\log(B/F)$ is highly significant compared to the equation with only $\log P$ ($n = 16$, $r = 0.928$, $s = 0.440$). However, $\log P$ and $\log(B/F)$ are themselves significantly correlated ($n = 16$, $r = 0.802$, $s = 0.708$). This point was not discussed by the authors. Use of binding to human serum albumin B/F gave slightly poorer correlations. Examination of plots of percentage binding to HSA versus atrial homogenate show families of curves depending upon charge, i.e., anionic, cationic, or neutral. Therefore, $\log(B/F)$ probably mimics specific binding effects not accounted for in $\log P$. [See also Franks and Lieb (*74*).]

The review by Seeman (*204*) gives the various membrane protective effects of anesthetics and tranquilizers and attempts an explanation of anesthetic activity. Seeman shows correlations of log of the concentration for nerve block (frog sciatic nerve) or the concentration for 50% antihemolysis versus log of the membrane–buffer partition coefficient P_{mb}. The correlation (see *204*, Fig. 9) for 71 miscellaneous agents is given in Eqs. (64) through (66):

$$\text{p}C = 1.20 + 1.15 \log P \qquad (64)$$

$$n = 71, \quad s = 0.340, \quad r = 0.959, \quad sd/sdm = 3.4\%$$

$$\text{p}C = 1.19 + 0.015MV \qquad (65)$$

$$n = 71, \quad s = 0.943, \quad r = 0.611, \quad sd/sdm = 9.5\%$$

$$\text{p}C = 0.90 + 1.03 \log P_{\text{mb}} + 0.0056MV \qquad (66)$$

$$n = 71, \quad s = 0.241, \quad r = 0.979, \quad sd/sdm = 2.4\%$$

The correlation between $\log P_{\text{mb}}$ and MV is significant but very low ($r = 0.449$). Addition of the MV term in Eq. (66) is highly significant (*22,24*). The larger and more lipophilic drugs are better anesthetics. The two-parameter model is superior to the one-parameter model shown by Seeman (*204*).

The above correlation shows the general trend of several chemical classes, but what about individual classes? For the series of 14 alcohols, we obtain the following correlation [benzyl,methyl to decyl (normal), *i*-pr, *t*-Am, and menthol] (Eqs. 67 and 68).

$$\text{p}NB = 1.05 + 1.14 \log P_{\text{mb}} \qquad (67)$$

$$n = 14, \quad s = 0.218, \quad r = 0.992, \quad sd/sdm = 3.8\%$$

$$pAH = 1.11 + 1.17 \log P_{mb} \tag{68}$$

$$n = 14, \quad s = 0.189, \quad r = 0.994, \quad sd/sdm = 3.2\%$$

Nerve block (NB) was correlated to antihemolysis (AH) by a coefficient of 0.888 and was used to fill in the two missing values (octanol and decanol for NB. For this series log P_{mb} and *MV* were correlated by 99.3%, making it impossible to differentiate between size and lipophilicity. However, log P_{mb} is statistically identical to that found by Hansch and Glave (*98*) for the average of 30 examples of polar molecules interacting with red blood cells obtained from various sources and causing either hemolysis or narcosis.

For eleven nonhydrogen-bonding inhalation anesthetics (H_2, Ne, Ar, Kr, Xe, N_2, CH_4, c-C_3H_6, SF_6, and CF_2CL_2) we obtain the trend expected from Mullin's rule.

$$pNB = 0.27 + 0.042MV \tag{69}$$

$$n = 11, \quad s = 0.145, \quad r = 0.970, \quad sd/sdm = 8.0\%$$

In this case, lipophilicity is not important.

Finally, for a series of 19 phenols (H, 4-OMe, 4-F, 3-NMe_2, 4-CO_2Me, 3-NO_2, 3-Me, 4-OEt, 4-Me, 2-Cl, 2,6-Me_2, 3,5-Me_2, 4-Cl, 2-CF_3, 4-Br, 2,4-Cl_2, 3-I, 4-*t*-Bu, and 3-Me-4Cl) we obtain Eq. (70), which shows the importance of hydrogen bonding (acidity) of phenolic OH. *MV* is fairly constant for this series.

$$pAH = 1.38 + 1.07 \log P_{mb} - 0.32fF - 0.47rR \tag{70}$$

$$n = 19, \quad s = 0.156, \quad r = 0.964, \quad sd/sd = 9\%$$

Again, the slope for log P_{mb} is as expected. The terms fF and rR are the (corrected) Wellcome values derived from the **F** and **R** of Swain and Lupton (*247*). The coefficients indicate that field and resonance donating substituents enhance anesthetic potency. Because electron-withdrawing substituents increase the acidity of phenols, these results suggest that the hydrogen-bonding properties of the phenolic OH may be more important in determining anesthetic potency. Compare Rogers and Davis (*191*) who studied alkyl and halo phenols above and below the phase transition temperature of DMPC liposomes.

It is evident that while the overall trend, as expressed by Eq. (66), can explain a large amount of the variation in different classes, individual classes do not interact in the same manner. The hydrogen-bonding but neutral alcohols depend mainly on lipophilicity (greater variation in bulk may show this to be an additional factor, but this cannot be detected with the present data set), whereas the hydrogen-bonding and acidic phenols require the addition of electronic effects (size variation is fairly constant in this series). Finally, the inhalation anesthetic gases respond to size alone.

We have used MV instead of log MV because MV (as MR) is thought to be proportional to free energy. Nonetheless, substitution of log MV in Eq. (66) gives virtually the same statistics ($s = 0.242$, $r = 0.980$, and $sd/sdm = 2.4\%$). Therefore, the difference is not critical in this particular instance.

The behavior of different classes of drugs precludes general correlations as those published by Seeman. A possible explanation for the differences observed between different classes might be the binding site within the membrane (*197*). For example, polar drugs would probably hydrogen-bond to the polar phosphatidyl head group, whereas nonpolar molecules would bind in the hydrophobic fatty acid chain. Seeman notes that anesthetic amines displace membrane-bound Ca^{2+}, generally depressing passive fluxes of cations. Neutral anesthetics generally increase membrane-bound Ca^{2+}, generally increasing passive fluxes. Schlieper (*203*) has found similar results in cholesterol-doped artificial membranes. Cation permeability was decreased by most of the basic amines (including β-blockers), except for quinidine and D-(−)-INPEA which increased the negative surface charge and decreased the permeability to anions. While anesthetics electrically stabilize membranes, they do so by fluidizing, swelling, and disordering the components of the membrane. Local anesthesia occurs at much higher concentrations of drug in membrane (about 0.04 mol/kg dry membrane, which is 0.3% of the volume of the membrane) than does general anesthesia [about 0.003 mol/kg or 0.02% of the membrane (*204*)].

Concentration of drug in membrane is clearly related to lipophilicity. However, Jain and Wu (*117*) have shown that for a series of 38 phenothiazines, equal concentrations in artificial lipid bilayers do not induce equal response (in this case, broadening of the phase transition profile in DSC by 50%). This observation was explained by assuming that the different phenothiazines were bound to different microhomogeneities in the lipid, which exists as an equilibrium of different gel and liquid crystalline phases. These microhomogeneities might be considered as pseudoreceptors (*117*).

A similar picture emerges from a study of substituted adamantane derivatives (*116*). Jain and co-workers (*118*) correlated the concentration of drug that induces 100% increase in phase transition width of dipalmitoyllecithin liposomes with either 50% or 8% antihemolysis for a collection of alcohols, local anesthetics, tranquilizers, and inhalant anesthetics.

The evidence for different binding sites, even in pure lipid membranes, tends to support our results obtained above on Seeman's data. Despite the evidence that equal concentrations of phenothiazines do not induce equal responses on the physical properties of membranes (*117*), activity and total binding is usually correlated by lipophilicity (*98,99*).

In contrast to these results, Franks and Lieb (*74*) found no evidence for perturbation of lipid bilayers by general anesthetics at clinical concentrations when examined by X-ray and neutron diffraction techniques. However, a good correlation of potency was obtained using 1-octanol partition coefficients. Using vegetable oil, hexadecane, or benzene gave families of curves, but 1-octanol gave only a single curve. The authors concluded that anesthetics probably do not act at a lipid receptor, but that the anesthetic receptor is probably protein or protein with closely associated lipid. The authors assumed that because 1-octanol is more polar than, e.g., hexadecane, the receptor must be more polar than the pure lipid.

Elonen (*67*) found that log *D* at pH 7.4 for amitriptyline, doxepin, nortriptyline, and protriptyline was correlated with the iv cardiotoxicity in mice. At low doses a sinus tachycardia and arrhythmias were observed, but as the dose increased bradycardia became dominant. Both mild to severe tachyarrhythmias after successive iv injections and local anesthetic effect on rabbit cornea at $2 \times 10^{-3}M$ were correlated by *n*-octanol–phosphate buffer distribution coefficients. The decrease in surface tension by 10 dynes/cm was uncorrelated with either biological parameter.

Epinephrine-induced ventricular automaticity (spontaneous beating) is antagonized by β-blockers, as expected, but it is also blocked by other drugs. A study of such agents by Molinengo (*169*) confirms the nonspecific action of such agents (urethane, phenylcarbinol, benzamide, acetanilide, acetylcholine, ephedrine, piperoxan, procainamide, ajamaline, emetine, atabrine, atropine, and quinidine). [See also Hellenbrecht and Gortner (*105*).]

ED_{50} was defined as the dose of drug that decreased the rate of contraction induced by 2×10^{-6} epinephrine by 50% in a rat heart ventricular strip preparation. Analysis of the dose-response curves showed that acetylcholine and ephedrine were different from the other eleven drugs tested. Omitting acetylcholine, Molinengo found significant correlation with log *MV* ($r = 0.964$) or log Sol ($r = 0.852$), where Sol is the aqueous solubility. Antiarrhythmic activity increases with increasing *MW* or decreasing Sol. The direct correlation with lipophilicity that is implied by these results was not tested by Molinengo.

Mathison and Morgan (*159,170*), Graeff *et al.* (*86*), and Engelmann *et al.* (*68*) include in their papers a qualitative discussion of the effects of lipophilicity in series **XXXVII–XXXIX**, respectively.

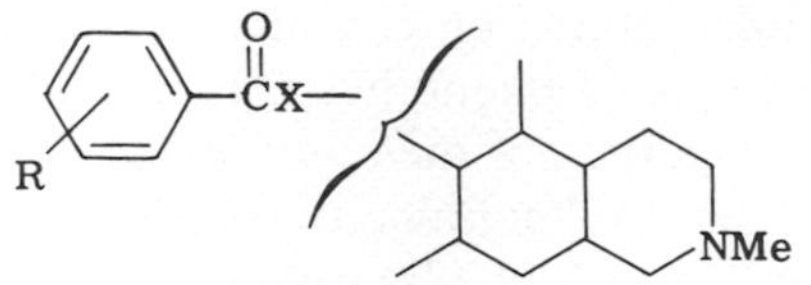

XXXVII

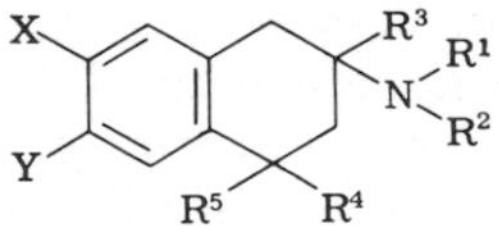

XXXVIII

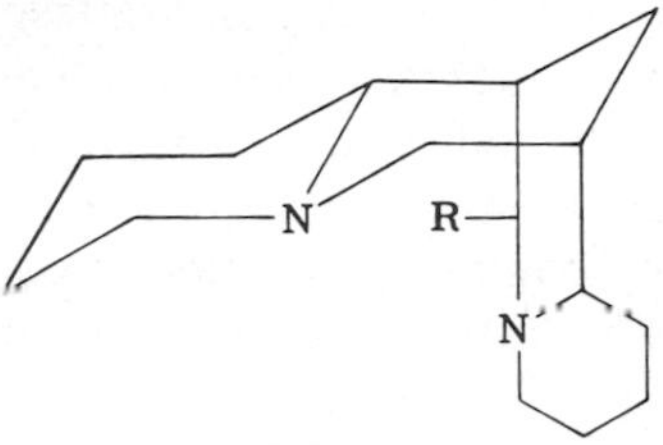

XXXIX

B. Effects on Enzymes

Grisham and Barnett (*89*) studied the effects of long-chain alcohols on membrane lipids and (Na^+/K^+)-ATPase (ATP pyrophosphatase) (lamb kidney). The alcohols (ethanol to octanol) have no direct effect on protein structure under these conditions but rather disrupt lipid structure by increasing membrane fluidity. [See also Puskin and Martin (*186*).] The more lipophilic the alcohol the greater the potency in inhibiting the enzyme and in disorienting a spin labeled androstanol, DH.

$$pC_{ATP} = -1.20 + 0.81 \log P \tag{71}$$

$$n = 6, \quad s = 0.080, \quad r = 0.998, \quad sd/sdm = 3.3\%$$

$$pC_{H} = -1.16 + 0.81 \log P \tag{72}$$

$$n = 6, \quad s = 0.098, \quad r = 0.997, \quad sd/sdm = 4.1\%$$

Unger and Chiang, (*252*) have obtained linear correlations for the inhibition of histamine release from rat mast cells with the lipophilicity of lipophilic amines (phenothiazines and tricyclic antidepressants) (Eq. 73) for binding co bovine serum albumin (BSA) (Eq. 74) and for inhibition of (rat brain) (Na^+/K^+)-ATPase (Eq. 75). The results tend to confirm the indirect action of such agents on (Na^+/K^+)-ATPase (*56,94*).

$$p(ED_{50} \times 10^{-3}) = 0.52 \log k' + 1.26 \tag{73}$$

$$n = 14, \quad s = 0.171, \quad r = 0.929, \quad sd/sdm = 10.7\%$$

$$-pK = 0.52 \log k' + 0.13\, pK_a + 1.31 \tag{74}$$

$$n = 7, \quad s = 0.059, \quad r = 0.980, \quad sd/sdm = 9.9\%$$

$$\text{logit } \% = 1.40 \log k' - 2.92 \qquad (75)$$

$$n = 9, \quad s = 0.269, \quad r = 0.962, \quad sd/sdm = 10.4\%$$

Log k' is obtained using an optimized HPLC system with an isotonic pH 7.4 1-octanol saturated phosphate buffer with added 4*mM* dimethyloctylamine on a persilated RP-18 column packing material; it is excellently correlated with shake–flask distribution coefficients using the same buffer system (without added dimethyloctylamine (DMOA), which suppresses adsorption retention). Logit % = log[%/(100 − %)] where % is the percentage of inhibition at $1 \times 10^{-4}M$.

The difference is slopes between Grisham and Barnett's (*89*) data (Eqs. 71 and 72) and these data cannot be ascribed to any single factor. The enzyme sources are different (rat brain versus lamb kidney) and because these are membrane bound enzymes, will most likely contain different lipids, if they are actually not isozymes of each other. The effect of various lipids on reconstituted (Na^+/K^+)-ATPase has been described (*84,124,208*). Lipophilic amines and alcohols may bind in somewhat different regions of the lipid. In fact, Unger and Chiang did not find great differences between three different mobile phases used in the HPLC study (*252*), in contrast to the other two biological systems examined (Eqs. 73 and 74).

Johnson and Schwartz (*119*) examined the effect of local anesthetics on isolated mitochondria, finding inhibition of K^+ transport, especially in the presence of histone. Histone and K^+ may together compete for an anionic binding site. The potency of local anesthetics increased with increasing lipophilicity.

Grobecker *et al.* (*90*) studied the inhibition of serotonin uptake by human platelets (a model membrane) by antiarrhythmic and sympatholytic drugs. However, the platelet model has been questioned for these drugs (*216*).

Further evidence that nonspecific agents can perturb enzyme activity comes from a study by Eletr *et al.* (*66*) who used adamatane to perturb artificial phospholipid vesicles prepared from *Saccharomyces cerevisiae*. Congruence of the transition temperature changes for both spin label motion and oxygen uptake show that the physical state of the membrane can influence enzyme activity. [See also Fourcans and Jain (*72*) and Sullivan *et al.* (*221*).]

C. Other Agents

Lin *et al.* (*143–146*) have used a quantum statistical approach to derive simple linear regression models to explain antiarrhythmic activity of di-

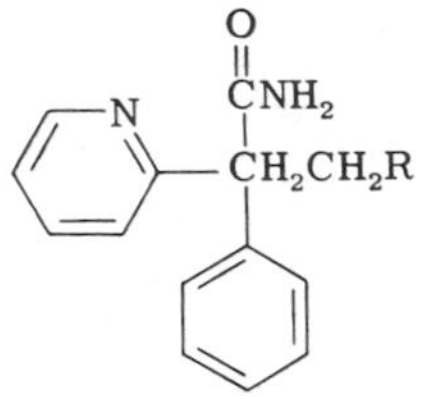

XL

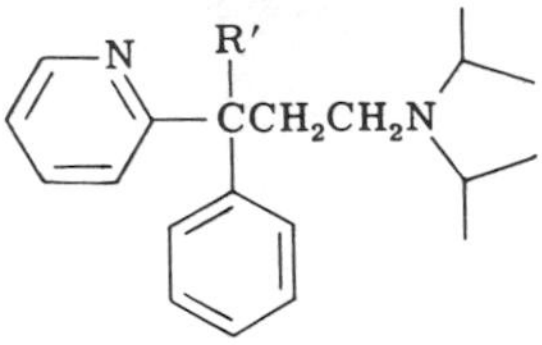

XLI

isopyramide derivatives **XL** and **XLI** against atrial arrhythmias in electrically stimulated right atria of dog or ventricular arrhythmias in unanesthetized dog with ligated coronary artery. If P is the relative potency compared to diisopyramide; $\nu_{C=O}$ is the IR shift of C=O; f_N is the frontier electron density on the nitrogen of the R group in **XL**, then Eq. (76) was derived (*145*) for compounds of type **XL** in the former model and Eq. (77) was derived (*146*) for **XLI** in the latter model. In this case π was found to be important.

$$\ln P = 105.86 - 0.06\nu_{C=O} - 2.46 f_N \tag{76}$$

$$n = 13, \quad s = 0.34, \quad r = 0.85$$

$$\ln AP = 26.04 + 0.85\pi - (14.65 \times 10^{-3})\nu_{C=O} \tag{77}$$

$$n = 15, \quad r = 0.86, \quad s = 0.25$$

AP is the mean maximal reduction in extrasystoles per mean effective dose. Neither of these equations is of particularly high precision.

Human plasma binding of 21 diisopyramide derivatives has been correlated with increasing measured lipophilicity at pH 7.4 ($r = 0.955$) (*46*). Measured lipophilicities gave higher correlation than calculated values ($r \doteq 0.94$).

The most interesting feature of this work is the derivation of a linear QSAR Model from a quantum statistical basis, rather than the application to this particular set of data. The low correlations obtained suggest further QSAR work may be in order. However, the experimental error in the data was not stated and this might account for these results.

Ehrhardt *et al.* (*65*) studied a series of 2,6-dichloro analogs of lidocaine for antiarrhythmic, local anesthetic, and antihypertensive activities. The activities were not correlated with each other. The antihypertensive effect was transient—although significant for some compounds—but could not be correlated with the parameters examined. Antiarrhythmic activity was taken as the concentration causing a 25% reduction in the difference between the resting beating rate and the maximally driven rate of isolated guinea pig atria. The local anesthetic activity was defined as the concentration causing a 15-sec delay in the blinking of a stimulated rabbit eye. Antiarrhythmic activity was correlated most simply by pK_a and the E_s of the para substituent [E_s (optimum) = 0.48] with $n = 18$, $r = 0.973$, and $s = 0.227$. Local anesthetic activity was increased by electron-donating, relatively insoluble, and lipophilic substituents ($n = 11$, $r = 0.998$, and $s = 0.11$). Compounds of similar solubility differed in lipophilicity.

Tenthorey *et al.* (*225*) obtained different results with a series of aminoxylidides of structure related to the proceding study. Antiarrhythmic activity was determined as the ED_{50} for protection of chloroform-induced tachyarrhythmias in mice; CNS toxicity (ataxia) in mice was also determined in order to obtain a QSAR for selectivity. The antiarrhythmic activity was correlated with log P (optimum) = 2.61 and $n = 18$, $r = 0.89$, and $s = 0.03$. Addition of pK_a was not statistically significant. Ataxia was correlated with log P (optimum) = 3.13 and $-pK_a$ with $n = 20$, $r = 0.92$, and $s = 0.04$. The importance of pK_a in the 2,6-dichloro analogs of lidocaine but lack of importance in the aminoxylidides was attributed (*225*) to differences in the pharmacological models and differences in the pK_a range of the compounds in the two series. The authors argued that both studies showed that the un-ionized form of the drug is unimportant in antiarrhythmic activity. Because the CNS toxicity was a function of penetration into the CNS, the therapeutic index was correlated by an equation that was a minimum in log P [log P (optimum) $\neq$ 2.3] and $+pK_a$. In other words, the safest compounds were those that were not near the log P = 2.3, whereas the most active were near 2.6. Because these are mutually exclusive requirements, the only factor left for increasing selectivity is pK_a, with the more strongly basic compounds being less toxic. This prediction was not tested by new syntheses.

D. Conclusions

Although there is a reasonable amount of material on QSAR effects (mainly lipophilicity) of anesthetics on membranes, there are relatively few studies on the antiarrhythmic effects of nonspecific agents per se. The effect of nonspecific agents on membranes and ionic fluxes is reasonably well understood on a macroscopic level, and some direct studies on the membrane-bound enzymes that are thought to be involved have been discussed. However, there are still many unanswered questions, particularly on the microscopic level. The exact sequence of events, the exact binding sites and so forth are all subjects of continuing investigation.

The problem is also one of pharmacological relevance. For example, Baum *et al.* (*26*) have studied the effect of 16 diverse drugs on 7 different antiarrhythmic models (maximal atrial following frequency, antagonism

TABLE II
Coded Activities for 16 Drugs in 8 Antiarrhythmic Models[a]

Drugs	Activities[b] OV	FF	AC	OU	EH	FI	LA	BP
Quinidine	4[c]	4	4	4	4	4	3	3
Procainamide	3	4	3	4	2	4	2	3
Lidocaine	3	2	3	4	3	3	3	1
Diphenylhydantoin	2	2	4	4	2	2	x	2
Propranolol	3	2	2	4	4	4	3	1
Promazine	3	3	4	4	4	2	4	4
Imipramine	3	4	4	3	4	2	4	4
Promethazine	2	2	3	3	4	1	4	3
Chlorpheniramine	3	3	4	3	3	2	3	3
Bretylium	2	2	3	1	1	4	1	−1
Phentolamine	4	4	4	3	4	3	3	2
Atropine	2	3	2	3	3	1	2	4
Meperidine	2	2	3	4	3	1	2	4
Lorazepam	1	2	1	2	2	1	x	2
Diazepam	1	1	1	2	1	1	x	2
Mephentermine	1	1	3	2	2	1	2	−1

[a] See Baum *et al.* (*26*) for further description.
[b] OV = overall rating; FF = maximal following frequency; AC = aconitine; OU = ouabain; EH = epinephrine–methylchloroform; FI = ventricular fibrillarory threshold; LA = local anesthetic relative to procaine (guinea pig wheal); BP = depressor activity in open-chest dogs.
[c] 4 = marked, 3 = moderate, 2 = slight, 1 = inactive, −1 = stimulate, x = not tested.

of aconitine, ouabain and epinephrine–hydrocarbon induced arrhythmias, and electrically induced ventricular fibrillation in anesthetized dogs, in addition to local anesthetic activity). Each drug was active in one or more of the models. Quabain, epinephrine–hydrocarbon, and aconitine arrhythmias were relatively nonspecific assays, whereas ventricular fibrillatory threshold was the most selective. Their summary data (*188*, Fig. 8) have been coded and is given in Table II. Either including or omitting the overall and blood pressure variables gives a similar cluster analysis (BMDP2M) for drugs, shown in Fig. 5a. Quinidine, phentolamine, chlorpheniramine, imipramine, and promazine form one cluster; promethazine, meperidine, atropine, propranolol, lidocaine, and diphenylhydantoin form a second cluster. Mephentermine, bretylium, and lorazepam and diazepam form the third, more distant cluster. Procainamide is somewhat unique, joining clusters one and two later on. Quinidine and procainamide are in different clusters primarily because of the low value of procainamide in both epinephrine–hydrocarbon and local anesthetic assays. These two assays are highly correlated (74%).

A cluster analysis of the assays is shown in Fig. 5b. The overall rating is

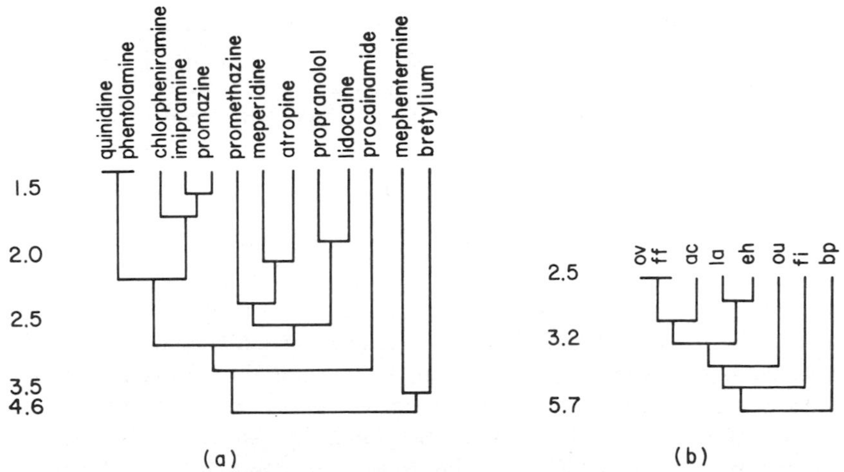

Fig. 5. BMDP2M Cluster analysis of Table II for (a) drugs and (b) antiarrhythmic models (see Table II for abbreviations). Numbers on left are amalgamation distances.

most closely associated with the maximal following frequency. Ventricular fibrillatory threshold is the most divergent, as is blood pressure. Finally, a principal compound analysis shows the following eigenvalues: 3.88, 1.77, 1.03, 0.78, 0.32, 0.12, 0.05, and 0.05, which show that there are four factors accounting for 93% of the variance (three factors account for 84%). The first factor contains about equal amounts of all components except ventricular fibrillatory threshold, which is the main component of factor two. Factor three is mainly aconitine and a negative ouabain, whereas factor four is maximal following frequency and blood pressure with negative epinephrine and local anesthetic activity.

These results show that existing drugs and methods studied are largely redundant (these data do not necessarily apply to the clinical situation, of course). The uniqueness of the ventricular fibrillatory threshold assay was not elucidated by the authors (*26*) but deserves further study. Local anesthetic activity is at least as good as other assays studied for measuring antiarrhythmic activity, and is quite similar overall to the epinephrine–hydrocarbon assay. Therefore, the general conclusions based on QSAR of anesthetic activity might be expected to be applicable for antiarhythmic activity.

V. INOTROPIC AGENTS

Agents for the treatment of cardiac failure were mainly limited to the cardiac glycosides in the past. Thomae has investigated a noncardiac glycoside and nonsympathomimetic agent AR-L 115 BS, designed with the help of QSAR. A large number of sympathomimetic agents of the dobutamine (Lilly) type (selective for force over rate of contraction) have been investigated recently, but no QSAR studies have appeared.

A. Cardiac Glycosides

A 1971 review (*7*) has summarized the putative mode of action of these compounds in terms of ionic flux: concentrations of digitalis causing inotropy cause only a moderate inhibition of (Na^+/K^+)-ATPase. This moderate inhibition of the Na^+ pump causes an enhanced intracellular Na^+ pulse over that normally occurring during membrane excitation. The link to intracellular free Ca^{2+} pulse is not yet known with certainty; however, the authors find this link to be plausible. Alternatively, either a decrease in intracellular K^+ or an increase in the Na^+/K^+ ratio following membrane excitation may be the key factor. Qualitative SAR and a model of the receptor have been presented recently (*228*).

Fullerton *et al.* (*81,192*) have attempted to correlate digitalis genin activity with structure. These compounds cause a moderate inhibition of membrane bound (Na^+/K^+)-ATPase (rat brain in this study). A series of 9 analogs (**XLII**: A = Me, CHO; B = H, OH; C = H, OH; D = H, OH)

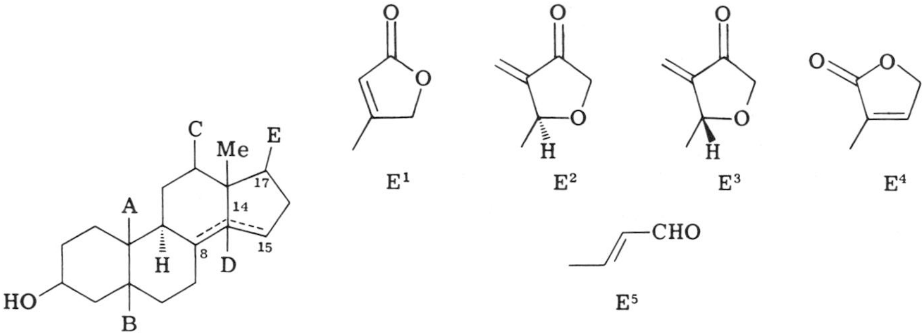

XLII

were studied. Rotation of the 17β side chain was studied by a version of CAMSEQ on the NIH PROPHET system starting from crystallographic coordinates. Ten-degree rotations using nonbonded and electrostatic potentials were used. No effect of the inclusion of H_2O was noted. Agreement was found between the calculated minima and crystallographic minima, therefore the crystallographic values were used in the next step. The PROPHET FITMOL program was used to superimpose structurally similar parts of the steroid backbone on the most active compound, digitoxigenin (**XLII**: A = Me; B = C = H; D = OH; E = E; saturated at positions 8 and 14) and to calculate various interatomic distances D (in Å), namely, carbonyl oxygens. A correlation was obtained with $+D$ (r = 0.997, $p = 0.0001$), suggesting that the enzyme binds the low energy conformer of each genin. The smaller D, the more strongly bound.

For this limited series, lipophilicity will not vary greatly and structural effects can dominate. However, the limited number of compounds and the fact that there are two subgroups with either high (about 5) or low (about 1) D means that this is essentially a two point correlation that limits the generality of the conclusions. It is an interesting integrated approach and inclusion of more compounds with intermediate D was planned by the authors for future work.

A similar approach was taken by Repke *et al.* (*188*) who investigated whether the permanent dipole moment of cardenolides was sufficient to explain biological activity. The *dpm* attraction relative to digitoxigenin was calculated from the crystal structure conformations and was correlated with log ID_{50} for (Na^+/K^+)-ATPase for eight analogs with $r = 0.95$. The larger the relative *dpm* attraction, the more potent the inhibitors.

An interesting study of cardiotoxic aglycons by the Minimal Steric Difference method of Simon has recently appeared (*207*).

A number of authors have discussed the importance of lipophilicity (*224*) or have presented pictorial models (*54,93,227,274*) along with qualitative discussions of SAR.

B. Other Nonsympathomimetic Agents

Austel and Kutter (*15,131*) have described the application of the theory of sets to drug design. Because new drugs must satisfy so many criteria (efficacy, safety, specificity, etc.), the authors stress the importance of the overall profile. The best drug is the one that satisfies multiple criteria. If the population of all drugs that satisfy a particular criterion is represented by an enclosed area, then the best drug will be located at the intersection of all relevant enclosed areas (the intersection of sets in a Venn diagram). The authors apply this logic to substructures as well. Thus they describe the discovery of Ar-L 115 (**XLIII**), a new cardiotonic agent under clinical investigation.

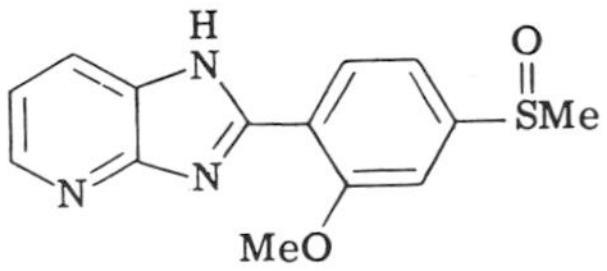

XLIII

The goals (profile) were higher intrinsic activity than cardiac glycosides, significantly higher therapeutic index (TI) compared to cardiac glycosides, no pronounced tachycardia at therapeutic doses, long duration of action, and oral activity. The universe of cardiotonic agents consisted of: steroids, phenylethylamines, peptides (glucagon), imidazoles (theophylline), and Ca^{2+} complexing compounds. Next, the systematic exclusion of subsets was applied. Steroids were considered unsuitable because of exhaustive literature work that has failed to improve upon the TI. Dobutamine was the only exception to the phenylethylamine class showing both duration of action and lack of tachycardia. This class was given low priority because of "experimental expense." Peptides were discarded because of problems of oral efficacy. Imidazoles were considered favorably, because aside from xanthines, other types have not been extensively investigated. Finally, Ca^{2+} antagonists were also considered favorably because some (not all) increased contractility (particularly the weakly complexing compounds).

On the basis of "chemical experience," the authors (*15,131*) chose **XLIV**

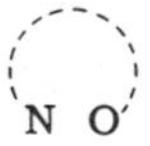

XLIV

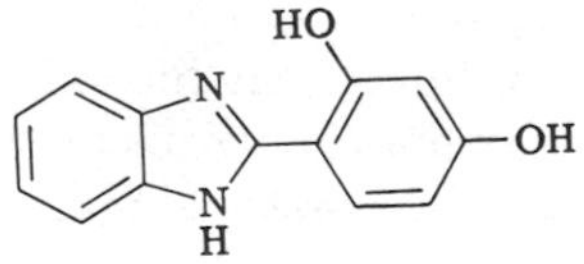

XLV

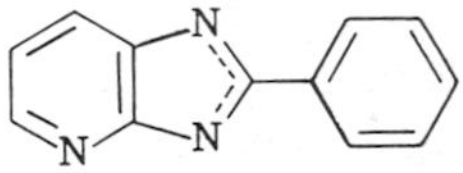

XLVI

as the Ca^{2+} pharmacophore. The authors then chose to examine the intersection of the imidazole set with the Ca^{2+} pharmacophore. Five subsets were defined on the basis of intuition, synthetic accessibility, and structural dissimilarity. Several examples of each subset were tested in the guinea pig atria. From this analysis only one lead was uncovered, which was also active *in vivo* (anesthetized cat model). The compound (**XLV**) had a higher intrinsic activity and TI than the cardiac glycosides and was not tachycardiac. It had a short duration of action and was not orally active, however. The relative potency was also low; it was not stated whether the compound was a Ca^{2+} antagonist. This lead was then optimized by looking at three substructural sets in order to define the pharmacophore more exactly. The imidazo[4,5-*b*]pyridines (**XLVI**) were found to be cardiotonic, and they extended the basic structure to this class. Further analysis showed that substitution on the imidazopyridine led to low relative potency and a further subset could be excluded. Another subset characterized by equilibrium protonation of the imidazole moiety was eliminated on the basis of obvious topological features, although these were not clarified.

Next, the 133 compounds examined thus far were subjected to a cluster analysis and divided into 20 classes on the basis of physicochemical properties. The following set of parameters were found to give a cluster of all actives: overall lipophilicity, *MR* of substituents on the outer part of the phenyl and the steric requirements of the ortho phenyl substituents (*16*). Electronic effects did not improve the classification. This analysis showed that a large substituent in the para position gave rise to lower activity. The

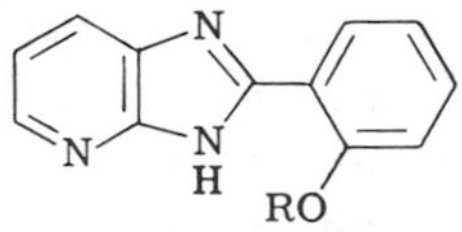

$\log P < 2.0$

XLVII

corresponding set could be excluded. Examples from each cluster were examined *in vitro* (rat atria) and *in vivo* (iv route in anesthetized cats). This interspecies comparison allowed nonether substituents in the ortho position to be excluded. Compounds with $\log P > 2$ were not long acting and allowed further exclusion. The resulting residue set could be described as **XLVII**. One of the members of the class, AR-L 115 BS, fulfilled the desired activity profile in both experimental animals and humans (another paper in the same volume).

Although this approach is rigorous, one can ask, is it logical? For example, the combination of the set of imidazoles with **XLIV**, the putative pharmacophore, should have led to a Ca^{2+} antagonist, but it was not stated that the Ar-L 115 had such a property (it may, but this is not the point). Furthermore, the construction of sets and intersection or exclusion of compounds is based on woefully sparce data. A compound may have the proper pharmacophore but be inactive for any number of reasons because of other properties of the molecule (absorption, distribution, metabolism, elimination, or interaction of pharmacophore with other parts of the molecule, for example).

C. Sympathomimetic Agents

Several qualitative discussions of sympathomimetic (adrenergic) stimulants and SAR have appeared (*134,244*), some with particular emphasis on conformational properties (*44,178*). Direct β-stimulants cause an increase in force (inotropic) and rate (chronotropic) of contraction of cardiac muscle. However, these agents also relax bronchi and uterine smooth muscle, decrease motility and tone of the alimentary tract, dilate blood vessels, decrease skeletal muscle spasm, stimulate glycogenolysis, glucolysis, lipolysis and secretion of insulin, and finally, inhibit the release of mast cell histamine and SRS-A, among other effects (*37*). Obviously, selectivity of action is a critical design criterion for sympathomimetics.

Direct β-stimulants increase inotropism and chronotropism of cardiac muscle, thereby increasing cardiac output, work, and myocardial oxygen consumption. This is accomplished by an increase in intracellular concentration of cyclic AMP in target tissues (*189,222*). β-Sympathomimetics bind to membrane receptors and activate adenylate cyclase via granine nucleotide binding (*223*). Adenylate cyclase catalyzes the conversion of ATP to cyclic AMP. The mechanism of action of cyclic AMP appears to involve the activation of a protein kinase which in turn regulates the activity of target enzymes via phosphorylation. The target enzymes are involved in the observed physiological response (Scheme III).

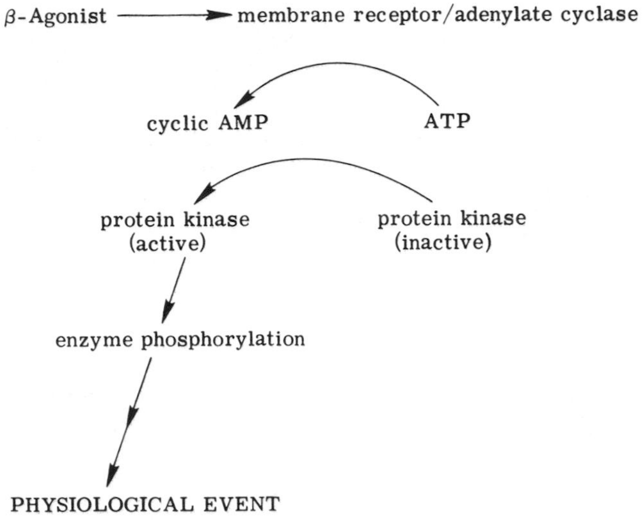

SCHEME III

The interaction of β-agonists with adenylate cyclase has been proposed (*27,244*) to involve a direct interaction of the agonist with ATP in the enzyme receptor. The charged NH^+ of the agonist neutralized the negative charge of the first phosphate, which is then subjected to nucleophilic attack by the 3-OH of the ribose, forming cyclic AMP and PP_i. The catechol OH (particularly the meta OH), aromatic portion, and aliphatic β-OH of the agonist serve to orient the molecule by specific binding. Substituents on the NH^+ bind to the adenine. This model is improbable because β-agonists bind to receptors located on the external surface of the plasma membrane and need not enter the cell to activate the adenylate cyclase (*189,222,223*).

Carlstrom *et al.* (*44*) summarized qualitative SAR conclusions based on X-ray, QM, and conformational and frozen rotomer analog studies (see **XLVIII**).

1. An aromatic six-membered ring system.
2. An extended ethylamine side chain approximately perpendicular to the ring system.
3. A positively charged tetracovalent nitrogen atom.
4. A hydrophilic and a hydrophobic side, i.e., with the hydroxyl group on the β-carbon atom cis to the meta phenolic hydroxyl group.
5. An *R* configuration at the β-carbon atom.

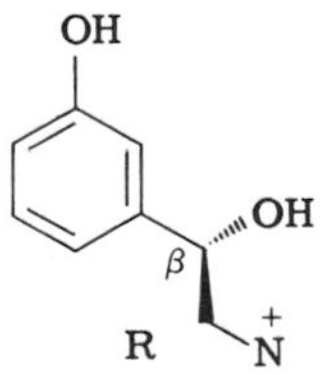

XLVIII

Bilezikian *et al.* (*34*) studied binding of over 50 catecholamines and analogs to turkey erythrocyte adenylate cyclase. Only qualitative SAR were attempted on this excellent collection of data.

A study of a number of β-agonists and blockers in isolated guinea pig atria and intact animal preparations has led to the proposal (*61*) of the existence of separate β-adrenergic chronotropic and inotropic receptors (*43*). Qualitative SAR showed (*61*) that the aliphatic nitrogen substituent of phenylephrine series (3-OH) (**XLIXa**), gave decreasing and then increasing selectivity with increasing chain length (or indistinguishably, lipophilicity). The synephrine (4-Oh) (**XLIXb**) series showed a similar tendency but was more selective for inotropic effects. The adrenaline (3,4-$[OH]_2$) (**XLIXc**) and terbutyline (3,5-$[OH]_2$) (**XLIXd**) series were not complete and no significant conclusions could be drawn.

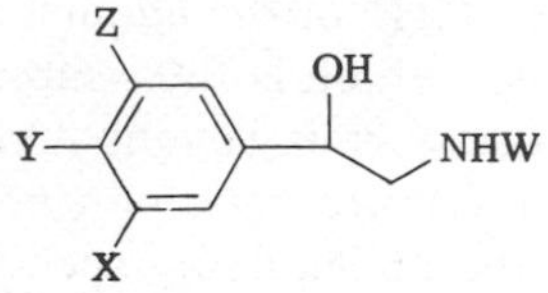

	X	Y	Z	W
a.	OH	H	H	Me
b.	H	OH	H	Me
c.	OH	OH	H	Me
d.	OH	H	OH	tBu

XLIX

Prastesi *et al.* (*181–183*) found that the selectivity of sympatholytics toward α- or β-adrenergic receptors is dependent upon the cationic head, namely, the inductive and steric effect of the alkyl group and hydrogen bonding or basicity of the nitrogen. Alpha (stimulation) reactivity is related to the acidity of the NH^+, aside from steric factors. Alpha effects are considered membrane effects and are primarily due to an interaction between the protonated base and a receptor chemical species ionic in nature, causing the breakup of a previously existing interaction (*183*). Beta (inhibition) reactivity was thought to be related to basicity of the nitrogen and to steric factors. Beta effects were metabolic (involving adenylate cyclase), and did not correlate with nonspecific lytic activity and the lipophilicity of the aromatic portion of the sympathomimetic. For series **L**, X,

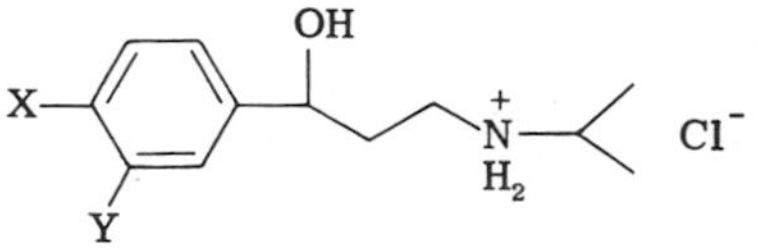

L

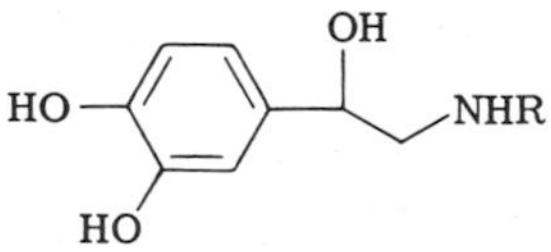

LI

Y = H, halo, alkyl, alkoxy, phenyl, or together rings C=CC=C or CCCC, the following equations were reported:

$$\mathrm{p}D_2' = 0.76 \sum \pi + 2.68 \tag{78}$$

$$\mathrm{p}A_2 = -0.84 \left(\sum \pi\right)^2 + 2.0 \sum \pi + 5.2 \tag{79}$$

$\mathrm{p}D_2'$ is the nonspecific binding (mean from rat vas deferens and intestine), $\mathrm{p}A_2$ is the agonist activity (mean guinea pig atria, calf tracheal, and rabbit intestine), $\Sigma\, \pi$ is the mean of the π values from phenoxyacetic, phenylacetic, and benzene systems. The quadratic expression was shown to possess considerable deviation about the parabola, due to other (unspecified) factors.

In a later study Pratesi *et al.* (*184*) found the following equations relating binding for **LI**:

$$pD_2^{\text{tracheal}} = 5.99 + 1.87E - 0.45E^2 \tag{80}$$

$$n = 9, \qquad r^2 = 0.977$$

$$pD_2^{\text{atrial}} = 6.64 + 3.24E - 1.09E^2 \tag{81}$$

$$n = 9, \qquad r = 0.977$$

where E is a steric term (pk and π not significant), that is, the ratio of the van der Waals volumes of the α to β moiety in R, where the N—C_α—C_β sequence is located.

George *et al.* (*82*) used Extended Hückel Theory to study the conformational properties of α- and β-adrenergic compounds. They concluded that the effect of aliphatic substitution on the nitrogen was not to influence conformation, but rather, for β-adrenergic activity through direct dispersion interactions on the receptor. Therefore, the nitrogen may not be required for activity. This observation was supported by the observation (*262*) that **LII** had modest β-adrenergic activity. α-Adrenergic activity involved hydrogen bond formation between the NH^+ and a sterically hindered receptor.

Mukherjee *et al.* (*173*) studied the qualitative SAR of 60 β-adrenergic compounds (**LIII**) on frog erythrocyte adenylate cyclase coupled β-adrenergic receptors. Both direct binding studies using inhibition of (−)-[^{3}H]alprenolol binding and the direct effects on the enzyme were measured. The two systems correlated (r = 0.95). For agonists, different SAR were found to determine receptor affinity and intrinsic activity. Affinity increased with larger substituents on the nitrogen, by a (−)-configuration of the β-OH and by a 3,4-$(OH)_2$ on the phenyl. Intrinsic activity was determined by phenyl substituents, a 3,4-$(OH)_2$ and also by (−)-β-OH. The authors do not discuss absolute configuration (R, S) requirements, only rotation (+, −). This is clearly in error.

These data have been subjected to SIMCA analysis in order to classify agonists, antagonists, or unclassified agents (*62,63*). SIMCA analysis is a principal components analysis of each class where a hyperbox is constructed about the defining hyperplane in order to define a region of maximum probability of class membership. Different numbers of variables may represent each class, but these are drawn from the same shopping list. In the agonist–antagonist example, agonists were classified by two principal components while antagonists were classified by one. A com-

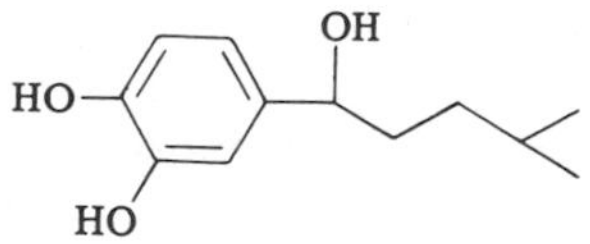

LII

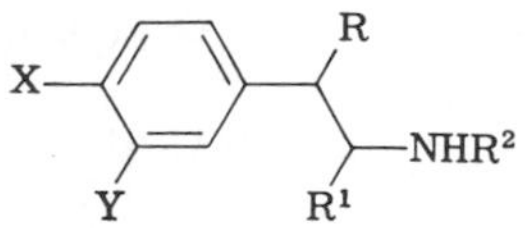

LIII

bined model with three principal components could describe both classes, using Hammett σ_p, Verloop L_p and B_p (B_4), Rekker f_{R_1} and f_{R_2}, Taft E_{s,R_2} and $\sigma^*_{R_2}$, the pK_a of the compound, and the pK_D for inhibition of alprenolol binding. On the basis of this model, 15/15 = 100% of agonists and 15/17 = 88% of antagonists were classified (i.e., 94% overall). When the inhibition of alprenolol binding constant was omitted, 13/15 = 87% of agonists and 15/17 = 88% of antagonists were correctly predicted (i.e., 88% overall). This level of prediction is often obtained in pattern recognition (PR) methods. One of the limits of SIMCA is a limit shared by all multivariate techniques, that the solution is limited to the substituent space chosen. Lack of a satisfactory solution is the usual criterion of adequacy of this substituent space. The SIMCA solution is considerably more detailed than the qualitative SAR given by the original authors (*173*). Similar levels of discrimination of agonist from antagonist activity for this data set has also been reported using molecular connectivity indices (*96*).

Tessel *et al.* (*226*) examined the effect of **LIV** on the maximal chronotropism of isolated guinea pig atria. The following QSAR was derived by stepwise regression using E_s, π, and σ:

$$Y = 30.59E_s + 35.42 \qquad (82)$$

$$n = 9, \qquad r = 0.843$$

Y is the maximum change in atrial rate from control, the numbers in parentheses are standard errors. Equation (85) is obtained for the maximum change in atrial rate in atria from pargyline pretreated guinea pigs.

$$Y' = 15.48E_s + 80.83 \qquad (83)$$

$$n = 9, \qquad r = 0.683$$

E_s is the only significant variable of those examined, but clearly Eq. (4) is inadequate because of low r. No QSAR was obtained in reserpine treated

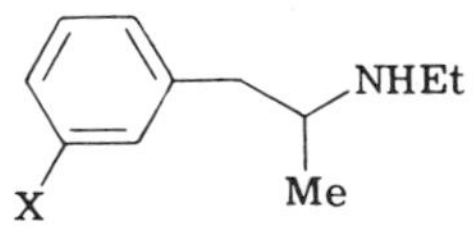

LIV

animals because only one compound showed chronotropism (X = OH). The drugs were therefore thought to be indirectly acting sympathomimetics, except for **LIV** (X = OH) by modulating the release of norepinephrine.

Mack and Bonisch (*152*) examined the partition properties of catecholamines and some of their metabolites and found a correlation with the log of the rate constants for efflux of O-methylated and deaminated metabolites of noradrenaline from perfused rat hearts ($n = 11$, $r = 0.856$) and rabbit aortic strips ($n = 5$, $r = 0.953$) with log G at pH 7.4. The influence of additional factors could not be excluded because of the low correlation coefficients.

A modified Free–Wilson analysis was performed by Ban and Fujita (*20*) on the nonepinephrine Uptake 1 and 2 inhibition of various sympathomimetic amines (**LV**) in rat heart. In addition to being a useful modification

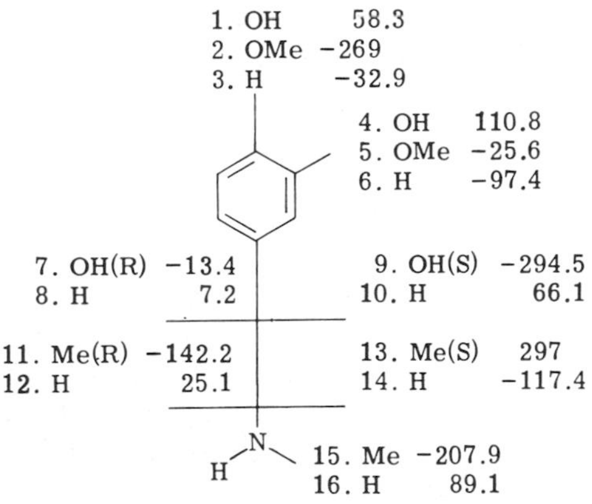

LV

of the Free–Wilson technique (*75*) this analysis was one of the first to attempt to handle optical activity in a quantitative manner by coding according to the absolute configuration. A "1" was used if the optical isomer presented a group to the putative receptor and a "0" was used if it did not; "0.5" was used for racemic compounds. The authors were able to obtain a reasonable solution and therefore concluded that norepinephrine uptake inhibition is subject to constant and additive activity contribution, which was taken to mean a constant stereoelectronic contribution. The conformations of the benzene ring and amino group were not expected to vary greatly, although minor changes might occur in compounds with bulky N-substituents. The large constant contributions of the ring OH suggests that these groups interact independently with the receptor site more strongly than with each other, whereas the constancy of the β-OH contribution does not necessarily mean that there is no intramolecular interaction with the α-amino group because this latter group is constant throughout the series.

Lukovits (*149*) obtained modified Free–Wilson group constants for the above and for several other sets of data (inhibition of phenylethanolamine *N*-methyltransferase, dopamine β-hydroxylase substrate activity, phenylethanolamine *N*-methyltransferase substrate activity, and antagonism of the pressor activity of epinephrine) and interrelated the group constants to one another ($r^2 \geq 0.8$). Only the antipressor activity failed to intercorrelate with any other series and phenylethanolamine *N*-methyltransferase substrate activity also did not correlate with inhibition of norepinephrine uptake. Although the author attempted to relate these results to putative molecular mechanisms, the small number of points upon which these correlations are based raises questions as to the validity of these conclusions.

Grunewald *et al.* (*55,263*) have applied QSAR techniques to the design of nonaromatic analogs of phenylethanolamine as inhibitors of phenylethanolamine *N*-methyltransferase.

D. Conclusions

Fullerton *et al.* (*81,192*) have an interesting line of investigation to pursue between conformational analysis and QSAR, but the work would benefit from the inclusion of considerably more analogs. Austel and Kutter (*15,16,131*) have an interesting methodological approach that should be verified against other types of activity. However, they have generalized concerning the nature of entire classes of compounds on the basis of only a few compounds.

QSAR studies in the area of β-agonists have been spotty. The data sets

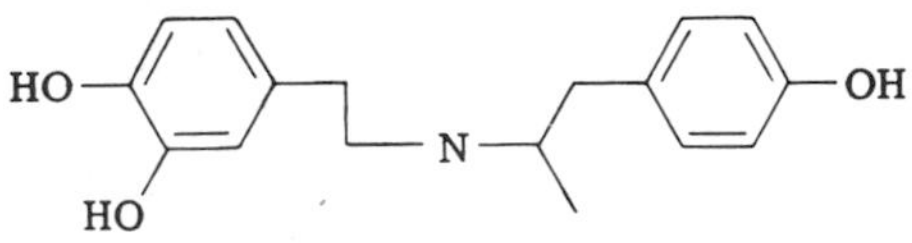

LVI

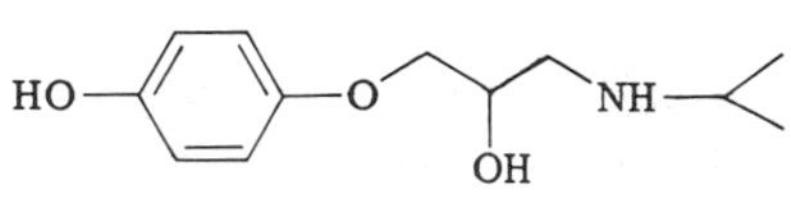

LVII

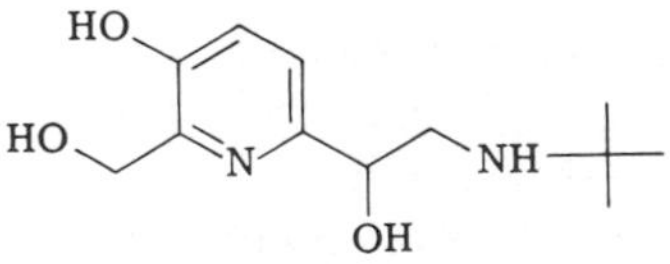

LVIII

are usually too small and have a too narrow structural variation to allow a completely satisfactory QSAR to be derived. Furthermore, the selectivity of these agents has only been addressed in a cursory fashion, and no unifying QSAR has been attempted. A further complication is the multiplicity of mechanisms, both indirect and direct, by which an agent can induce a chronotropic or inotropic effect, even within a given series of compounds (see Aviado [18] and discussions concerning **LVII**).

To data no QSAR work has appeared on the new generation of inotropic agents such as dobutamine (**LVI**) (*246*), prenalterol (**LVII**) (*43*), and pirbuterol (**LVIII**) (*19,205*), originally a bronchodilator.

VI. CONCLUDING REMARKS

It seems appropriate to attempt to tie this large collection of studies together at this point. Such a goal is frustrated in part because so many of the studies have been conducted *in vacuo*. Therefore, it is not appropriate to make sweeping generalizations as to the potential of the methods or the usefulness of particular predictions and models, nor is it appropriate to include the early primitive correlations that took $pC = a\pi + b\pi^2 + c\sigma + d$ too literally in the same way that some of the more modern approaches do.

In the area of β-blockers, the overall effort has certainly been worth the trouble. Not only is a fairly good picture of the β-receptor emerging, but one candidate (RS-51288) that was optimized with respect to three different types of activities has been taken into the clinic where it behaved as expected, although it was not as potent as one would have liked for commercial development (*47*). Unfortunately, the theoretical studies on depressivity have been a canard, inasmuch as the relevance of the *in vitro* studies and correlations to the clinical picture has been questioned.

A potent diuretic, muzolimine, was designed with the aid of QSAR techniques and a number of successful academic predictions have resulted from QSAR studies.

Some excellent work on clonidine-like antihypertensives has been published, and, again, a picture of the α-receptor is slowly emerging. QSAR has been instrumental in understanding the complicated mechanism of action of clonidine.

Antiarrhythmics have also benefited considerably from QSAR studies, particularly measurements of lipophilicity. Further study in this area may help to elucidate the nature of the membrane and electrical conduction. Understanding nonspecific effects can have a considerable impact on an understanding of the side effects of many drugs. A major difficulty, as in the case of the nonspecific effects of β-blockers, is the pharmacological relevance of the observations and correlations. Multivariate techniques have been helpful in detecting relevancy of particular assays.

In the area of inotropic agents the linking of conformational studies to QSAR has been useful, and a logic based method has produced a unique compound for clinical evaluation (Ar-L 115BS).

Therefore, despite the difficulties alluded to in the beginning concerning the pharmacodynamic nature of the biological activity, the QSAR approach has been instrumental in delivering no less than three clinical candidates. In addition, there have been many correct academic predictions and a considerable amount of understanding that would have been impossible without a systematic statistical model with which to evaluate data.

Acknowledgments. The author would like to thank Drs. R. Alvarez, R. Clark, C.-H. Lee, J. Muchowski, J. Pfister, J. Sims, and A. Strosberg for their help and comments on various sections of this work. Drs. V. Austel and P.B.M.W.M. Timmermans kindly provided preprints. Dr. J. Edwards provided the freedom to complete this review and many helpful comments. This is contribution number 571 from the Syntex Institute of Organic Chemistry.

REFERENCES

1. R. P. Ahlquist, *Am. J. Physiol.* **153,** 586 (1948).
2. R. P. Ahlquist, *Am. Heart J.* **97,** 137 (1979).
3. R. P. Ahlquist, *Am. Heart J.* **92,** 661 (1976).
4. R. P. Ahlquist, *Am. Heart J.* **93,** 117 (1977).
5. R. P. Ahlquist, *Am. Heart J.* **92,** 804 (1976).
6. H. Ahrens and J. Lauter, "Mehrdimensionale Varianzanlyse," Akademie-Verlag, Berlin, 1974.
7. T. Akera and T. M. Brody, *Life Sci.* **18,** 135 (1976).
8. S. Akiyama and H. Igisu, *Jpn. J. Pharmacol.* **29,** 144 (1979).
9. R. Alvarez, Inst. Biol. Sci., Syntex Res., Palo Alto, California, unpublished observations.
10. R. Alvarez and S. H. Unger, Insts. Biol. Sci. and Org. Chem., Syntex Res., Palo Alto, California, unpublished observations.
11. C. Appelgren, K. O. Borg, R. Elofsson, and K. A. Johansson, *Acta Pharm. Suec.* **11,** 325 (1974).
12. A. Aranda, *C. R. Acad. Sci. Ser. C* **276,** 1301 (1973).
13. E. J. Ariëns and A. M. Simonis, *in* "Beta-Adrenoceptor Blocking Agents" (P. P. Saxena and R. P. Forsyth, eds.), North-Holland Publ., Amsterdam, 1976.
14. D. Attwood and S. P. Agarwal, *J. Pharm. Pharmacol.* **31,** 392 (1979).
15. V. Austel and E. Kutter, *Arzneim.-Forsch.* **31,** 130 (1981).
16. V. Austel, E. Kutter, and W. Kalbfleisch, *Arzneim.-Forsch.* **29,** 585 (1979).
17. Australian Therapeutic Trial in Mild Hypertension, *Clin. Sci.* **57,** Suppl. 5, 499S (1979).
18. D. M. Avidao, "Sympathomimetic Drugs." Thomas, Springfield, Illinois, 1970.
19. N. A. Awan, J. Hermanovich, P. Skinner, and D. T. Mason, *Circulation* **60,** Supplement II, 229, Abstr. 895 (1979).

20. T. Ban and T. Fujita, *J. Med. Chem.* **12,** 353 (1969).
21. D. B. Barnett, E. L. Rugg, and S. R. Nahorski, *Nature (London)* **273,** 166 (1978).
22. A. M. Barrett, *J. Pharm. Pharmacol.* **21,** 241 (1969).
23. A. M. Barrett, *in* "Drug Design" (E. J. Ariëns, ed.), Medicinal Chemistry, Vol. III, p. 205. Academic Press, New York, 1972.
24. A. M. Barrett and V. A. Cullam, *Br. J. Pharmacol.* **34,** 43 (1968).
25. B. Basil, J. R. Clark, E. C. J. Coffee, R. Jordan, A. H. Loveless, D. L. Pain, and K. R. H. Wooldridge, *J. Med. Chem.* **19,** 399 (1976).
26. T. Baum, D. K. Eckfeld, A. T. Shropshire, G. Rowles, and L. L. Varner, *Arch. Int. Pharmacodyn.* **193,** 149 (1971).
27. B. Belleau, *Ann. N.Y. Acad. Sci.* **139,** 580 (1967).
28. B. G. Benfey, *Nature (London)* **256,** 745 (1975).
29. D. Bennet, R. Bal Con, J. Hoy, and E. Sowton, *Thorax* **25,** 86 (1970).
30. H. Bercher, W. Laass, E. Schultz, A. Grisk, and R. Franke, *Pharmazie* **34,** 336 (1979).
31. B. Berkoz, J. A. Edwards, and B. Lewis, *Am. Chem. Soc. Meet., 172nd, San Francisco, Calif.* Abstr. MEDI 014 (1976).
32. J. H. Biel and B. K. B. Lum, *Prog. Drug Res.* **10,** 46 (1966).
33. J. P. Bilezikian, A. M. Dornfeld, and D. E. Gammon, *Biochem. Pharmacol.* **27,** 1455 (1978).
34. T. P. Bilezikian, A. M. Dornfeld, and D. E. Gammon, *Biochem. Pharmacol.* **27,** 1445 (1978).
35. J. W. Black, *in* "Drug Responses in Man" (G. Wolstenholme and R. Porter, eds.), p. 111. Churchill, London, 1967.
36. P. A. Borea, A. Bonora, V. Bertolasi, and G. Gilli, *Arzneim.-Forsch.* **30,** 1613 (1980).
37. R. T. Brittain, C. M. Dean, and D. Jack, *Pharmacol. Ther.* **2,** 423 (1976).
38. J. Büchi and X. Perlia, *in* "Drug Design" (E. J. Ariëns, ed.), Medicinal Chemistry, Vol. III, p. 244. Academic Press, New York, 1972.
39. R. A. Burges and K. J. Blackburn, *Nature (London), New Biol.* **235,** 249 (1972).
40. A. Cammarata, *J. Med. Chem.* **15,** 573 (1972).
41. S. F. Campbell and J. C. Danilewicz, *Annu. Rep. Med. Chem.* **15,** 79 (1980).
42. E. Carlsson, B. Ablad, A. Brandstrom, and B. Carlsson, *Life Sci.* **11,** 953 (1972).
43. E. Carlsson, C.-G. Dahlöf, A. Hedberg, H. Persson, and B. Tångstrand, *Naunyn-Schmiedeberg's Arch. Pharmacol.* **300,** 101 (1977).
44. D. Carlstrom, R. Bergin, and G. Falkenberg, *Q. Rev. Biophys.* **6,** 257 (1973).
45. N. B. Chapman and D. J. Triggle, *J. Chem. Soc.* pp. 1385, 4835 (1963).
46. Y. W. Chien, H. J. Lambert, and T. K. Lin, *J. Pharm. Sci.* **64,** 961 (1975).
47. G. A. Christie, Syntex Res. Cent., Edinburgh, unpublished observations (1978).
48. R. Clarkson, *ACS Monogr.* No. 27, p. 1 (1976).
49. J. L. Coubeils, P. Courriere, and B. Pullman, *J. Med. Chem.* **15,** 453 (1972).
50. K. R. Courtney, *J. Pharmacol. Exp. Ther.* **213,** 114 (1980).
51. A. F. Crowther, R. Howe, and L. H. Smith, *J. Med. Chem.* **14,** 511 (1971).
52. R. H. Davies, *Int. J. Quantum Chem., Quantum Biol. Symp.* No. 6, p. 203 (1979).
53. R. H. Davies, *Int. J. Quantum Chem., Quantum Biol. Symp.* No. 4, p. 413 (1977).
54. C. S. Davis, and R. P. Halliday, *in* "Medicinal Chemistry" (A. Burger, ed.), 3rd ed., Part II, p. 1065. Wiley, New York, 1970.
55. D. P. Davis, R. T. Borchardt, and G. L. Grunewald, *J. Med. Chem.* **24,** 12 (1981).
56. P. W. Davis, and T. M. Brody, *Biochem. Pharmacol.* **15,** 703 (1966).
57. W. G. Davis, *J. Pharm. Pharmacol.* **22,** 284 (1970).
58. J. Dearden, *J. Pharm. Pharmacol.* **30,** 51P (1978).
59. A. P. deJong, and H. van Dam, *J. Med. Chem.* **23,** 889 (1980).

60. T. R. Dober, A. Kagen, and W. B. Kunnel, "The Framingham Heart Study," Natl. Heart Inst., Public Health Serv. U.S. Gov. Print. Off., Washington, D.C., 1966.
61. A. C. Dreyer, and J. Offermeier, *Pharmacol. Res. Commun.* **7,** 151 (1975).
62. W. J. Dunn, III, S. Wold, and Y. C. Martin, *J. Med. Chem.* **21,** 922 (1978).
63. W. J. Dunn, III, and S. Wold, *Biorg. Chem.* **9,** 505 (1980).
64. J. A. Edwards, B. Berkoz, G. S. Lewis, O. Halpern, J. H. Fried, A. M. Strosberg, L. M. Miller, S. Urich, F. Liu, and A. P. Roszkowski, *J. Med. Chem.* **17,** 200 (1974).
65. J.-D. Ehrhardt, B. Rouot, and J. Schwartz, *Eur. J. Med. Chem.—Chim. Ther.* **13,** 235 (1978).
66. S. Eletr, M. A. Williams, T. Watkins, and A. D. Keith, *Biochim. Biophys. Acta* **339,** 190 (1974).
67. E. Elonen, *Med. Biol.* **52,** 415 (1974).
68. K. Engelmann, W. Raake, and A. Petter, *Arzneim.-Forsch.* **24,** 59 (1974).
69. M. Erez, G. Schtacher, and M. Weinstock, *J. Med. Chem.* **21,** 982 (1974).
70. D. B. Evans, R. Fox, and F. P. Hauck, *Annu. Rep. Med. Chem.* **14,** 81 (1979).
71. J. D. Fitzgerald, *Clin. Pharmacol. Ther.* **10,** 292 (1969).
72. B. Fourcans and M. K. Jain, *Adv. Lipid Res.* **12,** 147 (1974).
73. J. E. Francis, *ACS Symp. Ser.* No. 27, p. 55 (1975).
74. N. P. Franks and W. R. Lieb, *Nature (London)* **274,** 339 (1978).
75. S. M. Free and J. W. Wilson, *J. Med. Chem.* **7,** 395 (1964).
76. W. Frishman, *Am. Heart J.* **97,** 663 (1979).
77. W. Frishman and R. Silverman, *Am. Heart J.* **97,** 797 (1979).
78. W. Frishman and R. Silverman, *Am. Heart J.* **98,** 119 (1979).
79. E. D. Frolich, *Hypertension* **1,** 547 (1979).
80. T. Fujita, *J. Med. Chem.* **16,** 923 (1973).
81. D. S. Fullerton, K. Yoshioka, D. C. Rohrer, A. H. L. From, and K. Ahmed, *Science* **205,** 917 (1979).
82. J. M. George, L. B. Kier, and J. R. Hoyland, *Mol. Pharmacol.* **7,** 328 (1971).
83. M. S. K. Ghouri and T. J. Haley, *J. Pharm. Sci.* **58,** 511 (1969).
84. S. L. Goodman, and K. P. Wheeler, *Biochem. J.* **169,** 313 (1978).
85. A. S. Graca and P. A. van Zwieten, *J. Pharm. Pharmacol.* **24,** 367 (1972).
86. D. M. Graeff, W. E. Johnson, C. D. St. Dennis, and A. R. Martin, *J. Med. Chem.* **14,** 60 (1971).
87. J. D. P. Graham and M. A. Karrar, *J. Med. Chem.* **6,** 103 (1963).
88. J. D. P. Graham and G. W. L. James, *J. Med. Chem.* **3,** 489 (1961).
89. C. M. Grisham and R. E. Barnett, *Biochim. Biophys. Acta* **311,** 417 (1973).
90. H. Grobecker, B. Lemmer, D. Hellenbrecht, and G. Wiethold, *Eur. J. Clin. Pharmacol.* **5,** 145 (1973).
91. C. Grunfeld and O. M. Rosen, *Pharmacologist* **13,** 256 (1971).
92. C. Grunfeld, A. P. Grollman, and O. M. Rosen, *Mol. Pharmacol.* **10,** 605 (1974).
93. T. W. Guntert and H. H. Linde, *Experientia* **33,** 697 (1977).
94. P. S. Guth and M. A. Spirtes, *Int. Rev. Neurobiol.* **7,** 231 (1964).
95. H.D.F.P. Cooperative Group, *J. Am. Med. Assoc.* **242,** 2562, 2572 (1979).
96. L. H. Hall, personal communication (1980).
97. C. Hansch and E. J. Lien, *Biochem. Pharmacol.* **17,** 709 (1968).
98. C. Hansch and W. R. Glave, *Mol. Pharmacol.* **7,** 337 (1971).
99. C. Hansch and W. J. Dunn, III, *J. Pharm. Sci.* **61,** 1 (1972).
100. W. P. Heilman, R. D. Heilman, J. A. Scozzie, R. J. Wayner, J. M. Gullo, and Z. S. Ariyan, *J. Med. Chem.* **22,** 671 (1979).
101. D. Hellenbrecht and K. F. Muller, *Experientia* **29,** 1255 (1973).

102. D. Hellenbrecht, B. Lemmer, G. Wiethold, and H. Grobecker, *Naunyn-Schmiedeberg's Arch. Pharmacol.* **272,** 211 (1973).
103. D. Hellenbrecht, K. F. Muller, and H. Grobecker, *Eur. J. Pharmacol.* **29,** 223 (1974).
104. D. Hellenbrecht and L. Gortner, *Naunyn-Schmiedeberg's Arch. Pharmacol.* **287S,** R32 (1975).
105. D. Hellenbrecht and L. Gortner, *Naunyn-Schmiedeberg's Arch. Pharmacol.* **287,** 227 (1975).
106. D. Hellenbrecht and J. Enenkel, *Naunyn-Schmiedeberg's Arch. Pharmacol.* **293S,** R22 (1976).
107. D. Hellenbrecht and L. Gortner, *Pol. J. Pharmacol. Pharm.* **28,** 625 (1976).
108. K. Hermannsen, *Br. J. Pharmacol.* **35,** 476 (1969).
109. W. Hoefke, W. Kobinger, and A. Walland, *Arzneim.-Forsch.* **25,** 786 (1975).
110. W. Hoefke, *ACS Symp. Ser.* No. 27, p. 27 (1976).
111. H. D. Höltje, *Arch. Pharm. (Weinheim, Ger.)* **309,** 480 (1976).
112. C. R. Honig and Y. S. Reddy, *J. Pharmaco. Exp. Ther.* **184,** 330 (1973).
113. H. Horstmann, E. Möller, E. Wehinger, and K. Meng, *ACS Symp. Ser.* No. 83, p. 125 (1978).
114. K. H. Hsieh, E. C. Jorgensen, and T. C. Lee, *J. Med. Chem.* **22,** 1038 (1979).
115. D. B. Jack, *Br. J. Clin. Pharmacol.* **11,** 402 (1981).
116. M. K. Jain, N. Y.-M. Wu, T. K. Morgan, Jr., M. S. Briggs, and R. K. Murray, Jr., *Chem. Phys. Lipids* **17,** 71 (1976).
117. M. K. Jain and N. Y.-M. Wu, *Biochem. Biophys. Res. Commun.* **81,** 1412 (1978).
118. M. K. Jain, N. Y.-M. Wu, and L. V. Wray, *Nature (London)* **255,** 494 (1975).
119. C. L. Johnson and A. Schwartz, *J. Pharmacol. Exp. Ther.* **167,** 365 (1969).
120. N. Kakeya, M. Aoki, A. Kamada, and N. Yata, *Chem. Pharm. Bull.* **17,** 1010 (1969).
121. N. Kakeya, N. Yata, A. Kamada, and M. Aoki, *Chem. Pharm. Bull.* **17,** 2000 (1969).
122. N. Kakeya, N. Yata, A. Kamada, and M. Aoki, *Chem. Pharm. Bull.* **17,** 2558 (1969).
123. N. Kakeya, N. Yata, A. Kamada, and M. Aoki, *Chem. Pharm. Bull.* **18,** 191 (1970).
124. H. K. Kimelberg and D. Papahadjopoulos, *J. Biol. Chem.* **249,** 1071 (1974).
125. W. Kobinger and Pichler, *Naunyn-Schmiedeberg's Arch. Pharmacol.* **291,** 175 (1975).
126. H. Kubinyi, *Prog. Drug Res.* **23,** 98 (1979).
127. V. M. Kulkarni, N. Vasanthkumar, A. Saran, and G. Govil, *Int. J. Quantum Chem., Quantum Biol. Symp.* No. 6, p. 153 (1979).
128. V. M. Kulkarni, *Curr. Sci.* **46,** 801 (1977).
129. G. Kunos, I. Vermes-Kunos, and M. Nickerson, *Nature (London)* **250,** 779 (1974).
130. E. Kutter and C. Hansch, *J. Med. Chem.* **12,** 647 (1969).
131. E. Kutter and V. Austel, *Arzneim.-Forsch.* **31,** 135 (1981).
132. W. Laass, H. Bercher, E. Schult, R. Franke, and A. Grisk, *Pharmazie* **34,** 334 (1979).
133. P. K. Lahiri and H. F. Hardman, *Arch. Int. Pharmacodyn.* **210,** 197 (1974).
134. A. M. Lands and T. G. Brown, Jr. *in* "Drugs Affecting the Peripheral Nervous System" (A. Burger, ed.), Vol. I, p. 399. Dekker, New York, 1976.
135. G. Leclerc, G.-G. Wermuth, F. Miesch, and J. Schwartz, *Eur. J. Med. Chem.—Chim. Ther.* **11,** 107 (1976).
136. G. Leclerc, A. Mann, C.-G. Wermuth, N. Bieth, and J. Schwartz, *J. Med. Chem.* **20,** 1657 (1977).
137. A. G. Lee, *Mol. Pharmacol.* **13,** 474 (1977).
138. C. Lemoulinier, J. M. Scheftel, G. Leclerc, C.-G. Wermuth, and J. C. Stoclet, *Eur. J. Med. Chem.—Chim. Ther.* **13,** 289 (1978).
139. A. Leo, P. Y. C. Jow, C. Silipo, and C. Hansch, *J. Med. Chem.* **18,** 865 (1975).
140. J. V. Levy, *J. Pharm. Pharmacol.* **20,** 813 (1968).

141. J. V. Levy, *Eur. J. Pharmacol.* **2,** 250 (1968).
142. E. J. Lien, M. Hussain, and G. L. Tong, *J. Pharm. Sci.* **59,** 865 (1970).
143. T. K. Lin, *J. Med. Chem.* **17,** 749 (1974).
144. T. K. Lin, *J. Med. Chem.* **17,** 151 (1974).
145. T. K. Lin, Y. W. Chien, H. B. Desai, and P. K. Yonan, *Chem. Pharm. Bull.* **24,** 2739 (1976).
146. T. K. Lin, Y. W. Chien, R. R. Dean, J. E. Dutt, H. W. Sause, C. H. Yen, and P. K. Yonan, *J. Med. Chem.* **17,** 751 (1974).
147. R. H. Lockwood and B. K. B. Lum, *Life Sci.* **14,** 73 (1974).
148. L. H. Loebis, *Arzneim.-Forsch.* **29,** 1853 (1979).
149. I. Lukovits, *Int. J. Quantum. Chem.* **20,** 429 (1981).
150. H. Lüllman, P. B. M. W. M. Timmermans, G. M. Weikert, and A. Ziegler, *J. Med. Chem.* **23,** 560 (1980).
151. B. Macchia, F. Macchia, and A. Martinelli, *Eur. J. Med. Chem.—Chim. Ther.* **15,** 515 (1980).
152. F. Mack and H. Bonisch, *Naunyn-Schmiedeberg's Arch. Pharmacol.* **310,** 1 (1979).
153. R. Maffei Facino and R. Lanzani, *Pharmacol. Res. Commun.* **11,** 433 (1979).
154. A. Makriyannis, *Abstr. Am. Chem. Soc. Meet.,* 177, *Honolulu* No. 95 (1979).
155. R. Mannhold, R. Steiner, W. Haas, and R. Kaufman, *Naunyn-Schmiedeberg's Arch. Pharmacol.* **302,** 217 (1978).
156. T. H. Maren, *J. Pharmacol. Exp. Ther.* **139,** 140 (1963).
157. A. Marques-Julio and E. M. Sellers, *Can. J. Hosp. Pharm.* **31,** 179 (1978).
158. Y. C. Martin, "Quantitative Drug Design. A Critical Introduction." Dekker, New York, 1978.
159. I. W. Mathison and P. H. Morgan, *J. Pharm. Sci.* **65,** 635 (1976).
160. W. L. Matier and W. T. Comer, *Annu. Rep. Med. Chem.* **14,** 61 (1979).
161. H. G. Mautner, C. Lorenc, P. Quain, J. K. Marquis, and I. Tasaki, *J. Med. Chem.* **23,** 282 (1980).
162. M. W. McCulloch, I. C. Medgett, M. J. Rand, and D. F. Story, *Br. J. Pharmacol.* **69,** 397 (1980).
163. D. G. McDevitt, *Drugs* **17,** 267 (1979).
164. C. M. Meerman-van Benthem, K. van der Meer, J. J. C. Mulder, P. B. M. W. M. Timmermans, and P. A. van Zwieten, *Mol. Pharmacol.* **11,** 667 (1975).
165. W. H. Miller, A. M. Dessert, and R. O. Roblin, Jr., *J. Am. Chem. Soc.* **72,** 4893 (1950).
166. K. P. Minneman and P. B. Molinoff, *Biochem. Pharmacol.* **29,** 1317 (1980).
167. E. Mizuta, K. Nishikawa, K. Omura, and Y. Oka, *Chem. Pharm. Bull.* **24,** 2078 (1976).
168. H. Moereels and J. P. Tollenaere, *J. Pharm. Pharmacol.* **27,** 294 (1975).
169. L. Molinengo, *Eur. J. Pharmacol.* **5,** 23 (1968).
170. P. H. Morgan and I. W. Mathison, *J. Pharm. Sci.* **65,** 467 (1976).
171. I. Moriguchi, Y. Kanada, and K. Komatsu, *Chem. Pharm. Bull.* **24,** 1799 (1976).
172. I. Moriguchi, K. Komatsu, and Y. Matsushita, *J. Med. Chem.* **23,** 20 (1980).
173. C. Mukherjee, M. G. Caron, D. Mullikin, and R. J. Lefkowitz, *Mol. Pharmacol.* **12,** 16 (1976).
174. E. J. Mylecharane and C. Raper, *Eur. J. Pharmacol.* **16,** 14 (1971).
175. W. G. Nayler, *J. Pharmacol. Exp. Ther.* **153,** 479 (1966).
176. P. Nuhn, J. Frenzel, and K. Arnold, *Pharmazie* **34,** 131 (1979).
177. P. N. Patil, *J. Pharm. Sci.* **59,** 1205 (1970).
178. P. N. Patil, J. B. LaPidiu, and A. Tye, *J. Pharm. Sci.* **59,** 1205 (1970).
179. Pomona College Medicinal Chemistry Project Data Listing, July 1980.
180. P. S. Portoghese, *Annu. Rev. Pharmacol.* **10,** 51 (1970).

181. P. Pratesi, *Proc. Int. Symp. Pharmacol. Chem.*, Florence, Italy, *1962* p. 435 (1963).
182. P. Pratesi and E. Grana, *Adv. Drug Res.* **2,** 127 (1965).
183. P. Pratesi, L. Villa, and E. Grana, *Farmaco* **21,** 409 (1966).
184. P. Pratesi, L. Villa, and E. Grana, *Farmaco* **30,** 315 (1975).
185. B. Pullman, J. L. Coubeils, P. Courriere, and J. P. Gervois, *J. Med. Chem.* **15,** 17 (1972).
186. J. S. Pushkin and T. Martin, *Mol. Pharmacol.* **14,** 454 (1978).
187. D. O. Rauls and J. K. Baker, *J. Med. Chem.* **22,** 81 (1979).
188. K. R. H. Repke, F. Dittrich, P. Berlin, and H. H. Portius, *Ann. N.Y. Acad. Sci.* **242,** 737 (1974).
189. G. A. Robison, R. W. Butcher, and E. W. Sutherland, "Cyclic AMP," Academic Press, New York, 1971.
190. R. Rodenkirchen, R. Bayer, R. Steiner, F. Bossert, H. Meyer, and E. Muller, *Naunyn-Schmiedeberg's Arch. Pharmacol.* **310,** 69 (1979).
191. J. A. Rogers and S. S. Davis, *Biochim. Biophys. Acta* **598,** 392 (1980).
192. D. C. Rohrer, D. S. Fullerton, K. Yoshioka, A. H. L. From, and K. Ahmed, *ACS Symp. Ser.* No. 112, p. 259 (1979).
193. G. M. Rosen and S. Ehrenpreis, *Arch. Int. Pharmacodyn. Ther.* **209,** 86 (1974).
194. O. M. Rosen, J. Erlichman, and S. M. Rosen, *Mol. Pharmacol.* **6,** 524 (1974).
195. A. P. Roszkowski, A. M. Strosberg, L. M. Miller, J. A. Edwards, B. Berkoz, G. S. Lewis, O. Halpern, and J. H. Fried, *Experientia* **28,** 1336 (1972).
196. S. H. Roth and P. Seeman, *Nature (London), New Biol.* **231,** 284 (1971).
197. S. H. Roth, *Annu. Rev. Pharmacol. Toxicol.* **19,** 159 (1979).
198. B. Rouot, G. Leclerc, C. G. Wermuth, F. Miesch, and J. Schwartz, *J. Med. Chem.* **19,** 1049 (1976).
199. B. Rouot, G. Leclerc, C.-G. Wermuth, F. Miesch, and J. Schwartz, *J. Pharmacol.* **8,** 95 (1977).
200. G. Satzinger, *Arzneim.-Forsch.* **27,** 1742 (1977).
201. Cited in A. K. Saxena and S. Ram, *Prog. Drug Res.* **23,** 199 (1979).
202. R. A. Scherrer and S. M. Howard, *ACS Symp. Ser.* No. 112, p. 507 (1979).
203. P. Schlieper, *Naunyn-Schmiedeberg's Arch. Pharmacol.* **287,** R33 (1975).
204. P. Seeman, *Pharmacol. Rev.* **24,** 583 (1972).
205. B. Sharma, J. Hoback, G. Francis, M. Hodges, R. W. Asinger, J. N. Cohn, and C. R. Taylor, *Circulation* **60,** II-229, Abstr. 896 (1979).
206. G. Shtacher, R. Rubinstein, and P. Somani, *J. Med. Chem.* **21,** 678 (1978).
207. Z. Simon, N. Dragomir, M. G. Plauchithiu, S. Holban, H. Glatt, and F. Kerek, *Eur. J. Med. Chem.—Chim. Ther.* **15,** 521 (1980).
208. M. Sinesky, F. Pinkerton, E. Sutherland, and F. R. Simon, *Proc. Natl. Acad. Sci.* U.S.A. **76,** 4893 (1979).
209. P. Singh and S. P. Gupta, *Indian J. Med. Res.* **69,** 804 (1979).
210. L. H. Smith, *J. Med. Chem.* **19,** 1119 (1976).
211. L. H. Smith, *J. Med. Chem.* **20,** 705 (1977).
212. L. H. Smith, *J. Med. Chem.* **20,** 1254 (1977).
213. L. H. Smith and H. Tucker, *J. Med. Chem.* **20,** 1653 (1977).
214. P. Somani, *J. Pharmacol. Exp. Ther.* **164,** 317 (1968).
215. A. R. Somerville and A. J. Coleman, Biochem. Dep., I.C.I. Pharm., Macclesfield, Cheshire, England cited in Refs. 48, 52, 53.
216. S. M. Stahl and H. Y. Meltzer, *Exp. Neurol.* **59,** 1 (1978).
217. A. M. Strosberg and A. P. Roszkowski, *Fed. Proc., Fed. Am. Soc. Exp. Biol.* **31,** 1991 (1972).

218. A. M. Strosberg, *Arch. Int. Pharmacodyn.* **222,** 200 (1976).
219. A. M. Strosberg, Inst. Pharmacol. Metab., Syntex Res., Palo Alto, California, unpublished observations.
220. H. Struyker Boudier, J. DeBoer, G. Smeets, E. J. Lien, and J. van Rossum, *Life Sci.* **17,** 377 (1975).
221. K. H. Sullivan, M. K. Jain, and A. L. Koch, *Biochim. Biophys. Acta* **352,** 287 (1954).
222. E. W. Sutherland, G. A. Robison, and R. W. Butcher, *Circulation* **37,** 279 (1968).
223. S. Swillens and J. E. Dumont, *Life Sci.* **27,** 1013 (1980).
224. K. Takiura, M. Yamamoto, Y. Miyaji, H. Takai, S. Honda, and H. Yuki, *Chem. Pharm. Bull.* **22,** 2451 (1974).
225. P. A. Tenthorey, A. J. Block, R. A. Ronfeld, P. D. McMaster, and E. W. Byrnes, *J. Med. Chem.* **24,** 798 (1981).
226. R. E. Tessel, J. H. Woods, R. E. Counsell, and G. P. Basmadjian, *J. Pharmacol. Exp. Ther.* **192,** 319 (1975).
227. R. Thomas, J. Boutagy, and A. Gelbart, *J. Pharm. Sci.* **63,** 1649 (1974).
228. R. Thomas, L. Brown, J. Boutagy, and A. Gelbart, *Circ. Res. Suppl.* **46,** I-167 (1980).
229. P. B. M. W. M. Timmermans and P. A. van Zwieten, *in* "The Pharmacology of Beta-Blocking Agents and its Relevance in Antihypertensive Treatment" (P. A. van Zwieten, ed.), p. 51. Exerpta Med. Found., Amsterdam, 1979.
230. P. B. M. W. M. Timmermans and P. A. van Zwieten, *Eur. J. Pharmacol.* **45,** 229 (1977).
231. P. B. M. W. M. Timmermans and P. A. van Zwieten, *Prog. Brain Res.* **47,** 391 (1977).
232. P. B. M. W. M. Timmermans, A. deJonge, J. C. A. van Meel, F. P. Slothorst-Grisdijk, E. Lam and P. A. van Zwieten, *J. Med. Chem.* **24,** 502 (1981).
233. P. B. M. W. M. Timmermans and P. A. van Zwieten, *Arch. Int. Pharmacodyn. Ther.* **228,** 237 (1977).
234. P. B. M. W. M. Timmermans, A. Brands, and P. A. van Zwieten, *Naunyn-Schmiedeberg's Arch. Pharmacol.* **300,** 217 (1977).
235. P. B. M. W. M. Timmermans and P. A. van Zwieten, *J. Med. Chem.* **20,** 1636 (1977).
236. P. B. M. W. M. Timmermans, P. A. van Zwieten, C. M. Meerman-van Benthem, K. van der Meer, and J. J. C. Mulder, *Arzneim.-Forsch.* **27,** 2266 (1977).
237. P. B. M. W. M. Timmermans, *Prog. Pharmacol.* **3** 25(1980).
238. B. Tinland, C. Decoret, and J. Badin, *Pharmacol. Res. Commun.* **4,** 195 (1972).
239. J. G. Topliss and M. D. Yudis, *J. Med. Chem.* **15,** 394 (1972).
240. J. G. Topliss and R. J. Costello, *J. Med. Chem.* **15,** 1066 (1972).
241. J. G. Topliss and M. D. Yudis, *J. Med. Chem.* **15,** 400 (1972).
242. J. G. Topliss and R. P. Edwards, *J. Med. Chem.* **22,** 1238 (1979).
243. N. M. Trieff, N. Venkatasubramanian, V. M. Sadagopa Ramanujam, T. R. Young, III, and B. Levy, *Tex. Rep. Biol. Med.* **34,** 315 (1976).
244. D. J. Triggle, *in* "Medicinal Chemistry" (A. Burger, ed.), p. 1235. Wiley, New York, 1970.
245. J. R. Trudell, *Anesthesiology* **46,** 5 (1977).
246. R. R. Tuttle and J. Mills, *Circ. Res.* **36,** 185 (1975).
247. S. H. Unger, *in* "Drug Design" (E. J. Ariëns, ed.), Medicinal Chemistry, Vol. IX, p. 47. Academic Press, New York, 1980.
248. S. H. Unger, K. Untch, B. Lewis, B. Berkoz, J. Edwards, A. Strosberg, R. Weissberg, and R. Alvarez, *in* "Chemical Structure–Biological Activity Relationships: Quantitative Approaches" (F. Darvas, ed.), p. 3. Akadémiai Kiadó, Budapest, 1980.
249. S. H. Unger, Ph.D. Thesis, MIT, Cambridge, Massachusetts, 1970.
250. S. H. Unger and C. Hansch, *J. Med. Chem.* **16,** 745 (1973).

251. S. H. Unger and C. Hansch, *Prog. Phys. Org. Chem.* **12,** 91 (1976).
252. S. H. Unger and G. H. Chiang, *J. Med. Chem.* **24,** 262 (1981).
253. U.S. Veterans Administration, Cooperative Study Group on Antihypertensive Agents, *J. Am. Med. Assoc.* **202,** 1028 (1967); **213,** 1143 (1970).
254. P. A. van Zwieten, *in* "The Pharmacology of Beta-Blocking Agents and its Relevance in Antihypertensive Treatment" (P. A. van Zwieten, ed.), p. 1. Excerpta Med. Found., Amsterdam, 1979.
255. P. A. van Zwieten and P. B. M. W. M. Timmermans, *J. Cardiovasc. Pharmacol.* **1,** 85 (1979).
256. P. A. van Zwieten and P. B. M. W. M. Timmermans, *Trends Pharmacol. Sci.* **1,** 39 (1979).
257. P. A. van Zwieten, *Br. J. Clin. Pharmacol.* **10,** 13S (1980).
258. D. E. Vatner and R. J. Lefkowitz, *Mol. Pharmacol.* **10,** 450 (1974).
259. E. M. Vaughan Williams, *Adv. Drug Res.* **9,** 69 (1974).
260. A. Verloop, W. Hoogenstraaten, and J. Tipker, *in* "Drug Design" (E. J. Ariëns, ed.), Medicinal Chemistry, Vol. VII, p. 165. Academic Press, New York, 1976.
261. P. Vermeij, *in* "The Pharmacology of Beta-Blocking Agents and its Relevance in Antihypertensive Treatment" (P. A. van Zwieten, ed.), p. 35. Exerpta Med. Found., Amsterdam, 1979.
262. L. Villa, V. Gerri, E. Grana, and O. Mastelli, *Farmaco, Ed. Sci.* **25,** 118 (1970).
263. W. C. Vincek, C. S. Aldrich, R. T. Borchardt, and G. L. Grunewald, *J. Med. Chem.* **24,** 7 (1981).
264. J. M. Walker and D. G. Beevers, *Drugs* **18,** 312 (1979).
265. A. Walland and W. Hoefke, *Naunyn-Schmiedeberg's Arch. Pharmacol.* **282,** R104 (1974).
266. D. F. Weetman, *Drugs Today* **13,** 261 (1977).
267. R. Weissberg, Inst. Pharmacol. Metab. Syntex Res., Palo Alto, California, unpublished observations.
268. C.-G. Wermuth, J. Schwartz, G. Leclerc, J. P. Garnier, and B. Rouot, *Clin. Ther.* **1,** 115 (1973).
269. G. Wiethold, B. Lemmer, D. Hellenbrecht, H. Grobecker, and D. Palm, *Naunyn-Schmiedeberg's Arch. Pharmacol.* **274,** R125 (1972).
270. G. Wiethold, D. Hellenbrecht, B. Lemmer, and D. Palm, *Biochem. Pharmacol.* **22,** 1437 (1973).
271. A. J. Wohl, *Mol. Pharmacol.* **6,** 195 (1970).
272. K. R. H. Wooldridge, *Chem. Ind.* (*London*) 478 (1980).
273. D. W. Woolley, *in* "The Transfer of Calcium and Strontium Across Biological Membranes" (R. H. Wasserman, ed.), p. 375 Academic Press, New York 1963.
274. A. Yoda and S. Yoda, *Mol. Pharmacol.* **11,** 653 (1975).
275. J. Zaggsma, *J. Med. Chem.* **22,** 441 (1979).
276. J. Zaggsma and W. T. Nauta, *J. Med. Chem.* **17,** 527 (1977).
277. J. Zaagsma and W. T. Nauta, *J. Med. Chem.* **17,** 507 (1974).
278. S. Zakhari, N. Pronayova, J. Drimal, and L. Molnar, *Bratisl. Lek. Listy* **62,** 678 (1974); *CA* **83,** 71485m (1975).

6

Antiallergic and Antiulcer Agents

RICHARD D. CRAMER III

I. INTRODUCTION

As a category, the QSAR of antiallergic and antiulcer agents is obviously a bit heterogeneous. Antiallergic therapy has been the ultimate objective of at least a dozen different approaches within recent years, and antiulcer therapy perhaps as many more. In these fields the pharmaceutical researcher usually has not had a thematically unifying objective such as "reduce blood pressure" or "kill microorganisms."

Yet such a diversity of pharmacological approach can make for a stimulating variety of topics to be reviewed. Certainly the following chapter includes some of the more clear-cut QSAR "success stories," either from a methodological or a clinical usage point of view. Also covered is a variety of molecular structures and drug design strategies.

QUANTITATIVE STRUCTURE–ACTIVITY
RELATIONSHIPS OF DRUGS

ISBN 0-12-695150-0

One recurring theme in this area is the strategy of seeking "end-organ antagonists," compounds that block an undesired effect of some natural messenger on some part of the body. Given this objective, many research groups have sought drug design insights by close study of the chemistry of the natural messenger itself. To embrace this work, I have assumed a broad definition of "QSAR," including any research where a serious effort to understand a structure–activity relationship in physicochemical terms seems to have been made. Thus quantum or classical molecular modeling and factor-analysis approaches are reviewed as well as the conventional substituent parameter–multiple regression techniques. Indeed, because this author has some working experience with these less common methods, an occasional attempt is made to draw a general lesson from some particular study.

II. HISTAMINE

Of these natural messengers, the most important within a chapter on antiallergic and antiulcer agents is clearly the histamine molecule (Fig. 1).

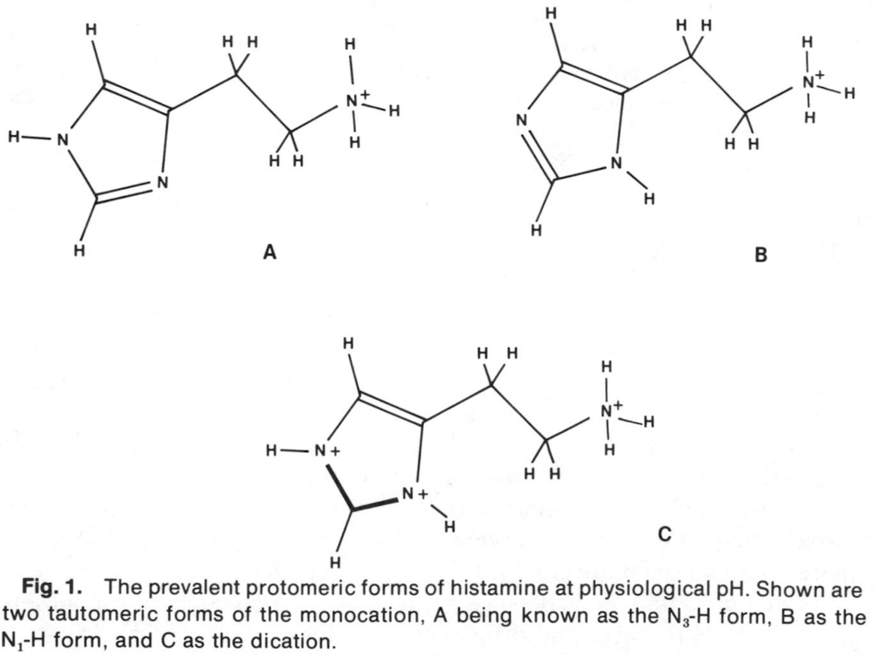

Fig. 1. The prevalent protomeric forms of histamine at physiological pH. Shown are two tautomeric forms of the monocation, A being known as the N_3-H form, B as the N_1-H form, and C as the dication.

The two best characterized actions of this physiological substance are the allergic response and the secretion of stomach acid. Drugs that block histamine-mediated components of the allergic response, the familiar antihistamines, are among the oldest of the mechanistically well characterized therapeutic agents, whereas the antiulcer action of the first agent found to block histamine-mediated stomach acid secretion, cimetidine, is a most recent reminder of the dramatic benefits that industrial pharmaceutical research can confer upon mankind. These two types of histamine response are said to be mediated by H_1 and H_2 receptors, respectively (*5*).

Although histamine itself consists of only eight skeletal atoms, it resembles many other physiological transmitters in being able to present a wide variety of shapes, or "pharmacophores," to a receptor. This protean nature of histamine arises from two of its properties (*17,18,36,47,101*). First, it has three basic nitrogens, each capable in principle of acquiring a proton and positive charge. As it happens, the ring nitrogens have similar proton affinities, and this similarity means that the neutral ring can also exist in two tautomeric forms of opposite dipole moment, denoted in Fig. 1 as forms A and B and designated in this review as the N_3-H and N_1-H forms, respectively. Second, the ring and amino nitrogens are attached by a freely rotating two-carbon chain, allowing the (possibly) charged centers to exist in a wide variety of relative geometries. The gauche and trans geometries of the N_3-H histamine monocation in Fig. 2 represent two such "conformeric" possibilities.

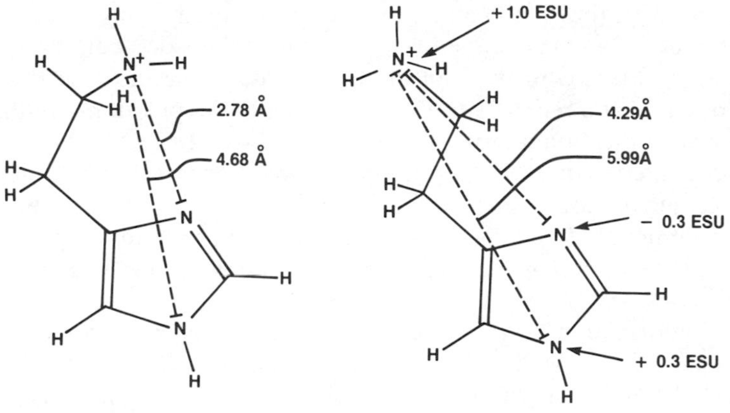

A B

Fig. 2. Two extreme conformers of the N_3-H monocation, showing the assumptions made for a classical calculation of their relative energy contents.

Because of the small differences of intrinsic energy content among the protomers and conformers of histamine, it is certain that the shape and charge state of histamine in a receptor environment could differ significantly from those for environments of histamine that are experimentally observed in solution or in a crystal. The energies of histamine–receptor binding (directly calculable from p*A* as 5–10 kcal/mol) are much greater than the relative energies of ring tautomers or of bond rotation in substituted ethanes (experimentally, up to 2 kcal/mol). And even if methods are ultimately found for studying the structure of a static histamine–receptor complex, there will still be the possibility that the dynamic process of receptor activation requires the protean nature of histamine. To put the latter argument differently, histamine must actually "do something" to its receptor because the interaction changes the state of the receptor. Because the receptor is a much bigger molecule than histamine, is it plausible that histamine can "do something" to the receptor without itself being "done to"? (*97*). See a counter example (β-agonist) below (*85*).

The foregoing arguments suggest that fundamental understanding of a histamine–receptor interaction might arise only from theoretical calculations of all the pharmacophoric possibilities for histamine and comparing these possibilities with those for related compounds tested for histamine agonism. Richards *et al.* (*98*) have taken some first steps in this direction. However, physical measurements are in general desirable to use to check present theoretical calculations, and in the particular case of histamine they might be helpful in reducing the number of protomeric forms to undergo calculation. Histamine is dibasic and has pK_a values at 37°C of 5.80 and 9.40 (*87*). The more acidic proton is associated with the ring and the less acidic with the side chain. Thus at a typical physiologic pH of 7.4, over 96% of histamine in aqueous solution is in the side-chain protonated monocation form. However, an increase or decrease of a pH unit, certainly possible at a receptor site, would bring the population of either the uncharged or dicationic form, respectively, above 10% (*44*). With regard to the dominant neutral ring form, NMR measurements and pK_a measurements on model compounds agree in assigning a 4:1 preference for the N_3-H protomer (*44,96*). In summary, physical data are consistent with any of four protomers of histamine being candidates for binding with a receptor.

The conformational preferences of the two major histamine monocations have been a subject of controversy (Table I). The relatively unsophisticated EHT quantum method predicts that the trans form is slightly more stable than the gauche form (*40,70,100*), a conclusion that is supported by NMR data in aqueous solution (*20,49,56,64*). But more sophisticated calculations, e.g., PCILO (*25,91*), assign greater stability to the

TABLE I
Quantum Calculations on the Conformation of the Histamine Monocation

Method	Species (position of ring H)	Energy (kcal/mol) (*trans*–*gauche*)[a]	Reference
EHT	N_3-H	~0.0	*70*
EHT	N_1-H	−1.0	*50*
CNDO	N_3-H	+3.7	
EHT	N_1-H	−1.0	
CNDO	N_3-H	+6.2	
CNDO, counterion	N_1-H, N_3-H	−0.5	*1*
PCILO	N_3-H	+11.0	*91*
ab initio (gaussian 70; STO3G)	N_3-H	+21.0	
PCILO	N_3-H + $4H_2O$	−3.0	
FSGO	N_3-H	+9.0	*105*

[a] Positive values imply a more stable gauche form.

trans form. Why does the unsophisticated quantum technique yield results in better agreement with experiment?

A completely unsophisticated calculation based strictly on Coulomb's law gives some insight into the situation. To a first approximation, one can view the N_3-H form of the histamine cation as a charge (side chain) next to a dipole (ring), the imino nitrogen being the negative end of the imidazole dipole (Fig. 2). There will be an attraction between the dipole and the cation, the magnitude of which is readily calculated by summing the individual electrostatic interactions using Coulomb's law (*61*):

$$E = \frac{332.0}{e}\left(\frac{q_1 q_2}{r_{12}} + \frac{q_1 q_2}{r_{13}}\right)$$

where q_1, q_2, and q_3 are the charges centered on the side-chain ammonium, the imino imidazole nitrogen, and the amino imidazole nitrogen, respectively; r_{12} and r_{13} are the distances between these centers; the number 332.0 converts the electrostatic units to kcal/mol; and e is the dielectric constant. Assuming q_1, q_2, q_3, r_{12}, and r_{13} to have the values shown in Fig. 2 and $e = 1$, as is implicit in most quantum chemical calculations, the Coulombic energy contents of the gauche and trans forms are −14.56 and −6.57 kcal/mol, respectively, the gauche thus being the more stable conformer by 7.99 kcal/mol. Because in classical terms any other (steric or torsional) contributions to a gauche–trans energy difference are relatively small, a quantum calculation should for these environmental assumptions also predict the gauche form to be the more stable. And as one would hope, the sophisticated more quantum methods do give the correct answer.

Why then do experimental measurements indicate the trans and gauche forms to be about equal in energy (according to NMR, a trans/gauche ratio of 54/46 in water)? The answer lies in the effect of the medium, which attenuates the electrostatic attractions of the charges. To continue these approximate calculations, the bulk dielectric constant of water is 78. If all Coulombic energies above are multiplied by 1/78, the electrostatic contribution favoring the gauche over the trans form is reduced to 0.10 kcal/mol, and steric and torsional factors could then be of equal or greater importance. The presence of a counterion (*1*) or of explicit solvent molecules (*91*) for the side-chain cationic nitrogen would also dampen the electrostatic gauche–trans energy difference to a greater or lesser extent depending on location.

Presumably the dielectric constant of the pharmacologically interesting environment, the histamine receptor, is somewhere between 1 and 78. Crystals tend to have bulk dielectrics of around 4 (*114*), and thus frequently encountered guesses from 3.5 to 10 seem reasonable. In summary, as in the case of the physical measurements on protomers, these and other (*88*) quantum calculations and measurements of histamine conformer populations serve only to confirm the idea that histamine could be binding to a receptor in many different ways.

A. H_1 Antagonists: Classical Antihistamines

The antihistaminic drugs used in the treatment of allergies are numerous and varied. Most structures are characterized by a basic tertiary amine separated by a two- or three-atom chain from a diarylmethane moiety. Some examples appear in Fig. 3. The two main objectives in drug design studies of these molecules are: synthesis of rotationally constrained molecules in hopes of identifying the "active conformation" of histamine itself at the H_1-receptor site; and QSAR studies intended to define the optimal substituent pattern for antagonism.

To draw inferences about histamine's active conformation from blockade of its effects by rigid analogs, one must assume that the rigid antagonists bind in an identifiably similar way to histamine. More specifically, one must identify the "primary cationic amine" and the "imidazole ring" with its "imine" or "amine" nitrogen in each antagonist and assume that these occupy the same relative receptor positions as do these elements in histamine. Such pharmacophoric identities must usually be based on substructural similarities, not shape or charge, and unavoidably include a subjective component. In the case of histamine and its antago-

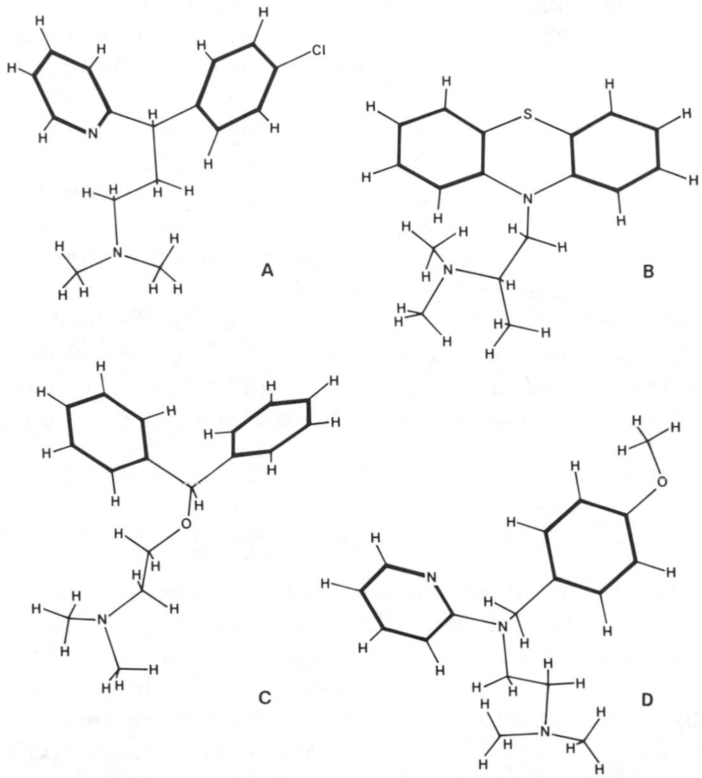

Fig. 3. Four classical H_1 antagonists in clinical use. Structure A is chlorpheniramine; structure B, promethazine; structure C, diphenhydramine; and structure D, pyrilamine.

nists, these identifications may seem relatively secure, but for example, all the most potent antagonists have a three- or four-carbon chain rather than the two-carbon chain of histamine.

Another reservation in the interpretation of these studies is the great lipophilicity of these antagonists, which lessens the difference in potency between receptor-mediated and nonspecific H_1 antagonism, whereas it increases the many other pharmacological activities (anticholinergic, antidopaminergic, etc.) that classical antihistamines so frequently exert. The nonspecific and receptor-mediated (competitive) antagonistic potencies even appear to be correlated, but this is in fact an artifact of the test system design (*109*). Because of all these reservations, the number of studies of rigid antagonists (*15,19,21,58*) are only perhaps most consistent with the proposition that histamine interacts with the H_1 receptor in a trans-like configuration. There is also a mild correlation between pA_2 and the proportion of trans rotamers in D_2O solution from NMR among a series of antihistamines that can be described as 1,2-disubstituted ethanes (*55*).

The most complete QSAR studies of analog series of H_1 antagonists have been done on diphenhydramine derivatives (Fig. 3B) substituted variously on the aryl rings. Early correlations involved the rate of hydrolysis of the benzhydryl ether (*73*) or UV and IR spectra (*93,94*). Multiparameter correlations, involving the classical trio of substituent parameters, π, σ, and E_s as well as several dummy parameters, have been carried out by several workers, most notably the Dutch school of Rekker and Nauta. Their equations are to be related to a model in which the less substituted ring binds to the receptor and the other ring is optimally placed for orbital overlap with the nitrogen. The best equation in their first study (*95*) is:

$$pA_2 = 0.35 \sum E_s^{o,m} + 0.68E_s^p - 0.46(E_s^p)^2 - 3.06\sigma_p' + 3.74 \qquad (1)$$

$$n = 16, \quad r = 0.960, \quad s = 0.294$$

where $E_s^{o,m}$ is the sum of the Taft steric parameters for all ortho and meta substituents, E_s^p the Taft parameter for the para substituent in the receptor-binding ring, and σ_p' is a Taft resonance parameter for the para substituent in the other ring. Potency decreases with the size of ortho and meta substituents, is optimal in the case of methyl in the para position of one ring, and is increased by electron donating (via resonance) substituents in the other para position. Unfortunately, one worries that the compounds on which this equation is based appear to have a high degree of colinearity among their substituent parameters, and thus firm conclusions are risky.

A second study treated variations in the alkyl substituents on the nitrogen end of diphenhydramines (*59*):

$$pA_2 = 1.38D + 2.8l - 0.42l^2 - 0.71\pi_n^+ - 1.25 \log P - 0.12 \qquad (2)$$

$$n = 27, \quad r = 0.928, \quad s = 0.370$$

where $D = 1$ if there is a 4-methyl group; l is a distance (Å) perpendicular to the main axis of the molecule; and π_n^+ is a difference between experimental and calculated log P values. As can be seen, the equation defines an optimal length and implies that increased hydrophilicity enhances activity. The latter interesting trend, taken with the absence of a lipophilicity effect in Eq. (1), suggests the possibility of discovering a potent antihistamine lacking the ability to cross the blood–brain barrier. Because antihistamines are used clinically to block peripheral allergic responses, and undesirable effects such as drowsiness are probably associated with CNS entry, such an agent would seem to have great therapeutic utility. One might also hope for greater selectivity vis-à-vis other receptors from less lipophilic H_1 antagonists.

The same group extended its QSAR work to a collection of seven different diarylalkylamine series (*95,113*), obtaining an "extended QSAR" correlating all data reported with an impressive r^2 of 0.928:

$$\begin{aligned} pA_2 = {} & 1.243(f_{\text{cis}}) + 1.19D_2 + 0.57D_3 + 0.38D_4 \\ & + 1.35D_5 + 0.93D_6 + 0.62D_7 + 5.19 \end{aligned} \tag{3}$$

$$n = 37, \quad \gamma = 0.963, \quad s = 0.332$$

The variance not accounted for by dummy parameters for each series is explained by a strong increase in H_1 antagonism with increased lipophilicity. However, there are inconsistencies between this and their previous studies. A minor problem noted in their paper is that for this study unsymmetrically substituted diphenhydramines were aligned so that the larger para substituent binds rather than hangs free as before. The serious problem is the omission of the 4-ethyl-, 4-isopropyl-, and 4-*tert*-butyldiphenhydramines from the extended QSAR, compounds whose steadily decreasing potency had in the previous study been responsible for the E_s^p term in Eq. (1). The extended QSAR, with its strongly positive correlation between potency and lipophilicity, would have overpredicted the activity of these congeners by factors of $\times 15$, $\times 250$, and $\times 16{,}000$, respectively. And no indication is given that these three compounds were omitted in the derivation of the new equation. This oversight is not easy to understand.

A series of 2-pyridylethylamines variously substituted on the nitrogen amine has been studied by Van den Brink and Lien (*109*). They find a somewhat better correlation with log(molecular volume) than with log P, but the two properties are so highly correlated within this data set that the difference is not significant. And a study by Kutter and Hansch (*75*) is noteworthy as an early use of the Taft E_s parameter in QSAR work.

B. Cimetidine: The H_2 Antagonist

Discovery of an effective treatment for ulcers was the result of a systematic search for a substance that would block the "second" histamine receptor, that is, the histamine-induced secretion of stomach acid not affected by classic antihistamines. The search, which involved a half dozen years of frustration for an entire laboratory before any tangible progress was made, is unusually well documented and has been carefully and candidly reviewed (*12,32a,46,48*), at least once as an example of "rational drug discovery" (*10*). Such a label could be questioned by a medicinal chemist of classical persuasion on the basis that a key discovery, lengthening the chain, is a very old practice and by a QSAR specialist because of the group's preference for attempting to vary just one property at a time rather than treat their data with multivariate computer methods. Luck surely played some role in the discovery of cimetidine, as indeed would have to be the case, given the present-day paucity of knowledge about drug action. On the other hand, the publication record indicates a consistent effort to understand drug action at the physicochemical level rather than the structurally or topologically descriptive level with which many synthetically trained medicinal chemists are content.

Given the task of designing an antagonist to a known natural transmitter, a reasonable approach would be to add a "secondary binding" site to a bulk tolerant position of the transmitting substance. This objective was the major factor in the synthesis of all the possible monomethylated histamines (*19,35,50*). Of these, 4-methylhistamine proved to be a selective H_2 agonist having 43% of histamine's H_2 potency but only 0.23% of histamine's H_1 activity. Kier had postulated that the H_1 receptor responds to trans, or fully extended, histamine and the H_2 to gauche histamine (*70,71*). The 4-methyl substituent sterically prevents the fully extended form, and thus its H_1 inactivity is generally consistent with Kier's postulate, although the trans conformer, which the 4-methyl group totally excludes, is a relative maximum having all histamine atoms in a plane, whereas Kier's "H_1 active form" is the local minimum with the α,β-carbon making a 120° dihedral angle with the ring (*45*). In any case, as discussed earlier, histamine can readily adopt a wide range of conformations, and the effect of the 4-methyl group might better be characterized as restricting the range of conformations rather than excluding a unique conformer. Richards and Ganellin used EHT to compute the range of conformations energetically excluded to 99% of histamine and 4-methylhistamine molecules (Fig. 4). The shaded area, representing the conformational difference between the two compounds, presumably contains an "H_1-essential" conformation (*41,99,100*). Similar conclusions have been reached in studies of the same two molecules using classical energy calculations (*65*).

The breakthroughs to an H_2 antagonist came with the successive discoveries of modest antagonism at high doses of the agonistic guanidine analog of histamine, enhancement of both effects with side-chain extension, and removal of the agonist property by replacing the charged guanidine by the still polar but uncharged thiourea moiety (Table II). These changes would seem to embody more of the perspiration of classical ap-

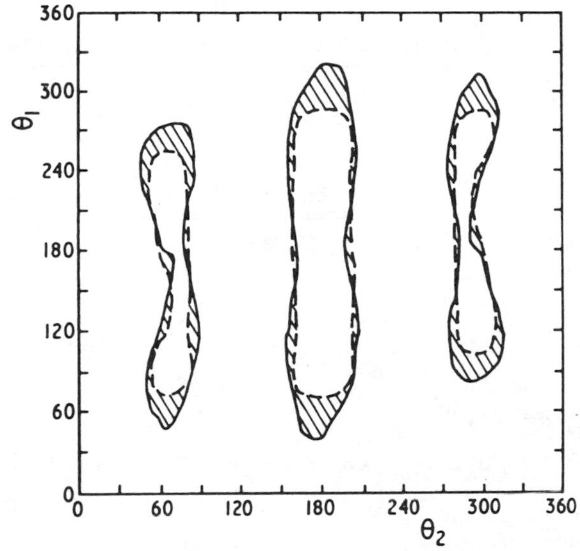

Fig. 4. Map of the conformations allowed to 4-methylhistamine (clear circled areas) and to histamine (clear plus hatched areas), where conformations up to 0.1 eV above the minimum are assumed to be allowed. The hatched area is the postulated H_1-essential region.

proaches than the inspiration of rational approaches. But from this point an unusually physicochemical orientation of the chemists involved is suggested by the steps that converted burimamide, a compound having the desired pharmacological profile but insufficient potency especially on oral administration, to cimetidine (*9*). First, it was assumed that the imidazole ring in a potent H_2 antagonist should have properties similar to the ring in histamine. But because the uncharged side chain of burimamide, in contrast to the charged histamine side chain, has little effect on the imidazole, the proportion of the N-H tautomer in burimamide is much lower than in histamine. To reproduce the inductive effect of the charge on the histamine tautomer populations, while keeping all other physical properties of burimamide as constant as possible, the second CH_2 in burimamide was replaced by S. Although S for CH_2 as a bioisosterism has been used next to aryl rings, especially in tricyclics, it has seldom if ever been used in the middle of a methylene chain. The S also enhances chain flexibility. The 4-methyl group that first produced a selective H_2 agonist also appears in metiamide, a clinically useful H_2 antagonist 10 times more potent *in vitro* than burimamide. Their central postulate, that steric and electronic influences dominate the effect of imidazole substituents on potency in this series (*39*), has been confirmed by a QSAR study reported in 1980 (*118*).

TABLE II
Some Key Compounds in the Development of H_2-Receptor Antagonists

Compound	Structure	Antagonist activity: *In vitro* K_B[a] ($\times 10^{-6}$ *M*)	Antagonist activity: *In vivo* ID_{50}[b] (μmol kg^{-1})
N^{α}-Guanylhistamine: the lead; a weakly active partial agonist	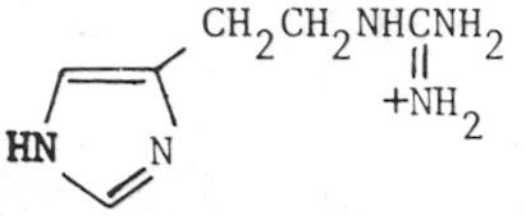	130	800
SK&F 91486: lengthening the side chain increases activity	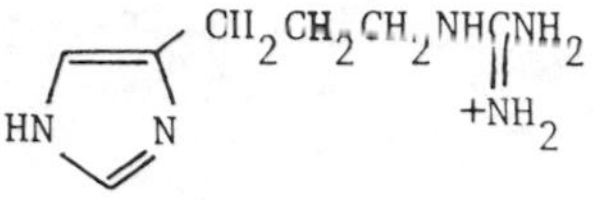	22	100
SK&F 91581: thiourea analog is much less active as an antagonist, but is not an agonist	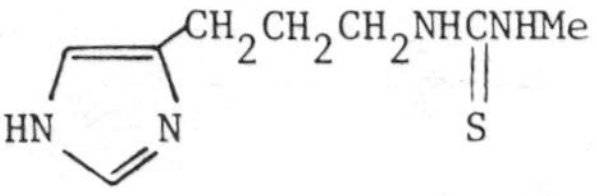	115	*c*
Burimamide: lengthening the side chain again dramatically increases antagonist activity	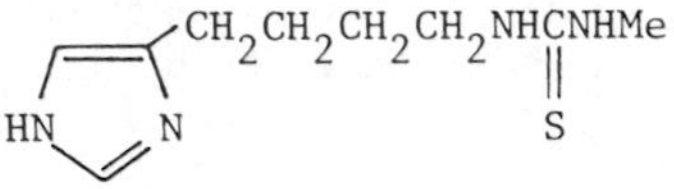	7.8	6.1
Metiamide: introducing S in the side chain and CH_3 in the ring alters imidazole tautomerism and increases activity	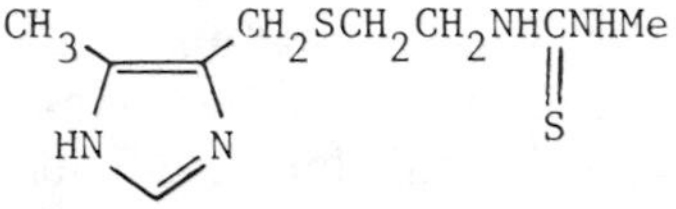	0.92	1.6
Guanidine isostere: replacing C=S by C=NH gives a basic side chain and reduces activity	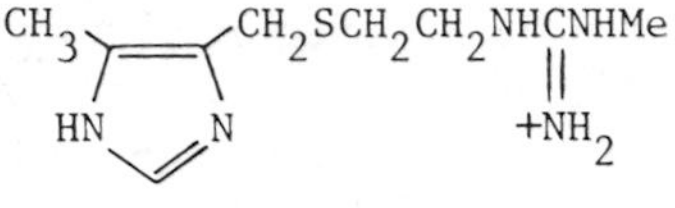	16	12
Cimetidine: introducing a CN substituent reduces basicity and increases activity	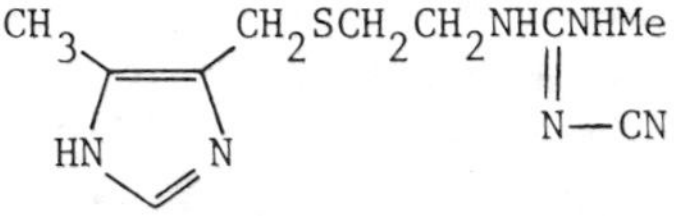	0.79	1.4

[a] Dissociation constant K_B determined *in vitro* on guinea pig right atrium against histamine stimulation.
[b] Activity *in vivo* as an antagonist of near maximal histamine stimulated gastric acid secretion in anesthetized rats, using a lumen perfused preparation. The ID_{50} is the intravenous dose required to produce 50% of inhibition.
[c] No antagonism seen up to an intravenous dose of 256 μmol kg^{-1}.

Perhaps the most convincing indication of the effects of physicochemical thinking on the development of cimetidine is the discovery of cyanoguanidine as a bioisostere for thiourea (*34*), in essence the replacement of =S by =NCN. The similarities in properties include tautomeric forms, pK_a values, N—C—N geometry, dipole moments, partitioning, and crystal packing geometries (*69*). However, NMR studies (*80*) confirm the existence of differences in the conformational states accessible to the two molecules, there being three possibilities for an *N,N'*-disubstituted thiourea but only two for the cyanoguanidine. Such differences could explain the unsuccessful application of this new bioisostere in other situations (*8*). Recent empirical calculations suggest that cimetidine has a tendency to "stack" the cyanoguanidine and imidazole adjacent to one another (*65,66*).

A boldly successful extrapolation of a structure–activity hypothesis was one outcome of work on a central H_2 receptor characterized by Green *et al.* (*52,53,115*). Hippocampus (a brain tissue) contains an adenylate cyclase whose activation by histamine is blocked competitively by cimetidine and D-LSD. Although D-LSD affects other central receptors at much lower concentrations, such that its notorious effects probably have some other molecular basis, nevertheless, the finding that L-LSD does not antagonize the hippocampal cyclase suggests that the histamine antagonism of D-LSD is receptor mediated. This raises a question—what commonality in structure between cimetidine and D-LSD might make them both H_2 antagonists?

Weinstein's answer to this question is shown in Fig. 5. An extended conformation of cimetidine can be overlayed on D-LSD as shown. The

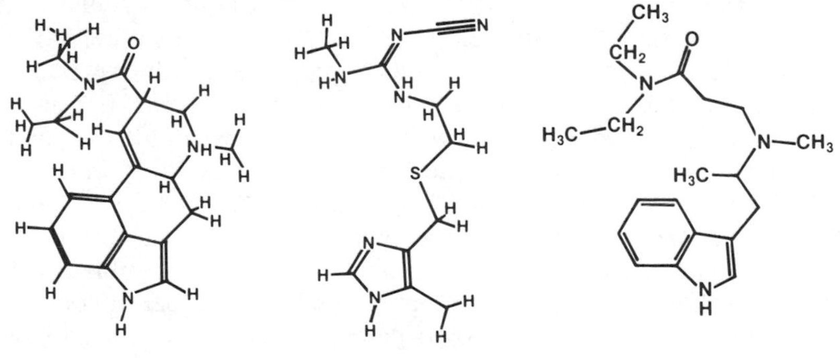

LSD Cimetidine SK&F 10856

Fig. 5. Three structures found to be antagonists of histamine-stimulated hippocampal adenyl cyclase, shown in conformations calculated to display similar electrostatic potentials.

similarity between the superposed structures is more convincing in the electrostatic potential maps, the iminoimidazole nitrogen of cimetidine and the vinylbenzo moiety of D-LSD both providing high electronegativity to the "left" side of their respective structures. However, the analogy is made most credible by a resulting successful prediction. In 1977 Weinstein described this theory to an SK & F (Philadelphia) audience and speculated that certain other structures would also antagonize the cyclase. Kaiser was able to supply him with one of the structures, previously synthesized as a serotonin antagonist, and in due course it was reported (*53*) that SK & F 10856 was, like cimetidine and D-LSD, indeed an antagonist of hippocampal histamine-stimulated adenylate cyclase.

III. PROSTAGLANDINS

A second class of physiological transmitters with therapeutic implications in both the antiallergic and antiulcer areas are the prostaglandins. Although a considerable investment has been made in attempts to prepare pharmacologically useful analogs of the prostaglandins, little work of a QSAR nature has been published, especially from the laboratories having the most active synthetic programs.

Prostaglandins are most certainly exceptionally flexible molecules when in solution. Evidence for this view includes the extreme difficulty of crystallizing the substances (lack of energetically preferred shapes means that an unusual amount of disorder must be overcome to form a crystal), the apparent dominance of packing forces in dictating chain conformations in those prostaglandin crystal structures that have been determined (*32,38,92,106*), and the paucity of rigidifying features such as rings or polar groups in their structures. Despite their flexibility in solution, the qualitative structure–activity relationships (*84,102*), most notably the profound effects of minor chain modifications, suggest that at their receptor sites prostaglandins must assume well-defined shapes. In principle one ought to be able to work backwards from energy calculations on the potential conformers of active and inactive analogs to an increasing knowledge of the receptor shape, as previously discussed for histamine. But in practice the prostaglandins are unattractive candidates for this approach, in part because of the challenging synthetic problems they present, but also because of the exceptionally large number of conformations potentially accessible to a prostaglandin. There are about 15 torsionally labile bonds in a typical prostaglandin excluding ring conformers. If we assume that any conformer pair differing by a 10° rotation about any of these bonds is distinguishable, there are 36 states for each of the 15 bonds, meaning 36^{15} or 2.2×10^{23} conformeric states to be explored. Even if we limit our interest to the possible "local minima," or staggered conformations for each bond, there are 3^{15} or 14,348,907 discrete shapes to be considered—about a week of computer time at the rate of 30 conformations/sec. It is evident that comparing the conformational habits of a few dozen prostaglandins is a major exercise.

These estimates of computing time should be sobering today for anyone considering conformational calculations for a molecule having more than about six rotatable bonds. Nevertheless, the future situation is not hopeless, particularly for structures having highly polar groups, such as peptides, in which electrostatic, directed interactions are well known to help in making conformations (such as α-helices and β-bends). much more energetically favorable. The computational challenge in this field is to improve our heuristics for recognizing these interactions. Indeed the information-carrying function of peptidal hormones would seem to require a relatively small number of actual shapes, for otherwise the intercellular communication involved would have to be extremely garbled and inefficient, adjectives certainly not characteristic of biological systems.

Despite the difficulties, three preliminary conformational calculations of prostaglandins have appeared, Hoyland and Kier tackling PGE_1 (*63*), Kothekar and Dutta $PGE_{2\alpha}$ (*74*), and Murakami and Akahori nine of the prostaglandins (*81–83*). As might be expected, none of these groups performed a complete study, Hoyland and Kier (*63*, p. 84) examining "over 400 conformations . . . felt [to] . . . include all the low-lying configurations," Kothekar and Dutta rotating only three of the bonds, and Murakami and Akahori apparently examining bond rotations only singly, not in combination. Rather different ranges of relative conformational energies were reported, about 2 kcal/mol below the all-trans reference state by Hoyland and Kier, 9 kcal/mol below the crystal state by Kothekar and Dutta, and 5 to 10 kcal/mol, depending on steric parameterization, by Murakami and Akahori. The latter two groups both appear to base their calculations on the widely used Scott–Scheraga parameterization (*103*) and thus these encouragingly high energy differences can be compared with those for peptides. Preliminary molecular orbital calculations for $PGF_{1\beta}$ have also been reported (*74*).

Physical measurements on prostaglandins tend to suggest that biologically active congeners prefer a conformation in which the two side chains, although forced to be trans where attached to the cyclopentane ring, interact as closely as possible. Probably because of the open loop between the trans chains at the ring end, the conformations are known as "hairpins" (Fig. 6). The most compelling evidence for chain interactions in ethanol solution are the circulor dichroism (CD) spectra of bis-chain

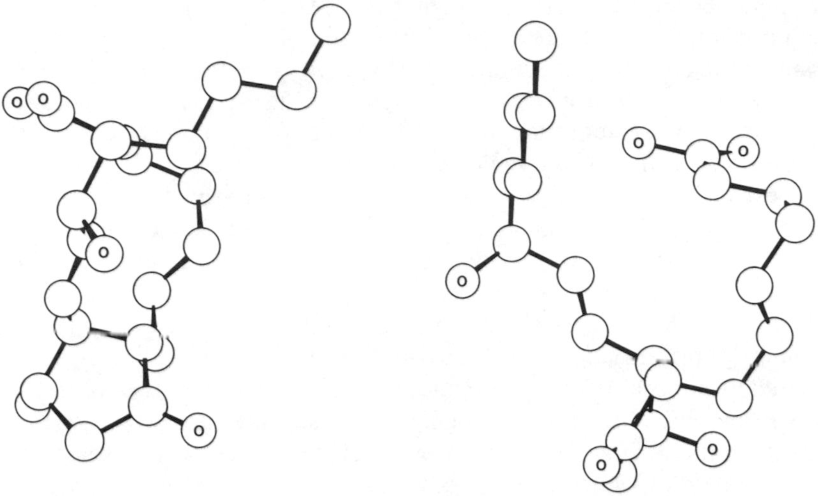

Fig. 6. Two views of a hairpin-like conformation of prostaglandin PGE_1.

unsaturated prostaglandins, for example $PGF_{2\alpha}$, which show nonadditive absorbances diagnostic of through-space interactions between the vinyl moieties. Less potent diastereomers 11-epi-$PGF_{2\alpha}$ and $PGF_{2\theta}$ show no evidence of such interactions (*3,78*).

IV. β-ADRENERGIC AGENTS

Another physiological transmitter therapeutically involved in treatment of the asthmatic response to allergans is adrenalin. Stimulants of the β-adrenergic receptor relax bronchial tissue and thus help the asthmatic sufferer to breathe. Quantitative drug design studies involving agonists or antagonists of other actions of epinephrine can be found elsewhere in this volume. The major objective in developing new bronchodilators is greater β_2-agonist selectivity, vis-à-vis both the α receptor and the β_1 receptor, than the prototype β-adrenergic agent isoproterenol (**I**). Many of the structural variations have been carefully reviewed (*68*). Explaining the ef-

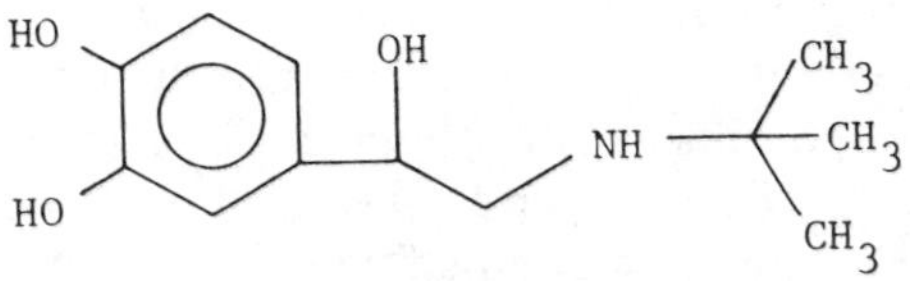

I

fects of different aromatic substituents on β_1 and β_2 receptors is an obvious challenge for the classical QSAR approach, and it is surprising how little work has been reported. Perhaps the parameters usually employed are not adequate for the task; this writer was unable to correlate more than 60% of the overall variation in 40 SK&F bronchodilators of structures related to **I**, using π, F, R, and E_s as parameters, and could not obtain any statistically significant rationalization of β_1/β_2 potency ratios (*27*).

Pratesi *et al.* (*90*) focused their attention on the other (*N*-alkyl) end of isoproterenol. By defining a parameter E to be the molecular volume ratio of a designated carbon (plus attachments β from the nitrogen) to all other carbons attached to the nitrogen, they obtained quadratic Eqs. (4) and (5), which rationalized 0.977 of the variation in both β_1 (atrial) and β_2 (tracheal) agonist potencies among mono-*N*-alkyl congeners of isoproterenol.

$$\text{Tracheal: } pD_2 = 1.87E - 0.45E^2 + 5.99 \qquad (4)$$

$$n = 7, \qquad r = 0.989$$

$$\text{Atria: } pD_2 = 3.24E - 1.90E^2 + 6.64 \qquad (5)$$

$$n = 7, \qquad r = 0.980$$

However, the hypothesis that isopropyl or *tert*-butyl are in some sense sterically optimal for β-receptor activation has long been obvious qualitatively, and it is not easy to see how this equation adds to our previous understanding.

The β-adrenergic agents have also been a subject for a new and potentially very useful method of data analysis, SIMCA pattern recognization (*33*). Dunn *et al.* have studied *in vitro* measurements of the affinity and intrinsic activity and the antagonist potency, toward the erythrocyte β-receptor, of 37 phenethylamines describable as analogs of isoproterenol. Their objectives are the ability to classify phenethylamines as β agonists, antagonists, or neither, as well as to predict the potency in either type of assay. The SIMCA mathematical model developed by Wold seems unusually well adapted to these joint objectives, and indeed a two-component model based on standard physicochemical parameters (pK_a, Hammett σ, Rekker f, and Verloop B and L) successfully identifies as agonist or antagonist 30 of the 32 unambiguously active substances. Because the physicochemical parameters have been reduced to two major components, either a graphical or a regression estimate of the antagonist and agonist potencies is possible, and from the graphs in the paper it would appear that correlations with r^2 in the range of 0.7 to 0.9 would be obtained for regression equations relating agonist or antagonist potency to the same two components used for classification. Such results are impressive, especially considering the ambitious objectives and the apparent lack of success by other QSAR workers with these data.

However, there are two related difficulties with this SIMCA application. The first is the highly nonintuitive and problem-dependent nature of the components produced by a SIMCA analysis. These components result from a principal-components analysis of the physicochemical parameters of compounds belonging to that class. To put the matter in terms of a similar study, the BC(DEF) derivation from physical properties (*28*), SIMCA produces a new set of BC(DEF) or principal components for each new set of compounds or problem. Certainly, it is impressive that SIMCA's components, however *ad hoc* their derivation may appear, can in this instance effect such class separations and potency correlations. But the components are not easily understood in chemical terms or rendered into a communicable physical model. The second difficulty is that because of the nonintuitive character of the components, one cannot tell how hard it would have been to devise criteria on the basis of intuition that would distinguish these antagonists from these agonists. Just how difficult is this problem for these data? A fair evaluation of this work will be possible only when predictions by the SIMCA model have been experimentally tested, an effort that is reportedly now underway (*116*).

A number of experimental and calculational studies of β agonists address the overall structural requirements for receptor activation. Richards and co-workers have invoked the "zipper" mechanism for β-receptor action, which holds that receptor–ligand activation is a cooperative process requiring molecular motions of both agonist and receptor (*100,101*). The zipper mechanism implies that a receptor agonist must have flexibility. The high potency of the relatively rigid β agonist (**II**) (*85*) suggests that the zipper mechanism cannot be universally valid.

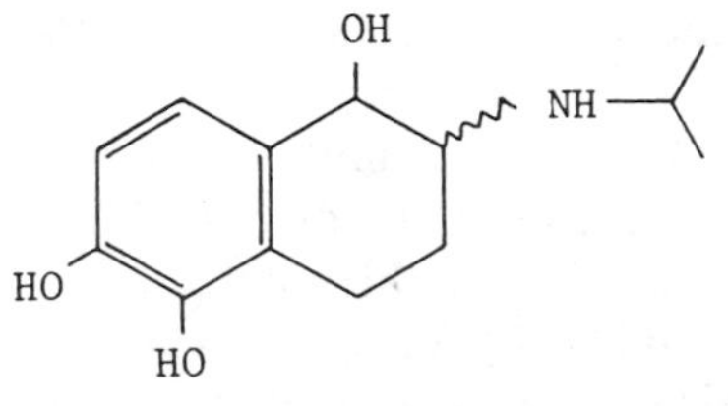

II

Two quantum chemical studies have attempted to define in electronic terms the differences between α and β agonists and between β agonists and antagonists, these being the issues that Pratesi *et al.* (*90*) and Dunn *et al.* (*33*), respectively, also addressed. George *et al.* consider several possible mechanisms for the influence of *N*-alkyl groups upon the α/β selectivity ratio of isoproterenol congeners (*51*) and, by conclusively eliminating effects on ethyl chain conformation and charge distribution (i.e., basicity) of the nitrogen, suggest that direct dispersion attraction between the alkyl group and the receptor plays a major role. Rather less successful is the attempt by Petrongolo *et al.* (*89*) to distinguish the β agonist isoproterenol from the β antagonists, INPEA (**III,** nifenalol) and doberol (**IV,** to-

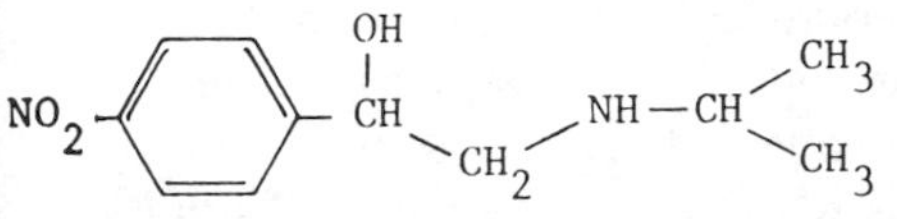

III

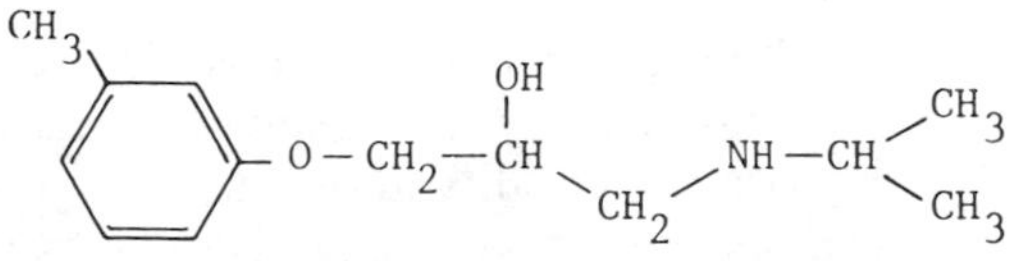

IV

liprolol), on the basis of electrostatic potential maps. As one might expect from classical Hammett substituent effect arguments, the maps for doberol and isoproterenol seem to resemble each other far more than either resembles the INPEA map.

Another related issue of current interest is to explain the similar pharmacological actions of the structurally different ethanolamine and oxypropanolamine side chains, exemplified in the INPEA and doberol side chains. Crystallographic and quantum chemical calculations are consistent with the proposition that the OCH_2 moiety (see **IV**) merely extends the domain of the aromatic moiety (*2,43*). However, because of the similarity in the effective patterns of aromatic substitution between the two different side chains, one is tempted to seek a conformation of the oxypropanolamine side chain that permits superposition of its aryl, hydroxy, and amine moieties with those of the ethanolamine side chain. NMR studies by Jen and Kaiser (*67*) indeed showed that in chloroform the cationic protomer of oxypropanolamines is internally hydrogen bonded; more detailed analysis led to the ingenious suggestion of a bicyclic conformer, many of the features of which are almost superimposable on phenylethanolamines. However, Zaagsma (*119*) has shown further that the nature of the counterion also affects these NMR spectra such that the seven-membered ring conformer must also be considered and in view of other evidence, particularly the IR evidence of hydroxyl hydrogen bonding as well, must probably be preferred to the bicyclic conformer.

V. REGULATORY PEPTIDES

Because of the combinatorial problem with multiple bond rotations, alluded to in connection with prostaglandins, it is particularly difficult at present to translate the backbone or topology of a peptide into a manageably small number of three-dimensional structures. This problem exists whether the chemist or computer is attempting the translation. However, peptide chemists seem especially receptive to computer technology or other formal methodology in rationalizing the results of previous syntheses and planning new ones. In the following section three applications of formal methodologies to the design of new peptides will be discussed.

Although somatostatin analogs are prepared mainly in a search for new diabetes therapy, a somatostatin agonist might also have antiulcer activity. This possibility allows us to highlight one of the current most elegant rational drug design successes, the simplification of somatostatin from its fourteen-peptide cycle to a seven-peptide cycle having improved efficacy by a group at Merck headed by Veber (*111,112*). This story can best be followed by reference to their conformational hypothesis shown as Fig. 7. A key observation was the enhanced *in vitro* potency of the 8-D-trytophan analog (inversion of the 8 amino acid), which suggested that the 7,8,9,10 residues might be forming the type **I** β turn indicated (*4*). NMR evidence confirmed the equatorial relationship thereby implied between the 8-tryptophan and 9-lysine side chains. Another set of data supporting the continuing mutual alignment shown for the backbone are the high potencies found upon replacement of Phe-6 and Phe-11 or Asn-5 and Thr-12,

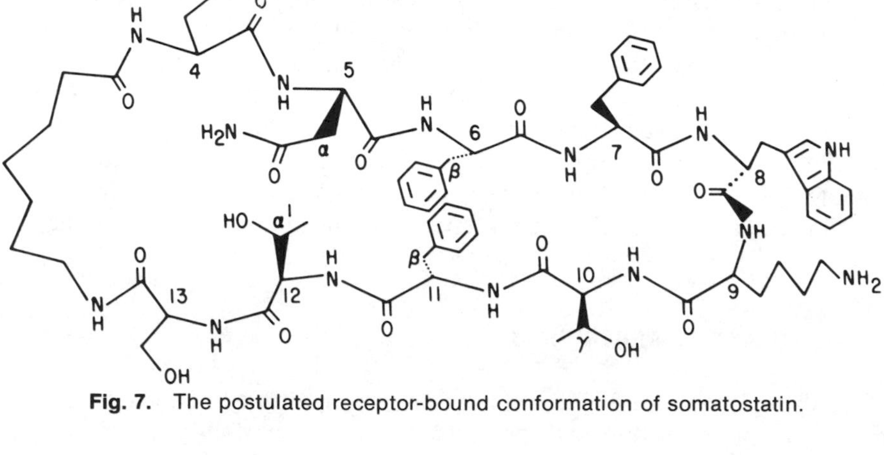

Fig. 7. The postulated receptor-bound conformation of somatostatin.

respectively, by a cysteine, whereas replacement of Phe-6 and Phe-11 by alanines abolishes activity. These results suggest that the interactions indicated between these groups in Fig. 7 do stabilize the cyclic conformer. It argues well for the power of the model that many of the active modifications that it inspired would have been contraindicated by the results of single residue replacements and that this "receptor active" conformation in general does not agree with a proposed conformation for somatostatin in solution. Merck scientists give substantial credit for this success (*110a*) to their computer molecular modeling system MMMS (*54*), which allowed them rigorous study of the implications of this productive conformational hypothesis.

The increasing number of X-ray determinations of immunoglobulin structures have inspired the design of peptides that would mimic or antagonize immunoglobulin binding. Hamburger (*57*) reported that injection of the pentapeptide Asp-Ser-Asp-Pro-Arg, a sequence in IgE that may be critical for its combination with mast cells and the subsequent allergic response, would block the Prausnitz–Kustner reaction in humans (allergic skin wheal produced by antibody injection followed 20 h later by antigen challenge). The Hamburger pentapeptide also inhibits *in vitro* the degranulation of mast cells induced by antigen–antibody complexes (*110*). Conformational studies of the pentapeptide (*62*) suggest that, despite the presence of 22 rotatable bonds, the proline residue and possibility of stabilizing attractions between the negative aspartate and positive arginine residues produces a single conformation some 20 kcal/mol more stable than any other.

Atassi *et al.* (*6,7,76,77,108*) have summarized a series of successful "surface-simulation syntheses." A surface-simulation synthesis involves (1) designation of residues on either an antigen (lysozyme) or antibody (vitamin K), preferably not directly linked, that may be critical for antigen–antibody combination; (2) synthesis of a peptide containing these residues, using glycine "spacers," if necessary, to achieve a sufficient spatial separation between residues; (3) observation that this peptide (typically in 100× excess) blocks antigen–antibody combination *in vitro*, whereas (4) control peptides having the same residues in different sequences are inactive, and (5) the surface simulator has no activity against other antibody–antigen reactions. Whether or not these results by themselves can be taken as conclusive proof that the binding residues have been correctly identified, they still constitute an example of truly *de novo* drug design. Considering the small proportion of a surface simulator that probably exists in a conformation suitable for binding, the potencies reported are not unimpressive.

VI. INHIBITORS OF THE PASSIVE CUTANEOUS ANAPHYLACTIC (PCA) RESPONSE

Disodium chromoglycate (**V**) exerts a prophylactic effect against allergic attacks in humans. Its mechanism of action is unclear, but it seems to inhibit the release of mediators such as histamine and SRS-A from mast cells. A simple animal model that demonstrates this action of DSCG is the passive cutaneous anaphylaxis (PCA) response in rats.

Because DSCG is neither particularly potent nor orally active, a number of companies have used the PCA rat model to screen for other compounds having a similar mode of action. From the dozens of structures that have been considered for clinical trial, it is evident that finding such compounds in the PCA rat is not difficult. However, few if any of these have been successful in the clinic, usually because of a lack of efficacy.

QSAR techniques have been valuable in optimizing the PCA rat potencies of the initial leads found by screening, and in the case of the pyraneamines (*29–31*) and the 2-phenyl-8-azapurinones (*11,14,24,60,117*), their use was directly responsible for potency enhancements of 100× or more. Other series of PCA inhibitors for which QSAR correlations have been reported are oxanilic acids and congeners (*23*), 8-azaxanthines (*26*), 9*H*-xanthen-9-one-2-carboxylic acids (*13*), and 4-hydroxy-3-nitrocoumarins (*22*). In this section, I will review the two QSAR success stories in particular detail and conclude by comparing all the QSAR in a search for regularities that may shed light on the test systems or on other QSAR applications. Structures appear in Table III.

The development of the pyranenamines began with 19 compounds that had been inspired by the "Topliss tree" scheme (*107*) for substituent selection. QSAR analysis of the data, first graphically and then by regression, yielded an extremely crude equation:

$$pI_{50} = -0.72 - 0.14\left(\sum \pi\right) - 1.35\left(\sum \sigma\right)^2 \qquad (6)$$

$$n = 19, \qquad r = 0.701, \qquad s = 0.47$$

which associated increased potency with greater hydrophilicity and unremarkable electronic influence ($\sigma = 0$). To extrapolate these trends, three multiply-substituted compounds were designed and synthesized. All were highly active, the most active being six times as active as any of the first 19. To pursue this breakthrough further, regression techniques were used to monitor results from a wide variety of hydrophilic substituents. Further refinement led through several stages to the design and synthesis of one compound (Table III, Structure A, X, Y = 3,5-$NHCOCHOHCH_2OH$) a

TABLE III
Antiallergic Series in Which QSAR Correlations Were Found Between Activity and the Properties of X and Y

Properties correlating with increased PCA potency	Structure/series	References
A. Low π (optimum = -5.0?); hydrogen bond donating groups of specified structure; $\Sigma\sigma \simeq 0$, but electron-withdrawing groups in the 5-position desirable	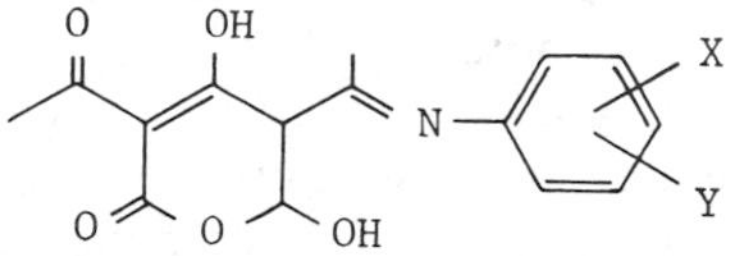	*29,30,31*
B. For ortho X: small size; good hydrogen bond accepting characters; possible π optimum; low π (= 2.0?) and high R of 5 substituents	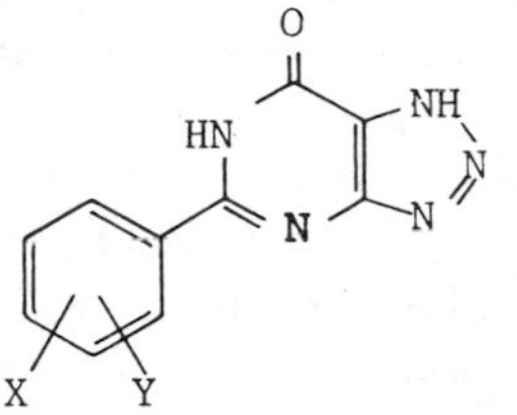	*11,14,24, 60,117*
C. Energy of the LUMO (lowest unoccupied antibinding π orbital) bond	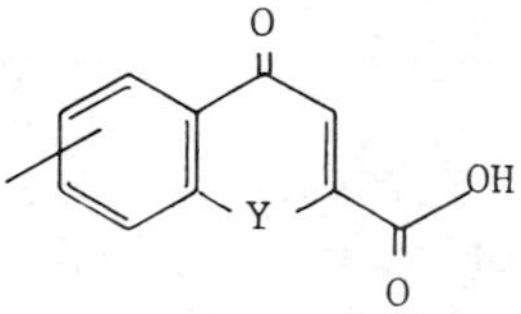	*23*
D. Optimal π (R^2 or R^1) = 0.0; increasing E_s	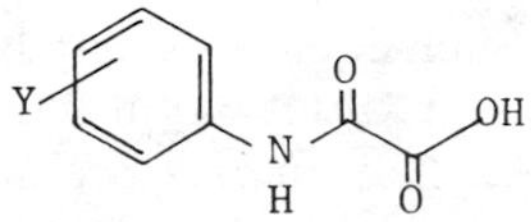 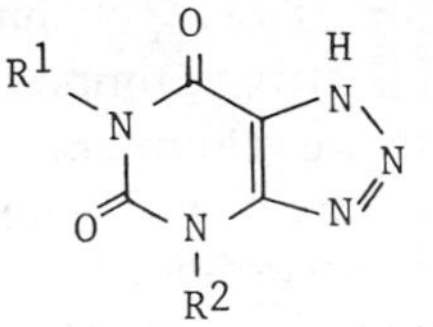	*26*
E. Increasing E_s; decreasing *MR*; "fat, stubby" R	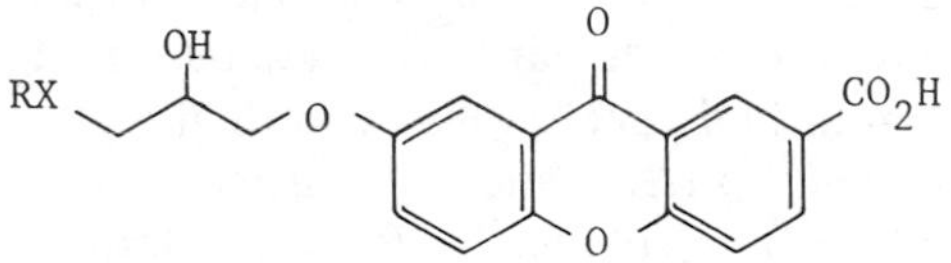	*13*
F. High HOMO; low π	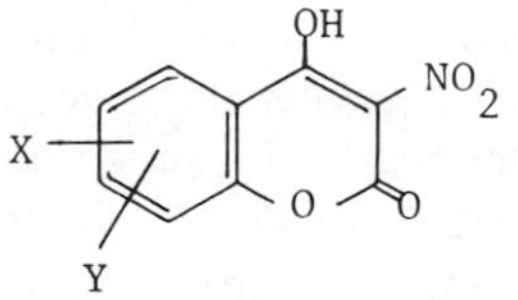	*22*

thousand times more potent than either Intal or any of the original 19 compounds. At this writing, another series member (X = 3-NH_2; Y = 4-OH) is still undergoing clinical efficacy trials.

Several features of the pyranenamine development make this story an exceptionally clear-cut illustration of the value of QSAR techniques. First, very large enhancements in potency were obtained within a series that in the view of many observers had already been optimized after the first 19 compounds were tested. Second, the basic hypothesis that increasing hydrophilicity produces increased potency was a consistent indicator of potency for more than 80 compounds, most more active than the original 19. Finally, it is difficult to believe that many of the most active compounds would have been synthesized anyway in the absence of the guiding hypothesis; their structures were too unusual and their synthesis too difficult.

There may also be lessons in this story for the QSAR practitioner. It is surely odd that such a crude equation proved to be such a robust, or reliable, predictor of so many biological potencies. No doubt we were lucky, but another reason for the robustness of our equation may be the unusually great variety of substituent properties and arrangements represented among the 19 compounds on which the equation was based. These were H; 2-, 3-, and 4-Cl; 2-, 3-, and 4-OH; 4-F; 4-NO_2; 4-COOMe; 4-Me; 2-NH_2; 4-$N(Me)_2$; 3-4-Cl_2; 3,5-$(CF_3)_2$; 2,6-Cl_2; 2,6-$(OH)_2$; and 4-pyridyl. By contrast, far too many of the other QSAR discussed in this chapter were based on variations at one position and/or of one structural type, usually alkyl or halogen. Such equations may be reasonable predictors of the properties of other similar variations at the same position, but usually the originator of the QSAR had much more ambitious objectives. A related dubious QSAR practice is that of "polishing" equations, i.e., obtaining higher r^2, by dropping ill-fitting compounds with little apparent justification. The pyranenamine development story suggests that the greater benefits can sometimes arise from fitting poorer equations to a much greater variety of data. Perhaps some clever QSAR practitioner can devise a new "r^2," one that compares the variance explained by the equation to the total possible variation in substituent properties rather than to the variation in biological potency actually observed.

The second QSAR success story, due to Wooldridge *et al.* (*11,14,24,60,117*), involves the PCA rat activity of 2-phenyl-8-azapurin-6-ones. Its most active product [Table III, Structure B, X = 2-OPr; Y = 5-$SO_2NH(t)Bu$] is equipotent with the most active pyranenamine.

Series development commenced with observation of DSCG-like activity (log potency = −2.0, relative to DSCG) in compound **V**, followed by the discovery that an 8-aza modification eliminated undesirable side ef-

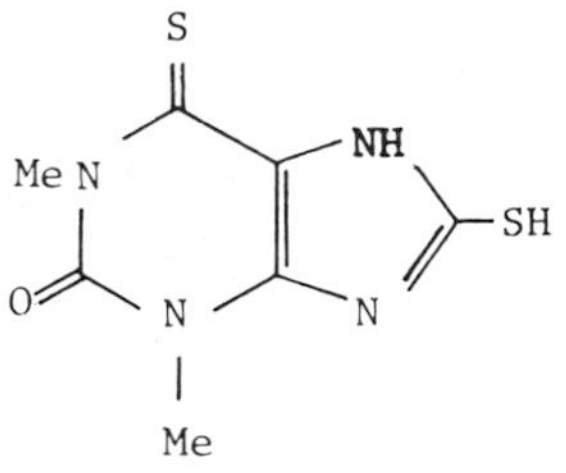

V

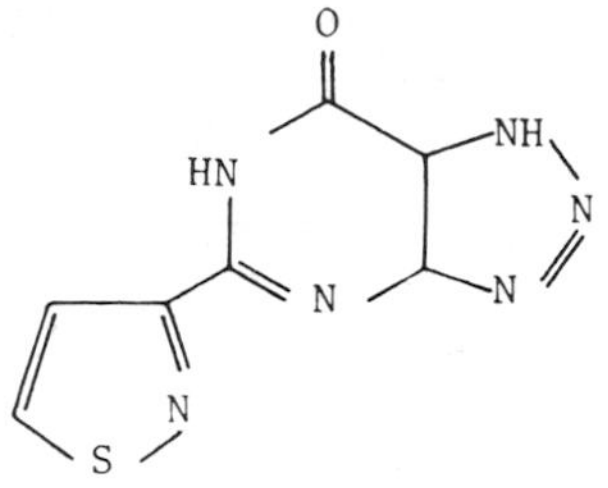

VI

fects and raised potency (−0.7). Activity in the 8-azaxanthines increased with the size of 3-substituents and has an optimal π of 0, the most active compound (R^1 = CH_3, R^2 = p-methoxybenzyl) having a potency of 0.0. Further testing of related 8-azapurines yielded **VI**, which has a potency of 0.6. QSAR analysis of the obvious follow-up series, 2-phenyl-8-azapurin-6-ones, ultimately produced two key trends:

$$\log(MW \times I) = 0.013\ \Delta\bar{\nu} + 1.125E_s + 1.045 \quad (7)$$

$$n = 35, \qquad r = 0.828, \qquad s = 0.415$$

One focused on the 2′ position of the phenyl, activity increasing with an IR frequency probably related to its H-bond donating properties but decreasing with local bulk (Taft E_s), and culminated with the 2′-propoxy derivative, potency = 1.6 and clinically active on aerosol administration. The other trend involved the 5′ position, where potency increased with hydrophilicity and with R (electron withdrawing via resonance) and produced the 2′-propoxy-5′-SO_2NH_2 derivative, potency = 2.3. The hypothesis that the oxygens should be shielded brought about the final enhancement to 3.0.

Thus series development appears to have passed through several iterations of the following sequence: (1) identify trend, (2) extrapolate trend as far as possible, and (3) cast about in search of a new trend. Although this method of series development is perhaps a less convincing demonstration of QSAR potential than is the pyranenamine series, because many key potency enhancements resulted more from casting about than from trend extrapolation, it may be a much better role model for other medicinal chemists because the number of situations in which really extensive extrapolation of a trend is possible do not seem to be numerous.

A remarkably high correlation coefficient (r^2 = 0.96) was obtained by Cheney *et al.* (*23*), of Upjohn, between PCA antiallergic potency and the energy of the lowest unoccupied antibonding molecular π orbital, in a series of 13 compounds related to oxanilic acids:

$$-\ln ED_{50} = -64.4E_a + 29.0 \quad (8)$$

$$n = 13, \quad r = 0.98, \quad s = 0.37$$

Indeed, the standard error of the residual (0.37) is substantially smaller than the biological variability estimate (0.95) (note the use of natural instead of base 10 logarithms.) This "too good" fit is one of several indications that the authors might have been seeking a high correlation coefficient more than an accurate and general model of reality. The compound set seems both wider in overall structural variety and less numerous in substituent variation than is typical in industrial lead optimization, and the authors occasionally use phrases such as "molecules under consideration" and "series . . . was selected" (*23*, p. 936), which suggest to me that their 13 compounds were winnowed from a much larger group. Finally, although the authors list several reasonable assumptions in deriving a charge-transfer rationalization of their equation, there is another implicit assumption that seems hard to accept: steric factors (differences in molecular shape) do not affect the binding energy of the charge-transfer complex.

Because I am something of an agnostic with respect to the value of applying necessarily approximate molecular orbital methods to molecules of this complexity, I attempted to see how well one might have done fitting these activities with conventional physicochemical parameters. The following equation was obtained:

$$-\ln ED_{50} = 9.14 + (4.33 \pm 1.47) \sum F \quad (9)$$

$$r = 0.90, \quad s = 0.88$$

where ΣF is the sum of Swain–Lupton–Unger "field" effects of all substituents present.

Both equations have much the same implications for further synthesis, suggesting that loading the phenyl ring with even more elctron-withdrawing groups would steeply enhance potency. However, one would really need more data for a wider variety of substituents before placing great confidence in this conclusion. The statistical quality of the LUMO equation is much greater, but the superiority has little practical significance inasmuch as both equations explain "too much" of the variance based on the cited experimental errors averaging about 1.0.

In Table III appear all the lead structures and reported QSAR trends among series of compounds that have been tested for PCA inhibition in the rat. One unusual feature that most of the studies have in common is the tendency for activity to increase with substituent hydrophilicity, a trend certainly opposite to most hydrophilicity trends whether *in vivo* or *in vitro,* as is discussed elsewhere in this book. The only important exception to this "hydrophilicity rule" is the oxanilic acid series, in which lipophilicity seems for the data cited to have no effect, both according to Cheney *et al.* and in my reanalysis. Why do so many different series of compounds behave in such an unusual way in this particular assay? More precisely, does this dependence reflect specific receptor binding or some aspecific feature of the PCA rat test system itself? Because the same correlation is found for so many different lead structures, particularly in the pyranenamines where the hydrophilicity effect is relatively position independent, my speculation is that there is some aspecific feature of the route of administration or of mast cells that promotes the potency of hydrophilic compounds.

There appears to be some structural commonality between the 5 positions of the phenyl rings in pyranenamines and 2-phenyl-6-azapurin-6-ones. (A 5 substituent is defined only for a 2- or 3-substituted phenyl.) In both series electron-withdrawing and hydrophilic 5 substituents seem to produce strong and positionally selective enhancements of potency. This may indicate a common geometry of receptor binding for the two phenyl rings. In contrast, the Upjohn oxanilic acids have a positionally nonspecific increase in potency with electron-withdrawing character.

VII. MISCELLANEOUS STUDIES

Five studies employing relevant methodologies did not fall into any of the preceding categories, three involving antiulcer and two antiallergic

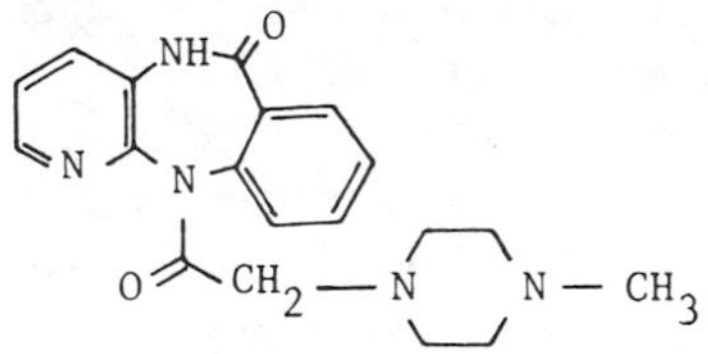

VII

therapies. Eberlein *et al.* (*37*) designed an antiulcer agent, pirenzepine (**VII**), to be a compound with the overall shape of psychotropic tricyclics but with physicochemical properties that would prevent it from entering the CNS. The trick was to replace lipophilic structural features with hydrophilic ones, yielding a compound with a log(distribution coefficient) of −0.64.

Bustard and Martin (*16*) sought a combination of features common to six structurally diverse compounds known to have antiulcer effects, deciding that a necessary, but not sufficient, condition might be two heteroatoms separated by 3.7 ± 0.2 Å, one having a lone pair and the other a π-electron or otherwise conjugated electronic configuration. Kier and George constructed a conformation for the secretory agent gastrin tetrapeptide (Try-Met-Asp-Phe-NH_2) by joining the EHT-calculated low energy residues (30° scan) end-to-end (*72*), a conformation that finds some NMR support (*42*).

Novinson *et al.* (*86*) found rough correlations between substituent π values and phosphodiesterase inhibition among a series of alkylpyrazolopyrimidines. Finally, Bowden and Wooldridge (*11*) obtained a respectable correlation between the bronchodilator potency of some alkyl 6-thioxanthines and Newman "six-numbers," in essence finding a superiority for "fat, stubby" alkyl substitutents that could also be expressed using the Taft E_s parameter.

VIII. CONCLUSION

The diversity of successful approaches to the rational design of antiallergic and antiulcer agents is impressive. However, it would be a bold scientist indeed who would deny the continuing role of luck in drug discovery. Indeed, the skimpy state of knowledge about the mechanics of drug–receptor interaction, both in particular cases and in general, will for the foreseeable future continue to make fortune a critical ingredient of successful pharmaceutical research.

Yet there is a proverb in technology: "Chance favors the prepared mind." If one has studied the chemical properties of his molecules and has made a serious attempt, computer aided or not, to construct relationships between activity and structure using structural descriptors more fundamental than "meta-chloro is good," then one is more likely to make a better molecule. At least one is less likely to make "more of the same" inadvertently. Knowing your molecules (*48*) or rigorously pursuing the implication of one's statistical (*30,79*) or three-dimensional molecular model (*110a*) is certainly a dominant theme in recent drug discovery success stories.

REFERENCES

1. R. J. Abraham and D. Birch, *Mol. Pharmacol.* **11,** 663 (1975).
2. H. L. Ammon, A. Balsamo, B. Macchia, F. Macchia, D. B. Howe, and W. E. Keefe, *Experientia* **31,** 644 (1975).

3. N. H. Andersen, P. W. Ramwell, E. M. K. Leovey, and M. Johnson, *Adv. Prostaglandin Thromboxane Res.* **1,** p. 271, (1976).
4. B. H. Arison, R. Hirschmann, and D. F. Veber, *Bioorg. Chem.* **7,** 447 (1978).
5. A. S. F. Ash and H. O. Schild, *Br. J. Pharmacol. Chemother.* **27,** 427 (1966).
6. M. Z. Atassi and C. L. Lee, *Biochem. J.* **171,** 419 (1978).
7. M. Z. Atassi and W. Zablocki, *J. Biol. Chem.* **252,** 8784 (1977).
8. D. E. Beattie, R. Crossley, A. C. W. Curran, and A. E. Lawrence, *J. Med Chem.* **20,** 718 (1977).
9. J. W. Black, G. J. Durant, J. C. Emmett, and C. R. Ganellin, *Nature* (*London*) **248,** 65 (1974).
10. A. Boucherle, S. Casadio, F. Favier, and H. Cousse, *Lyon Pharm.* **29,** 79 (1979).
11. K. Bowden and K. R. H. Wooldridge, *Biochem. Pharmacol.* **22,** 1015 (1973).
12. R. W. Brimblecombe, W. A. M. Duncan, G. J. Durant, J. C. Emmett, C. R. Ganellin, G. B. Leslie, and M. E. Parsons, *Gastroenterology* **74,** 339 (1978).
13. J. A. Bristol, R. Alekel, J. Y. Fukunaga, and M. Steinman, *J. Med. Chem.* **21,** 1327 (1978).
14. B. J. Broughton, P. Chaplin, P. Knowles, E. Lunt, S. M. Marshall, D. L. Pain, and K. R. H. Wooldridge, *J. Med. Chem.* **18,** 1117 (1975).
15. A. Burger, M. Bernabe, and P. W. Collins, *J. Med. Chem.* **13,** 33 (1970).
16. T. M. Bustard and Y. C. Martin, *J. Med. Chem.* **15,** 1101 (1972).
17. D. Carlstrom, R. Bergin, and G. Falkenberg, *Q. Rev. Biophys.* **6,** 257 (1973).
18. A. F. Casy, *Annu. Rep. Prog. Chem.* **70,** 477 (1974).
19. A. F. Casy and R. R. Ison, *J. Pharm. Pharmacol.* **22,** 270 (1970).
20. A. F. Casy, R. R. Ison, and N. S. Ham, *Chem. Commun.* p. 1343 (1970).
21. A. F. Casy and A. P. Parulkar, *Can. J. Chem.* **47,** 423 (1969).
22. M. Charton and J. Royer, *Res. Commun. Chem. Pathol. Pharmacol.* **23,** 341 (1979).
23. B. V. Cheney, J. B. Wright, C. M. Hall, H. G. Johnson, and R. E. Christofferson, *J. Med. Chem.* **21,** 936 (1978).
24. S. J. Cline and D. J. Hodgson, *J. Am. Chem. Soc.* **102,** 6285 (1980).
25. J. L. Coubeils, P. Courriere, and B. Pullman, *C. R. Hebd. Seances Acad. Sci., Ser. D* **272,** 1813 (1971).
26. C. J. Coulson, R. E. Ford, E. Lunt, S. Marshall, D. L. Pain, I. H. Rogers, and K. R. H. Wooldridge, *Eur. J. Med. Chem.—Chim. Ther.* **9,** 313 (1974).
27. R. D. Cramer, III, unpublished observations (1975).
28. R. D. Cramer, III, *J. Am. Chem. Soc.* **102,** 1837 (1980).
29. R. D. Cramer, III, *CHEM TECH* p.744 (1980).
30. R. D. Cramer, III, K. M. Snader, C. R. Willis, L. W. Chakrin, J. Thomas, and B. M. Sutton, *J. Med. Chem.* **22,** 714 (1979).
31. R. D. Cramer, III, K. M. Snader, C. R. Willis, L. W. Chakrin, J. Thomas, and B. M. Sutton, *in* "Drugs Affecting the Respiratory System" (D. L. Temple, ed.), p. 159. Am. Chem. Soc., Washington, D.C., 1980.
32. W. L. Duax and J. W. Edmonds, *Prostaglandins* **3,** 201 (1973).
32a. W. A. M. Duncan and M. E. Parsons, *Gastroenterology* **78,** 620 (1980).
33. W. J. Dunn, III, S. Wold, and Y. C. Martin, *J. Med. Chem.* **21,** 922 (1978).
34. G. J. Durant, J. C. Emmett, C. R. Ganellin, P. D. Miles, M. E. Parsons, H. D. Prain, and G. R. White, *J. Med. Chem.* **20,** 902 (1977).
35. G. J. Durant, J. C. Emmett, C. R. Ganellin, A. M. Roe, and R. A. Slater, *J. Med. Chem.* **19,** 923 (1976).
36. G. J. Durant, C. R. Ganellin, and M. E. Parsons, *J. Med. Chem.* **18,** 905 (1975).
37. W. Eberlein, G. Schmidt, A. Reuter, and E. Kutter, *Arzneim.-Forsch.* **27,** 356 (1977).
38. J. W. Edmonds and W. L. Duax, *Prostaglandins* **5,** 275 (1974).

39. J. C. Emmett, C. R. Ganellin, M. J. Graham, and F. H. Holloway, *Agents Actions* **9,** 27 (1979).
40. L. Farnell, W. G. Richards, and C. R. Ganellin, *J. Theor. Biol.* **43,** 389 (1974).
41. L. Farnell, W. G. Richards, and C. R. Ganellin, *J. Med. Chem.* **18,** 662 (1975).
42. J. Feeney, G. C. K. Roberts, and A. S. V. Burgen, *in* "Molecular and Quantum Pharmacology" (F. Bergmann and B. Pullman, eds.), p. 45. Reidel Publ., Dordrecht, Netherlands, 1974.
43. M. Gadret, J. M. Leger, A. Carpy, and H. Berthod, *Eur. J. Med. Chem.—Chim. Ther.* **13,** 367 (1978).
44. C. R. Ganellin, *J. Pharm. Pharmacol.* **25,** 787 (1973).
45. C. R. Ganellin, *J. Med. Chem.* **16,** 620 (1973).
46. C. R. Ganellin, *J. Appl. Chem. Biotechnol.* **28,** 183 (1978).
47. C. R. Ganellin, *Annu. Rep. Med. Chem.* **14,** 91 (1979).
48. C. R. Ganellin, *J. Med. Chem.* **24,** 913 (1981).
49. C. R. Ganellin, E. S. Pepper, G. N. J. Port, and W. G. Richards, *J. Med. Chem.* **16,** 610 (1973).
50. C. R. Ganellin, G. N. J. Port, and W. G. Richards, *J. Med. Chem.* **16,** 616 (1974).
51. J. M. George, L. B. Kier, and J. R. Hoyland, *Mol. Pharmacol.* **7,** 328 (1971).
52. J. P. Green, C. L. Johnson, H. Weinstein, and S. Maayani, *Proc. Natl. Acad. Sci. U.S.A.* **74,** 5697 (1977).
53. J. P. Green, H. Weinstein, and S. Maayani, *in* "QuaSAR" (G. Barnett, M. Trsic, and R. Willette, eds.), NIDA Research Monograph, No. 22, p. 38. Natl. Inst. Drug Abuse, Rockville, Maryland, 1978.
54. P. Gund, J. D. Andose, J. B. Rhodes, and G. M. Smith, *Science* **208,** 1425 (1980).
55. N. S. Ham, *J. Pharm. Sci.* **65,** 612 (1976).
56. N. S. Ham, A. F. Casy, and R. R. Ison, *J. Med. Chem.* **16,** 470 (1973).
57. R. N. Hamburger, *Science* **189,** 389 (1975).
58. P. E. Hanna and A. F. Ahmed, *J. Med. Chem.* **16,** 963 (1973).
59. A. V. Harms, W. Hespe, W. T. Nauta, R. F. Rekker, H. Timmerman, and J. de Vries, *in* "Drug Design" (E. J. Ariëns, ed.), Vol. VI, p. 2. Academic Press, New York, 1975.
60. A. Holland, D. Jackson, P. Chaplen, E. Lunt, S. Marshall, D. Pain, and K. Wooldridge, *Eur. J. Med. Chem.—Chim. Ther.* **10,** 447 (1975).
61. A. J. Hopfinger, "Conformational Properties of Macromolecules," p. 49. Academic Press, New York, 1973.
62. A. J. Hopfinger, personal communication (1978).
63. J. R. Hoyland and L. B. Kier, *J. Med. Chem.* **15,** 84 (1972).
64. R. R. Ison, *in* "Molecular and Quantum Pharmacology" (F. Bergmann and B. Pullman, eds.), p. 56. Reidel Publ., Dordrecht, Netherlands, 1974.
65. E. A. Jauregui, M. R. Estrada, L. S. Mayorga, and G. M. Ciuffo, *J. Mol. Struct.* **54,** 257 (1979).
66. E. A. Jauregui, M. R. Estrada, L. S. Mayorga, G. M. Ciuffo, R. R. Ibanez, and M. B. Santillen, *J. Mol. Struct.* in press (1983).
67. T. Jen and C. Kaiser, *J. Med. Chem.* **20,** 693 (1977).
68. C. Kaiser, *in* "Drugs Affecting the Respiratory System" (D. L. Temple, ed.), p. 251. Am. Chem. Soc., Washington, D.C., 1980.
69. B. Kamenar, K. Prout, and C. R. Ganellin, *J. C. S. Perkins II* p. 1734 (1973).
70. L. B. Kier, *J. Med. Chem.* **11,** 441 (1968).
71. L. B. Kier, *J. Pharm. Pharmacol.* **21,** 93 (1969).
72. L. B. Kier and J. M. George, *J. Med. Chem.* **15,** 384 (1972).
73. E. Knobloch, F. Macha, O. Exner, and M. Protiva, *Collect. Czech. Chem. Commun.* **19,** 976 (1954).

74. V. Kothekar and S. Dutta, *Int. J. Quantum Chem.* **15,** 481 (1979).
75. E. Kutter and C. Hansch, *J. Med. Chem.* **12,** 647 (1969).
76. C. L. Lee and M. Z. Atassi, *Biochem. J.* **159,** 89 (1976).
77. C. L. Lee and M. Z. Atassi, *Biochem. J.* **167,** 571 (1977).
78. E. M. K. Leovey and N. H. Andersen, *J. Am. Chem. Soc.* **97,** 4148 (1975).
79. Y. C. Martin, *J. Med. Chem.* **24,** 229 (1981).
80. R. C. Mitchell, *J. C. S. Perkin II* p. 915 (1980).
81. A. Murakami and Y. Akahori, *Chem. Pharm. Bull.* **22,** 1133 (1974).
82. A. Murakami and Y. Akahori, *Chem. Pharm. Bull.* **25,** 2870 (1977).
83. A. Murakami and Y. Akahori, *Chem. Pharm. Bull.* **25,** 3155 (1977).
84. K. C. Nicolaou and J. B. Smith, *Annu. Rep. Med. Chem.* **14,** 178 (1979).
85. M. Nishakawa, M. Kanno, H. Kuriki, H. Sugihara, M. Motohashi, K. Itoh, O. Miyashita, Y. Oka, and Y. Sanno, *Life. Sci.* **16,** 305 (1975).
86. T. Novinson, J. P. Miller, M. Scholten, R. K. Robins, L. N. Simon, D. E. O'Brien, and R. B. Meyer, Jr., *J. Med. Chem.* **18,** 460 (1975).
87. T. B. Paiva, M. Tominaga, and A. C. M. Paiva, *J. Med. Chem.* **13,** 689 (1970).
88. P. F. Periti, *Pharmacol. Res. Commun.* **2,** 309 (1970).
89. C. Petrongolo, B. Macchia, F. Macchia, and A. Martinelli, *J. Med. Chem.* **20,** 1645 (1977).
90. P. Pratesi, L. Villa, and E. Grana, *Farmaco Ed. Sci.* **30,** 315 (1975).
91. B. Pullman and J. Port, *Mol. Pharmacol.* **10,** 360 (1974).
92. I. Rabinowitz, P. Ramwell, and P. Davison, *Nature (London), New Biol.* **233,** 88 (1971).
93. R. F. Rekker and W. T. Nauta, *Arzneim.-Forsch.* **20,** 1572 (1970).
94. R. F. Rekker and W. T. Nauta, *Recl. Trav. Chim. Pays-Bas* **87,** 1099 (1968).
95. R. F. Rekker, W. T. Nauta, T. Bulstma, and C. G. Waringa. *Eur. J. Med. Chem.—Chim. Ther.* **10,** 577 (1975).
96. W. F. Reynolds, I. R. Peat, M. H. Freedman, and J. R. Lyerla, *J. Am. Chem. Soc.* **95,** 328 (1973).
97. W. G. Richards, D. G. Aschman, and J. Hammond, *J. Theor. Biol.* **52,** 223 (1975).
98. W. G. Richards, R. Clarkson, and C. R. Ganellin, *Philos. Trans. R. Soc. London, Ser. B* **272,** 75 (1975).
99. W. G. Richards and C. R. Ganellin, *in* "Molecular and Quantum Pharmacology" (F. Bergmann and B. Pullman, eds.), p. 391. Reidel Publ., Dordrecht, Netherlands, 1974.
100. W. G. Richards, J. Hammond, and D. G. Aschman, *J. Theor. Biol.* **51,** 237 (1975).
101. W. G. Richards, J. Wallis, and C. R. Ganellin, *Eur. J. Med. Chem.—Chim. Ther.* **14,** 9 (1979).
102. T. K. Schaaf, *Annu. Rep. Med. Chem.* **12,** 182 (1977).
103. R. A. Scott and H. A. Scheraga, *J. Chem. Phys.* **45,** 2091 (1966).
105. G. Simons and E. R. Talaty, *J. Am. Chem. Soc.* **99,** 2407 (1977).
106. A. L. Spek, *Acta Crystallogr., Sect. B* **B33,** 816 (1977).
107. J. G. Topliss, *J. Med. Chem.* **15,** 1006 (1972).
108. S. S. Twining and M. Z. Atassi, *J. Biol. Chem.* **253,** 5259 (1978).
109. F. G. Van den Brink and E. J. Lien, *Eur. J. Pharmacol.* **44,** 251 (1977).
110. N. Vardinon, Z. Spirer, M. Fridkin, J. Schwartz, and S. Ben-Efram, *Acta Allergol.* **32,** 291 (1977).
110a. D. F. Veber, *in* "Peptides: Structure and Biological Function" (E. Gross and J. Meiehofer, eds.), Pierce Chem. Co., Rockford, Illinois, 1981.
111. D. F. Veber, F. W. Holly, W. J. Paleveda, R. F. Nutt, S. J. Bergstrand, M. Torchiana, M. S. Glitzer R. Saperstein, and R. Hirschmann, *Proc. Natl. Acad. Sci. U.S.A.* **75,** 2636 (1978).

112. D. F. Veber and R. Saperstein, *Annu. Rep. Med. Chem.* **14,** 209 (1979).
113. C. G. Waringa, R. F. Rekker, and W. T. Nauta, *Eur. J. Med. Chem.—Chim. Ther.* **10,** 349 (1975).
114. R. C. Weast, "Handbook of Chemistry and Physics," 58th ed., p.E-58. CRC Press, Cleveland, Ohio, 1977.
115. H. Weinstein, D. Chou, C. L. Johnson, S. Kang, and J. P. Green, *Mol. Pharmacol.* **12,** 738 (1976).
116. S. Wold, personal communication (1980).
117. K. R. H. Wooldridge, *Proc. Int. Symp. Med. Chem., 5th,* p. 427 (1976).
118. R. C. Young, J. C. Emmett, C. R. Ganellin, G. Durant, and A. M. Roe, *Proc. Int. Symp. Med. Chem., 9th,* Torremolinos, Spain, p. 222 (1980).
119. J. Zaagsma, *J. Med. Chem.* **22,** 441 (1979).

7

Nonsteroidal Antiinflammatory and Antiarthritic Drugs

PETER GUND AND NORMAN P. JENSEN

I. INTRODUCTION

The methodology of QSAR was developed in the early 1960s by Hansch and Fujita (*42*) and Free and Wilson (*34*) at about the same time that nonsteroidal antiinflammatory drugs (NSAIDs) became established as an important field of research (*73,76*). Therefore it is not surprising that QSAR studies were not reported for such compounds until 1970 (*24,26*). Since that time a large number of papers have been published in this field, cov-

QUANTITATIVE STRUCTURE–ACTIVITY
RELATIONSHIPS OF DRUGS

ISBN 0-12-695150-0

TABLE I
References to Assays Used in Deriving QSAR Equations for Antiinflammatory and Antiarthritic Drugs

	In vitro tests					
In vivo tests	No *in vitro* data	Prostaglandin synthesis	Plasma binding	Oxidative phosphorylation	Clotting or erythrocyte stabilization	Complement inhibition
No *in vivo* data	—	(*23*)	(*80,85*)	(*79,80,83*)	(*16,44*)	(*1,45,46,93*)
Edema carrageenan kaolin, or adjuvant induced	(*3,5,9,18,28,30,32,37,47, 51,58–60,62,63,65*)	(*11,38,39,47,82*)	(*38,39*)	(*84*)	(*52,53*)	—
Analgesia	(*12,15,19,20,26,28,41*)	(*11*)	—	—	—	—
UV erythema	(*67,81*)	—	—	—	—	—
Ulcerogenicity	(*70*)	—	—	—	—	—
LD_{50}	(*62*)	—	—	—	—	—

ering a large variety of QSAR techniques applied to a multitude of structure classes tested in numerous *in vitro* and *in vivo* assays (Table I). These papers may be differentiated as "QSAR methodology" and "QSAR application" studies. Methodology papers, which are common in this field, emphasize a particular statistical procedure and use the structure–activity data primarily as a test of validity of that procedure. Application papers utilize such correlations for assay evaluation or for prediction, synthesis, and testing of new compounds; unfortunately, there are not many papers of this type. A number of papers fit neither of these categories but instead report a more or less typical regression analysis correlation and attempt to extract some generalization about the activity of a class of compounds. In the absence of additional experimentation such generalizations are of limited value to the practicing medicinal chemist, thus these papers may be termed "QSAR speculation" papers.

Although studies of all three categories are reviewed in this chapter, we have tried to highlight information useful to the medicinal chemist. Following a brief review of types of assays used, studies are grouped according to the major NSAID structure classes.

II. MEASURING ANTIINFLAMMATORY ACTIVITY

Defining the scope of antiinflammatory and antiarthritic drug agents in any context is a difficult and complex task. Published QSAR studies are primarily confined to what are commonly called nonsteroidal antiinflammatory drugs (NSAIDs), nonnarcotic analgesics, or aspirin-like drugs. There have been some QSAR studies based on *in vitro* immunological assays, but these are sufficiently unrelated to warrant their discussion separately at the end of this chapter.

A. *In Vivo* Assays

The classical, empirical elements of inflammation are "redness, swelling, heat, and pain" (*90*). These elements are the basis for most of the standard *in vivo* laboratory assays used to determine activities of NSAIDs. Redness is the basis for the UV erythema assay (*91*). Swelling is the quantity measured in the very widely used carrageenan foot edema assay (*59,92*). Heat can be equated to pyresis assays in which NSAIDs are active, and pain is the basis of various assays that demonstrate the peripheral and nonnarcotic analgesic activity of NSAIDs. Of these four basic kinds of assays only the antipyretic assay has not been used as the basis for QSAR studies on NSAIDs (see Table I).

Regression analysis techniques have been employed to assess the relevance of these *in vivo* assays to clinical dose of antiinflammatory drugs (*59,67*). In the first such study (*59*), for 15 acidic NSAID enolic compounds, which included aspirin, fenamates, and several arylacetic acids, an attempt was made to correlate the clinical dose with acidity (pK_a), partition coefficient (P_c), half-life of drugs in human plasma ($t_{1/2}$), and the ED_{50} in the carrageenan foot edema (CFE) assay. Multilinear regression analysis using Eq. (1) indicated that the B_2, B_3, and B_4 factors were not statistically significant and the relation could therefore be reduced to Eq. (2), giving a direct relationship between the widely used CFE assay and clinical dose. This study also showed a lack of correlation between pK_a, Pc, and ED_{50} in the CFE assay.

$$\log(\text{clinical dose}) = B_0 + B_1 \log(ED_{50}) + B_2 t_{1/2} + B_3 pK_a + B_4 \log P_c \quad (1)$$

$$\log(\text{daily clinical dose, mg}) = 0.97 \log(ED_{50}, \text{mg/kg}) + 0.96 \quad (2)$$

$$n = 13, \qquad r = 0.88$$

There was found to be a weak correlation between pK_a and $t_{1/2}$ in humans, and a lower pK_a was associated with a longer $t_{1/2}$. It was also noted that these NSAIDs, which are representative of commercially successful NSAIDs, all have pK_a values that fall in a fairly narrow range (5.3–7.9). This observation, that a specific range of weak acidity is a desirable property in NSAIDs, is reinforced by studies that show that acidic NSAIDs, but not nonacidic NSAIDs, accumulate preferentially in inflamed tissues (*36*). A second study (*67*) compared the older UV erythema assay (*91*) with the CFE assay. For a group of 12 commercial NSAIDs, the correlation coefficient was $r = 0.81$ for relating $\log(ED_{50})$ in CFE to log(clinical dose), while the corresponding correlation for the UV erythema assay was less significant ($r = 0.71$). In Eq. (3), used for these correlations, the slope coefficient B_1 for CFE was 0.86, whereas the coefficient for the erythema was a much lower 0.54—again indicating the superiority of the CFE assay.

$$\log(\text{clinical dose}) = B_0 + B_1 \log(ED_{50} \text{ of } \textit{in vivo} \text{ assay}) \quad (3)$$

Although this study would seem to imply that the CFE assay is preferable to the UV erythema assay for finding clinically useful drugs, such reasoning is somewhat circular because most of the 12 tested drugs were probably found via the widely used CFE assay. As suggested by the authors (*67*), the data could mean that the mechanisms of the CFE and erythema assays are different or contain different components.

Besides assays measuring edema, pyresis, analgesia, and erythema, one other type of assay—for ulcerogenicity—is commonly used for NSAIDs. Empirically this side effect is generally found at the same level as desirable activity and mechanistically it has been suggested that this effect cannot be dissociated from antiinflammatory action (*36*). One study, which will be discussed later in terms of specific structural classes, used regression analysis methods to correlate ulcerogenic activity with physical parameters (*70*).

B. *In Vitro* Assays

A variety of *in vitro* assays have been used to assess the activity of NSAIDs, and in many cases QSAR studies have been used to compare *in*

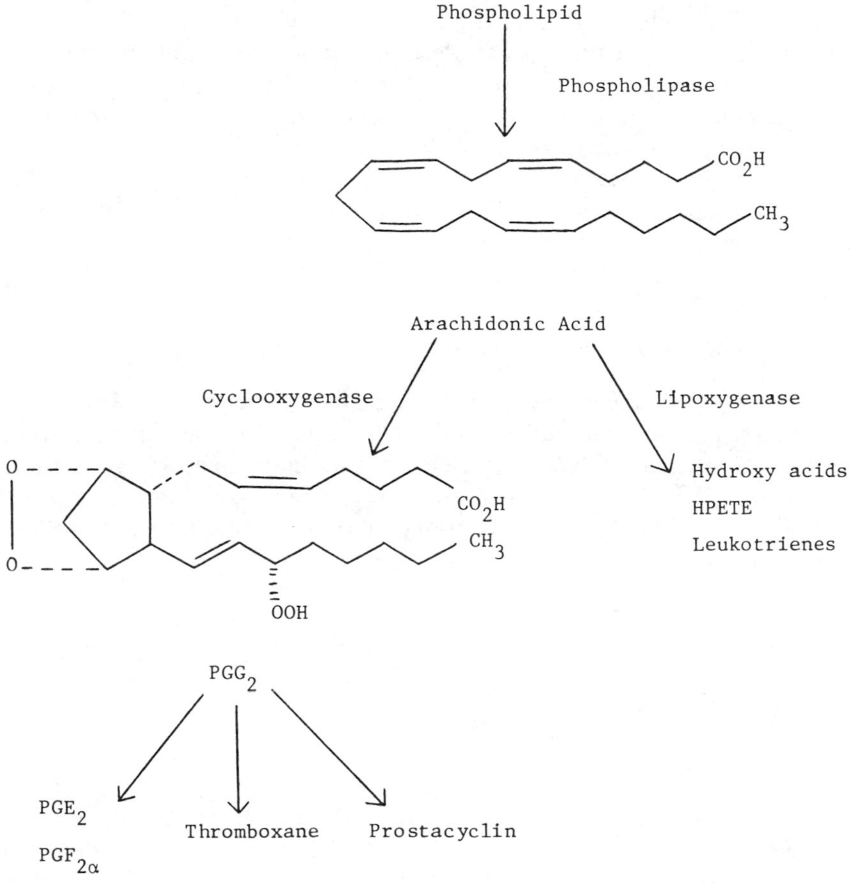

CHART I

vivo and *in vitro* results for a given class of compounds (see Table I). Unlike the *in vivo* assays already discussed, use of an *in vitro* assay raises the question of mechanistic relevance. The question of the mechanism of action of NSAIDs is controversial and by no measure a settled question (*8,29,35,77,87*). Since the discovery in 1971 that aspirin and NSAIDs inhibit prostaglandin synthesis (*86*), or more specifically the enzyme cyclooxygenase (Chart I), this mechanism has drawn the greatest attention and has led to a great deal of study of arachidonic acid metabolism as a component of inflammation (*54*). In spite of this attention, and even acceptance of this mechanism to the point where NSAIDs are sometimes clinically classified as inhibitors of prostaglandin synthesis (*64*), Brune *et al.* (*8*) have listed eight other mechanisms proposed in the literature. To these eight could be added influencing the plasma binding of corticosteroids (*27*), inhibition of cell migration (*7,61,89*), raising cAMP concentrations in leukocytes (*22*), possible modulation of phospholipids (*33,74*) or the lipoxygenase pathway of arachidonic acid metabolism (*78,88*) and, as reviewed by Famaey (*29*) and Kuehl and Egan (*54*), a mechanism that encompasses the modulation of free radicals and activated oxygen species. There are also compounds with antiinflammatory activity that have been reported to stimulate prostaglandin synthesis (*35,55*). Of these many *in vitro* possibilities, five basic types have been used in QSAR studies of NSAIDs (Table I).

C. *In Vitro–In Vivo* Correlations

Because of the uncertainty of the mechanism of action of NSAIDs, it is of interest that several studies have been directed toward quantitatively correlating *in vitro* with *in vivo* assays for antiinflammatory, antipyretic, and analgesic action. Thus in a series of 2-phenyl-1,3-indanones (**I**), no correlation could be found between the inhibition of oxidative phosphorylation and activity in the CFE assay (*84*). For a small series of six anthra-

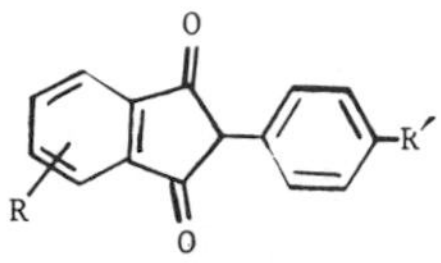

I

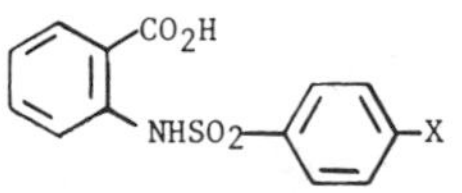

II

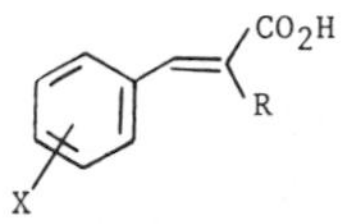

III

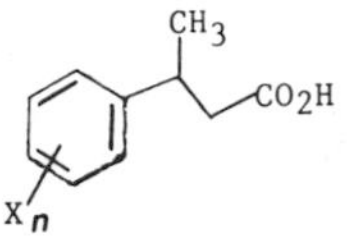

IV

nilic acid derivatives (**II**), a reasonable qualitative correlation is claimed between the CFE assay and inhibition of heat-induced hemolysis of erthyrocytes—although ED_{50} values are not reported for the latter assay (*5*). In a study of cinnamic acids (**III**), inhibition of kaolin-induced edema only partly corresponded to the *in vitro* results of stabilization of erythrocytes to hypotonic hemolysis (*53*). More success was obtained in correlating erythrocyte stabilization with *in vivo* activity in kaolin- and adjuvant-induced edema for a series of β-aryl-*n*-butyric acids (**IV**) (*52*). In this study the *in vivo* assays of kaolin-induced edema (Eq. 4) and adjuvant-induced edema (Eq. 5) predict an optimal π of about 3 to 5. On the other hand, an *in vitro* assay for the stabilization of erythrocyte membranes to hypotonic hemolysis (Eq. 6) predicts a linear dependence on π. If, however, the two most lipophilic compounds are dropped from the kaolin edema analysis (Eq. 4), then Eq. (7) is obtained, which constitutes the ascending limb of the parabola described by Eq. (4). The parallelism between this restricted *in vivo* correlation (Eq. 7) and the *in vitro* correlation (Eq. 6) is evident. The authors suggest that stabilization of erythrocyte membrane is a suitable criterion for the kaolin edema inhibition, but at lipophilicities greater than optimal other factors (most likely drug transport) interfere with *in vivo* activity. It also should be noted that Eqs. (4) and (5) predict that the optimally active compound in this series (**IV**) is insufficiently active compared with the standard (*52*).

β-Arylbutyric acids (**IV**):

$$\log I^{K} = (0.28 \pm 0.12)\pi - (0.05 \pm 0.02)\pi^2 - 0.50 \pm 0.13) \quad (4)$$

$$n = 18, \quad r = 0.886, \quad s = 0.078$$

$$\log I^{F} = (0.62 \pm 0.40)\pi - (0.10 \pm 0.06)\pi^2 - (1.06 \pm 0.50) \quad (5)$$

$$n = 13, \quad r = 0.879, \quad s = 0.137$$

$$\log(1/C) = (0.21 \pm 0.06)\pi + (0.22 \pm 0.20)\sigma + (3.06 \pm 0.10) \quad (6)$$

$$n = 17, \quad r = 0.971, \quad s = 0.052$$

$$\log I^{K} = (0.18 \pm 0.04)\pi + (0.25 \pm 0.12)\sigma - 0.48 \pm 0.05) \quad (7)$$

$$n = 16, \quad r = 0.982, \quad s = 0.031$$

The relationship of *in vitro* prostaglandin synthase inhibition to *in vivo* assays has been examined by several groups (*11,24,38,39,47,82,94*). Ziel and Krupp (*94*) found a close and statistically significant correlation of PG-synthetase inhibition and antipyretic and analgesic assays for seven different commercial NSAIDs. In contrast to these results, a study of 2-aryl-1,3-indandione derivatives (*82*) (**I**) yielded Eq. (8) relating π and σ to inhibition of PG synthetase, but for this single structure class no correlation could be found between this inhibitory activity and *in vivo* antiinflammatory activity. The most disappointing aspect of this lack of correlation was that the most potent PG synthetase inhibitor of the series (**I** with phenyl-substituted 3,5-dichloro) was virtually without antiinflammatory activity.

2-Aryl-1,3-indanones (**I**):

$$\log(1/ID_{50}) = 0.40\pi + 1.64\sigma + 3.47 \quad (8)$$

$$n = 24, \quad r = 0.912, \quad s = 0.239$$

In order to better correlate PG-synthetase activity with antiinflammatory activity in rat-foot edema, Gryglewski (*38*) devised the value Q (Eq. 9), which is large when a compound binds poorly to albumin and/or is a good PG-synthetase inhibitor.

$$Q = \frac{ID_{50} \text{ displacement of ANS from albumin}}{ID_{50} \text{ PG synthetase}} \quad (9)$$

ANS is 1-anilino-8-naphthalene sulfonate

The ratio Q was correlated with the PG-synthetase inhibitory activity of four commercial acidic NSAIDs, namely, indomethacin (**V**), mefanamic acid (**VI**), phenylbutazone (**VII**), and aspirin (**VIII**) with $R = 0.9991$.

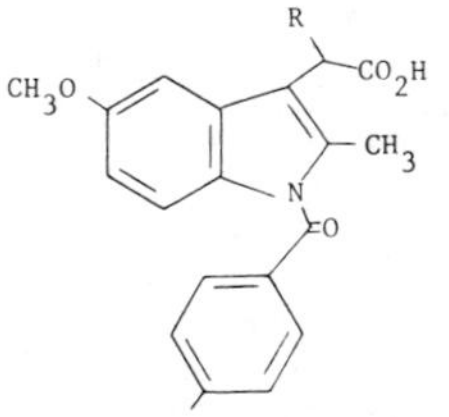

V

a R = H = indomethacin
b R = CH_3

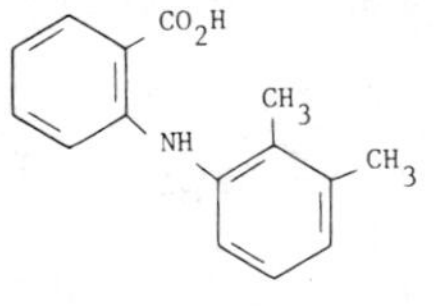

VI

Mefanamic Acid

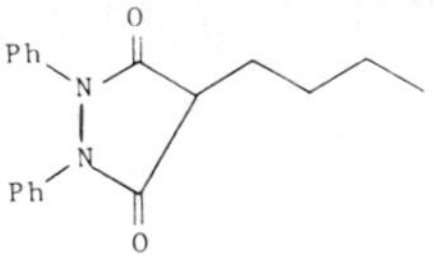

VII

Phenyl Butazone

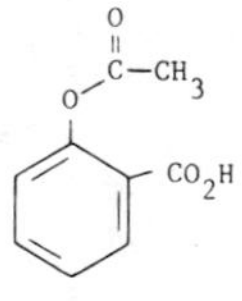

VIII

Aspirin

Gryglewski *et al.* (*39*) successfully used this same comparison for a series of anthranilic acid derivatives (**IX**). In this small group of compounds ($n = 7$) there was poor correlation ($r = 0.44$) of PG-synthetase inhibitory activity with carrageenan foot edema activity, whereas the combined ratio Q correlated well with the antiinflammatory assay ($r = 0.96$). In a very limited series of five indoprofen analogs (**XI**) Eq. (10) was derived (*11*) for the relation of PG-synthetase inhibitory activity to partition coefficient K_p, but no relationship was found between PG-synthetase inhibitory activity and antiinflammatory activity (carrageenan-induced edema and granuloma pouch). These authors, however, noted that for indomethacin (**V**), phenylbutazone (**VII**), and indoprofen (**X**: $r = CH_3$) *in vitro* and *in vivo* activity correlate well (*11*). They made the observation that each of

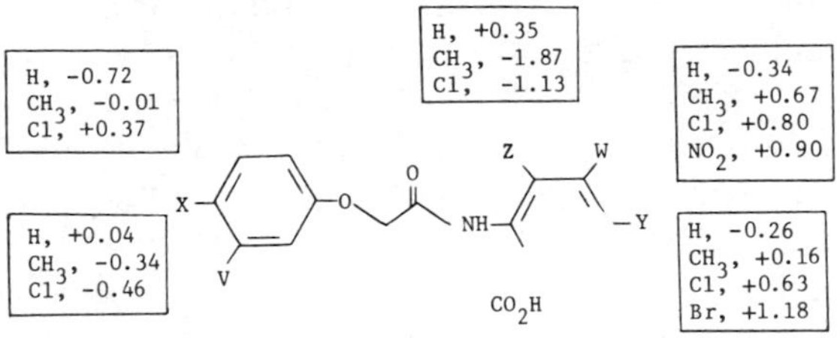

IX

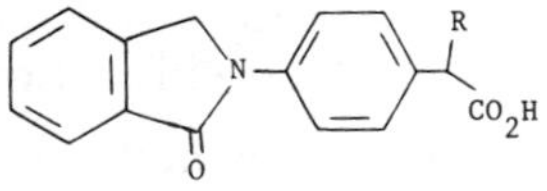

X

R = CH_3 = Indoprofen

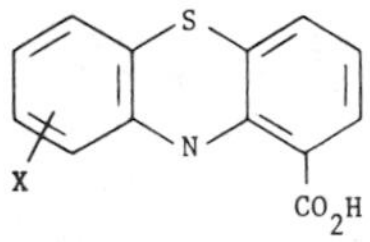

XI

these compounds is the result of selection on the basis of *in vivo* test results. Thus transport and metabolic problems were minimized for the selected compounds and the basis of their mechanism of action, namely, inhibiting PG-synthetase activity, is undisguised. For the series of indoprofen analogs (**X**), the lack of such correlation is attributed to masking effects, especially plasma binding (*11*).

Indoprofen analogs (**X**):

$$\log IC_{50} = -0.49 \log K_p + 2.19 \tag{10}$$

$$n = 5, \qquad r = 0.97$$

Another study (*47*) of a series of anthranilic acids, cyclized to give phenothiazines (**XI**), attempted to relate activity in the carrageenan foot edema assay to PG-synthetase inhibition. For this class of compounds Eq. (11) was derived, which could be improved by the addition of log P factors to give Eq. (12).

Phenothiazines (**XI**):

$$\text{CFE Activity} = (0.35 \pm 0.27)\ \text{PG inhibition} - 1.51 \tag{11}$$

$$n = 14, \qquad r = 0.613, \qquad s = 0.511$$

$$\text{CFE Activity} = (0.45 \pm 0.27)\ \text{PG inhibition} + (0.86 \pm 0.27) \log P - (0.14 \pm 0.04)(\log P)^2 - 2.23 \tag{12}$$

$$n = 14, \qquad r = 0.696, \qquad s = 0.509$$

Despite the low r-values and high s-values, an F-test for statistical significance of Eq. (11) gives a 0.975 confidence level, which represents the best correlation we have found of these two activities for a series of analogs. The log P_0 of 3.1 for Eq. (12) also seems to be in the range found to be optimal for other acidic NSAIDs.

On the other hand, there have been difficulties in relating *in vitro* PG-synthetase inhibition results to *in vivo* antiinflammatory activity. Thus DiPasquale and Mellace (*24*) attempted to correlate the *in vivo* activities of 11 acidic NSAIDs plus hydrocortisone in assays of analgesia, edema, ulcerogenicity, and protection against the effects of intravenous injection of arachidonic acid. (The latter assay was chosen as a direct *in vivo* measure of PG-synthetase inhibitory activity.) In this study all the acidic NSAIDs were found to be protective against the effects of injected arachidonic acid, but no correlation could be found between results in the arachidonic acid assay and the ulcerogenic, edema, or analgesic assays. Furthermore, no potency correlations could be found between the *in vivo* arachidonic acid assay and *in vitro* PG-synthetase inhibition—again pointing up the problems in transferring *in vitro* results into predictions of *in vivo* activities.

III. SALICYLATES

Because the use of salicylates derived from willow bark to deaden pain dates back to prebiblical times, it is fitting that the first published QSAR on NSAIDs deals with salicylates (*44*). In this early (1970) study, *in vitro* fibrinolytic (blood-clot preventing) activity was studied for a series of 49 salicylic acids (**XII**: R = H). Equation (13), based only on lipophilicity,

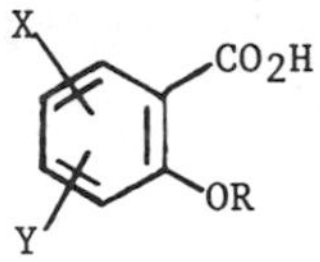

XII

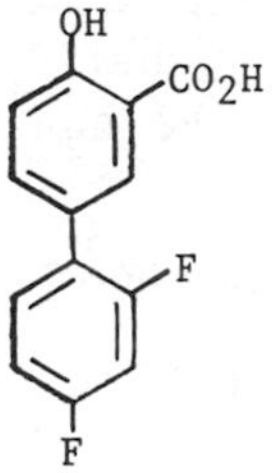

XIII: Diflunisal

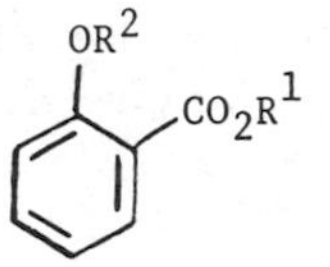

XIV

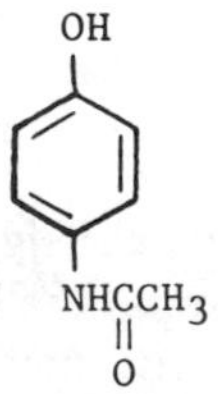

XV: Paracetimol (Acetomenophen)

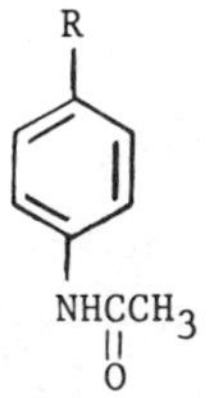

XVI

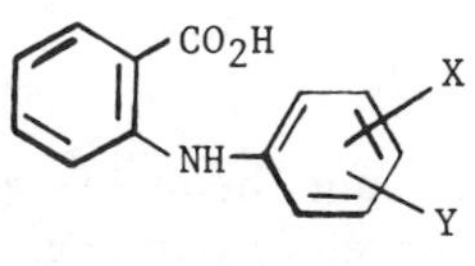

XVII

and Eq. (14), slightly improved by adding electronic and steric factors, were obtained. Both equations indicate that very high lipophilicity enhances activity. In fact, as is pointed out by the authors, the reliability of predicting ideal log P by Eq. (14) is suspect because no compounds in the high lipophilicity range were tested. For a smaller group of 13 of these salicylic acids, fibrinolytic activity in a more "*in vivo*-like" plasma clot test (*44*) gave Eq. (15), which predicts an ideal log P of 5.9.

Salicylic acids (**XII**: R = H):

$$\log(1/C) = (0.51 \pm 0.06) \log P - (0.08 \pm 0.25) \tag{13}$$

$$n = 49, \quad r = 0.929, \quad s = 0.203.$$

$$\log(1/C) = 0.98 \log P - 0.06(\log P)^2 - (0.21 \pm 0.19)\sigma + (0.22 \pm 0.14)E_s^o - (1.21 \pm 0.86) \tag{14}$$

$$n = 49, \quad r = 0.946, \quad \log P_o = 8.4(6.3\text{–}41.0), \quad s = 0.184$$

$$\log(1/C) = 0.93 \log P - 0.08(\log P)^2 - (0.77 \pm 1.12) \tag{15}$$

$$n = 13, \quad r = 0.94, \quad s = 0.161, \quad \log P_o = 5.9(4.9\text{–}30)$$

Although fibrinolytic activities may not be the best *in vitro* assay for gauging antiinflammatory activity, it is interesting that an analogous tendency was found for hydrophobic substituents at the carbon-5 position to increase activity in the antiinflammatory assays used in the development of the most potent known salicylate, diflunisal (**XIII**) (*41*).

In 1977 Dearden reported a study of a series of aspirins by regression analysis methods using platelet aggregation (*16*), analgesic activity (*17*), and antiinflammatory (rat-paw edema) activity (*18*) as the biological readout. In the first of these papers (*16*), which describes *ex vivo* platelet aggregation after *in vivo* dosing with the drugs, a relationship with R_M (a chromatographic measure of lipophilicity) (*6*) was derived (Eq. 16), which predicts an optimal lipophilicity corresponding to an R_M of -0.32. Using the phenylquinone writhing assay as a measure of analgesia, a visual interpretation of the graphic relationship between potency and π was suggested (*17*) to indicate a double parabola with optimal π values of about 0 and 2.5. A more quantitative relationship was obtained when the rat-paw edema assay was used with these aspirin derivatives (*18*). In this case, Eq. (17) was devised, which again demonstrated lipophilicity to be of concern. More interestingly, improved Eqs. (18) and (19) could be obtained for all compounds except 4-substituted analogs and for 4-substituted analogs, respectively. The authors interpreted the lower activity of 4-substituted analogs to be the consequence of an undesirable steric effect. In agreement with this theory they were able to derive an even better equation (Eq. 20) for all the analogs by adding Verloop steric factors for 4-substituents.

Acetylsalicylic acids (**XII**: R = Ac):

$$\log(1/ED_{50}) = -9.06R_{\mathrm{M}} - 28.77R_{\mathrm{M}}^{2} + 3.57 \quad (16)$$

$$n = 15, \quad r = 0.846, \quad s = 0.227$$

$$\log(1/ED_{50}) = 1.03 \log P - 0.20(\log P)^{2} + 1.82 \quad (17)$$

$$n = 28, \quad r = 0.812, \quad s = 0.243, \quad \log P_{\mathrm{o}} = 2.6$$

4-Substitution excluded:

$$\log(1/ED_{50}) = 1.03 \log P - 0.20(\log P)^{2} + 1.96 \quad (18)$$

$$n = 20, \quad r = 0.951, \quad s = 0.118, \quad \log P_{\mathrm{o}} = 2.6$$

4-Substituted derivatives:

$$\log(1/ED_{50}) = 1.03 \log P - 0.21(\log P)^{2} + 1.58 \quad (19)$$

$$n = 8, \quad r = 0.934, \quad s = 0.146, \quad \log P_{\mathrm{o}} = 2.5$$

All substituents:

$$\log(1/ED_{50}) = 1.03 \log P - 0.20(\log P)^{2} - 0.05L_{(4)} - 0.24B_{2(4)} + 2.29 \quad (20)$$

$$n = 28, \quad r = 0.966, \quad s = 0.113, \quad \log P_{\mathrm{o}} = 2.6$$

Because of the empirical and mechanistic connection between ulcerogenicity and antiinflammatory potency (*36,70*), it is worth comparing Eq. (20) with Eq. (21) derived by Rainsford (*70*) for the ulcerogenicity of a series of 10 aspirin analogs. While these two equations are reasonably consistent in predicting optimal log *P* (2.6 versus 2.0), the ulcerogenicity-based Eq. (21) also indicates a strong preference for electron-donating substituents. Furthermore, and in contrast to Dearden's work in which 4-substituents were found to be sterically unfavorable, Rainsford found that 3-substituted analogs were the odd class. Dropping out 3-substituted analogs gave Eq. (22) of considerably increased reliability.

Acetylsalicylic acids (**XII**: R = Ac):

$$\log(1/C_{10}) = (1.21 \pm 0.79) \log P - (0.30 \pm 0.16)(\log P)^{2} - (0.76 \pm 1.34)\sigma - (0.08 \pm 0.95) \quad (21)$$

$$n = 10, \quad r = 0.613, \quad s = 0.708, \quad \log P_{\mathrm{o}} = 2.0$$

3-Substitution excluded:

$$\log(1/C_{10}) = (4.21 \pm 1.06)\log P - (1.08 \pm 0.27)(\log P)^2 - (1.78 \pm 0.85)\sigma - (2.34 \pm 0.95) \quad (22)$$

$$n = 7, \quad r = 0.870, \quad s = 0.494, \quad \log P_0 = 1.9$$

In treating salicylates rather than aspirins, Rainsford separates analogs into 3-, 4-, and 5-substituted series to get Eqs. (23), (24), and (25), respectively. Equation (25) was improved by excluding diflunisal (**XIII**), giving Eq. (26). Equations (23) through (26) are consistent with the Eqs. (17) through (22), derived for aspirins in requiring a log *P* in the 2–4 range, but are dramatically different than Eqs. (21) and (22) in requiring electron-withdrawing rather than electron-donating substituents.

Salicylic acids (**XII**: R = H):

3-Substituted:

$$\log(1/C_{10}) = (0.47 \pm 0.48)\log P - 0.16(\pm 0.08)(\log P)^2 + (0.39 \pm 0.34)\sigma - (0.34 \pm 0.70) \quad (23)$$

$$n = 7, \quad r = 0.907, \quad s = 0.216, \quad \log P_0 = 1.5$$

4-Substituted:

$$\log(1/C_{10}) = -(4.25 \pm 0.33)\log P + (0.73 \pm 0.05)(\log P)^2 + (5.19 \pm 0.55)\sigma + (6.82 \pm 0.65) \quad (24)$$

$$n = 6, \quad r = 0.995, \quad s = 0.047, \quad \log P_0 = 2.9$$

5-Substituted:

$$\log(1/C_{10}) = +(2.13 \pm 0.48)\log P - (0.37 \pm 0.09)(\log P)^2 + (1.07 \pm 0.34)\sigma - (2.99 \pm 0.70) \quad (25)$$

$$n = 6, \quad r = 0.910, \quad s = 0.084, \quad \log P_0 = 2.8$$

5-Substituted, excluding diflunisal (**XIII**):

$$\log(1/C_{10}) = +(4.63 \pm 2.77)\log P - (0.84 \pm 0.52)(\log P)^2 + (1.45 \pm 0.54)\sigma - (6.29 \pm 3.66) \quad (26)$$

$$n = 5, \quad r = 0.927, \quad \log P_0 = 2.8$$

Such a dramatic difference between aspirins and salicylates could be rationalized by the well-discussed (*75*) difference between the action of most NSAIDs on PG-synthetase inhibition compared to aspirin, which has actually been shown to acetylate the cyclooxygenase enzyme. In contrast to the difference between salicylates and aspirins shown by the separate Eqs. (*21*) through (26) in the ulcerogenicity studies (*70*), Mager was able to correlate the antiinflammatory activity of a combined series of 5 salicylates and 10 aspirins (**XIV**: R^1 = OR or NHR, R^2 = H or acetyl) by Eq. (27) (*60*). This equation is strongly dependent on the electronic term, which corrects Hammet's σ values for negative resonance interaction with para substituents, and is less dependent on lipophilicity.

Salicylates and acetylsalicylates (**XIV**):

$$\log(1/C_{10}) = 0.91(\sigma - \Delta R^{+}) - 0.15\pi - 0.18\pi^2 + 1.10 \qquad (27)$$

$$n = 15, \qquad r = 0.886$$

Because optimal π is predicted to be -0.42 by this equation, and because π_0 for aspirin or salicylic acid in this sytem is -0.37 (by comparison, log P values for aspirin and salicylic acid are 1.23 and 2.26, respectively) (*70*) it appears that Eq. (27) requires a somewhat lower lipophilicity than in the relationship developed for analogs with substituents on the 3, 4, and 5 positions. Although no claim is made that QSAR methods were instrumental in the development of the series correlated by Eq. (27), it is of interest that the most active analog, both by prediction of Eq. (27) and by observation *in vivo*, is **XIV** (R^1 = OPh-4-NHAc, R^2 = acetyl), which is an ester of aspirin with 50% increased potency. This most active analog is also a derivative of paracetamol (**XV**), a drug of low analgesic and antipyretic activity, which is generally not considered to be antiinflammatory.

In a quite different approach, Franke (*32*) described a principal component analysis of antiinflammatory activity (carrageenan edema, Wistar rats) of 14 disubstituted salicylic acids as a function of time after application of drug (3, 4, and 5 hours). The data could be correlated with two components, the first of which (U_1) was time independent, and the second of which (U_2) was time dependent. Component U_1 further correlated with molar refractivity and the presence of a free carboxyl group and was claimed to represent a receptor binding effect. Component U_2 correlated with two "pharmacokinetic constants," derived on the assumption that activity varies with time by a first-order kinetic process, and suggested that the second component represents a dynamic effect on the activity.

IV. Phenols

Phenolic compounds are not generally thought of as belonging to the class of NSAID, but Dewhirst (*23*) has summarized several pieces of evidence supporting such a designation. In particular, he has pointed out that many phenols have PG-synthetase inhibitory activity, and he has derived regression analysis equations correlating the *in vitro* ID_{50} versus PG-synthetase (more correctly, cyclooxygenase) activities with σ and π for certain subclasses of phenols. These equations (28–30) are all very similar in predicting increased activity with increased lipophilicity and increased electron-donating ability of substituents. Unfortunately, the 44 compounds used to derive Eqs. (28–30), although reasonably numerous, represent a narrow range of π and σ values. Of the 44 only two compounds have positive σ and only two have negative π for the contributions of the substituent.

Alkylphenols:

$$\log(1/ID_{50}) = 0.28\pi - 4.27\sigma + 3.00 \quad (28)$$

$$n = 20, \qquad r = 0.92$$

2-Alkoxyphenols:

$$\log(1/ID_{50}) = 0.77\pi - 0.25\sigma + 3.95 \quad (29)$$

$$n = 6, \qquad r = 0.99$$

Other 2-substituted phenols:

$$\log(1/ID_{50}) = 0.30\pi - 0.60\sigma + 3.58 \quad (30)$$

$$n = 8, \qquad r = 0.99$$

As noted above, paracetamol (**XV**) is not considered an antiinflammatory drug, but its PG-synthetase inhibitory activity has been demonstrated. Furthermore, a greater inhibitory effect was found against brain than against spleen PG synthetase, and the potency variations were related to paracetamol's antipyretic and analgesic activities (via brain PG-synthetase inhibition) (*31*). The assumption that paracetamol needs the phenolic group for *in vivo* activity as an analgesic is, however, wrong. In a series of three papers (*15,19,20*) on the analgesic properties of paracetamol analogs, in which the phenol was replaced by other substituents (**XVI**), it was shown that such diverse groups as nitro and methyl—and even hydrogen—replaced the phenolic group with a gain in activity. In this series of compounds lipophilicity as measured by buccal absorption (*19*), π (*15,19*), or R_M (*20*) was found to correlate with analgesia. The best correlation was with buccal absorption as given by Eq. (31), in which A/U is the ratio of absorbed to unabsorbed drug. The other measures of lipophilicity gave similar relationships with analgesic activity, as would be expected from Eqs. (32) and (33), which correlate buccal absorbtion and ΔR_M with π for this series of compounds.

4-Substituted acetanilides (**XVI**):

$$\log(1/ED_{50}) = (2.80 \pm 0.44)A/U - (1.99 \pm 0.32)(A/U)^2 - (0.44 \pm 0.12) \quad (31)$$

$$n = 16, \quad F_{2,12} = 4.86, \quad (F_{2,12}[\alpha,0.05] = 3.89)$$

$$\%\ \text{absorbtion} = (23.73 \pm 1.15)\pi + (27.37 \pm 0.71) \quad (32)$$

$$n = 16, \quad F_{1,14} = 427.6, \quad (F_{1,14}[\alpha,0.001] = 17.14)$$

$$\Delta R_M = (0.83 \pm 0.04)\pi + (0.02 \pm 0.02) \quad (33)$$

$$n = 16, \quad F_{1,14} = 528.6, \quad (F_{1,14}[\alpha,0.001] = 17.14)$$

V. ANTHRANILIC ACIDS

Anthranilic acids, especially the *N*-phenyl members of this series, which are also known as fenamates (**XVII**), are relatively old NSAIDs. The first QSAR studies on this series of drugs were published by Terada and co-workers (*79,80*). In this work the authors were able to correlate *in vitro* activity as measured by log K (binding to bovine serum albumin) and $\log(1/C)$ (for uncoupling of phosphorylation) with π by means of Eqs. (34) and (35). If the drug is bound to serum in neutral form, then the equation was modified by first deriving the relationship of Eq. (36) for pK_a and substituting into Eq. (37) to get Eq. (38) for K_n (the neutral binding constant), in which σ is an important factor.

Fenamates (**XVII**):

$$\log K = (0.14 \pm 0.06)\pi + (5.59 \pm 0.05) \quad (34)$$

$$n = 8, \quad r = 0.927, \quad s = 0.054$$

$$\log(1/C) = (0.51 \pm 0.12)\pi + (3.53 \pm 0.11) \quad (35)$$

$$n = 13, \quad r = 0.947, \quad s = 0.160$$

$$\log K_a = (0.74 \pm 0.39)\sigma - 4.14 \pm 0.10) \quad (36)$$

$$n = 6, \quad r = 0.935, \quad s = 0.076$$

$$\log K_n = \log K + \log[(K_a + [H^+])/[H^+]] \simeq \log K + \log K_a - \log[H^+] \quad (37)$$

$$\log K_n = 0.74\sigma + 0.14\pi + 8.45 \quad (38)$$

Rainsford (*70*) also considered the role of pK_a on activity of seven fenamates as ulcerogenic agents. Equation (39), based only on lipophilicity, was considerably improved by the addition of pK_a giving Eq. 40.

Fenamates (**XVII**):

$$\log(1/C_{10}) = (3.53 \pm 1.98) \log P - (0.85 \pm 0.42)(\log P)^2 - (3.30 \pm 2.24) \quad (39)$$

$$n = 7, \quad r = 0.771, \quad s = 0.316, \quad \log P_o = 2.1$$

$$\log(1/C_{10}) = (1.46 \pm 0.28) \log P - (0.40 \pm 0.06)(\log P)^2 - (0.55 \pm 0.16)\mathrm{p}K_a + (1.20 \pm 0.72) \quad (40)$$

$$n = 7, \quad r = 0.944, \quad s = 0.039, \quad \log P_o = 1.8$$

In one of the few Free–Wilson treatments of NSAIDs, Gryglewski and co-workers (*39*) analyzed 21 analogs in the anthranilic acid series, depicted as structure **IX**. This structure also shows the activity contributions derived for various substituents at positions V–Z. The significance of these values are relatively high ($n = 21$, $R = 0.9552$, and $F = 10.42$), and, using these results as a basis, compound **IX** (X = Br, Y = Cl) was prepared and found to have a $\log(1/C)$ of 6.38 compared with a calculated $\log(1/C)$ of 6.53. This is considerably higher than the observed $\log(1/C)$ of 4.98 for the parent system. (The calculated value requires that bromine substitution at X enhances activity by 0.77; although this activity contribution is reasonable, it is missing from the paper. The test compound also is unsubstituted at W, although the analysis suggests that any substitution at this position would be highly favorable.) The optimally substituted compound by the above analysis (**IX**: X = Cl, V = Z = H, W = NO_2, Y = Br), which would be expected to be much more active (calculated $\log[1/C] = 7.82$), was not reported.

The *in vivo* antiinflammatory activity of the test compound (**IX**: X = Br, Y = Cl) was disappointingly as low as aspirin. The lower than expected potency, as discussed earlier, has been attributed to high plasma binding.

In another series of anthranilic acids of structure **XVIII**, the relation-

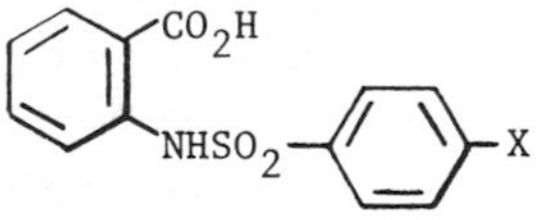

XVIII

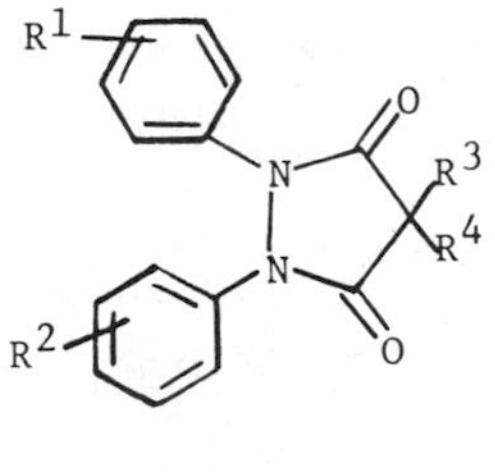

XIX

ship described by Eq. (41) was obtained for antiinflammatory activity in the carrageenan rat-paw assay (*5*). As pointed out by the authors, the fairly good correlation with π is somewhat suspect because of the narrow range of σ examined. They suggest that a parabolic relationship might arise if X substituents of higher lipophilicity were included.

N-benzenesulfonylanthranilic acids (**XVIII**):

$$\log(1/I_{50}) = (0.44 \pm 0.34)\pi + 0.22 \pm 0.27) \qquad (41)$$

$$n = 5, \qquad r = 0.92, \qquad s = 0.11$$

VI. ENOLIC COMPOUNDS

Examples of enolic NSAID are not numerous, but this structural class does contain some important drugs. Phenylbutazone (**XIX**: $R^1 = R^2 = R^3 = H$, $R^4 = n$-butyl), which has been in commerce for 30 years, is the best known drug of this class. Although no equations were derived to express their results numerically, some early workers (*69*) examined the relationship of a numbr of physicochemical properties to $t_{1/2}$ in man and dogs for 16 compounds in the series represented by structure **XIX** ($R^4 = H$). From these data it was suggested that a pK_a in the range 4.5–5.5 favored long $t_{1/2}$, and a pK_a in the range 2.3–3.1 was associated with short $t_{1/2}$. Besides noting these trends, the authors advise on the basis of their data that it may be erroneous to reject a series of drugs based on a clinical trial of only one analog. Some 10 years later, a group of 24 compounds of the type **XIX** ($R^4 = H$) were the subject of a regression analysis study (*63*) in which antiinflammatory activity in a kaolin-induced rat-paw edema assay was correlated with lipophilicity. After excluding several compounds that were inactive, and two in which $R^1 = R^2 = CH_3$ or Cl, Eq. (42) was obtained, which predicts log P_0 of 0.68. Other models using steric or electronic parameters did not improve the equation. Free–Wilson treatment of the substituents was also attempted without success.

In contrast to the results of Eq. (42), which indicates the importance of lipophilicity, for a narrower class of phenylbutazone derivatives (**XIX**: R^3 = butyl, $R^4 = H_2NCH_2$-substituted phenyl), Mager and co-workers (*60*) have found that log P terms did not improve Eqs. (43) and (44), which they obtained at 3- and 4-h readings of activity in the carrageenan edema assay. Comparison of these equations shows that after 3 h only a relative surface tension factor (ϵ is the parachor/molar volume) is needed, whereas at 4 h an electronic term improves the equation. The authors interpret the emergence of dependence on an electronic factor as a consequence of drug–enzyme interactions, causing drug degradation.

Phenylbutazones (**XIX**)

$$\log(1/C) = (0.77 \pm 0.37) \log P - (0.57 + 0.26)(\log P)^2 - 2.10 \quad (42)$$

$$n = 16, \quad r = 0.798, \quad s = 0.255, \quad \log P_0 = 0.68$$

$$3\text{ h: } y_1 = -104.28 \log \xi + 244.92 \quad (43)$$

$$n = 9, \quad r = 0.89$$

$$4\text{ h: } y_2 = -62.54 \log \xi - 22.342\sigma_R + 177.96 \quad (44)$$

$$n = 9, \quad r = 0.96$$

Van der Berg and collaborators have correlated the physicochemical properties of a number of 2-aryl-1,3-indandiones (**I**) with their activities as uncouplers of oxidative phosphorylation (*83*), stabilization of bovine albumin (BSA) against heat denaturation (*85*), and as inhibitors of PG synthetase (*82*). In each of these cases a fairly significant equation was obtained for a reasonably large number of derivatives (Eqs. 8, 45, and 46). Equation (46), which is the least significant, could be improved by splitting the analogs into groups of ortho-, meta-, and para-substituted derivatives; as discussed above, these results were somewhat academic in interest, because for this class of compounds *in vitro* activities had no meaningful relationship to *in vivo* potency.

1-Aryl-1,3-indandiones (**I**):

Uncoupling (D = 1 for ortho substituent, 0 for others):

$$\log(1/C_{50}) = -0.47\pi - 0.26\sigma - 0.72D + 3.86 \quad (45)$$

$$n = 44, \quad r = 0.974, \quad s = 0.158, \quad F = 246.64$$

Stabilization of BSA (D = as in Eq. 45):

$$\log Inh = 0.18\pi + 0.12\sigma + 0.05E_s^M - 0.45D + 1.32 \quad (46)$$

$$n = 44, \quad r = 0.854, \quad s = 0.133, \quad F = 26.16$$

In a later study of the 2-phenyl-1,3-indandione system (**I**) Badin and co-workers (*3*) used CNDO calculations to examine the effect of changes in R and R′ on antiinflammatory activity. They were able to separate 14 of 17 of these analogs into three groups that showed increased biological activity with increased π-bond character of the 2–3 bond. Eight heterocyclic modifications of type **XX** were then prepared in which substituents and atoms were changed in the 2 and 3 positions. The *in vivo* activities of all of these newly synthesized analogs (except for **XX**: Z = N, Y = Ph, X = C) were lower than the parent indandione, but the eight new analogs could again be separated into three groups. Compounds with X—Z bond indices >0.60 were the most active, whereas those <0.59 were less active.

The group of compounds represented by structure **XXI**, which contains the Japanese drug Bucolome (R^1 = cyclohexyl, R^3 = H, R^5 = butyl), has been the subject of a rather thorough Free–Wilson analysis (*62*). Although this study is clearly after the fact with respect to the develop-

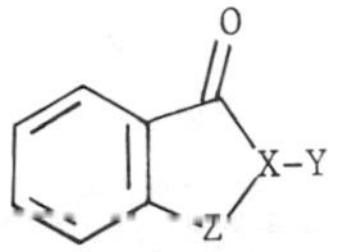

XX

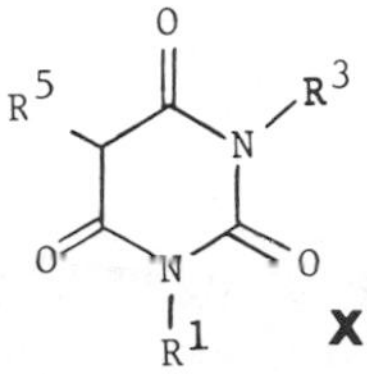

XXI

ment of Bucolome, it is praiseworthy because not only are activities treated by QSAR methods but toxicity is given an equal and parallel treatment, allowing conclusions to be drawn about optimal therapeutic indices. A toxicity model was obtained, using all 49 available analogs, that had a correlation constant of 0.739 (s = 0.234, F = 2.40). This could be improved to 0.879 (s = 0.169, F = 6.08) by exclusion of nine analogs in which R^5 is identical to or closely resembles R^1 or R^3. Activities were measured in ovalbumin, dextran, and carrageenan rat-foot edema assays. The carrageenan assay results, used in the same model as used for the toxicity studies, yielded results with a correlation coefficient of 0.958 (n = 49, s = 0.161, F = 11.03). The final conclusion gleaned from this study was that Bucolome is among the best NSAID in therapeutic index. A more provocative conclusion was that replacing the butyl in the R^5 position with methyl or ethyl would lower toxicity but not antiinflammatory activity. Both these analogs were among the previously prepared 49. The methyl analog was about one-fourth as toxic as Bucolome but was not reported as tested in the carrageenan assay and was less potent in the ovalbumin induced edema assay.

VII. CARBOXYLIC ACIDS

The carboxylic acids contain an important subgroup, the arylacetic acids. Seven of eight prostaglandin-affecting NSAIDs that are listed as marketed in the United States, and greater than 75% of the 42 antiinflammatories listed as marketed outside the United States or under clinical investigation (*64*), fall into this very important subclass. It is therefore remarkable that only five QSAR studies (*11,51,58,65,70*) on compounds of this class could be found in the literature. Of these five studies only two (*11,70*) deal with series represented by the drugs on Nickander's list (*64*).

Furthermore, both of these two studies are post facto reports that clearly had no part in the successful development of the drugs involved.

An early QSAR study used regression analysis to find a relationship between π and human buccal absorption for a group of 31 carboxylic acids of which 18 were phenylacetics (*58*). Equation (*47*) was obtained, which predicts an optimal log P_0 of 4.19. This is only in fair agreement with a log P_0 of 2.8 obtained for the antiinflammatory activity of a series of 22 phenylacetic acids by a discriminant analysis treatment (*65*).

Phenylacetic acids

$$\log(\%\ \text{Abs}) = 1.29 \log P - 0.15(\log P)^2 + 0.66(\text{p}K_a - 6.0) - 0.01 \quad (47)$$

$$n = 31, \quad r = 0.968, \quad s = 0.138, \quad \log P_0 = 4.19$$

A group of 28 4-benzyloxyphenylacetic acids (**XXII**) was tested for antiinflammatory activities in both the kaolin and adjuvant edema assays (*51*). Use of regression analysis gave Eq. (48) for the kaolin data and Eq. (49) for the adjuvant data. From these equations it was concluded that an

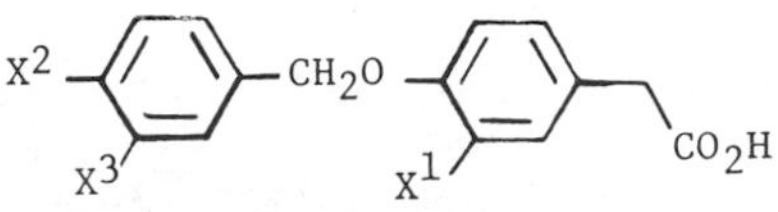

XXII

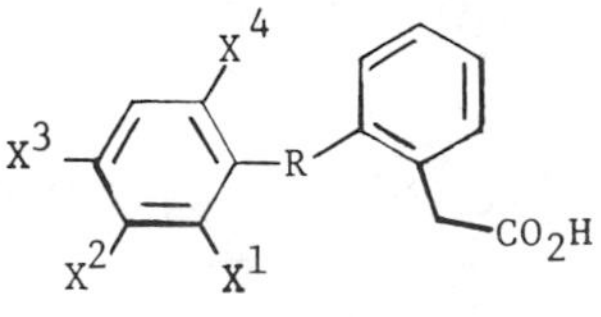

XXIII

optimum is reached when $\Sigma\ \pi$ is in the range of 0.6 to 1.1 and that of the 3 substituents tried at X^1 (OCH_3, CH_3, Cl), chlorine (with the largest σ value) was best. On this basis **XXII** (X^1 = Cl, X^2 = X^3 = H) was chosen as a candidate for further development. The impressiveness of this regression analysis study is weakened by the fact that simple inspection of the activities of the 28 analogs also leads to the selection of the same compound, which is the most active compound in both assays. The study would have benefited from postanalysis synthesis and testing of compounds predicted to have high activity; particularly of analogs having strongly electron-withdrawing groups at X^1 (e.g., No_2 or CN).

4-Benzyloxyphenylacetic acids (**XXII**):

$$\log(1/Act) = (0.61 \pm 0.25) \sum \pi - (0.30 \pm 0.10) \left(\sum \pi\right)^2 \pm (0.27 \pm 0.26)\sigma \text{ (for } X^1) - (0.41 \pm 0.15) \quad (48)$$

$$n = 28, \quad r = 0.909, \quad s = 0.080, \quad F = 37.88, \quad \sum \pi_0 = 1.01$$

$$\log(1/Act) = (0.24 \pm 0.22) \sum \pi - (0.19 \pm 0.12) \left(\sum \pi\right)^2 + (0.51 \pm 0.29)\sigma \text{ (for } X^1) - (0.26 \pm 0.15) \qquad (49)$$

$$n = 25, \quad r = 0.841, \quad s = 0.099, \quad F = 16.93, \quad \sum \pi_0 = 0.63$$

Rainsford (*70*) in his ulcerogenicity studies has treated three different arylacetic acid classes, as depicted by structure **XXIII** (diclofenac: R = NH, $X^2 = X^3 = H$, $X^1 = X^4 = Cl$ and analogs); by structures **XXIV**

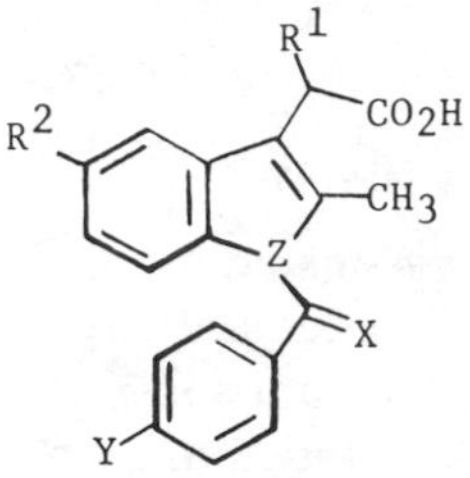

XXIV

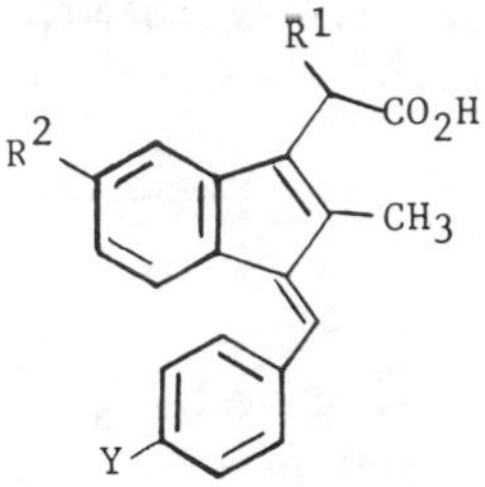

XXV

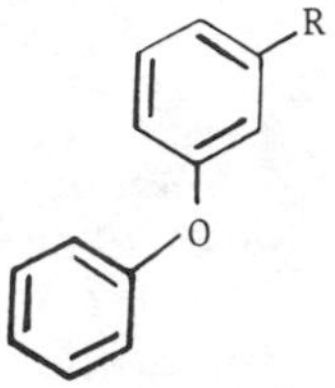

XXVI

and **XXV** together, a series that contains indomethacin (**V**) and sulindac (**XXV**: R^1 = H, R^2 = F, Y = $\overset{O}{\overset{\uparrow}{S}}$—$CH_3$); and by fenoprofen (**XXVI**: R = $CH(CH_3)CO_2H$) and analogs. As seen from Eqs. (50) through (52), reasonably good correlation with log *P* was found for all three series, but the log P_0 values of 0.75, −1.8, and 1.90 cover such a range that any generalizations about optimal log *P* for arylacetic acids as a class are not possible. As in other studies, it would be interesting to derive QSAR relationships based on antiinflammatory activities for these compounds to compare with Rainsford's QSAR relationships describing the serious toxic effect of ulcerogenicity. Such a combined approach is more desirable, because establishing optimal parameters for toxicity is not a drug development objective by itself but is only useful in conjunction with optimizing antiinflammatory activities.

Clofenacs (**XXIII**):

$$\log(1/C_{10}) = (1.78 \pm 0.48) \log P - (1.19 \pm 0.28)(\log P)^2 + (1.05 \pm 0.27) \qquad (50)$$

$$n = 6, \quad r = 0.884, \quad \log P_0 = 0.75$$

Indomethacins and sulindacs (**XXIV** and **XXV**):

$$\log(1/C_{10}) = (26.04 \pm 9.20) \log P + (7.27 \pm 2.84)(\log P)^2 - (0.24 \pm 0.29)\mathrm{p}K_a + (21.87 \pm 8.00) \quad (51)$$

$$n = 6, \quad r = 0.925, \quad s = 0.435, \quad \log P_0 = -1.8$$

Fenoprofens (**XXVI**):

$$\log(1/C_{10}) = -(4.67 \pm 1.13) \log P + (1.23 \pm 0.33)(\log P)^2 + (4.44 \pm 0.87) \quad (52)$$

$$n = 5, \quad r = 0.926, \quad s = 0.20, \quad \log P_0 = 1.90$$

Two QSAR studies have been published on aryl-*n*-propionic acids (*9,52*). In the first study, both multiple regression analysis and Free–Wilson techniques were utilized (*9*). For a set of 33 analogs of type **XXVII** ($n = 2$, $R^2 = H$), Eq. (53) represents the best correlation covcring the en-

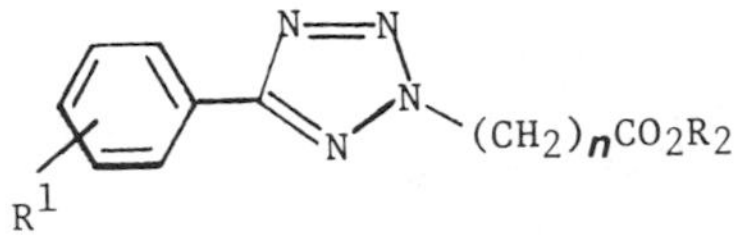

XXVII

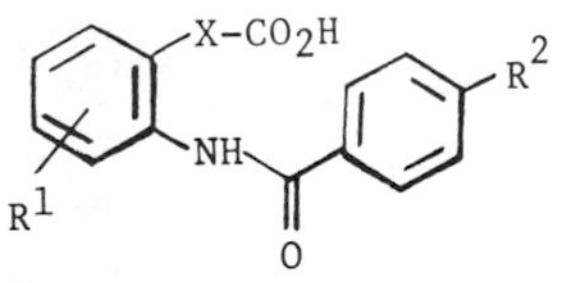

XXVIII

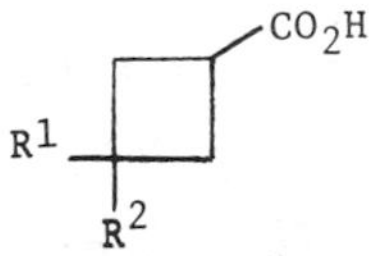

XXIX

tire set of compounds. However, by dropping nitro compounds that are thought to be easily metabolized, and excluding two analogs with R^1 = 4-methyl or 4-trifluoromethyl, Eq. (54) of improved correlation was obtained. Improved equations could also be obtained by splitting the compounds into meta-substituted (Eq. 55) and para-substituted (Eq. 56) analogs. That the electronic effect of the para substituents in Eq. (56) can completely disappear in Eq. (54) simply by the exclusion of a few analogs has been interpreted by the authors to be due to the presence of a real but small electronic effect that is masked by the stronger lipophilic factor in Eqs. (54) and (55). This lipophilicity is expressed by a π_0 of 0.8, which in this system corresponds to $\log P_0$ of 1.4. In their Free–Wilson treatment, an original set of 27 analogs was reduced to 25 by elimination of some lipophilic dibromo analogs, giving an equation having $r = 0.931$, $s = 0.16$, and $F = 12.90$. For **XXVII**, R^1 ranks Br > Cl > H > NO_2 and $n = 2$ is better than $n = 3$. Both the regression analysis and Free–Wilson results predict the most active analogs but fail to provide ideas for the synthesis of more active compounds. The difference in meta and para substituents, however, suggested that steric and geometrical effects were important, which led to further synthesis in these series (*10*). In contrast, Kuchar's QSAR studies of the β-aryl-*n*-butyric acids (**IV**) (*52*), led to the conclusion that optimal activity as defined by Eqs. (4) and (5) would not yield a compound of potency as high as their standard, 3-chloro-4-benzyloxyphenylacetic acid (**XXII**: X^1 = Cl, $X^2 = X^3$ = H), and further synthesis was therefore considered fruitless.

Other carboxylic acids

Tetrazolylpropionic acids (**XXVII**: $n = 2$, R^2 = OH):

$$\log(AI) = 0.42\pi - 0.22\pi^2 + 0.61 \tag{53}$$

$$n = 33, \quad r = 0.697, \quad s = 0.27, \quad \pi_0 = 0.95$$

$$\log(AI) = 0.48\pi - 0.31\pi^2 + 0.73 \tag{54}$$

$$n = 28, \quad r = 0.851, \quad s = 0.20, \quad \pi_0 = 0.77$$

Meta R^1:

$$\log(AI) = 0.58\pi - 0.37\pi^2 + 0.63 \tag{55}$$

$$n = 16, \quad r = 0.945, \quad s = 0.16, \quad \pi_0 = 0.78$$

Para R^1:

$$\log(AI) = 0.77\sigma_m - 0.85\sigma_p^2 + 0.58 \tag{56}$$

$$n = 14, \quad r = 0.841, \quad s = 0.14$$

The Kuchar group has also examined a series of cinnamic acids (**III**) (*53*) in a study of doubtful practical utility. Starting with 34 analogs of structure **III** with R = H, CH_3, Et, or Pr and only one X substituent, they were able to derive. Eq. 57, (*D* is a "dummy" variable for the number of hydrogens on the double bond, and Δp*K* is 4.96 − p*K*) for the activity in stabilizing erythrocyte membranes *in vitro*.

Cinnamic acids (**III**):

$$\log(1/C) = 0.33 \sum \pi + 1.57\Delta pK + 0.28D + 0.31E_s + 4.23 \tag{57}$$

$$n = 30, \quad r = 0.951, \quad s = 0.141$$

Using these results, they predicted that para X should be higher alkoxy and meta X should be halogen. Using these predictions, 10 new derivatives were prepared, several of which were more active than any of the first set of analogs. Practical success was, however, limited by poor correlation of these *in vitro* results with *in vivo* activity, as expressed in the kaolin-induced rat-foot edema assay; all of the analogs showed low levels of *in vivo* activity.

A limited number of analogs of the type **XXVIII** (R^1 = H, X = OCH_2) have been reported (*26*) to give Eq. (58) when an *in vivo* phenylquinone writhing assay is used for measuring analgesic potency. Several other variations of **XXVIII** were made, but only this small set of 11 compounds (from a total of 56 analogs) were reported to yield a significant regression analysis equation. In addition to four ortho-substituted analogs, which had to be excluded, two more analogs with R_2 = 4-OH and 4-CH_3SO_2 were also apparently left out because of lack of testing. This is unfortunate since the remaining 11 compounds contained no examples with R^2 having positive π values. In spite of such possible criticism, this study contains a useful discussion of the task of getting reproducible quantitative biological data—a prerequisite for good QSAR studies and a difficulty that is not often discussed. In this study, when the authors had trouble getting satisfactory quantitative data with the carrageenan edema assay, they switched to the phenylquinone writhing assay which, in their hands, was more reproducible.

Phenoxyacetic acids (**XXVIII**: R^1 = H, X = OCH_2):

$$\log(1/ID_{50}) = 0.55\pi - 2.14 \qquad (58)$$

$$n = 11, \qquad r = 0.87$$

Another report, in which analgesic and antiinflammatory assays were examined as the basis of QSAR regression analysis data, is a French study (*28*) on the cyclobutane analogs **XXIX**. A group of 12 compounds were tested in both of these assays and the results from oral administration of the drugs yielded Eq. (59) (δ_{NMR} is the NMR shift of the acidic proton and T_s is a formally introduced value equal to 1 for R^1, R^2 = H and equal to 1/2 for R^1 = H) from the carrageenan assay antiinflammatory data and Eq. (60) from the phenylquinone analgesic assay. On the basis of these equations eight more analogs were prepared. Although none of the new derivatives were very active in the antiinflammatory assay, considerable enhancement of analgesic activity was realized. By letting R^1 = H (which lowers T_s from 1 to 1/2) and substituting R^2 with groups high in π (e.g., cyclopentyl and cyclohexyl), analgesic activity was raised threefold with no increase in toxicity. Lack of success with the antiinflammatory data led this same group to reexamine these data by multicomponent analysis in a later paper (*37*). This technique allowed separating the analogs into three classes, of which only 4-alkyl substituted derivatives gave a simple correlation with π and a steric effect.

Cyclobutanecarboxylic acids (**XXIX**):

$$\log(1/C_{50}) = 0.08\delta_{\mathrm{NMR}} - 1.08T_s + 2.70 \quad (59)$$

$$n = 12, \quad r = 0.91, \quad s = 0.255, \quad F = 21.8$$

$$\log(1/C_{50}) = -0.04\delta_{\mathrm{NMR}} + 0.23\pi^2 - 0.50T_s + 2.71 \quad (60)$$

$$n = 12, \quad r = 0.79, \quad s = 0.272, \quad F = 4.44$$

VIII. CONFORMATIONAL STUDIES OF ARALKANOIC ACIDS

It appears that standard QSAR techniques have not been notably successful in correlating activities or predicting better analogs. Among the commercially important arylacetic acids, experience is perhaps typified by a study of more than 350 analogs of indomethacin (**Va**) (*73*), in which no simple relationships could be found between biological activity and protein binding, solubility, distribution coefficient, or acidity. A later study also reports difficulty in obtaining statistically significant correlations in this series (*40*).

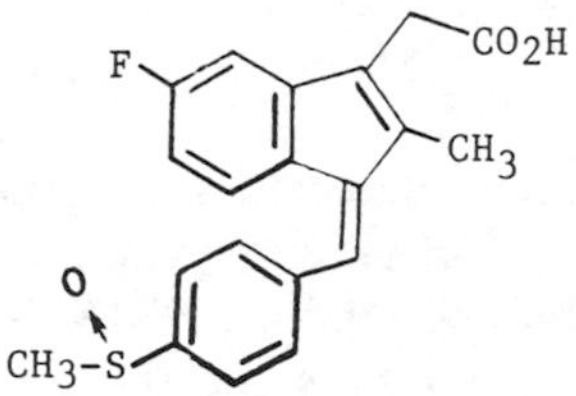

XXX

On the other hand, stereochemistry was shown to be very important, with the (+)-(*S*)-α-methyl isomer being much more active than the (−)-*R* enantiomer (*73*). Furthermore, the (*Z*)-1-arylidenylindene-3-acetic acids (**XXX**) were highly active, with exactly parallel substituent effects in the two series. As a consequence of these conformational and configurational relationships, a hypothetical "receptor site" for antiinflammatory indomethacin analogs was postulated (*73*) as shown in Fig. 1. The trough accommodated the *p*-chlorophenyl group of **Va**, which according to X-ray analysis (*50*) was tilted with respect to the indole ring.

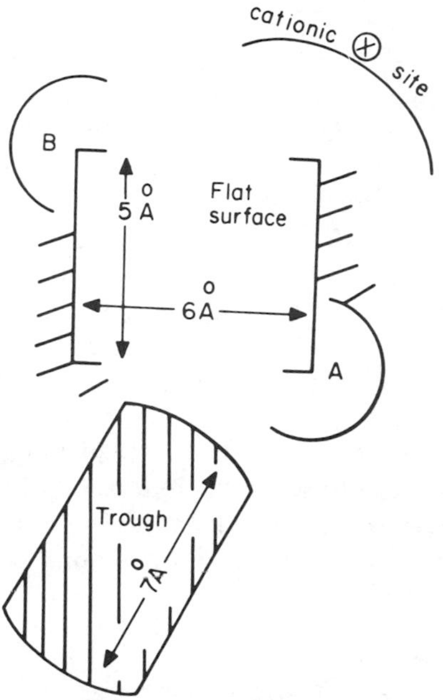

Fig. 1. Hypothetical synthetase binding site. From Shen (*73*), with permission.

Later, when it became clear that NSAIDs exert at least part of their antiinflammatory effect by inhibiting prostaglandin synthesis, Shen *et al.* (*74*) proposed that this indomethacin binding site model represented the prostaglandin synthetase binding site. In the same year Scherrer (*72*) proposed a modified receptor site, which, by placing the carboxyl binding site coplanar with one of the ring binding sites, accommodated salicylates as well as arylacetates. In another review that same year, Gryglewski (*38*) noted that most NSAIDs investigated to that date would fit the hypothetical Shen receptor model.

At about the same time, Demerson *et al.* (*21*) rationalized the SAR in a

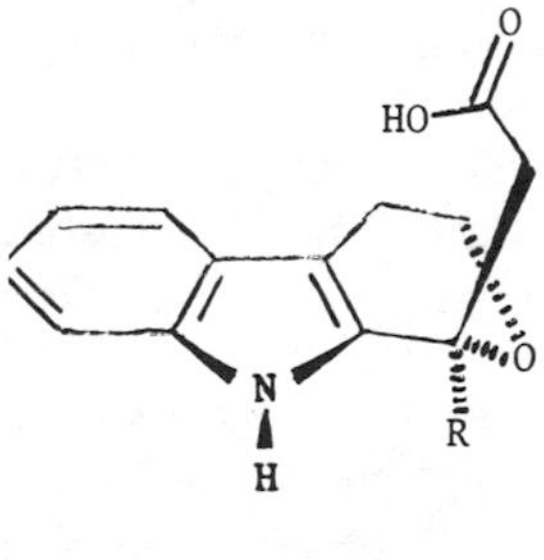

XXXI

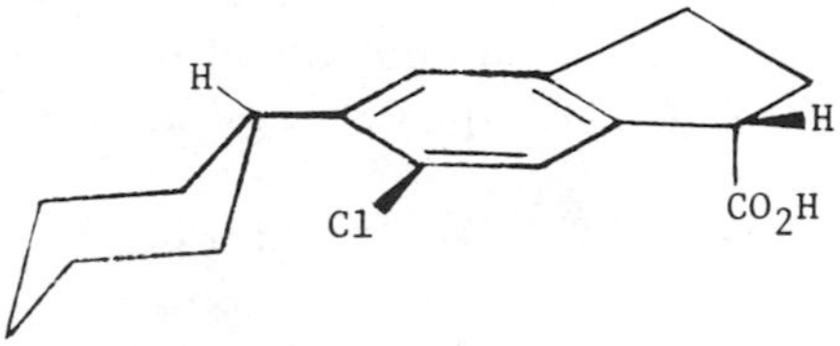

XXXII

series of pyrano[3,4-*b*]indoleacetic acids, culminating in the highly active prodolic acid (**XXXI**: R = *n* -Pr) by proposing a bioactive conformation having the acetic acid chain above the pyranoindole nucleus for optimal interaction with an antiinflammatory receptor. However, because the stereochemistry of the active isomer was not determined, the picture of the receptor site remained somewhat hazy.

In the same year Kamiya *et al.* (*49*) determined by X-ray diffraction the absolute stereochemistry and preferred conformation of (+)-6-chloro-5-cyclohexylindan-1-carboxylic acid (d-TAI-284, **XXXII**). They suggested that this drug could fit the same receptor site as indomethacin, and noted that antiinflammatory activity resides in the *S* isomer for most of these drugs.

Langlois *et al.* (*57*) used theoretical (classical and quantum mechanical) and experimental methods to study the related (methylcyclohexyl)phenylpropionic acids (**XXXIII**). They discovered that compounds with methyl at the 1-axial, 2-axial, and 2-equatorial positions were quite active and

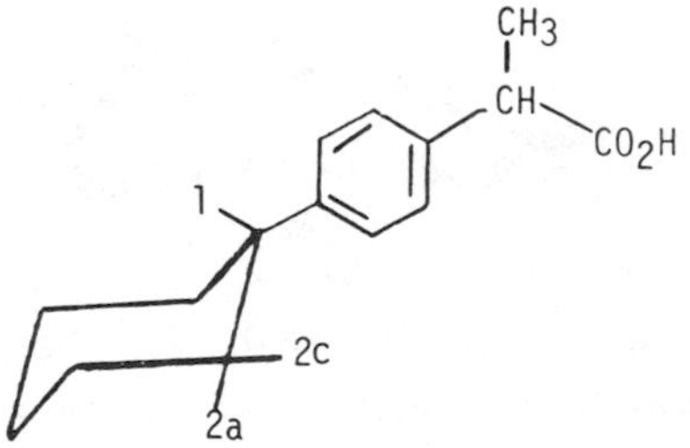

XXXIII

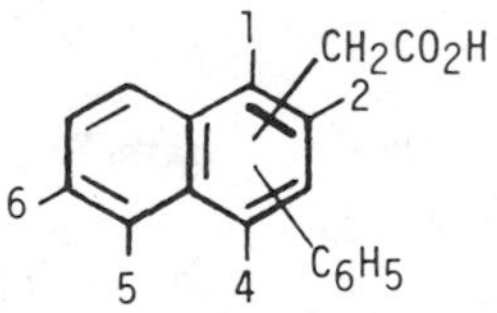

XXXIV

concluded that the conformation of the cyclohexane ring was not important. Similarly, Kaltenbronn (*48*) found some positional variation tolerated in phenylnaphthaleneacetic acids (**XXXIV**); 4- and 5-phenyl substitution gave equally high antiinflammatory activity in the nephthalene-1-acetic acid series, whereas 5- and 6-phenyl substituted derivatives were equally efficacious in the (slightly less active) naphthalene-2-acetic acid series.

Dive *et al.* (*25*) performed a systematic conformational analysis of eight arylacetic acid antiinflammatory drugs, including indomethacin, tolmetin, ketoprofen, fenoprofen, and some experimental drugs, by the Complete Neglect of Differential Overlap Self Consistent Field Molecular Orbital (CNDO-SCF-MO) method. For general structures **XXXV** and **XXXVI** and torsion angles τ_1(1-2-3-4), τ_2(2-3-4-5), τ_3(5-6-7-8), and τ_4(6-7-8-9), all active compounds shared a low energy acetic acid side-chain conformation having $\tau_3 = 90°$, $\tau_4 = -90°$. Rigid indane-1-carboxylic acids are fixed in a

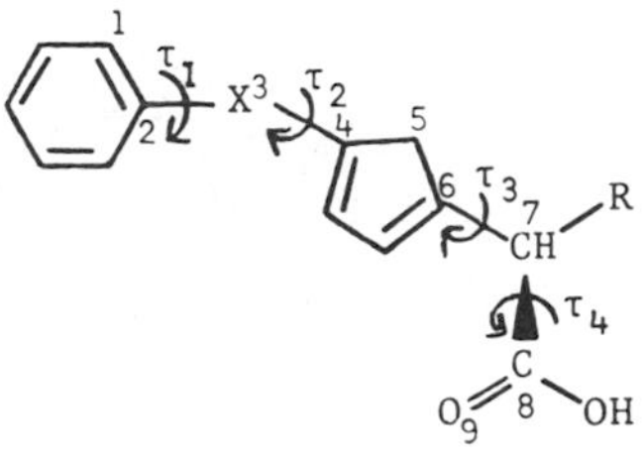

XXXV

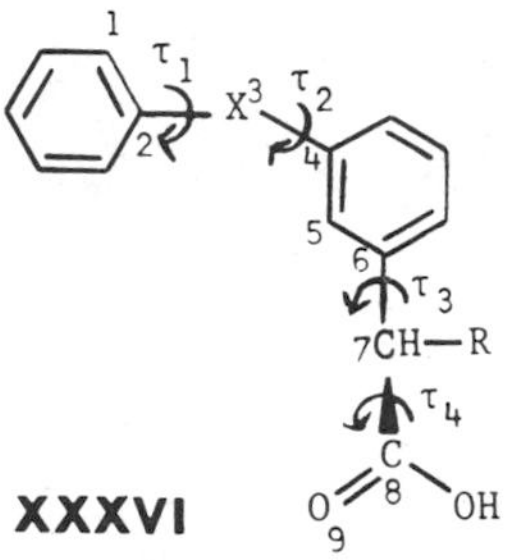

XXXVI

comparable conformation. Furthermore, although no common low-energy value of τ_2 was found for all compounds, a conformation having $\tau_2 \approx 135°$ was accessible to all members and was tentatively assigned to the bioactive conformation. Finally, energy was optimal for $\tau_1 \geq 90°$. For confirmation of the importance of an optimal τ_2 value, the authors noted the excellent activity of the (*Z*)-2 ($\tau_2 \sim 150°$) isomer of sulindac (**XXX**), and the low activity of the (*E*)-2 isomer. To show the importance of τ_1, they pointed to the inactive (*66*) **XXXVII** ($\tau_1 \approx 0$). Several other classes of NSAIDs were also found to fit the proposed conformational constraints.

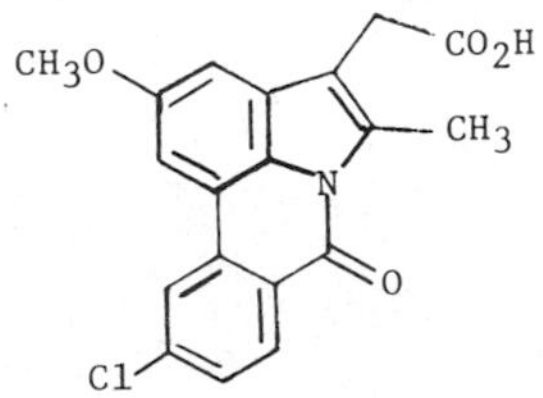

XXXVII

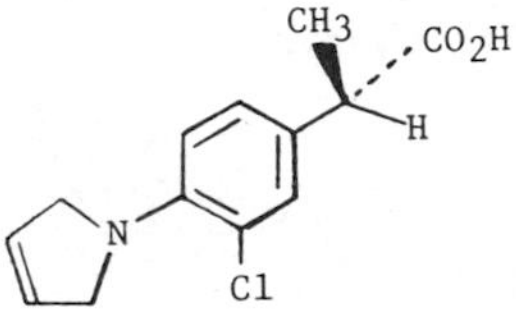

XXXVIII

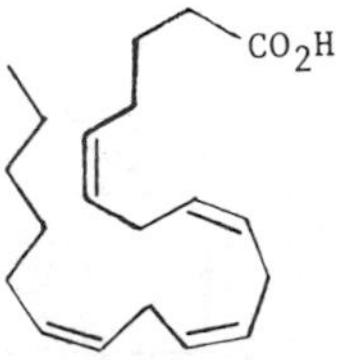

XXXIX

Independently Gund and Shen (*40*) performed a similar conformational analysis of indolylacetic acid model systems and of pirprofen (**XXXVIII**) by CNDO and classical mechanical methods. They also investigated the hypothesis that arachidonic acid (**XXXIX**), the natural substrate of the prostaglandin cyclooxygenase enzyme that most NSAIDs inhibit, could fit a receptor analogous to Shen's postulated indomethacin binding site. Since arachidonic acid possesses five threefold and nine sixfold rotatable single bonds, or a possible 10^6 all-staggered conformations, no attempt was made to find the lowest energy form. Rather, a CPK model of **XXXIX** was folded to find a conformation that resembled indomethacin and that would fit the same binding site. Such a conformation was found, which had the additional feature of "explaining" the mechanism of stereospecific conversion of **XXXIX** to the prostaglandin cyclic endoperoxide, PGE_2 (Fig. 2). Figure 3 illustrates the shape and functionality of **XXXIX**

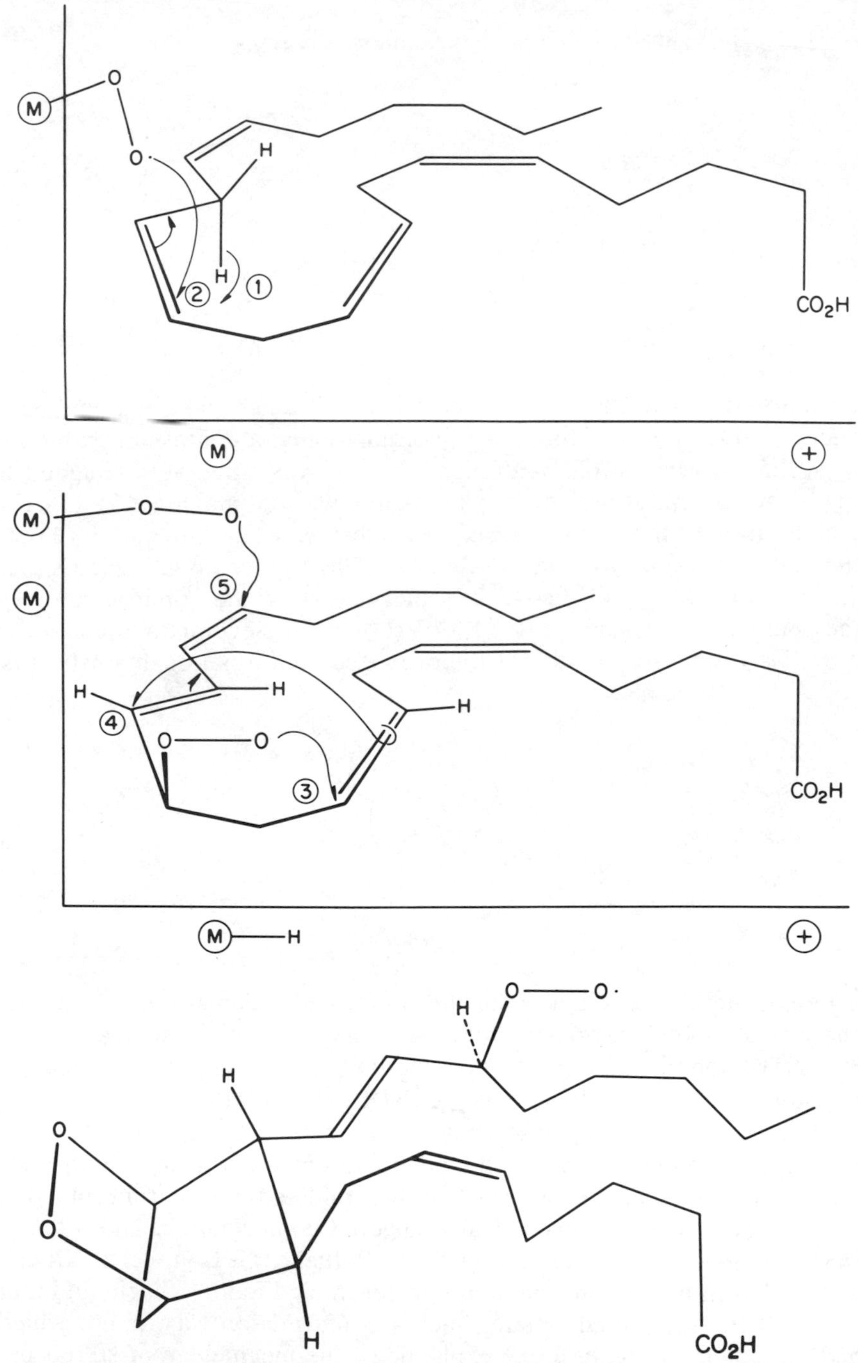

Fig. 2. Proposed mechanism of PGG formation from arachidonic acid. From Gund and Shen (*40*), with permission.

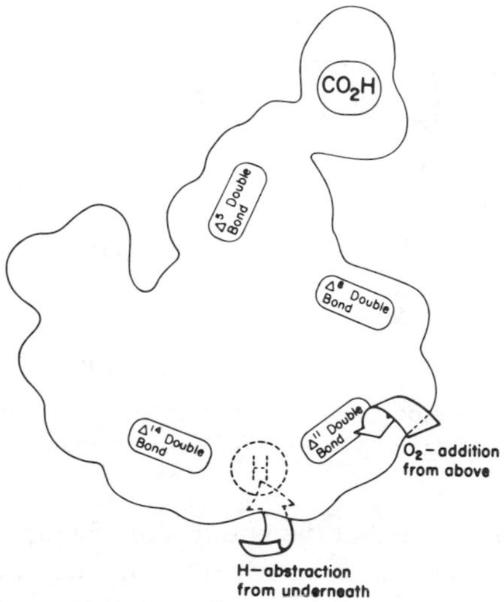

Fig. 3. Model of the fatty acid substrate binding site of prostaglandin synthetase. From Gund and Shen (*40*), with permission.

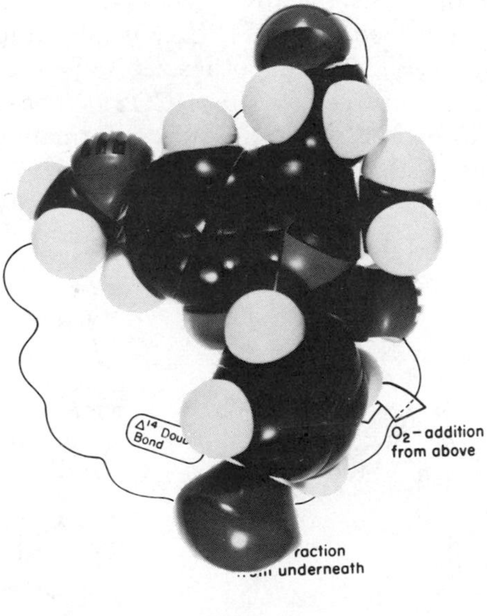

Fig. 4. Binding of indomethacin to the fatty acid binding site model. From Gund and Shen (*40*), with permission.

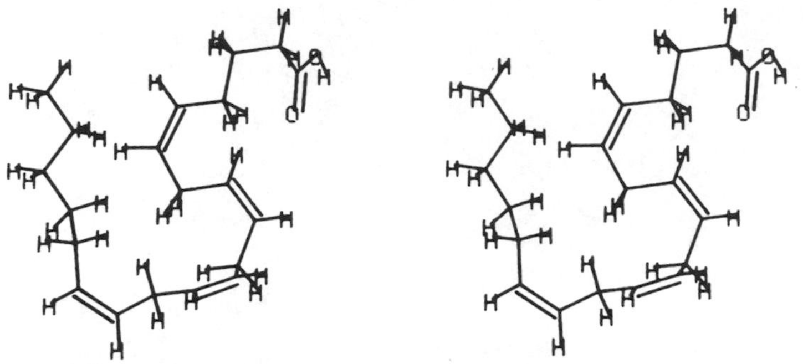

Fig. 5. Proposed receptor bound conformation of arachidonic acid (**XXXIX**) (Stereoscopic view). From Gund and Shen (*40*), with permission.

that must be accommodated at the active site. Figure 4 indicates how indomethacin (**Va**) fits the same receptor site. Figure 5 shows a stereoscopic view of the proposed receptor-bound conformation of arachidonic acid (**XXXIX**), whereas Fig. 6 shows the X-ray conformation of indomethacin (**Va**) to emphasize the structural similarities.

In a recent communication, Salvetti *et al.* (*71*) started from the all-transoid conformation of arachidonic acid (except the double bonds, which are cis) and performed a constrained conformational energy search by a combination of consistent force field and Perturbatic Configuration Interaction using Localized Orbitals (PCILO) calculations. Their final low energy conformation (Fig. 7) is hypothesized to be the form that binds to the "hydrophobic cyclooxygenase site (HCOS)." These authors favor this model for the following reasons. (1) Their conformation was substantially lower in strain energy than the Gund and Shen (*40*) model, although the latter could be strain minimized to a conformation only 1.0 kcal higher in

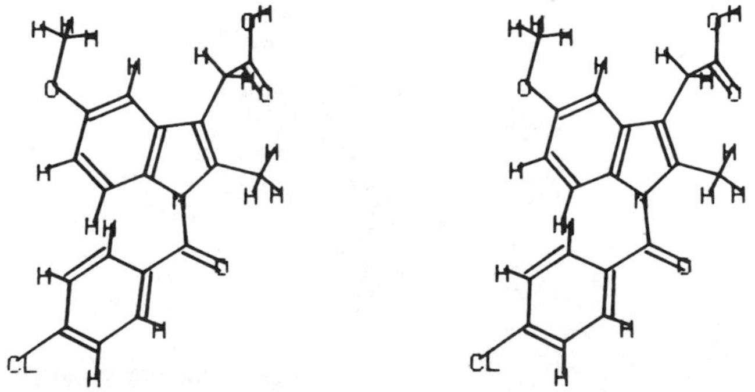

Fig. 6. Crystal conformation of indomethacin (**Va**) (Stereoscopic view). From Gund and Shen (*40*), with permission.

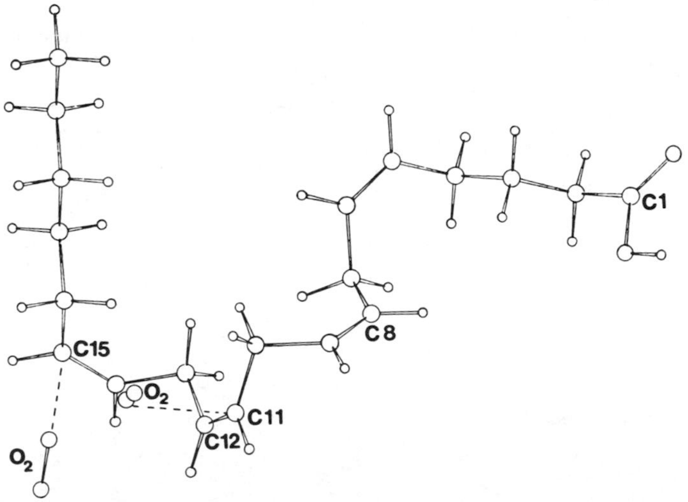

Fig. 7. Hypothesized cyclooxygenase binding conformation of arachidonic acid showing direction of approach of the oxygens. From Salvetti *et al.* (*71*), with permission.

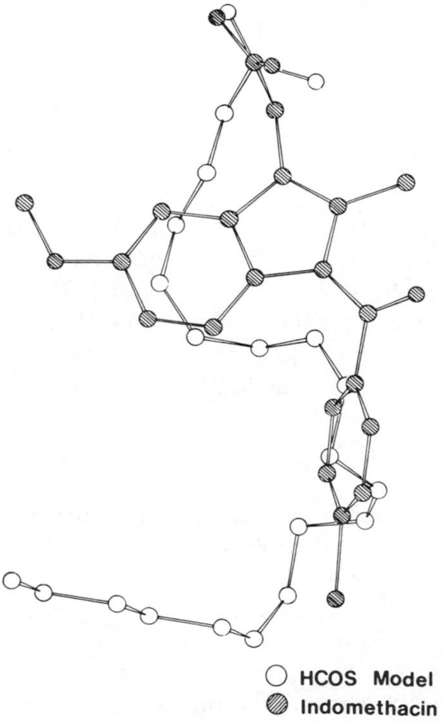

Fig. 8. Superposition of hypothesized cyclooxygenase binding conformation of arachidonic acid with the crystal structure of indomethacin. From Salvetti *et al.* (*71*), with permission.

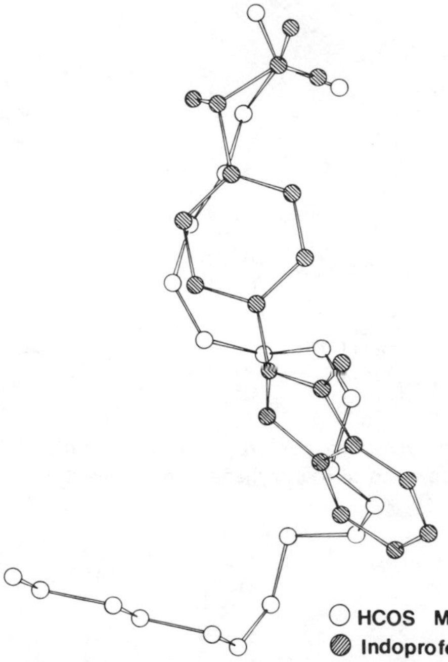

Fig. 9. Superposition of hypothesized cyclooxygenase conformation of arachidonic acid with one of two calculated low energy forms of indoprofen. From Salvetti *et al.* (*71*), with permission.

energy than their preferred conformation. (2) The Salvetti *et al.* conformation allowed unhindered approach of both oxygens from the observed direction, whereas the Gund and Shen model showed some hindrance (actually the second oxygen must be added in a later step, so only accessibility to the first oxygen would appear to be relevant to the starting conformation). (3) The atoms that join to form a ring are close together (4.1 Å), as they are in the Gund and Shen model. (4) The Salvetti *et al.* conformation resembles the geometry of an ultimate product, PGE_2, as determined by X-ray diffraction (this would appear to be irrelevant, inasmuch as arachidonic acid is converted by this enzyme to PGG_2, which in turn is converted—by another enzyme—to PGE_2). (5) The Salvetti *et al.* conformation gives a good superposition with the crystal structure of indomethacin (Fig. 8) and a different good superposition with one of two low-energy forms of (*S*)-indoprofen (Fig. 9). It will be interesting to see if this model proves useful for new drug design.

Courriere *et al.* (*14*) has studied the conformation of antiinflammatory fenamates, niflumic acid, and bisnaphtholic acids by the PCILO method. Calculation of distances between crucial functional atoms in the preferred conformations have suggested that the fenamates and niflumic acid could fit the same receptor site, but the bisnaphtholic acids (e.g., **XL**) appear not be suited to fit this receptor.

Appleton and Brown (*2*) have proposed an alternative model, which they call a template, for compounds interacting at the cyclooxygenase receptor site. They argue that a peroxy radical intermediate (**XLI**), which occurs before cyclization of arachidonic acid, must be bound in the "looped" conformation shown. This same arrangement of atoms occurs in most of the highly active NSAIDs—for example, 2(*S*)-(3-chloro-4-

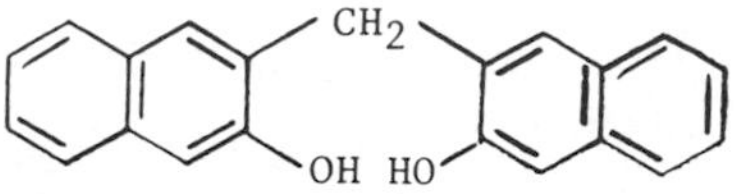

XL

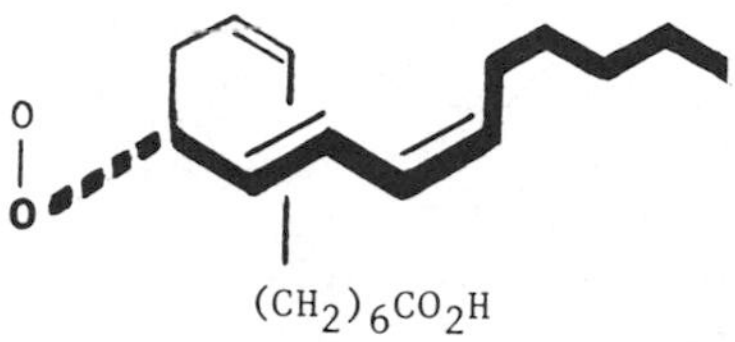

XLI

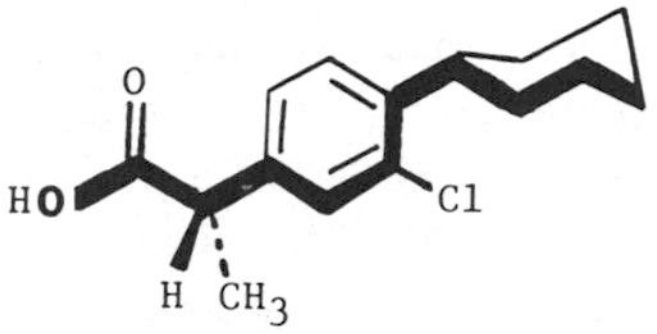

XLII

cyclohexylphenyl)propionic acid (**XLII**)—if one assumes that the arylacetic acid carboxyl may bind to the same site as the peroxy radical oxygen of **XLI**. Although the correlation of substrate carboxyl with NSAID carboxyl in the Shen (*74*) and Scherrer (*72*) models seems reasonable, Appleton and Brown report that this assumption led to difficulties in accommodating the rest of the structure of the NSAIDs to these models. These latter authors list a large number of NSAIDs that fit their template and claim that this model led to the preparation of novel, potent NSAIDs.

Dewhirst (*23*) has recently shown that phenolic compounds may be potent cyclooxygenase inhibitors and that they may also be accommodated by the Appleton and Brown template model.

In summary, for the antiinflammatory arylacetic and arylpropionic acids, it has proved remarkably difficult to obtain valid correlations with common physicochemical parameters, and much of the small success in these correlations has been in series with relatively uninteresting activity. On the other hand, a multitude of chemically diverse structures, showing a small number of common structural features, may exhibit potent activity. In efforts to understand this paradox, chemists have studied the conformations of these active compounds by crystallographic analysis, theoretical calculations, spectroscopy, synthesis and testing of conformationally restricted analogs, and manipulation of Corey-Pauling-Koltum (CPK) models. They have found that most potent NSAIDs can attain a reduced number of conformations. On the basis of these conformational results, several models for the prostaglandin cyclooxygenase receptor site have been proposed. Although discovery of the detailed receptor site ultimately may be possible by protein crystallography or enzyme labeling studies, in the meantime these models have proved useful for the preparation of novel, specifically acting NSAID.

IX. MISCELLANEOUS STRUCTURES

Although most NSAIDs are weakly acidic, there are a few nonacidic or weakly basic structures that demonstrate antiinflammatory activity and QSAR methods have also been applied to this class. A report in the Hungarian literature (*30*) derived Eq. (61) on the basis of nine analogs of structure **XLIII**. Using this equation, the authors then sought new analogs with substituents having Taft's σ^* values in the 0.08–0.32 range and π in the 0.90–3.90 range. Success was claimed for at least one of the new analogs of undisclosed structure. Testing for this series of analogs (**XLIII**) was done at 300 mg/kg in a rat-paw edema assay. Even at that high level only two compounds had greater than 30% inhibition and, not surprisingly, many analogs were toxic.

Indazoles (**XLIII**):

$$\%\ \text{inhibition} = 105.1\sigma^* - 256.0(\sigma^*)^2 + 19.60\pi - 4.88\pi^2 + 5.37 \quad (61)$$

$$n = 9, \qquad r = 0.92, \qquad s = 17.38$$

Tinland and Badin (*81*) have examined a series of 2,2-dimethyl-1,2-dihydroquinolines (**XLIV**) by a variety of QSAR methods. A Free–Wilson treatment of 18 analogs gave a correlation coefficient of 0.96 and F value of 188, but the results were not much more specific than what could be seen by inspection—which was that substitution at several positions resulted in loss of activity in a UV erythema assay. Regression analysis methods were also used to correlate activity with CNDO/2 and EHT calculated electronic charges at atoms 1 to 10. One of the best equations obtained was Eq. (62) in which CNDO/2-calculated charge densities Q_7 and Q_2 as well as π^2 were found to give a fairly good correlation. As noted by the authors, substituents with $\pi < 0$ would be desirable and such substituents were notably lacking from the original series. However, no synthesis to test this suggestion was reported.

Dihydroquinolines (**XLIV**):

$$A_{\mathrm{obs}} = -31.1\pi^2 - 265.1Q_7 - 1526.6Q_2 + 7002.4 \quad (62)$$

$$n = 15, \quad r = 0.92, \quad s = 9.0$$

For a relatively large number of analogs related to structure **XLV**, Hansch regression analysis was reported to have been unsuccessful (*13*). For a selected group of 11 analogs of **XLV**, Eq. (63) was obtained, which indicated the desirability of electron-donating R substituents and which gave a π_0 of 0.76 (*12*). Unfortunately, no significant improvements in activity could be predicted on the basis of this equation because several of the prepared compounds had substituents in the optimal range.

Imidazopyridones (**XLV**):

$$\log(1/C) = -1.50\sigma^* + 0.64\pi - 0.43\pi^2 + 2.01 \quad (63)$$

$$n = 11, \quad r = 0.91, \quad \pi_0 = 0.76$$

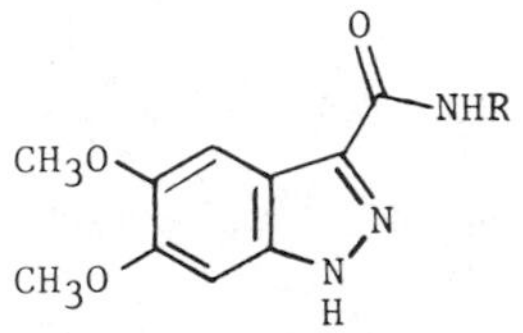

XLIII

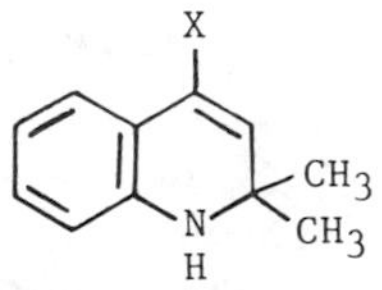

XLIV

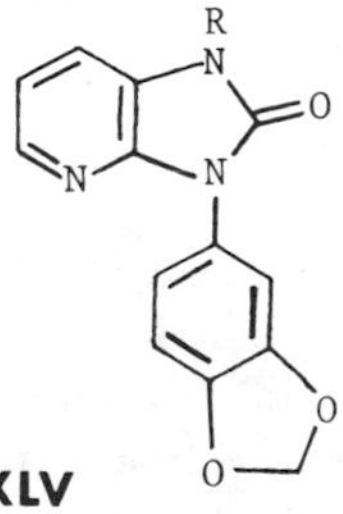

XLV

X. IMMUNOREGULANT AGENTS

An immunoregulant approach to agents such as antirheumatics is still in its infancy. As has been observed, "Apart from a few exceptions (e.g., cyclooxygenase inhibitors) SAR of antirheumatic drugs have not been investigated" (*4*, p. 187). The use of QSAR methods is understandably even more rare. In spite of these uncertainties in developing drugs via immunoregulant approaches, the possibility of doing so prompted Hansch and co-workers to publish a series of papers (*43,45,46,56,93*) on the use of QSAR in immunochemistry. Of these reports, three of them (*45,46,93*) deal with QSAR studies on *in vitro* inhibition of complement by benzylpyridinium compounds (**XLVI**) and benzamidines (**XLVII**). (Complement is a term used to describe a group of proteolytic enzymes that are required for destructive lysis of cells when they are "recognized" by antibodies as foreign.) In autoimmune diseases such as rheumatoid arthritis, modulation at this point in the self-destructive process has long been considered as a possible therapeutic approach, and a considerable number of inhibitors of the entire complement system, as well as of individual enzymes of the system, have been reported (*68*). Although very little correlation has been established between *in vitro* complement inhibition and *in vivo* activ-

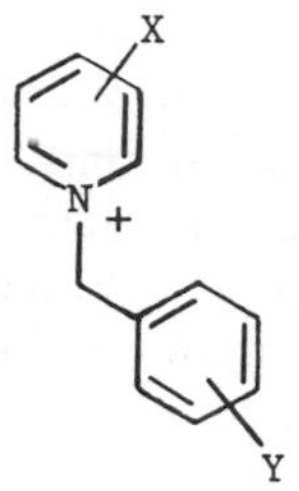

XLVI

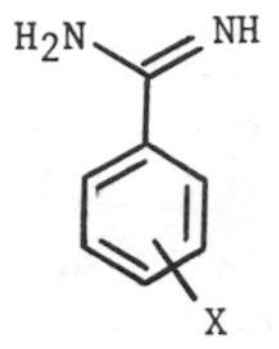

XLVII

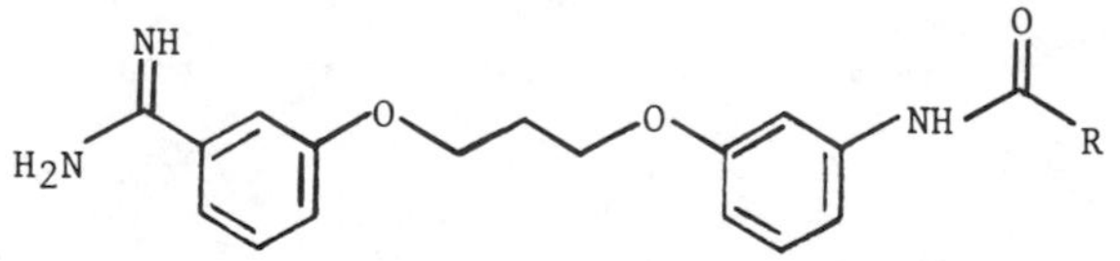

XLVIII

ity relevant to immune diseases such as rheumatoid arthritis, the possibility of being able to work with an enzyme system relevant to these diseases certainly heightens interest in these studies.

The Hansch study (*45*) of the multiple regression analysis of structures **XLVII** draws on data for 108 of these compounds as published by B. R. Baker. For this large numbr of analogs (claimed as a record by Hansch) he was able to derive Eq. (64) by the introduction of a number of "indicator" variables D_j for specific structural elements. The most active compounds were derivatives **XLVIII** (R = 4-$PhSO_2F$ and 4-$NHPhNO_2$). Hansch concludes that Eq. (64) should allow one to make compounds 10 times more active than were previously prepared, without using the toxic SO_2F functional group, and that these compounds might be valuable for *in vivo* studies. Testing of these predictions, however, was not reported.

Benzamidines (**XLVII**):

Whole complement

$$\log(1/C) = (0.15 \pm 0.03)MR_{1,2} + (1.07 \pm 0.13)D_1 + 0.52 \pm 0.28)D_2 + (0.43 \pm 0.14)D_3 + 2.43 \quad (64)$$

$$n = 108, \quad r = 0.935, \quad s = 0.258$$

C1s

$$\log(1/K_i) = (0.41 \pm 0.22)\pi - (1.11 \pm 0.75)R + (2.99 \pm 0.29) \quad (65)$$

$$n = 14, \quad r = 0.82, \quad s = 0.45$$

Plasmin

$$\log(1/K_i) = (0.25 \pm 0.12)\pi - (1.11 \pm 0.43)R + (3.23 \pm 0.16) \quad (66)$$

$$n = 14, \quad r = 0.79, \quad s = 0.26$$

A few years later a second study of benzamidines (**XLVII**) was reported by other workers (*1*) whose aim was to utilize QSAR methods to probe similarities and differences of several proteolytic enzymes. Instead of using the whole complement cascade only purified C1s was used and was compared to other proteolytic enzymes such as thrombin, plasmin, and trypsin. For the complement component C1s, Eq. (65) was obtained, whereas Eq. (66) was found for plasmin. Comparison of inhibition constants for these enzymes yielded little information about enzyme specificity and structure.

Hansch's two papers on benzylpyridine inhibitors of complement (*46,93*) are especially interesting because they represent, at least in a formal sense, a test of QSAR predictability. Data for both papers was again drawn from published work of B. R. Baker, but data on two different sets of analogs were considered independently. Equation (67), derived on the basis of the first 69 analogs can be tested to see how well it predicts the activities of the second set of 66 analogs. Prediction success, as Hansch discusses (*46*), can be measured in several ways, but as a group the second set of derivatives may be described as well predicted. Such judgment is supported by Eq. (68), which included all 132 compounds with only very small changes in the constants. Another way to examine predictibility is to examine the nine analogs from the second group of compounds that were predicted to be most active by Eq. (67). If one were to make those nine analogs in order of their predicted potency, starting with the one predicted to be most potent, six analogs would have to be prepared before a new analog was obtained that actually was more active. This new analog would then represent a fourfold increase in activity over the best derivative in the first set of 69. One question that this comparison raises is whether a sixth analog would often be prepared after five failures.

Benzylpyridinium ions (**XLVI**):

$$\log(1/C) = (0.18 \pm 0.04)(\pi - 1) + (0.46 \pm 0.14)(\pi - 2) + (1.01 \pm 0.28)(\sigma^+ - 1) + (0.72 \pm 0.12)(D - 1) + (2.50 \pm 0.13) \quad (67)$$

$$n = 69, \quad r = 0.939, \quad s = 0.198$$

$$\log(1/C) = (0.16 \pm 0.03)(\pi - 1) + (0.38 \pm 0.11)(\pi - 2) + (0.91 \pm 0.25)(\sigma^+ - 1) + (0.71 \pm 0.10)(D - 1) + (2.58 \pm 0.10) \quad (68)$$

$$n = 132, \quad r = 0.945, \quad s = 0.213$$

XI. SUMMARY

It appears that there has been considerable use of QSAR methods in the handling of data generated for antiinflammatory and antiarthritic drugs. However, substantially less useful information has been generated. It must be admitted that there are several different criteria for gauging success in the use of QSAR. Perhaps the most demanding standards are the ones that most synthetic medicinal chemists would like to see fulfilled. In this ideal case a method such as multiple regression analysis would be applied to analogs already prepared. The results would then suggest further analogs that would be prepared and subsequently found to be so much more advantageous that a commercially useful drug would eventually follow. This scenario has not even been remotely approached for an NSAID. As noted in the above discussion of commercially important arylacetic acids, there is a negligible overlap between the very numerous NSAIDs that have reached the stage of clinical trials (*64*) and structures that were developed with the aid of published QSAR studies. This is not to say that these successful drugs have not been included in QSAR studies (*11,36,38,40,47,59,62,63,67,69,73,94*), but rather that these studies all appear to be "after the fact" with respect to the medicinal chemical development of these drugs.

Even if the criterion of commercial success is not applied, as Hansch has noted (*46*), "there are relatively few examples in the literature where the formulation of a QSAR has been followed up by the synthesis of new derivatives to check up on the predictive value of correlation equations" (p. 1089). There are a few examples in the antiinflammatory and antiarthritis drug field in which this measure of success is claimed (*28,30,39,46,53*) but only one of these references (*28*) describes a significant increase in *in vivo* activity. More convincing is a quite limited form of success in which investigators concluded on the basis of QSAR that they had reached a maximum of activity for a given series and thus did not need to prepare more analogs (*9,12,52*).

In spite of the apparent lack of success and paucity of practical use of QSAR methods in the development of antiinflammatory and antiarthritic drugs, attempts to correlate activity and measurable physical parameters will certainly continue. It appears from the papers in this field that the practicing medicinal chemist is generally not using QSAR techniques to guide NSAID drug development, and the QSAR practitioners are often not convincing the synthetic chemist of the utility of the correlations obtained. It is perhaps normal that a relatively young and mathematically based discipline takes time to be fully appreciated by the older, well established field of medicinal chemistry. We may look forward, however, to a merging of these disciplines, to the testing and refining of preliminary QSAR by scientists of other disciplines, and ultimately to the routine use of QSAR methodology and conclusions by the practicing medicinal chemist.

REFERENCES

1. J. M. Andrews, D. P. Roman, Jr., D. H. Bing, and M. Cory, *J. Med. Chem.* **21,** 1202 (1978).
2. R. A. Appleton and K. Brown, *Prostaglandins* **18,** 29 (1979).
3. J. Badin, A. Merle, G. Descotes, B. Tinland, and C. Bacques, *Eur. J. Med. Chem.—Chim. Ther.* **11,** 533 (1976).
4. I. L. Bonita, M. J. Parham, J. E. Vincent, and P. C. Bragt, *Prog. Med. Chem.* **17,** 185 (1980).
5. R. F. Borne, R. L. Peden, I. W. Waters, M. Weiner, R. Jordan, and E. A. Coats, *J. Pharm. Sci.* **63,** 615 (1974).
6. C. B. C. Boyle and B. V. Milborrow, *Nature (London)* **208,** 537 (1965).
7. K. A. Brown and A. J. Collins, *Br. J. Pharmacol.* **64,** 347 (1978).
8. K. Brune, M. Glatt, and P. Graf, *Gen. Pharmacol.* **7,** 27 (1976).
9. R. T. Buckler, *J. Med. Chem.* **15,** 578 (1972).
10. R. T. Buckler, H. E. Hartzler, E. Kurchacova, G. Nichols, and B. M. Phillips, *J. Med. Chem.* **21,** 1255 (1978).
11. R. Ceserani, M. Ferrari, G. Goldaniga, E. Moro, and A. Buttinoni, *Life Sci.* **21,** 223 (1977).
12. R. L. Clark and P. Gund, unpublished observations (1975).
13. R. L. Clark, A. A. Pessolano, T. Y. Shen, D. P. Jacobus, H. Jones, V. J. Lotti, and L. M. Flataker, *J. Med. Chem.* **21,** 965 (1978).
14. P. Courriere, R. Lacroix, and J. P. Poupflin, *Eur. J. Med. Chem.—Chim. Ther.* **14,** 17 (1979).
15. J. C. Dearden, J. H. Collett, and E. Tomlinson, *Experientia, Suppl.,* **23,** p. 37 (1976).
16. J. C. Dearden and E. George, *J. Pharm. Pharmacol.* **29,** Suppl. 74P (1977).
17. J. C. Dearden and E. George, *in* "Quantitative Structure–Activity Analysis" (R. Franke and P. Oehme, eds.), p. 101. Akademie-Verlag, Berlin, 1978.
18. J. C. Dearden and E. George, *J. Pharm. Pharmacol.* **31,** Suppl. 45P (1979).
19. J. C. Dearden and E. Tomlinson, *J. Pharm. Pharmacol.* **23,** Suppl., 73S (1971).
20. J. C. Dearden and E. Tomlinson, *J. Pharm. Pharmacol.* **24,** Suppl., 115P (1972).
21. C. A. Demerson, L. G. Humber, T. A. Dobson, and R. R. Martel, *J. Med. Chem.* **18,** 189 (1975).
22. D. A. Deporter, C. J. Dunn, and D. A. Willoughby, *Br. J. Pharmacol.* **65,** 163 (1979).

23. F. E. Dewhirst, *Prostaglandins* **20,** 209 (1980).
24. G. DiPasquale and D. Mellace, *Agents Actions* **7,** 481 (1977).
25. G. Dive, C. L. Lapiere, and G. Leroy, *Bull Soc. Chim. Belg.* **86,** 73 (1977).
26. D. J. Drain, M. J. Daly, B. Davy, M. Horlington, J. G. B. Howes, J. M. Scruion, and R. A. Selway, *J. Pharm. Pharmacol.* **22,** 684 (1970).
27. V. G. Engelhardt, *Arzneim.-Forsch.* **28,** 1714 (1978).
28. R. Escale, J. P. Girard, P. Vergnon, G. Grassy, J. P. Chapat, and R. Granger, *Eur. J. Med. Chem.—Chim. Ther.* **12,** 501 (1977).
29. J. P. Famaey, *Gen. Pharmacol.* **9,** 155 (1978).
30. D. Ferenc, M. László, and B. László, *Mag. Kem. Lapja,* **30,** 208 (1975).
31. R. J. Flower and J. R. Vane, *Nature (London)* **240,** 410 (1972).
32. R. Franke, *Farmaco, Ed. Sci.* **34,** 545 (1979).
33. R. C. Franson, D. Eisen, R. Jesse, and C. Lanni, *Biochem. J.* **186,** 633 (1980).
34. S. M. Free and J. W. Wilson, *J. Med. Chem.* **7,** 395 (1964).
35. E. M. Glenn, B. J. Bowman, and N. A. Rohloff, *Agents Actions* **9,** 257 (1979).
36. P. Graf, M. Glatt, and K. Brune, *Experientia* **31,** 951 (1975).
37. G. Grassy, R. Escale, J. P. Chapat, J. C. Rossi, and J. A. Girard, *Eur. J. Med. Chem.—Chim. Ther.* **14,** 493 (1979).
38. R. J. Gryglewski, *in* "Prostaglandin Synthetase Inhibitors" (H. J. Robinson and J. R. Vane, eds.), p. 33. Raven, New York, 1974.
39. R. J. Gryglewski, Z. Ryznerski, M. Gorczyca, and J. Krupinska, *Adv. Prostaglandin Thromboxane Res.* **1,** 117 (1976).
40. P. Gund and T. Y. Shen, *J. Med. Chem.* **20,** 1146 (1977).
41. J. Hannah, W. V. Ruyle, H. Jones, A. R. Matzuk, K. W. Kelly, B. E. Witzel, W. J. Holtz, R. W. Houser, T. Y. Shen, and L. H. Sarett, *Br. J. Clin. Pharmacol.* **4,** 7S (1977).
42. C. Hansch and T. Fujita, *J. Am. Chem. Soc.* **86,** 1616 (1964).
43. C. Hansch and P. Moser, *Immunochemistry* **15,** 535 (1978).
44. C. Hansch and K. N. Von Kaulla, *Biochem. Pharmacol.* **19,** 2193 (1970).
45. C. Hansch and M. Yoshimoto, *J. Med. Chem.* **17,** 1160 (1974).
46. C. Hansch, M. Yoshimoto, and M. H. Doll, *J. Med. Chem.* **19,** 1089 (1976).
47. J. W. Horodniak, E. D. Matz, D. T. Walz, R. D. Cramer, III, B. M. Sotton, C. E. Berkoff, J. E. Zarembo, and A. D. Bender, *Drugs Exp. Clin. Res.* **2**(1), 35 (1977).
48. J. S. Kaltenbronn, *J. Med. Chem.* **20,** 596 (1977).
49. K. Kamiya, Y. Wada, and M. Nishikawa, *Chem. Pharm. Bull.* **23,** 1589 (1975).
50. T. J. Kistenmacher and R. E. Marsh, *J. Am. Chem. Soc.* **94,** 1340 (1972).
51. M. Kuchař, B. Brůnová, V. Rejholec, J. Grimová, and O. Němeček, *Collect. Czech. Chem. Commun.* **42,** 1723 (1977).
52. M. Kuchař, B. Brůnová, V. Rejholec, and J. Grimová, *Eur. J. Med. Chem.—Chim. Ther.* **13,** 363 (1976).
53. M. Kuchař, B. Brůnová, V. Rejholec, Z. Roubal, J. Grimová, and O. Němeček, *Collect. Czech. Chem. Commun.* **40,** 3345 (1975).
54. F. A. Kuehl, Jr. and R. W. Egan, *Science* **210,** 978 (1980).
55. F. A. Kuehl, Jr., J. L. Humes, R. W. Egan, E. A. Ham, G. C. Beveridge, and C. G. Van Arman, *Nature (London)* **265,** 170 (1977).
56. E. Kutter and C. Hansch, *Arch. Biochem. Biophys.* **135,** 126 (1969).
57. M. Langlois, M. Rapin, J. P. Meingan, T. V. Van, J. Maillard, C. Guillonneau, C. Maloizel, H. N. Nguyen, R. Morin, C. Manuel, and C. Mazmanian, *Eur. J. Med. Chem.—Chim. Ther.* **11,** 493 (1976).
58. E. Lien, R. T. Koda, and G. L. Tong, *Drug Intell. Clin. Pharm.* **5,** 38 (1971).
59. J. G. Lombardino, I. G. Otterness, and E. H. Wiseman, *Arzneim.-Forsch.* **25,** 1629 (1975).

60. P. P. Mager, J. Metzner, M. Paintz, and U. Wenzel, *Sci. Pharm.* **48,** 7 (1980).
61. S. C. R. Meacock and E. A. Kitchen, *J. Pharm. Pharmacol.* **31,** 366 (1978).
62. E. Mizuta, N. Suzuki, Y. Miyake, M. Nishikawa, and T. Fujita, *Chem. Pharm. Bull.* **23,** 5 (1975).
63. P. Moser, K. Jakel, P. Krupp, R. Menasse, and A. Sallmann, *Eur. J. Med. Chem.—Chim. Ther.* **10,** 613 (1975).
64. R. Nickander, F. G. McMahon, and A. S. Ridolfo, *Annu. Rev. Pharmacol. Toxicol.* **19,** 469 (1979).
65. A. Ogino, S. Matsumura, and T. Fujita, *J. Med. Chem.* **23,** 437 (1980).
66. D. R. Olson, W. J. Wheeler, and J. N. Wells, *J. Med. Chem.* **17,** 167 (1974).
67. I. G. Otterness, E. H. Wiseman, and D. J. Gans, *Agents Actions* **9,** 177 (1979).
68. R. A. Patrick and R. E. Johnson, *Annu. Rep. Med. Chem.* **15,** 193 (1980).
69. J. M. Perel, M. M. Snell, W. Chen, and P. G. Dayton, *Biochem. Pharmacol.* **13,** 1305 (1964).
70. K. D. Rainsford, *Agents Actions* **8,** 587 (1978).
71. F. Salvetti, A. Buttinoni, R. Ceserani, and C. Tosi, *Eur. J. Med. Chem.—Chim. Ther.* **16,** 81 (1981).
72. R. A. Scherrer, *in* "Antiinflammatory Agents: Chemistry and Pharmacology" (R. A. Scherrer and M. W. Whitehouse, eds.), Vol. 1, p. 29. Academic Press, New York, 1974.
73. T. Y. Shen, *Top. Med. Chem.,* **1,** 29 (1967).
74. T. Y. Shen, E. A. Ham, V. J. Cirillo, and M. Zanetti, *in* "Prostaglandin Synthetase Inhibitors" (H. J. Robinson and J. R. Vane, eds.), p. 19. Raven, New York, 1974.
75. T. Y. Shen, *in* "Prostaglandins and Thromboxanes" (F. Berti, B. Samuelsson, and G. P. Velo, eds.), p. 111. Plenum, New York, 1977.
76. T. Y. Shen, *J. Med. Chem.* **24,** 1 (1981).
77. M. J. H. Smith, *Agents Actions* **8,** 427 (1978).
78. J. E. Smolen and G. Weissmann, *Biochem. Pharmacol.* **29,** 533 (1980).
79. H. Terada and S. Muraoka, *Mol. Pharmacol.* **8,** 95 (1972).
80. H. Terada, S. Muraoka, and T. Fujita, *J. Med. Chem.* **17,** 330 (1974).
81. B. Tinland and J. Badin, *Farmaco. Ed. Sci.* **29,** 886 (1974).
82. G. Van den Berg, T. Bultsma, and W. T. Nauta, *Biochem. Pharmacol.* **24,** 1115 (1975).
83. G. Van der Berg, T. Bultsma, R. F. Rekker, and W. T. Nauta, *Eur. J. Med. Chem.—Chim. Ther.* **10,** 242 (1975).
84. G. Van den Berg and W. T. Nauta, *Biochem. Pharmacol.* **24,** 815 (1975).
85. G. Van den Berg, R. F. Rekker, and W. T. Nauta, *Eur. J. Med. Chem.—Chim. Ther.* **10,** 408 (1975).
86. J. R. Vane, *Nature (London), New Biol.* **231,** 232 (1971).
87. J. R. Vane, *Agents Actions* **8,** 430 (1978).
88. J. R. Walker and W. Dawson, *J. Pharm. Pharmacol.* **31,** 778 (1979).
89. J. R. Walker, M. J. H. Smith, and A. N. Ford-Hutchinson, *Agents Actions* **6,** 602 (1976).
90. D. A. Willoughby, *Endeavour* **2,** 57 (1978).
91. C. V. Winder, J. Wax, V. Burr, M. Been, and C. E. Rosiere, *Arch. Int. Pharmacodyn.* **116,** 261 (1958).
92. C. A. Winter, E. A. Risley, and G. W. Nuss, *Proc. Soc. Exp. Biol. Med.* **111,** 544 (1962).
93. M. Yoshimoto, C. Hansch, and P. Y. C. Jow, *Chem. Pharm. Bull.* **23,** 437 (1975).
94. R. Ziel and P. Krupp, *Int. J. Clin. Pharmacol.* **12,** 186 (1975).

8

Agents Affecting the Central Nervous System

JAMES Y. FUKUNAGA AND
JOEL G. BERGER

I. INTRODUCTION

Ideally, a QSAR study of a structurally specific series of drugs will relate the interaction of a drug molecule with a receptor as a function of one or several physicochemical parameters. The effect of this interaction is expressed as a biological or pharmacological response. For *in vivo* systems, QSAR studies are of necessity complicated by the fact that the drug molecule once administered to an intact animal must be delivered to its receptor, and factors such as absorption, distribution, and metabolism become important. A particular problem exists in the evaluation of CNS-active drugs in *in vivo* systems due to a physiological barrier that insulates CNS tissues from the effects of small molecules present in the blood.

QUANTITATIVE STRUCTURE–ACTIVITY
RELATIONSHIPS OF DRUGS

ISBN 0-12-695150-0

This "blood–brain barrier" results from the very closely packed nature of the cells of the blood vessels that perfuse the CNS, as well as from the presence of large numbers of astroglial cells that surround these blood vessels and interpose themselves between the blood vessels and neuronal cells. Thus the transport of small molecules from the blood to neuronal tissue becomes largely a function of the properties of the cell membrane. Small, hydrophilic, charged molecules would not be expected to pass through cellular membranes, but neutral lipophilic ones would. Molecules that are highly lipophilic might become trapped in a cell membrane and thus may also never reach a neuronal binding site. Thus it is not surprising, as shown by Hansch (*27*), that a number of QSAR of CNS-active drugs show a parabolic dependence on log *P* having the optimal value of about 2. This relationship must, therefore, be kept in mind when one considers the design of CNS-active drugs.

Meyer and Overton's work on the narcotic actions of small organic molecules laid the foundations for modern QSAR techniques. These early studies were reevaluated by Hansch (*27*), using octanol–water partition coefficients, and are not covered here. This chapter covers the work between 1970 and 1981. The broad area has been divided into sections, each dealing with a specific pharmacological effect.

II. ANALGESICS

Opium extracts have long been recognized for their analgesic actions. For the past three decades, considerable efforts were made to find analgesics that eliminated the dependence liability of the opiates. Some of the early work resulted in the synthesis of compounds structurally related to the opiate alkaloids; one such compound is codeine.

For esters of 14-hydroxycodeinone (**I**) tested by the tail clip method, Lien *et al.* (*41*) derived Eqs. (1) and (2) where MW is molecular weight. The $\log(MW_R)$ term in Eq. (2) is significant at the 90% level and is believed to reflect a nonspecific van der Waals type drug–receptor interaction.

$$\log(RA) = -0.34(\log P)^2 + 2.19 \log P - 1.75 \quad (1)$$

$$n = 13, \quad r = 0.960, \quad s = 0.307, \quad \log P_0 = 3.23$$

$$\log(RA) = -0.20(\log P)^2 + 0.58 \log P + 2.92 \log(MW_R) - 3.41 \quad (2)$$

$$n = 13, \quad r = 0.973, \quad s = 0.267, \quad \log P_0 = 1.43$$

The analgesic activity of the benzomorphans (**II**) determined in mice by the hot-plate technique was analyzed using the Free–Wilson (F–W)

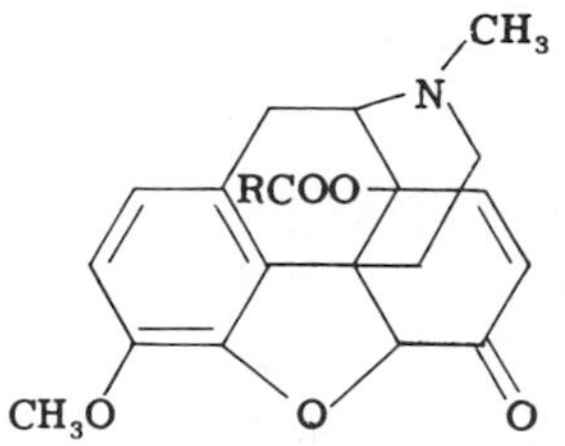

I

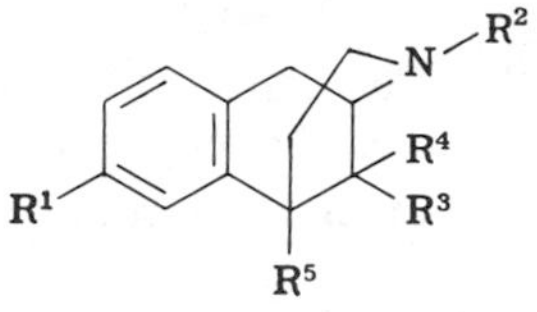

II

method (*37*). (The parent structure of the benzomorphans was proposed after analyzing the structures of various narcotic analgesics (*46*). These bezomorphans contain the pharmacophores essential for analgesic activity.) For 99 compounds a correlation coefficient of 0.893 was obtained. Thirteen dextrorotary compounds were removed from the F–W matrix; $r = 0.909$ resulted. Another 16 compounds were eliminated because these contained substituents with one occurrence in the matrix. The F–W correlation coefficient for the remaining 70 compounds was 0.879. The F–W coefficients for these 70 compounds show four substituents, R^2 = isobutyl, R^3 = acetate or OH, and R^5 = OH, resulting in decreased analgesic activity relative to the corresponding H compounds.

If one considers the benzomorphans to be a "stripped" model of the opiate narcotics, then the *N*-alkylnormeperidines (**III**) represent the base structure. The QSAR of this series was reported by Lien *et al.* (*41*). Eq. (3) was derived for nine compounds. BA is biological activity, $\log P_{\mathrm{app}}$ is

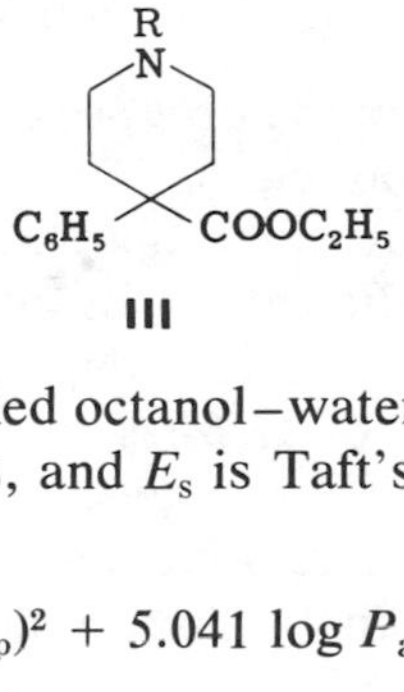

III

the experimentally determined octanol–water partition coefficient uncorrected for ionization effects, and E_s is Taft's steric parameter corrected for hyperconjugation.

$$\log(BA) = -0.854(\log P_{\mathrm{app}})^2 + 5.041 \log P_{\mathrm{app}} + 2.246E_s - 0.563 \quad (3)$$

$$r = 0.994, \quad s = 0.051, \quad \log P_0 = 2.95$$

In contrast to the structurally well-defined series represented by Eqs. (1–3), Jacobson *et al.* (*31*) analyzed the antinociceptive activities of a diverse series of drugs, including among others, morphine, fentanyl, and methadone. Equation (4), showing the correlation between rat hot-plate data and $\log P$, is not as good as Eqs. (1–3) on the basis of regression statistics ($r < 0.90$ and large standard deviation).

$$\log(1/C) = 3.457 + 0.209 \log P \tag{4}$$

$$n = 10, \quad r = 0.46, \quad s = 1.22$$

These authors determined the affinities of the 10 compounds for a narcotic receptor in rat brain homogenates and used the affinities, $\log(1/B)$, as a parameter in regression analysis Eq. (5).

$$\log(1/C) = 4.254 + 1.107 \log(1/B) + 0.317 \log P \tag{5}$$

$$n = 10, \quad r = 0.91, \quad s = 0.62$$

They did not identify the physicochemical parameters that influence the relative drug–receptor affinities.

Since a reasonable correlation exists between biological activity and binding affinity, a method for calculating the binding strength is desirable. Johnson (*36*) analyzed the *in vitro* binding of an extensive, diverse series of drugs. Log *P*, *MW*, and *MR* (molar retractivity) were used as continuous variables. These variables were factored into 10 regiochemically distinct areas in an attempt to derive a quantitative stereochemical receptor-binding relationship. Correlations between affinity and log *P*, *MW*, *MR*, and combinations of these, including quadratic terms, did not result in a significant equation. The regional fragmental variables, however, identified physicochemical parameters that significantly influenced binding affinity. One such equation (6) is

$$\log(BA) = -11.9 + 2.9MW + 21.1(W_{\mathrm{H}}) - 8.4(W_{\mathrm{B}}) + 13.1(W_{\mathrm{a}}) \tag{6}$$

$$n = 42, \quad r = 0.879$$

MW is the molecular weight of the drug scaled by 100 and W_{i} is the molecular weight of the fragment in region i.

All of these studies show that lipophilicity, as measured by the octanol–water partition coefficient, is not solely responsible for the variation in biological activities. It is interesting to note that the steric size expressed in terms of *MW*, E_s, or *MR* has an important role in determining relative biological activities. The analysis of binding affinities and their importance in accounting for relative activities indicate the need for a better understanding of the analgesic receptor.

III. GENERAL INHALATION ANESTHETICS

General inhalation anesthetics have attracted the interest of many researchers. In this section QSAR of general anesthetics, characterized as those gaseous compounds that induce sleep in animals, are discussed.

Local anesthetics, such as lidocaine, are omitted from discussion. Unlike the narcotic studies of Meyer and Hemmi (*46a*) and Overton (*51a*) on congeneric series of alcohols and ketones, general anesthetics do not have a well-defined pharmacophore.

Mice are the usual test animals, dosing being done in sealed containers to control the atmosphere rigorously. Partial pressures or concentrations of the test anesthetic are measured, which either induces sleep or blocks the animals' righting reflex.

Glave and Hansch (*25*) reported one of the first QSAR for general anesthetics. Their best equation for a series of aliphatic ethers is:

$$\log(1/C) = -0.221(\log P)^2 + 1.038 \log P + 21.16 \tag{7}$$

$$n = 26, \quad r = 0.966, \quad s = 0.101, \quad \log P_0 = 2.35$$

(Two ethers were omitted in formulating Eq. 7.) Using connectivity indices (X), Di Paolo (*14*) formulated Eq. (8) for these same ethers:

$$\log(1/C) = -0.230(^1X)^2 + 1.865(^1X) - 0.365 \tag{8}$$

$$n = 28, \quad r = 0.986, \quad s = 0.063.$$

Miller *et al.* (*47*) found an excellent correlation between anesthetic potencies and olive oil–gas partition coefficients. A plot of potency against partition coefficient was presented and a correlation coefficient of $r = 0.944$ was reported (*28*). For this series of compounds, Eq. (9) was formulated.

$$\log(1/P) = 1.166 \log P + 1.88I - 2.106 \tag{9}$$

$$n = 30, \quad r = 0.947, \quad s = 0.438.$$

Inclusion of a quadratic term in log P results in a slightly better equation ($r = 0.956$, $\log P_0 = 2.7$), although confidence limits on the ideal lipophilicity could not be determined.

These 30 gases include the noble gases helium, neon, argon, and krypton along with hydrogen, nitrogen, and sulfur hexafluoride. The indicator variable I parameterizes those compounds having a polar hydrogen or a basic oxygen, which can conceivably act as hydrogen bond donors or acceptors.

For those compounds where connectivity indices could be calculated, Di Paolo *et al.* (*16*) reported Eq. (10).

$$\log(1/P) = 0.496(^0X^1) + 10.30Q_H - 0.807 \tag{10}$$

$$n = 29, \quad r = 0.966, \quad s = 0.278$$

In an analysis of the anesthetic activities of ethers, ketones, and alkanes connectivity indices were again used (*15*) (Eq. 11).

$$\log(1/C) = -1.487({}^4X_p^2) - 8.539({}^1X)^{-1} + 2.895 \tag{11}$$

$$n = 27, \quad r = 0.943, \quad s = 0.170$$

Using partition coefficients, Jeppson (*14*) reported Eq. (12), (13), and (14) for these same compounds.

Ethers:

$$\log(1/C) = -0.09(\log P)^2 + 0.64 \log P + 1.67 \tag{12}$$

$$n = 7, \quad r = 0.955, \quad s = 0.450, \quad \log P_o = 3.56$$

Alkanes:

$$\log(1/C) = -0.09(\log P)^2 + 0.76 \log P + 0.74 \tag{13}$$

$$n = 12, \quad r = 0.91, \quad s = 0.192, \quad \log P_o = 4.33$$

Ketones:

$$\log(1/C) = -0.09(\log P)^2 + 0.49 \log P + 2.18 \tag{14}$$

$$n = 7, \quad r = 0.906, \quad s = 0.309, \quad \log P_o = 2.70$$

The anesthetic activities of halogenated alkanes were analyzed. Equation (15) was formulated (*13*).

$$\log(AD_{50}) = 5.98 - 2.20(P_o) - \delta_1(0.6H_{a1} - 0.43) - \delta_2(0.49H_{a2} - 0.16) \tag{15}$$

$$n = 45, \quad r = 0.988, \quad s = 0.20$$

P_o is not the partition coefficient of the compounds; rather, it parameterizes a nonpolar factor derived from partition coefficients. H_{a1} accounts for the total electron demand on the hydrogens; S_i are indicator variables. Using connectivity indices (*17*) the best equation for these halogenated compounds is Eq. (16):

$$\log_e(AD_{50}) = 5.19 - 0.993({}^0X^v) - 1.13Q_{H_1} - 1.12Q_{H_2} - 0.800Q_{H_3} \tag{16}$$

$$n = 45, \quad r = 0.976, \quad s = 0.271$$

The variable Q_H is a measure of the total C—H bond polarity and is estimated from the inductive effects of halogens.

Inspection of the activities of these halogenated alkanes revealed a discrepancy in the $\log(AD_{50})$ used in the QSAR analysis. These AD_{50} values were reevaluated and, using log P values calculated from fragment values, a new equation (17) was formulated.

$$\log_{10}(1/AD_{50}) = -0.10(\log P)^2 + 0.88 \log P + 0.51I + 0.18 \quad (17)$$

$$n = 45, \quad r = 0.62, \quad s = 0.494, \quad \log P_o = 4.4$$

(The indicator variable, I, was used for those compounds containing a hydrogen that could participate in hydrogen bonding.)

Theories on the mechanism of actions of general inhalation anesthetics should account for the QSAR reported in this section. These theories should also provide clues about the possible sites of actions. One such theory states that anesthesia occurs when a hydrophobic region expands beyond a critical volume. Such a mechanism would be sensitive to the pressure of the administered anesthetic. Miller *et al.* (*48*) investigated the high pressure effects of helium on the anesthetic potencies of neon, argon, nitrous oxide, tetrafluoromethane, and sulfur hexafluoride. These studies demonstrated the existence of two distinct sites of actions, the first being a hydrophobic region that is not particularly sensitive to pressure. A second site shows increased sensitivity to pressure and characterizes a region corresponding to hyperactivity when inhalation anesthetics are administered.

An attempt to pinpoint the physiological site of action was the objective in a study by Franks and Lieb (*22*). The effects of gaseous anesthetics on lipid bilayers were investigated. Using X-ray and neutron diffraction methods, no perturbation of the lipid bilayer structures was observed. ESR experiments, however, indicate that lipid bilayers are disordered, albeit minimally, by anesthetics (*52*). It appears reasonable to conclude, therefore, that structural modifications of cellular membranes by clinical concentrations of anesthetics are not solely responsible for anesthesia. The site of action is lipophilic in character and resembles octanol more so than it does benzene. Further, a protein, or membrane-bound protein, is a component of the anesthetic site of action, a conclusion that is similar to that suggested by Simon *et al.* (*60*).

Hansch concluded that general anesthetics acted at a lipophilic site inasmuch as log P was an important variable in his equations. For those equations involving connectivity indices, ${}^1X^v$ emerged as an important variable. Kier and Hall (*38*) have shown that a significant linear relationship exists between this connectivity index and octanol–water partition coefficients.

In addition to the lipophilic component of the active site, there exists an important polar component. This polar component is described by the indicator term in Eq. (9) and the Q_H terms in Eq. (17). Specifically, these terms are used to describe those anesthetics having covalently-bonded polar hydrogens.

A physical interpretation of this polar character is of interest. Years ago Pauling suggested that general aneshetics could disrupt the extensive hydrogen-bonded network found in liquid water, and smaller networks could be formed around the dissolved anesthetic (*26*). Recent results from infrared (*45,50,66*) and NMR (*7*) studies indicate that general anesthetics having polar, acidic hydrogens can form hydrogen bonds to amides or disrupt existing hydrogen bonds to amides. Such a phenomenon may account for the discrete H-polar terms in the QSAR equations.

IV. ANTIDEPRESSANTS

Since the discovery of the mood-elevating effect of iproniazid (*58*), significant effort has been expended in the search for antidepressants with increased efficacy. Almost simultaneously with the discovery of its effects on mood, it was found that iproniazid was a potent inhibitor of the enzyme monoamine oxidase (MAO) (*69*). Large series of hydrazines and hydrazides have since been tested as MAO inhibitors in the hope of producing inhibitors that would be useful as antidepressants.

Fujita (*23*) has formulated QSAR for 11 series of MAO inhibitors in both *in vitro* and *in vivo* tests. Three parameters, π, σ, and E_s, are the dominant physicochemical properties used to account for the relative orders of bioactivities. The 11 series include phenyl, benzyl- and phenethylhydrazines, propargylamines (pargylines), tryptamines, cyclopropylamines, and β-carbolines. Although both positive and negative coefficients result for the lipophilicity term, only positive coefficients were obtained for the electronic and steric terms.

Johnson (*35*) has formulated QSAR for *in vivo* potencies of aryl hydrazide MAO inhibitors (**IV**). The activity analyzed was the increase in rat brain serotonin levels brought about by the test drug using Marsilid (iproniazide, **IVa**) as the reference standard (Marsilid Index, M.I. = 100). For 23 compounds in this series, Eq. (18) was obtained:

$$\text{M.I.} = -3900Q_0 + 5579 \tag{18}$$

$$n = 23, \quad r = 0.619, \quad s = 53.2$$

Q_0 is the π-electron density of the carbonyl oxygen calculated by CNDO/2. A subset of the 23 compounds was analyzed using available Hammett σ values, and Eq. (19) was formulated.

$$M.I. = 88.25 + 83.37\sigma \tag{19}$$

$$n = 10, \quad r = 0.804, \quad s = 31.4$$

For these hydrazides partition coefficient log P was not a significant determinant of relative activity.

Equation (20) was formulated for aryloxyacethydrazides (**V**), acting as MAO inhibitors (*24*).

$$pI_{50} = -26.5\ \Delta EDP - 0.634\ \Delta pK_{a_2} + 0.307E_{S6} + 5.46 \tag{20}$$

$$n = 23, \quad r = 0.962, \quad s = 0.163$$

EDP is the half-wave potential for oxidation, pK_{a_2} is a measure of the relative basicity of nitrogen and E_{S6} is Taft's steric parameter.

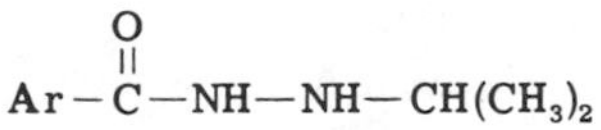

IV

IVa: Marsilid(iproniazid)
Ar = 4-pyridyl

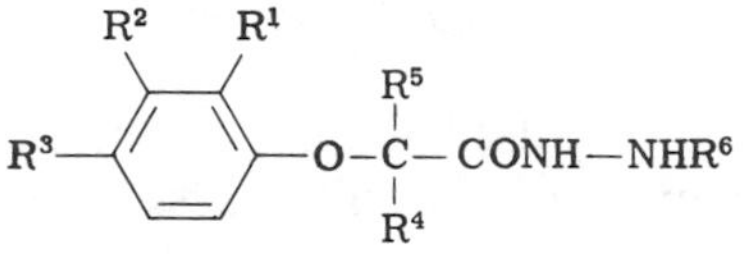

V

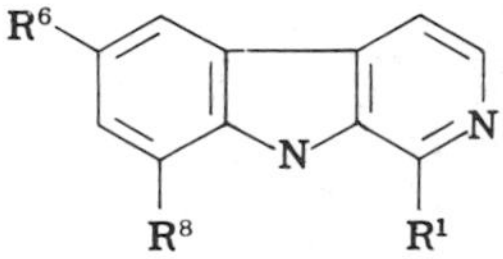

VI

For this series of compounds the steric parameter associated with R_6 has a direct effect on the basicity of the nitrogen atom to which it is attached. Larger R_6 groups lower basicity and increase inhibitory activity.

The activities of a set of β-carboline MAO inhibitors (**VI**) was analyzed, using quantum mechanical indices (*65*).

$$\begin{aligned} pI_{50} = {} & 31.806 + 11.782Q_9 + 140.546S_9^e + 14.405Q_6 \\ & + 18.199S_6^e + 42.378Q_5 - 28.496S_5^e \\ & + 22.284Q_{13} - 101.543S_{13}^e + 63.959S_8^e \end{aligned} \tag{21}$$

$$n = 13, \quad r = 0.999, \quad s = 0.042$$

The *Q* and *S* terms are the net atomic charges and superdelocalizability indices, respectively.

In considering the above equation, it was concluded that only the indole portion of the β-carboline is involved in formation of an enzyme (Michaelis) complex, whereas the pyridine nitrogen is required for inhibitory activity.

A clear picture emerges from these analyses of MAO inhibitors. Lipophilicity, as measured by log *P* or π does not constitute an important factor in determining the relative inhibition of MAO by these compounds. Charge densities, either calculated by quantum chemical techniques or inferred by Hammett σ values seem to be the dominant factors for inhibition of the enzyme. Size, expressed by Taft's E_s parameter, decreases the inhibitory potencies of these compounds.

Brodie *et al.* (*6*) discovered that iproniazide inhibition of the enzyme (MAO) responsible for degrading sympathomimetic amines produced elevated brain levels of serotonin and norepinephrine. This implied that a possible etiology of mental depression is a functional deficit of sympathomimetic amines. Further, compounds that reversed this deficiency by blocking the reuptake of released sympathomimetic amines by neuronal cells may exhibit antidepressant activity. Many novel chemical series have been synthesized and tested *in vitro* as reuptake inhibitors.

One such series, the phthalanes (**VII**) has been studied by QSAR (*4*). Both *in vitro* inhibition (pI_{50}) of serotonin uptake by blood platelets and *in vivo* potentiation [log(1/*C*)] of 5-hydroxytryptamine syndrome were studied. The correlation between these two bioactivities is low ($r = 0.21$). Free–Wilson analysis of pI_{50} (55 compounds) and log(1/*C*) (36 compounds) gave excellent correlations (r = 0.89 and 0.92, respectively. The activities were also analyzed using classical Hansch techniques. For the *in vitro* inhibition of serotonin uptake by blood platelets, Eq. (22) was derived in which **F** is the Swain and Lupton field effect.

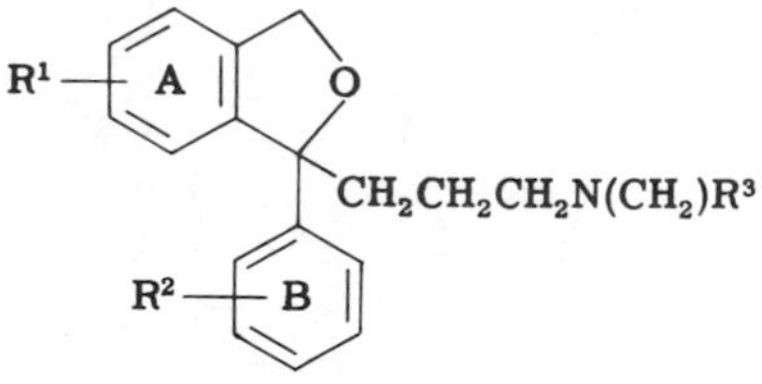

VII

$$pI_{50} = -1.062 + 0.154\pi_{\text{total}} + 1.605\mathbf{F} \quad (22)$$

$$n = 36, \qquad r = 0.85$$

Equations (23) and (24) best correlated *in vivo* activity (potentiation of serotonin syndrome in mice) with physicochemical parameters.

$$\log(1/C) = 0.080 - 1.556\pi_a - 1.826\mathbf{R}_b + 1.643\mathbf{F}_b + 1.989\pi_{\text{total}} \quad (23)$$

$$n = 35, \qquad r = 0.73$$

$$\log(1/C) = 0.168 + 0.445\pi_a + 1.578\mathbf{F}_b + 1.001D \quad (24)$$

$$n = 35, \qquad r = 0.72$$

The subscripts a and b refer to substituents in ring A or B, $D = 1$ for tertiary amines, and $D = 0$ for secondary amines.

As in the case of MAO inhibitors, electronic factors again seem to be important. Although lipophilic terms appear in these equations, no clear interpretation can be offered. Despite the poor correlation between pI_{50} and $\log(1/C)$, the results of the QSAR analysis indicate that similar receptors are involved.

V. CONVULSANTS AND ANTICONVULSANTS

Anticonvulsants are useful for the control of epileptic seizures. Several compounds of varying structures are currently in use. The structural class **VIII** has been summarized by Woodbury and Fingl (*68*). Other classes in-

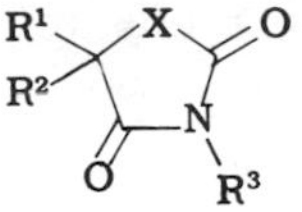

VIII

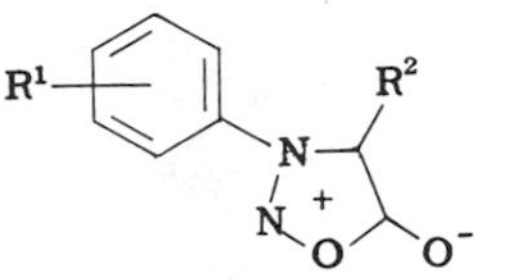

IX

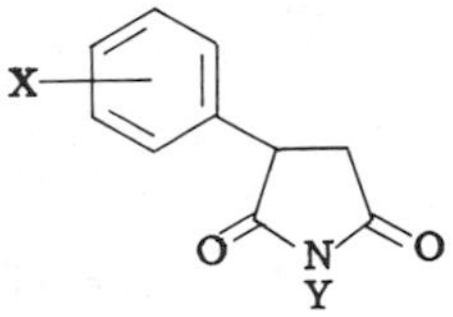

X

clude benzodiazepines and sydnones. The laboratory tests utilized in identifying anticonvulsant drugs are antagonism of pentylenetetrazole (PTZ) induced convulsions and electroshock convulsions.

Franke *et al.* analyzed the anti-PTZ activities of sydnones (**IX**) in mice (*21*). For seven compounds, the best single parameter equation is (25):

$$\log(1/ED_{50}) = 0.66\pi_{p,1} - 2.06 \qquad (25)$$

$$n = 7, \quad r = 0.944, \quad s = 0.115$$

They reported a significant two-parameter equation (27) also.

$$\log(1/ED_{50}) = 0.71\pi_1 - 0.64E_{s_1} \qquad (26)$$

$$n = 7, \quad r = 0.983, \quad s = 0.079$$

The phenylsuccinimides (**X**) prevent seizures due to electrical shock in mice. A three-parameter equation (27) was derived for the relative biological activities (*40*),

$$\log(1/ED_{50}) = -0.35\pi_X^2 + 1.03\pi_X - 0.17\mathbf{F} + 3.23 \qquad (27)$$

$$n = 15, \quad r = 0.970, \quad s = 0.079, \quad X_o = 0.83\text{–}2.81$$

where **F** is the Swain–Lupton field parameter.

The QSAR of 16 currently prescribed anticonvulsants were reported (*42*). These compounds were screened in the electroshock and pentylenetetrazole tests in mice. The 16 compounds include barbiturates, phenylsuccinimides, and benzodiazepines. Equations (29) through (33) emerged as the best, where μ is the dipole moment).

Maximal electroshock:

$$\log(1/C) = 0.65 \log P - 0.13\mu + 2.79 \quad (28)$$

$$n = 16, \quad r = 0.879, \quad s = 0.348$$

Pentylenetetrazole seizure:

$$\log(1/C) = -0.30(\log P)^2 + 0.85 \log P - 0.63\mu + 4.14 \quad (29)$$

$$n = 12, \quad r = 0.915, \quad s = 0.227, \quad \log P_0 = 1.42$$

For 7-substituted 1,4-benzodiazepines, the following equations resulted.

Maximal electroshock test:

$$\log(1/C) = -0.26\pi^2 + 0.36\pi + 0.95\sigma + 3.66 \quad (30)$$

$$n = 11, \quad r = 0.824, \quad s = 0.418, \quad \pi_0 = 0.70$$

Pentylenetetrazole test:

$$\log(1/C) = -0.31\pi^2 + 0.14\pi + 1.29\sigma + 4.56 \quad (31)$$

$$n = 10, \quad r = 0.867, \quad s = 0.470, \quad \pi_0 = 0.23$$

Minimal electroshock test:

$$\log(1/C) = -0.22\pi^2 + 0.081\pi + 0.98\sigma + 3.26 \quad (32)$$

$$n = 10, \quad r = 0.827, \quad s = 0.326, \quad \pi_0 = 0.18.$$

The anticonvulsive potentials of two series of benzodiazepines were studied, using multiple regression techniques. For 52 compounds, active in the pentylenetetrazole test in mice, Blair and Webb (*5*) reported, among others, Eq. (33), where μ is the dipole moment.

$$\log 1/C = -0.50\mu + 3.26 \quad (33)$$

$$n = 52, \quad r = 0.621, \quad s = 0.866$$

Addition of π was not significant, whereas q_0, the calculated charge densities of carbonyl oxygen, gave a statistically significant equation.

An interesting correlation between the rate of borohydride reduction (k_2) of 11 different 1,4-benzodiazepines and anti-PTZ activity in mice was formulated,

$$ED_{50} = 5.40 - 0.88 \log k_2 \qquad (34)$$
$$n = 11, \qquad r^2 = 0.99$$

suggesting a possible involvement of the carbonyl group at the receptor site (*57*).

In a related finding, the anti-PTZ activity of a series of benzodiazepines showed a highly significant correlation with the electron density in the π orbital at the aromatic carbon adjacent to the amide function (*43*).

Lactams and thiolactams are structural analogs of the anticonvulsants, yet exhibit epileptogenic effects. Lien *et al.* measured the convulsive activities and quantitatively correlated the acute lethal toxicity (log $1/C$) with physicochemical parameters (Eq. 35) (*40a*).

$$\log(1/C) = -0.59(\log P)^2 + 1.34 \log P + 0.58\mu - 0.012 \qquad (35)$$
$$n = 10, \qquad r = 0.935, \qquad s = 0.240, \qquad \log P_0 = 1.13$$

β-Lactams produce epileptic-like discharges in brain cortex tissues (*61*). QSAR analyses indicate that convulsive activity correlates significantly with lipophilicity (Eqs. 36 and 37) (see also Chapter 3, this volume).

Aliphatic penicillins:

$$\log(1/C) = 0.313 \log P - 0.43 \qquad (36)$$
$$n = 5, \qquad r = 0.993$$

Aromatic penicillins:

$$\log(1/C) = 0.118 \log P - 0.720 \qquad (37)$$
$$n = 8, \qquad r = 0.512$$

The convulsant and anticonvulsant activities of different series of compounds demonstrate the difficulties in trying to obtain a drug having a highly selective CNS activity. In both instances lipophilicity plays such an important part that other factors need to be considered. Electronic factors, such as σ (Eqs. 2 and 3) or other factors not yet considered, may be the difference that causes one series of compounds to possess anticonvulsant activity, whereas it causes another structurally analogous series to be epileptogenic.

VI. NEUROLEPTICS

The earliest attempts to relate physicochemical parameters to pharmacological activity in the neuroleptics were performed on the phenothiazines. These studies centered on some properties peculiar to the phenothiazines and have been summarized (*55*).

The first systematic attempt to relate physicochemical descriptors to activity in a congeneric series of neuroleptic compounds is due to Tollenaere and co-workers (*63*). Thus for a series of 10-piperazinodibenzo-[*b,f*]thiepins (**XI**) the best equation for relating activity in the iv mouse rotating rod test and four parameters is Eq. (38):

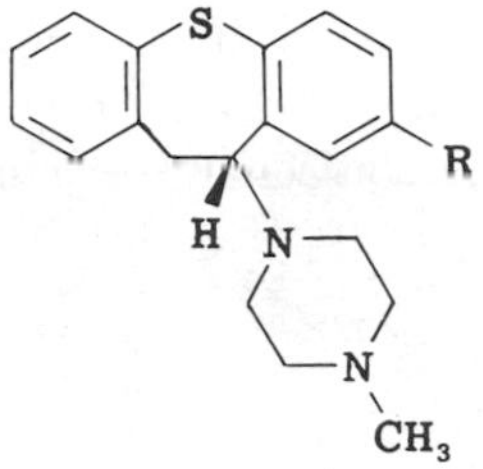

XI

$$pED_{50} = 0.698\sigma_p + 0.347E_s + 0.0458U_T - 0.00059U_T^2 \qquad (38)$$

$$n = 17, \quad r = 0.965, \quad s = 0.128$$

where σ_p is the Hammett constant, E_s the steric parameter, and U_T the molar volume of the substituent R. It is of interest to note that for this pharmacological property, the lipophilic parameter π is not important, and that use of σm leads to inferior equations. This suggests that the R substituent exerts an electronic effect on a position para to it, namely the sulfur atom. The appearance of the terms E_s, U_T, and U_T^2 indicates the importance of steric requirements for acitivty in this series, and foreshadowed the later findings of enantioselectivity of neuroleptic activity found with (+)octoclothepin (**XI**: R = Cl) (*33,53*) as well as several other different structural classes (*10,11,30,56,67*).

Although the rotating rod test is a measure of ataxia, which is neither specific for neuroleptics nor generally seen in all classes of neuroleptics, the authors maintain that Eq. (38) resembles those used to describe more typical properties of neuroleptics such as antiemetic, jump box, and cataleptogenic activity.

The relationship between detailed three-dimensional structural parameters and neuroleptic activity has also been analyzed recently (*64*). Information on molecular structure is obtained experimentally in the solid state (X-ray crystallography) or in solution (high resolution NMR). Low energy conformers may be identified by use of quantum chemical techniques. For flexible molecules, the most prominent objection to this type of treatment of QSAR is that the conformation in the above aggregation states may not correspond to the conformation required to express an effect at a receptor. Obviously, the most useful information of this type would result from studies on conformationally restricted molecules having specific neuroleptic properties.

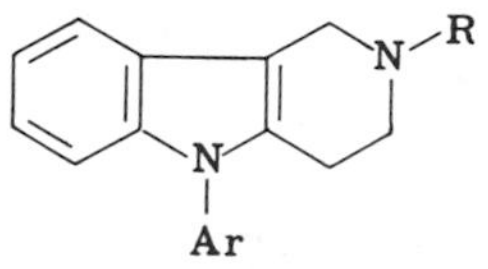

XII

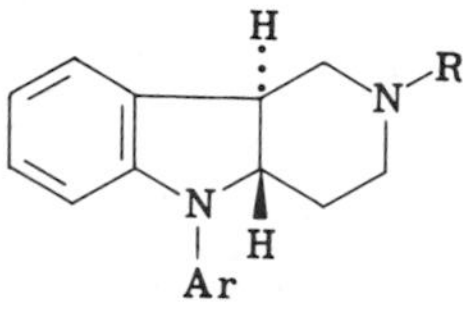

XIII

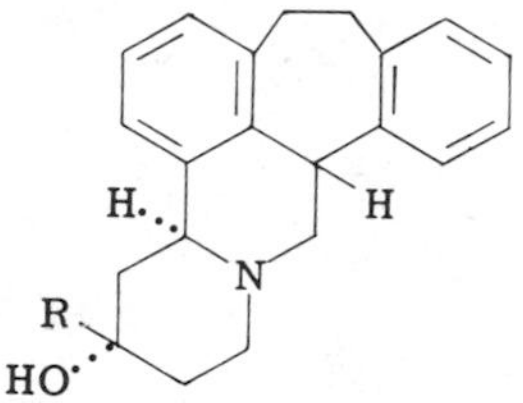

XIV

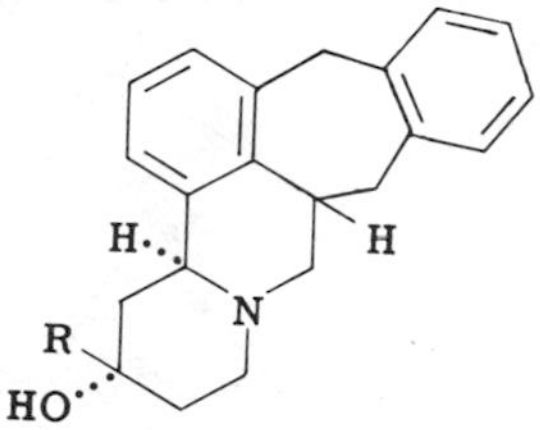

XV

Recently, several conformationally well-defined polycyclic series of neuroleptics (**XII–XV**) have been described (*3,8,29,44,54*). Comparisons of the X-ray crystallographically derived conformations of several flexible neuroleptics have been made with dexclamol (**XIV:** R = *i* − Pr), and certain common features were observed (*49,62*). However, a detailed examination of the molecular geometry of **XII–XV** has lead to the development of a receptor map for neuroleptic drugs in which a quintessential pharmacophoric pattern is defined (*29,54*). The salient features of this model (Fig. 1) are a planar aromatic binding site (K-L-M-N) and a cationic binding site (D) 0.6–0.9 Å above the plane of the aromatic site and 5.1–6.4 Å from the center of the aromatic binding region. It is of interest to note that the conformationally flexible neuroleptics will fit this model by adopting the "S-shape" proposed by Janssen (*32*), but that these conformations are not the ones derived from crystallographic data. It is expected that this model will lead to the rational design of new drugs of this type having the requisite pharmacophore.

VII. PSYCHOTOMIMETICS

The extraordinary work of Shulgin and co-workers (*59*) provided the rare opportunity to study the effects of physicochemical parameters on psychotomimetic activity in man. The activities of several hallucinogenic

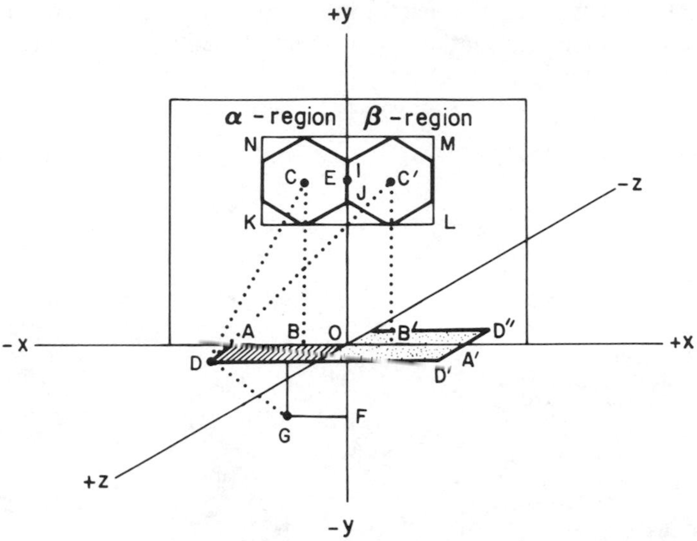

Fig. 1. Representation of primary binding sites on the dopamine receptor derived from measurements of Dreiding models of the B conformers of (+)-butaclamol (**XIV:** R = *tert*-butyl) and (+)-isobutaclamol (**XV:** R = *tert*-butyl). Key distances are: O–E = B′–C′ = 4.7 Å; A–D = A′–D′ = A″–D″ = 0.9 Å; A–B = A′–B′ = 2.0 Å; A–B′ = 4.4 Å; D–C = 6.4 Å; D–G = 2.6 Å; A–O = A′–O′ = 3.2 Å; K–L = M–N = 4.8 Å; N–K = M–L = 2.4 Å; O–F = 1.8 Å; F–G = 1.7 Å. Reprinted with permission from Philipp *et al.* (*54*). Copyright © 1979 American Chemical Society.

agents relative to mescaline (*59*) was expressed in terms of the molar mescaline unit (*MMU*).

Hallucinogenic potency of a series of phenethylamines and amphetamines showed a significant correlation with the partition coefficient (Eq. 39) (*1*).

$$\log(MMU) = 3.15 \log P - 0.50 \log P^2 - 3.17 \quad (39)$$

$$n = 26, \quad r = 0.79, \quad s = 0.41, \quad \log P_o = 3.14$$

Connectivity indices have also been used in a study of a series of amphetamines (*39*). The best equation from this study is Eq. (40).

$$\log(MMU) = 45.16/({}^3X_p) + 1.288({}^6X_p) - 4.298({}^4X^V_{pc}) - 5.592 \quad (40)$$

$$n = 23, \quad r = 0.920, \quad s = 0.251$$

The induced contraction of sheep umbilical artery has been shown to be a useful *in vitro* assay of hallucinogenic activity (*19,20*). Employing this test, the activity of substituted phenethylamines has been analyzed. An excellent fit was derived using a cubic term in log P (Eq. 41) (*51*),

$$\log(RBR) = 0.23 - 0.89 \log P + 0.95(\log P)^2 - 0.16(\log P)^3 \quad (41)$$

$$n = 15, \quad r = 0.98, \quad s = 0.13, \quad \log P_o = 3.41$$

in which RBR represents the ED_{50} mescaline/ED_{50} test compound. (This optimal log P coincides well with that derived from Eq. 39.) Hammett's σ_p was not important. Inclusion of molar refraction (MR) as a measure of steric bulk resulted in an equation having a higher correlation coefficient than a first-order equation in log P alone (Eq. 42).

$$\log(RBR) = 0.354 - 0.043MR + 0.501 \log P \quad (42)$$

$$n = 17, \quad r = 0.81, \quad s = 0.39$$

The ionization potentials of a varied set of psychotomimetic amines were measured and utilized as variables in QSAR analysis (*18*). Equation (43) was formulated showing the correlation between MMU (molar activity of a test compound relative to mescaline) and IP_1 (first ionization potential expressed in electron-volts). Addition of IP_2 does not produce a better correlation;

$$\log(MMU) = -2.37(IP_1) + 19.53 \quad (43)$$

$$n = 11, \quad r = 0.86$$

however, inclusion of a log P terms does (Eq. 44).

$$\log(MMU) = -1.48(IP_1) + 0.78 \log P + 11.15 \quad (44)$$

$$n = 11, \quad r = 0.94$$

A recent receptor study indicates that both serotonin (5-HT) and D-lysergic acid diethylamide (LSD) label the postsynaptic 5-HT receptor in rat brain, showing that 5-HT is specific for the agonist state of the receptor and that LSD labels both agonist and antagonist states (*2*).

The displacement of tritiated serotonin and tritiated LSD from cerebral cortex membrane by four structurally diverse classes of compounds has been analyzed using regression techniques (*9*). For displacement of serotonin a parabolic relationship with log P was observed (Eq. 45), but a log(molecular weight) term was needed for the displacement of LSD (Eq. 46).

$$\log(1/IC_{50}) = -0.330(\log P)^2 + 1.39 P + 6.181 \quad (45)$$

$$n = 14, \quad r = 0.873, \quad s = 0.766, \quad \log P_o = 2.11$$

$$\log(1/IC_{50}) = -0.171(\log P)^2 + 0.980 \log P + 3.283 \log \mathrm{MW} - 2.206 \quad (46)$$

$$n = 26, \quad r = 0.929, \quad s = 0.559, \quad \log P_o = 2.87$$

It is of interest to note that for both of these parabolic equations, a higher optimal log P was obtained for LSD indicating a greater degree of hydrophobic interaction in its displacement. In terms of receptor topography, this finding led to the postulation of two conformationally related binding sites differing in the relationship of accessory sites to the primary binding site. The one for the agonist (5-HT) appears less hydrophobic than the one for antagonists (e.g., methylsergide and cyproheptadine). LSD, with an intermediate lipophilicity, thus acts as an agonist–antagonist.

Ionization potentials were also used in an analysis of D-LSD binding (Eq. 47) and D-LSD displacement (Eq. 48) in rat brain homogenates by a structurally diverse series of drugs that included alkyl and polyalkoxytryptamines and amphetamines and LSD (*18*).

$$pIC_{50} = -3.81(IP_1) - 1.64(IP_2) + 47.78 \quad (47)$$

$$n = 10, \quad r = 0.85$$

$$pED_{50} = -2.79(IP_1) - 1.93(IP_2) + 43.36 \quad (48)$$

$$n = 7, \quad r = 0.97$$

IC_{50} is the concentration of drug required to inhibit binding of D-LSD by 50%, ED_{50} is the dose required to displace 50% of bound D-LSD, and IP_1 and IP_2 are the first and second ionization potentials of test drug. It may be seen that smaller IP values result in more potent drugs in both cases, and indicate an important role for complexation of the aromatic portion of the drug at the receptor site.

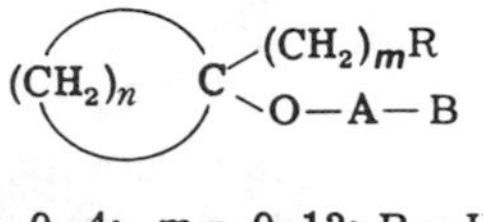

n = 0-4; m = 0-12; R = H or aryl

XVI

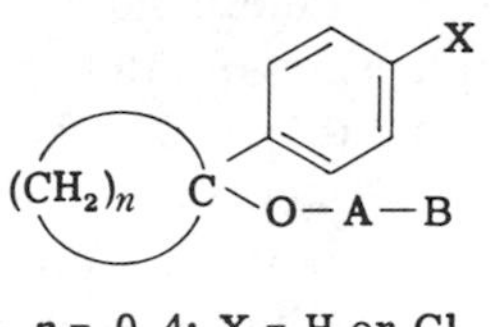

n = 0-4; X = H or Cl

XVII

The psychostimulant properties of substituted cycloalkoxyalkylamines (**XVI** and **XVIII**) in white mice were measured (*12*). A is n alkyl chain and B contains a basic nitrogen. Although the equations were not reported, the following statistics were available:

$n = 10, \quad r = 0.906 \quad$ for π as the independent variable

$n = 20, \quad r = 0.928, \quad s = 0.117 \quad$ for a Free–Wilson analysis

These studies on psychostimulant activities quite conclusively show that lipophilicity is an important determinant and that, where available, the ideal lipophilicity is relatively high (log $P_0 = 3$). Of special interest is the apparent importance of a cubic term in log P.

VIII. OVERVIEW

Some of the important physicochemical properties that have emerged as determinants of the different types of CNS activities are shown in Table I. Steric size or bulk and electronic effects are not as well-defined as lipophilicity. We have grouped MR, MW, and U_T with E_S for size. Quantum chemical indices as well as pK_a are classified under electronic effects. These three factors are the most common variables used in multiple regression analyses of relative biological activity.

Inspection of Table I shows the tremendous overlap of physical properties influencing the various types of CNS effects. It is obvious that, within a series of compounds targeted for a specific CNS activity, increased potency cannot be achieved simply by varying on property only. Hence several properties within a series must be monitored if multiple regression analysis is to be an effective method for selecting congeners.

Hansch (*27*) has suggested that log $P_0 \approx 2$ is the ideal lipophilicity for drugs to pass the blood–brain barrier. We have collected log P values (Table II) where available within this chapter to see if this approximation is still reasonable. The overall mean log P_0 is 2.8; however, log P_0 varies significantly from one pharmacological class to another.

TABLE I
Properties Affecting Relative CNS Activities

Activity	Lipophilicity	Size	Electronic effects
Analgesia	X	X	
Anesthesia	X		X
Antidepressant		X	X
Convulsants	X		
Anticonvulsant	X		X
Neuroleptic		X	X
Psychotomimetic	X	X	X

TABLE II
Calculated Ideal Lipophilicities[a]

Equation number	Activity	Log P_0
1	Analgesia	3.23
2	Analgesia	1.43
3	Analgesia	2.95
7	Anesthetic	2.35
12	Anesthetic	3.56
13	Anesthetic	4.33
14	Anesthetic	2.70
18	Anesthetic	4.40
30	Anticonvulsive	1.42
36	Convulsive	1.13
40	Psychotomimetic	3.14

[a] Overall: mean = 2.79, s.d. = 1.02, range = 1.13–4.40

The equations in this chapter are useful for rationalizing the relative orders of biological activities within a series and for predicting the activities of compounds not yet made. They cannot, however, be readily used for uncovering new lead compounds. Part of this limitation arises because there is no effective way of determining *a priori* what fundamental structural features are necessary for eliciting a particular pharmacological effect. As biochemical techniques for identifying, isolating, and characterizing receptors improve, efforts to design compounds that are highly specific for a given receptor will undoubtedly be undertaken. These equations could then be used as starting points for congener selection.

REFERENCES

1. C. F. Barfknecht, D. E. Nichols, and W. J. Dunn, III, *J. Med. Chem.* **18,** 208 (1975).
2. J. P. Bennett and S. H. Snyder, *Mol. Pharmacol.* **12,** 373 (1976).
3. J. G. Berger, U.S. Patent No. 3,991,199 (1976).
4. A. J. Bigler, K. P. Bogeso, A. Toft, and V. Hansen, *Eur. J. Med. Chem.—Chim. Ther.* **12,** 289 (1977).
5. T. Blair and G. A. Webb, *J. Med. Chem.* **20,** 1206 (1977).
6. B. B. Brodie, A. Pletscher, and P. A. Shore, *J. Pharmacol. Exp. Ther.* **116,** 9 (1956).
7. J. M. Brown and P. A. Chaloner, *Can. J. Chem.* **55,** 3380 (1977).
8. F. T. Bruderlein, L. G. Humber, and K. Voith, *J. Med. Chem.* **18,** 185 (1975).
9. Y. L. Chan, E. J. Lien, and J. C. Shih, *in* "QUASAR" (G. Barnett, M. Trsic, and R. Willette, eds.), NIDA Res. Monogr., No. 22, p. 103. Natl. Inst. Drug Abuse, Rockville, Maryland, 1978.

10. N. Chaudhuri, T. J. Ball, and N. Finch, *Experientia* **33,** 575 (1977).
11. S. S. C. Chiu and R. D. Rosenstein, *J. C. S. Chem. Commun.* p. 491 (1979).
12. F. Darvas, Z. Budai, L. Pesocz, and I. Kosoczky, *Res. Commun. Chem. Pathol. Pharmacol.* **12,** 243 (1975).
13. R. H. Davies, R. D. Bagnall, and W. G. M. Jones, *Int. J. Quantum Chem., Quantum Biol. Symp.* No. 1, p. 201 (1974).
14. T. Di Paolo, *J. Pharm. Sci.* **67,** 564 (1978).
15. T. Di Paolo, *J. Pharm. Sci.* **67,** 566 (1978).
16. T. Di Paolo, L. B. Kier, and L. H. Hall, *Mol. Pharmacol.* **13,** 31 (1977).
17. T. Di Paolo, L. B. Kier, and L. H. Hall, *J. Pharm. Sci.* **68,** 39 (1979).
18. L. N. Domelsmith and K. N. Houk, *in* "QUASAR" (J. Barnett, M. Trsic, and R. Willette, eds.), NIDA Res. Monogr., No. 22, p. 423. Natl. Inst. Drug. Abuse, Rockville, Maryland, 1978.
19. D. C. Dyer, *J. Pharmacol. Exp. Ther.* **188,** 336 (1974).
20. D. C. Dyer and D. W. Grant, *J. Pharmacol. Exp. Ther.* **184,** 366 (1973).
21. R. Franke, E. Gabler, and P. Oehme, *Acta Biol. Med. Ger.* **32,** 545 (1974).
22. N. P. Franks and W. R. Lieb, *Nature (London)* **274,** 339 (1978).
23. T. Fujita, *J. Med. Chem.* **16,** 923 (1973).
24. P. Fulcrand, G. Berge, J. Castel, A.-M. Noel, P. Chevallet, and H. Orzaleski, *C. R. Hebd. Seances Acad. Sci., Ser. C.* **284** 49 (1977).
25. W. R. Glave and C. Hansch, *J. Pharm. Sci.* **61,** 589 (1972).
26. L. S. Goodman and A. Gilman, "The Pharmacological Basis of Therapeutics," 5th ed., p. 57. Macmillan, New York, 1975.
27. C. Hansch, *Acc. Chem. Res.* **2,** 232 (1969).
28. C. Hansch, A Vittoria, C. Silipo, and P. Y. C. Jow, *J. Med. Chem.* **18,** 546 (1975).
29. C. A. Harbert, J. J. Plattner, W. M. Welch, A. Weissman, and B. K. Koe, *Mol. Pharmacol.* **17,** 38 (1980).
30. L. G. Humber, F. T. Bruderlein, and K. Voith, *Mol. Pharmacol.* **11,** 833 (1975).
31. A. E. Jacobson, W. A. Klee, and W. J. Dunn, III, *Eur. J. Med. Chem.—Chim. Ther.* **12,** 49 (1977).
32. P. A. J. Janssen, *in* "The Neuroleptics" (D. P. Bobon, P. A. J. Janssen, and J. Bobon, eds.), Modern Problems of Pharmacopsychiatry, Vol. 5, p. 33. Karger, Basel, 1970.
33. A. Jaunin, T. J. Petcher, and H. P. Weber, *J. C. S. Perkin II* p. 186 (1977).
34. R. Jeppson, *Acta Pharmacol. Toxicol.* **37,** 56 (1975).
35. C. L. Johnson, *J. Med. Chem.* **19,** 600 (1976).
36. H. Johnson, *in* "QUASAR" (G. Barnett, M. Trsic, and R. Willette, eds.), NIDA Res. Monogr., No. 22, p. 146. Natl. Inst. Drug Abuse, Rockville, Maryland, 1978.
37. R. Katz, S. F. Osborne, and F. Ionescu, *J. Med. Chem.* **20,** 1413 (1977).
38. L. B. Kier and L. H. Hall, "Molecular Connectivity in Chemistry and Drug Research," p. 158. Macmillan, New York, 1976.
39. L. B. Kier and L. H. Hall, *J. Med. Chem.* **20,** 1631 (1977).
40. J. Lapszewicz, J. Lange, S. Rump, and K. Walczyna, *Eur. J. Med. Chem.—Chim. Ther.* **13,** 465 (1978).
40a. E. J. Lien, L. L. Lien, and G. L. Tong, *J. Med. Chem.* **14,** 846 (1971).
41. E. J. Lien, G. L. Tong, D. B. Srulevitch, and C. Dias, "QUASAR" (G. Barnett, M. Trsic, and R. Willette, eds. NIDA Res. Monogr., No. 22, p. 186. Natl. Inst. Drug Abuse, Rockville, Maryland, 1978.
42. E. J. Lien, R. C. H. Liao, and H. G. Shinouda, *J. Pharm. Sci.* **68,** 463 (1979).
43. R. W. Lucek, W. A. Garland, and W. Dairman, *Fed. Proc., Fed. Am. Soc. Exp. Biol.* **38,** 541 (1979).

44. G. R. Marshall, C. D. Barry, H. E. Bosshard, R. A. Dammkoehler, and D. A. Dunn, *in* "Computer-assisted Drug Design" (E. C. Olson and R. E. Christoffersen, eds.), ACS Symposium Series, No. 112, p. 219. Am. Chem. Soc., Washington, D.C., 1979.
45. R. Massuda and C. Sandorfy, *Can. J. Chem.* **55,** 3211 (1977).
46. For an example of the history and chemistry of these agents, see E. L. May, *J. Med. Chem.* **23,** 225 (1980).
46a. K. H. Meyer and H. Hemmi, *Biochem. Z.* **277,** 39 (1935).
47. K. W. Miller, N. D. M. Paton, E. B. Smith, and R. A. Smith, *Anesthesiology* **36,** 339 (1972).
48. K. W. Miller, M. W. Wilson, and R. A. Smith, *Mol. Pharmacol.* **14,** 950 (1978).
49. H. Moereels and J. P. Tolleneare, *Life Sci.* **23,** 459 (1978).
50. A. Nagyrevi and C. Sandorfy, *Can. J. Chem.* **55,** 1593 (1977).
51. D. E. Nichols, A. T. Shulgin, and D. C. Dyer, *Life Sci.* **21,** 569 (1977).
51a. E. Overton, "Studien uber die Narkose," Fischer, Jena, Germany, 1901.
52. K.-Y. Pang, L. M. Braswell, L. Chang, T. Sommer, and K. W. Miller, *Mol. Pharmacol.* **18,** 84 (1980).
53. T. J. Petcher, J. Schmutz, H. P. Weber, and T. G. White, *Experientia,* **31,** 1389 (1975).
54. A. H. Philipp. L. G. Humber, and K. Voith, *J. Med. Chem.* **22,** 768 (1979).
55. W. P. Purcell, *Int. J. Quantum Chem., Quantum Biol. Symp.* No. 2, p. 191 (1975).
56. D. C. Remy, K. E. Rittle, C. A. Hunt, P. S. Anderson, B. H. Arison, E. L. Englehart, R. Hirschmann, B. J. Clineschmidt, V. J. Lotti, P. R. Bunting, R. J. Ballentine, N. L. Papp, L. Flataher, J. J. Witoslaski, and C. A. Stone, *J. Med. Chem.* **20,** 1013 (1977).
57. O. M. Sadagopa Ramanujam and N. M. Trieff, *J. Pharm. Pharmacol.* **30,** 542 (1978).
58. I. J. Selikoff, E. H. Robitzek, and G. G. Ornstein, *Q. Bull. Sea View Hosp.* **13,** 17 (1952).
59. A. T. Shulgin, T. Sargent, and C. Naranjo, *Nature (London)* **221,** 537 (1969).
60. S. A. Simon, T. J. McIntosh, P. B. Bennett, and B. B. Shrivastev, *Mol. Pharmacol.* **16,** 163 (1979).
61. P. Sobotka and J. Safanda, *J. Mol. Med.* **1,** 151 (1976).
62. J. P. Tolleneare and H. Moereels, *Gazz. Chim. Ital.* **108,** 419 (1978).
63. J. P. Tollenaere, H. Moereels, and M. Protiva, *Eur. J. Med. Chem.—Chim. Ther.* **11,** 293 (1976).
64. J. P. Tollenaere, H. Moereels, and M. H. J. Koch, *Eur. J. Med. Chem.—Chim. Ther.* **12,** 199 (1977).
65. F. Tomas and J. M. Aullo, *J. Pharm. Sci.* **68,** 772 (1979).
66. G. Trudeau, K. C. Cole, R. Massuda, and C. Sandorfy, *Can. J. Chem.* **56,** 1681 (1978).
67. W. M. Welch, F. E. Ewing, C. A. Harbert, A. Weissman, and B. K. Koe, *J. Med. Chem.* **23,** 1823 (1980).
68. D. M. Woodbury and E. Fingl, *in* "The Pharmacological Basis of Therapeutics" (L. S. Godman and A. Gilman, eds.), 5th ed., p. 204. Macmillan, New York, 1975.
69. E. A. Zeller, J. Barsky, J. R. Fouts, W. F. Kirchheimer, and L. S. Van Orden, *Experientia* **8,** 349 (1952).

9

Steroids and Other Hormones

MANFRED E. WOLFF

I. INTRODUCTION AND SCOPE

The examination of the relationship between chemical constitution and biological activity of hormonal substances is as old as the history of hormones themselves inasmuch as the course of their isolation was monitored by bioassay procedures. Further interest in this topic has been stim-

ISBN 0-12-695150-0

ulated by the hope of obtaining modified hormones useful as drugs. It is not surprising, therefore, that some of the earliest attempts at any quantitative approaches to structure–activity relationships were initiated in the thyromimetic area by Bruice *et al.* (*16*) and in the antiinflammatory steroids by Fried and Borman (*39*).

In the recent past the term *hormone* has been broadened considerably owing to the emergence of many neural and local or tissue hormones including the prostaglandins and the other members of the arachidonic acid cascade. This chapter, however, will be restricted to the classical endocrine hormones including the steroids, the peptide hormones, and thyroxine. Of these, the steroids are by far the most widely investigated using QSAR techniques. Linear free-energy techniques have been applied not only to the pharmacological activity of steroids but also to simpler processes such as absorption and receptor affinity. Moreover, the conformation of steroids has been investigated extensively by X-ray analysis as well as by molecular modeling techniques such as energy minimization and quantum mechanical calculations. For these reasons, the steroids will be considered first in this chapter, and the more limited studies carried out on other hormones will be treated afterward.

The structure and numbering for the pregnane ring system are shown.

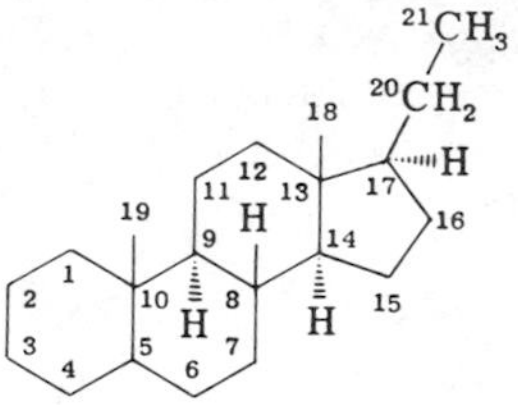

Abbreviated names for steroids discussed in this chapter are shown in Table I.

II. STEROIDS

A. QSAR of Processes Affecting Steroid Activity

As pointed out by Lee *et al.* (*69*), the major difficulty in QSAR studies that attempt to relate the structure of steroids to their pharmacological activity is the oversimplification inherent in relating animal pharmacology to simple physicochemical vectors. Gross pharmacological results represent the sum of a number of part processes including absorption, drug distribution, drug metabolism, receptor affinity, and intrinsic activity. These processes have been schematized by Chu (*23*) (Fig. 1).

TABLE I
Names of Steroids in This Chapter

Common name	Chemical nomenclature
Betamethasone	9-Fluoro-11β,17,21-trihydroxy-16β-Methylpregna-1,4-diene-3,20-dione
Cortexolone	17,21-Dihydroxypregn-4-ene-3,20-dione
Corticosterone	11β,21-Dihydroxypregn-4-ene-3,20-dione
Cortisol	11β,17,21-trihydroxypregn-4-ene-3,20-dione
Cortisone	17,21-Dihydroxypregn-4-ene-3,11,20-trione
Deoxycorticosterone	21-Hydroxypregn-4-ene-3,20-dione
21-Deoxydexamethasone	9-Fluoro-11β,17-dihydroxy-16α-Methylpregna-1,4-diene-3,20-dione
Dexamethasone	9-Fluoro-11α,17,21-trihydroxy-16α-methylpregna-1,4-diene-3,20-dione
Dichlorisone	9,11β-Dichloro-17,21-dihydroxypregn-4-ene-3,20-dione
Flumethasone	6α,9α-Difluoro-16α-methyl-11β,17,21-trihydroxy-1,4-pregnadiene-3,20-dione
Fluocinolone	6α,9-Difluoro-11β,16α,17,21-tetrahydroxypregna-1,4-diene-3,20-dione
Fluocinolone acetonide	6α,9-Difluoro-11β,21-dihydroxy-16α,17-[(1-methylethylidene)bis(oxy)]pregna-1,4-diene-3,20-dione
6α-Fluorocortisol	6α-Fluoro-11β,17,21-trihydroxypregn-4-ene-3,20-dione
9α-Fluorocortisol	9-Fluoro-11β,17,21-trihydroxypregn-4-ene-3,20-dione
6α-Fluoro-16α-hydroxycortisol	6α-Fluoro-11β,16α,17,21-tetrahydroxypregn-4-ene-3,20-dione
9α-Fluoroprednisolone	9-Fluoro-11β,17,21-trihydroxypregna-1,4-diene-3,20-dione
Flurandrenolide	6α-Fluoro-11β,21-dihydroxy-16α,17-[(1-methylethylidene)bis(oxy)]pregn-4-ene-3,20-dione
Nandrolone	17β-Hydroxyestr-4-en-3-one
Paramethasone	6α-Fluoro-11β,17,21-trihydroxy-16α-methylpregna-1,4-diene-3,20-dione
Prednisolone	11β-17,21-Trihydroxypregna-1,4-diene-3,20-dione
Prednisone	17,21-Dihydroxypregna-1,4-diene-3,11,20-trione
Progesterone	Pregn-4-ene-3,20-dione
Triamcinolone acetonide	9-Fluoro-11β,21-dihydroxy-16α,17-[(1-methylethylidene)bis(oxy)]pregna-1,4-diene-3,20-dione

In a QSAR study that attempts to analyze animal pharmacology, a particular parameter, such as π, will probably have a different effect on each process. The regression coefficient for each such variable, therefore, will be the net average of the effect of a parameter on all of these activities. Obviously, the study of individual processes is therefore preferable.

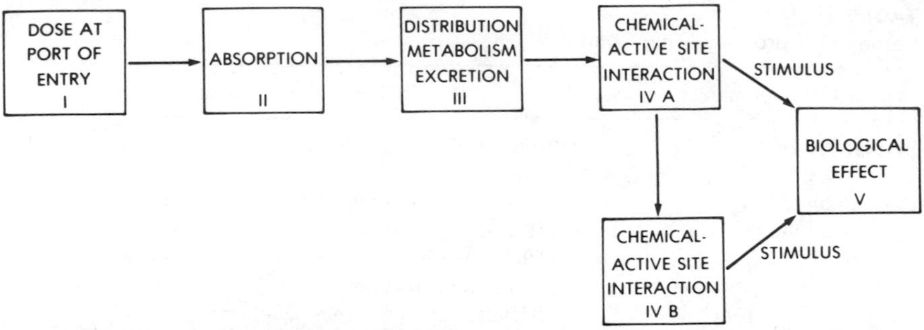

Fig. 1. General scheme for hormone analog action *in vivo.* Phase I involves the dose of the chemical administered and the route and site of administration. Phase II deals with the absorption of the drug. Phase III is concerned with the distribution, metabolic conversion (both bioactivation and detoxification), and excretion of the chemical. Phase IVA deals with the induction of a stimulus by the interaction of the chemical with the active site(s). Phase IVB involves the induction of the stimulus after a series of chemical–active site interactions. Phase V deals with the stimulus producing a biological effect (a process that is compound independent). From Chu (*23*), with permission.

Some of these have been investigated by QSAR techniques and will be considered in the following section.

1. Absorption

a. Intestinal Absorption. In their examination of the absorption of steroids by the perfused rat small intestine, Schedl and Clifton (*91*) demonstrated a close relationship between the absorption of the steroid

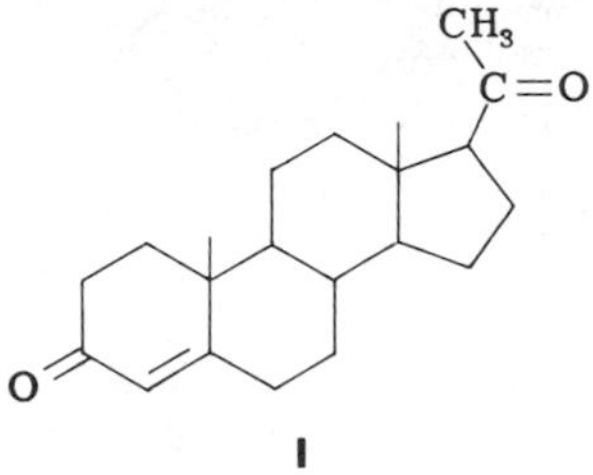

I

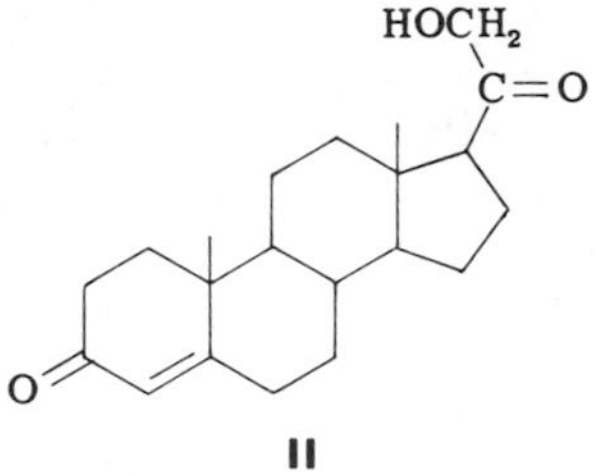

II

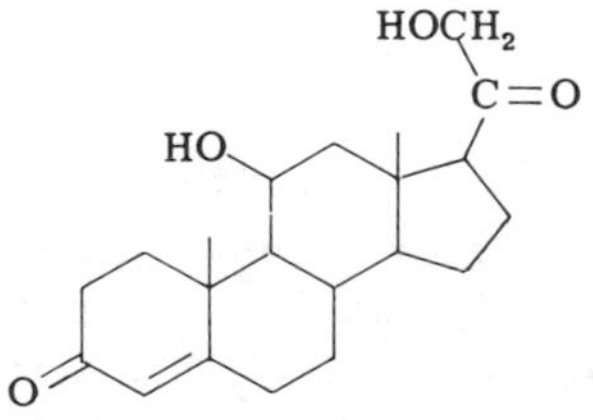

III

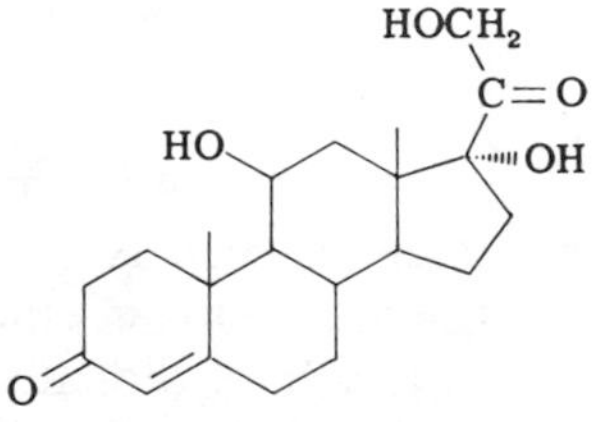

IV

TABLE II
Quantitation of Steroid Absorption by Perfused Rat Small Intestine

Steroid	Number of OH groups	% absorption[a]	Log % absorption	Calculated % absorption[b]	Calculated log % absorption[b]
Progesterone (**I**)	0	93.9	1.97	117.5	2.07
Deoxycorticosterone (**II**)	1	83.7	1.92	67.6	1.83
Corticosterone (**III**)	2	46.5	1.67	46.8	1.59
Cortisol (**IV**)	3	21.0	1.32	20.9	1.35
Triamcinolone (**V**)	4	11.5	1.06	11.5	1.11

[a] Absorption data from Schedl and Clifton (*91*).
[b] From Eq. (1).

and its polarity. The least polar compound in the investigation, progesterone (**I**), is absorbed almost completely, whereas the introduction of hydroxyl groups reduces the extent of absorption (Table II). Because all of the compounds in the study contain 21 carbon atoms and two carbonyl groups, the major difference between them affecting polarity is the number of hydroxyl groups that they contain. Therefore, I have carried out a linear regression of the log of the percent of absorption on the number of hydroxyl groups (Σ OH) giving Eq. (1):

$$\log(\text{percent absorption}) = 2.07 - 0.24 \sum \text{OH} \quad (1)$$

For this equation $r^2 = 0.95$, indicating that 95% of the variance in the data is accounted for by the relationship. Although the intestinal absorption of these important drugs is thus readily correlated with their physical properties and therefore appears to proceed by a diffusion-controlled process rather than by active transport, these figures have no relationship to relative oral clinical potencies. Thus it seems likely that the rate of intestinal absorption is not a controlling factor in the activity of many or, possibly, any steroids. Hüttenrauch and Keiner (*48*) examined the relationship of the solubilities of some anabolic steroids in water or artificial intestinal fluid to their anabolic and androgenic activities. They obtained the relationship shown in Eq. (2):

$$\%\ \text{Rel. Act.} = 208 \log(\text{sol})(\mu\text{g/liter}) - 183 \quad (2)$$

for a series of seven compounds and attributed the increase in activity of the more water-soluble compounds to an increase in speed of dissolution.

b. Corneal Penetration. A major factor in the ophthalmic utility of a medicinal agent is its ophthalmic bioavailability after intraocular administration. Schoenwald and Ward (*95*) developed a model for the optimization of corneal permeability based on molecular modification. They studied the relationship between the 1-octanol–water partition coefficient and the permeability of various structurally related steroids across an excised rabbit cornea and were able to calculate the permeability coefficient (in cm/sec) for each steroid. For 11 steroids, the log of the permeability coefficient ($\log P_{\text{perm}}$) was related to the log of the partition coefficient (Fig. 2) by a second degree polynomial (Eq. 3),

$$\log(P_{\text{perm}}) = -0.28(\log P)^2 + 1.7 \log P - 7.0 \quad (3)$$

giving an optimum $\log P_0$ value of 2.9 (close to dexamethasone acetate). This dependence of penetration rates upon 1-octanol–water partition coefficients apparently is due to the necessity for the drug to penetrate the lipid layers of the cornea.

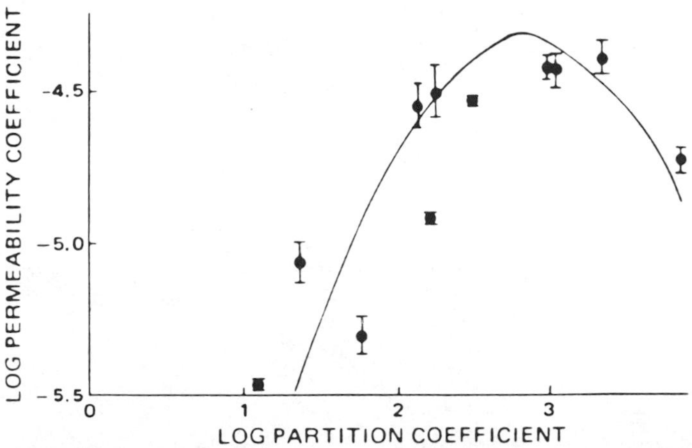

Fig. 2. Computer-generated curvilinear relationship between the log permeability coefficient of 11 labeled steroids and their respective log octanol–water partition coefficient, From left to right, the steroids are prednisolone, hydrocortisone, dexamethasone, fluorometholone, triamcinolone acetonide, prednisolone acetate, cortexolone, deoxycorticosterone, dexamethasone acetate, testosterone, and progesterone. The vertical bars represent 1 SD. From Schoenwald and Ward (*95*), with permission.

c. Percutaneous Absorption. Most steroids are active upon topical administration. For example, using ^{14}C-labeled steroids it has been shown (*71*) that cortisol (**IV**) and triamcinolone (**V**) are absorbed from a topical

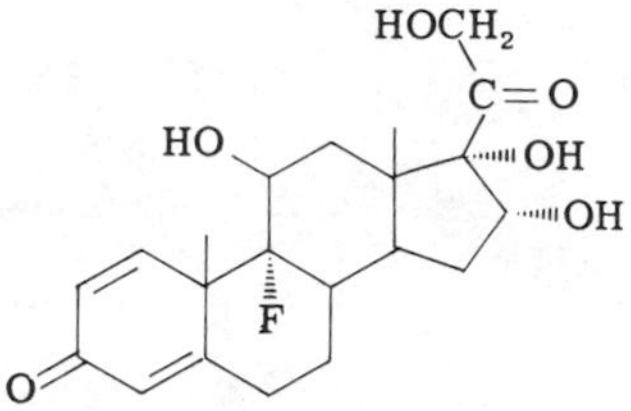

V

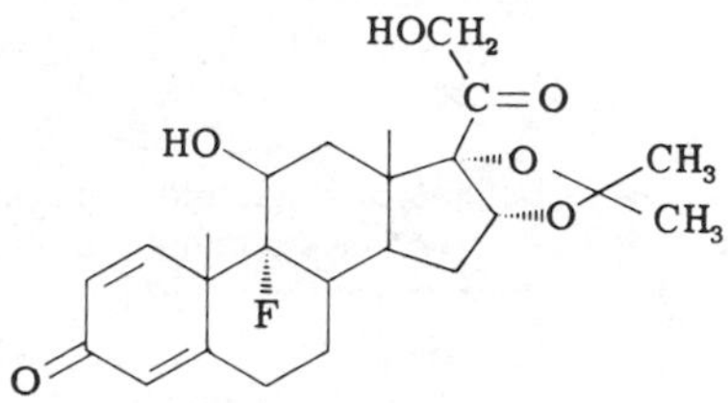

VI

site of application and that the radioactivity appears in the urine. In the early 1960s Demos *et al.* (*30*) made the surprising observation that triamcinolone acetonide (**VI**) is 10 times as active topically as triamcinolone itself but only equiactive systemically. This appears to be due to the partition coefficient of the compound and can be quantified using QSAR techniques. As pointed out by Popper and Watnick (*85*), to be topically effective the steroid must penetrate the keratin layer of the stratum corneum of the skin before it can exert its effect on the squamous cell layer of the epidermis. But to reach the general circulation and produce systemic

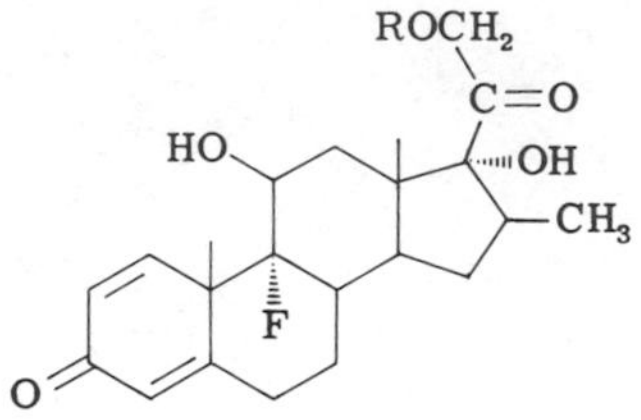

VII **a** R = H
b R = $P(O)(ONa)_2$
c R = Ac
d R = COC_3H_7
e R = COC_4H_9
f R = COC_5H_{11}
g R = $COC_{15}H_{31}$

side effects, the steroid must later penetrate the barrier between the epidermis and the dermis. Thus for a useful topical agent it is desirable for the compound to remain in the epidermis and to migrate only slowly into the dermis. This property is fostered by the presence of lipophilic groups and by the absence of hydroxyl groups in the steroid. The evaluation of a number of 21-esters of betamethasone (**VIIa–g**) was carried out by MacKenzie and Atkinson (*70*) (Table III). I have fitted the π value of the C-21 group to a second-degree polynomial to give the plot shown in Fig. 3, indicating that, as in the case of corneal absorption, the percutaneous absorption has a roughly parabolic dependency on the partition coefficient of the steroid.

TABLE III
Relative Potencies of Betamethasone and Some of Its 21-Esters in Antiinflammatory Vasoconstriction Assays against Fluocinolone Acetonide

Compound	Approximate π value of C-21 group	Relative potency[a,b]
Betamethasone alcohol (**VIIa**)	−1.12	0.8
Betamethasone 21-disodium phosphate (**VIIb**)	−5[c]	0.9
Betamethasone 21-acetate (**VIIc**)	−0.95	18
Betamethasone 21-butyrate (**VIId**)	0.05	85
Betamethasone 21-valerate (**VIIe**)	1.05	26
Betamethasone 21-hexanoate (**VIIf**)	1.55	123
Betamethasone 21-palmitate (**VIIg**)	6.05	0.1

[a] Data from McKenzie and Atkinson (*70*).
[b] Fluocinolone acetonide = 100.
[c] Estimated value.

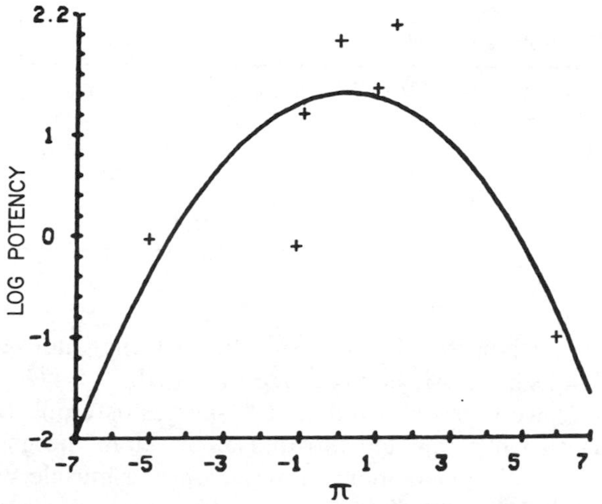

Fig. 3. PROPHET plot showing approximate parabolic dependency of betamethasone ester activity on π.

d. Absorption from Injection Sites. As pointed out by Counsell and Brueggemeir (*26*), two factors are involved in the increase in androgenic and anabolic potency and in the prolongation of action brought about by changes in the esterifying acid of steroid esters. These factors were already identified by Gould *et al.* (*43*) who surmised that esterifying acids that are hydrolyzed with exceptional difficulty give androgens of inferior activity and that the more oil-soluble esters give compounds of superior utility. Studies by James (*52*) and James *et al.* (*55*) indicate that the effect of various aliphatic esters of testosterone on rat prostate and seminal vesicle is correlated with the lipophilicity of the esterifying acid and the rate of ester hydrolysis by liver esterase. It was concluded that the ease of hydrolysis controls the weight of the target organs, whereas

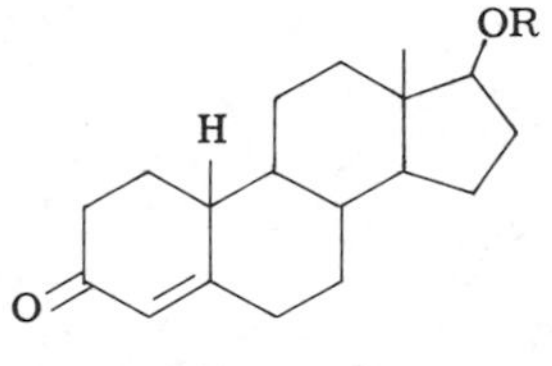

VIII **a** R = H
b R = $C_6H_5CH_2CH_2CO$
c R = $C_9H_{19}CO$
d R = $CH_3(CH_2)_7CH{=}CH(CH_2)_7CO$

TABLE IV
Half-Times of Nandrolone Esters[a]

Compound	Rat gastrocnemius (h)	Rat blood (h)
Nandrolone (**VIIIa**)	0.62	—
Nandrolone phenpropionate (**VIIIb**)	25.0	0.78
Nandrolone decanoate (**VIIIc**)	130.0	3.47
Nandrolone oleate (**VIIId**)	504.0	33.5

[a] Data from Van der Vies (*108*).

lipophilicity is responsible for the duration of the androgenic effect. These conclusions had also been reached by Van der Vies (*108*) and Overbeek *et al.* (*81*) who also showed that 19-nortestosterone (nandrolone) esters (**VIIIa–d**), when injected intramuscularly into the gastrocnemius muscle of the rat, disappear more slowly from the muscle with increasing chain length of the esterifying acid. Half-times in the muscle *in vivo* are shown in Table IV.

It is not surprising, therefore, that the activity of testosterone esters can be related quantitatively to the partition coefficient of the compounds. Moreover, a significant relationship exists between the Hansch π values and the R_M values for such esters (*11*) (Table V) and between π and R_M

TABLE V
Relationship of R_M to π and Hemolytic Activity[a]

Equations	n	r	s
(a) $R_M(Me_2CO) = -0.509 + 0.728R_M(MeOH)$	14	0.993	0.051
(b) $R_M(Me_2CO) = -0.143 + 0.288\pi$	14	0.964	0.119
(c) $R_M(MeOH) = 0.496 + 0.394\pi$	14	0.981	0.118
(d) $\log(BR) = 1.289 + 0.766R_M(Me_2CO)$	14	0.622	0.431
(e) $\log(BR) = 1.502 + 1.561R_M(Me_2CO) - 1.723R_M^2(Me_2CO)$	14	0.954	0.173
(f) $\log(BR) = 0.922 + 0.537R_M(MeOH)$	14	0.594	0.443
(g) $\log(BR) = 0.087 + 2.716R_M(MeOH) - 1.020R_M^2(MeOH)$	14	0.949	0.183
(h) $\log(BR) = 1.192 + 0.209\pi$	14	0.577	0.450
(i) $\log(BR) = 1.155 + 0.172\pi - 0.169\pi^2$	14	0.944	0.189

[a] Data from Biagi *et al.* (*11*).

generally (*37,50*). Again, the free energy of solution in water of steroids is a function of the number of methylene groups in the molecule (*56*). The best rationalization of the relationship between structure and activity is provided by Eqs. (e) and (f) in Table V, which account for 91 and 90% of the variation, respectively, in biological activity on the basis of R_M. Similar results were obtained by James *et al.* (*54*). Furthermore, Eq. (i) in Table V accounts for the hemolytic activity in terms of π. Biagi *et al.* (*11,12*) expanded their studies to data obtained in the capon's comb test (*101*). They obtained the relationship

$$\log(BR) = 0.416R_M + 0.295 \tag{4}$$

for a series of testosterone esters. The results could be explained on the basis of slower absorption from the site of administration with increasing lipophilic character. This work was confirmed by James (*52*) who later (*53*) extended the correlation to the time of maximum effect (t_M) in rats:

$$\log t_M = 0.310R_M + 0.173 \tag{5}$$

$$n = 6, \qquad r = 0.983, \qquad s = 0.034$$

The formate ester was excluded from the series. Chaudry and James (*20*) examined the anabolic activities of normal fatty acid esters (butyrate to undecanoate) of nandrolone (**VIII**) in the rat. The results, when compared to the water–ethyl oleate distribution coefficient, gave the binomial in Eq. (6).

$$\log(BR) = 7.33 \log P - 0.36 \log P^2 - 17.8 \tag{6}$$

$$n = 7, \qquad r = 0.970, \qquad s = 0.064$$

James *et al.* (*55*) studied these data further in an effort to determine if the utilization of the hydrolysis constant of the ester could improve the correlation. They were frustrated in this by the fact that the hydrolysis constant is highly cross-correlated with the R_M values, and therefore no conclusion could be drawn.

In 1982 Draffehn *et al.* (*33*) reported the examination of the R_M values of nearly 100 steroids having hetero substituents, using reversed-phase thin layer chromatography. The ΔR_M values of substituents were calculated and correlated with different linear free-energy parameters of hydrophobicity (π_{Ar}, π_{Al}, and V_I). The calculation of hydrophobicity by such an incremental system was found to be subject to error because of the influence of neighboring groups on the ΔR_M value of a given substituent. This effect was explained in terms of the disturbance of the hydration envelope around a given substituent by different neighboring groups, a phenomenon that also leads to changes in R_M value depending on the composition of the mobile phase. A new hydrophobic parameter, D' was developed to obviate these difficulties. An alternative explanation for the neighboring group effects by hydroxy groups on ΔR_M values was given by Schneider and Lewbart (*94*) who concluded that it is due to intramolecular hydrogen bonding.

Zeelen (*120*) found that the activity of ten 17α-substituted progesterone derivatives in the subcutaneous Clauberg test was well accounted for by the equation

$$\log A = -0.56\pi - 0.64E_s + 0.68 \quad (7)$$

$$n - 10, \quad r = 0.97$$

It was concluded that the negative coefficient of π is best explained by assuming slower release of the more lipophilic compounds from injection sites, whereas E_s represents the steric effect of the 17α-group in blocking metabolism of the compounds by 20-ketoreductases. The receptor affinity is not affected by these modifications.

Zeelen (*122*) recommended the use of the Fibonacci search techniques (*18*) to solve the problem of selecting proper esterifying acids for testosterone ester production from hundreds of available acids. In this way the preparation of 6 or 7 compounds is sufficient to locate the maximum of a series of 20 or 33 compounds, respectively.

2. Distribution: Protein Binding

Steroids are bound to transport proteins primarily by hydrophobic forces. Shown in Fig. 4 is the recalculation by Wolff *et al.* (*116*) of the re-

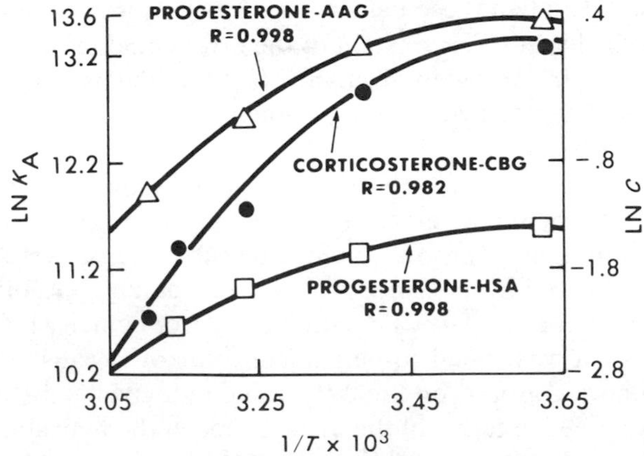

Fig. 4. Corticosterone–CBG plot of ln C versus $1/T$ (T in K); progesterone–AAG plot of ln K_A versus $1/T$ (T in K); progesterone–HSA plot of ln K_A versus $1/T$ (T in K). From Wolff *et al.* (*116*), with permission.

TABLE VI
Calculated Values of the Enthalpic and Entropic Terms for Steroid Binding to Plasma-Binding Proteins as Analyzed by a Second Degree Polynomial Fit to the Data Points[a]

System	Temperature (°C)				
	0	5	10	15	20
Human CBG corticosterone					
ΔH[b]	2,200	320	2,700	−5,000	−7,200
ΔS[c]	48	38	30	21	13
Human Serum Albumin (HSA) (progesterone)					
ΔH[b]	2,400	520	−1,250	−3,000	−4,700
ΔS[c]	37	30	23	16	10
Serum α_1-acid protein (AAG)[a] (progesterone)					
ΔH[b]	1,354	−2,888	−6,980	−11,100	−14,740
ΔS[c]	42	29	12	0.6	−12.5

[a] From Wolff *et al.* (*116*). The data for CBG are from Westphal (1967), those for AAG are from Ganguly *et al.* (*41a*), and those for HSA are from Westphal (*110a,111*). The polynomial functions employed were as follows: corticosterone–glucocorticoid receptor, $1.62 \times 10^7(1/T^2) + 1118.000(1/T) - 195 = \ln K_a$; progesterone HSA, $-4.58 \times 10^6(1/T)^2 + 32900(1/T) - 47.5 = \ln K_a$; progesterone–AAG, $-7.07 \times 10^6(1/T)^2 + 50{,}600(1/T) - 47.5 = -9.43 \times 10^6(1/T) - 77 = \ln K_a$; and corticosterone–CBG, $\ln C = -9.43 \times 10^6(1/T)^2 = 6.8 \times 10^4(1/T) - 122.34$.
[b] cal/mol.
[c] e.u.

lationship of the equilibrium association constant to $1/T$ for three steroid–protein binding systems (*111*): progesterone (**II**) with human serum albumin, corticosterone (**III**) with corticosterone-binding globulin (CBG), and progesterone (**II**) with α-acid glycoprotein (AAG). Unlike the results for many simple association reactions, the plot of $\ln K_A$ as a function of $1/T$ is not a straight line. The enthalpy change, ΔH, determined from the slope of the second-degree polynomial least squares fitted to the data points, decreases as the temperature increases. The entropy change, ΔS, also decreases as the temperature increases (Table VI). These temperature influences are those to be expected for a process driven by the hydrophobic effect and are not in agreement with the recent suggestions that hydrogen bonds and van der Waals forces are principally responsible for steroid protein binding (*75,78*). Scholtan (*96*) already concluded that the binding of steroid hormones to human serum albumin as well as to RNA is mainly due to hydrophobic binding. These workers found that the introduction of hydrophobic alkyl groups and halogen atoms into the steroid ring strengthens protein binding, whereas this interaction is weakened through the substitution of polar carbonyl, hydroxyl, and cyano groups for hydrogen. Unsaturation in the steroid ring increases the binding. Not only are binding affinity and π virtually proportional to each other (*97*), but protein binding is proportional by R_M values, indicating that protein binding depends linearly on the lipophilic character of the molecule (*41*). The ultrafilterable fraction *BR*, which is inversely proportional to the protein bound fraction, is related to R_M by Eq. (8).

$$BR = -0.672R_M + 2.290 \tag{8}$$

$$n = 9, \quad r = 0.964, \quad s = 0.094$$

Because protein binding leads to loss of biological activity (*99*), this effect is of clear importance.

3. Receptor Affinity

There is a growing body of evidence that indicates that induction of protein synthesis mediates the action of hormones on growth, differentiation, and metabolism in target tissues. In the case of the steroids, the initial events involve binding of the steroid to a steroid-specific receptor protein and attachment of the resulting complex to the genome. Cytoplasmic receptors characterized by specificity in binding steroid hormones with high affinity have been demonstrated for all of the physiological steroids. Thus, in principle, it is possible to study drug–receptor affinity as a single part process by the use of QSAR techniques.

The glucocorticoid receptor from rat liver cytosol has been purified to 85% homogeneity as the steroid–receptor complex with triamcinolone acetonide (**VI**). It consists of a single polypeptide chain with a molecular weight of 89,000 and a Stokes radius of 6.0 nm, and it has one ligand binding site per molecule (*119*).

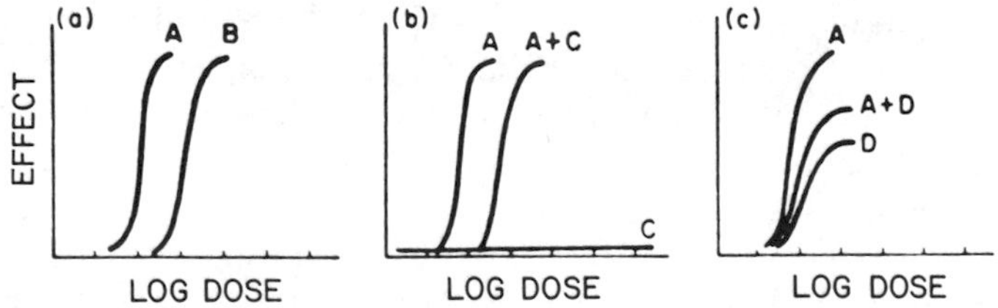

Fig. 5. Examples of dose-response curves of agonists and partial agonists. (a) Drugs A and B are agonists; they have equal efficacies, but A has 10 times the affinity of B. (b) Drug C is a competitive antagonist of drug A. It may have a high affinity, but it exhibits negligible efficacy. The degree of displacement of the curve for A in the presence of C depends on the concentration of C relative to its dissociation constant. (c) Drug D is a partial agonist. It may have an affinity of the same order of magnitude as that of agonist A, but its efficacy is less than that of A. The intermediate curve results if a dose of a mixture of A and D is administered. The exact shape and position of the intermediate curve depend on the ration of the concentrations of A and D. From Mautner (*72*), with permission.

TABLE VII
Receptor Binding and Biological Activity in Progestational Steroids[a]

Compound	Receptor binding	Clauberg activity
6α-Me-Progesterone	26	150
6-Cl-17α-OAc-Δ^6-Progesterone	50	6000
6α-Me-17α-OAc-Progesterone	90	5500
Fluoroprogesterone	130	200
19-Norprogesterone	168	600
Progesterone	100	100

[a] From Smith *et al.* (*100*).

The affinity of the hormone for such a receptor is not necessarily related directly to the pharmacological efficacy of the hormone analog. Two reasons underlie this behavior. First, compounds that are agonists, partial agonists, or antagonists may all have equivalent affinity for the receptor (Fig. 5). Second, some other process, such as exceptionally rapid or slow metabolic destruction, can also affect the overall pharmacological activity of the compound. An example is seen in the data of Smith *et al.* (*100*), relating to the progesterone receptor (Table VII). Whereas 6-substituents and the 16α-acetoxy group actually decrease the receptor binding of progesterone, the progestational (Clauberg) activity is markedly enhanced. This important effect may be due to decreased metabolic inactivation, although more data are needed to establish this. Even groups such as the 19-nor modification, which substantially increase receptor binding, increase biological activity only by a factor of six; whereas the most powerful enhancing groups (Table VII) raise activity by a factor of 60. Notwithstanding the lack of an obligatory direct relationship between receptor binding and biological activity, the question of a quantitative relationship between chemical constitution and receptor binding is of great interest, since receptor binding is a *sine qua non* for biological activity. Therefore, attempts have been made to derive quantitative expressions for the relationship of chemical structure to receptor binding for both the steroid hormones and the thyroid hormones, as described in the following sections.

In a systematic study of the thermodynamics of binding of 29 different corticoids to the receptor of rat hepatoma cells Wolff *et al.* (*116*) formulated a concept of the nature of the steroid–receptor interaction that rationalizes the thermodynamic properties of the steroid–receptor binding process and affords a basis for predicting the binding affinity of any glucocorticoid derivative. The temperature dependency of binding of corticosterone to the rat hepatoma cell (HTC) receptor was determined and a second-degree polynomial equation was fitted to the data points obtained

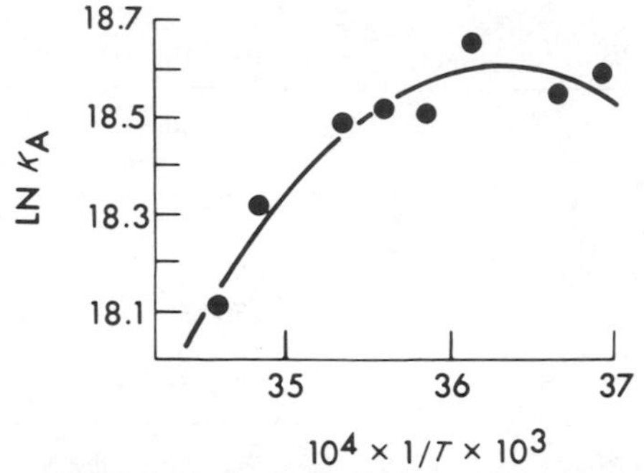

Fig. 6. Plot of ln K_A versus $1/T$ for corticosterone binding to the rat HTC cell glucocorticoid receptor (T in K.) From Wolff *et al.* (*116*).

(Fig. 6). The enthalpic and entropic terms of binding were calculated (Table VIII). As was the case for the other steroid–protein interactions already cited (Section III,A,2,a) changes in both the enthalpy and entropy of binding decreased as the temperature was increased, leading to the conclusion that the steroid receptor binding forces are mainly hydrophobic in character. Both the steroid and receptor are extensively hydrated, and the displacement of water molecules upon binding is a principal driving force. This is reflected by the negative change in heat capacity (ΔC_p), positive ΔS, and negative ΔH upon association, which are characteristic of the hydrophobic effect. Similar conclusions were drawn on the same basis in the case of the interaction of insulin with its receptor (*109*). From the temperature dependence of the rate constant (Fig. 7) the enthalpy of activation was found to be 12.8 kcal/mol and the entropy of activation to be 17.2 e.u., indicating that the driving force for the formation of the transition state is also the hydrophobic effect. It is noteworthy that if the formation of hydrogen bonds and other oriented struc-

TABLE VIII

Calculated Values of the Enthalpic and Entropic Terms for Corticosterone Binding to the Rat HTC Glucocorticoid Receptor[a]

	Temperature (°C)				
Term	0	5	10	15	20
ΔH^b	1200	0	−1000	−2200	−3200
ΔS^c	29	24	20	15	12

[a] Taken from Wolff *et al.* (*116*). The polynomial function employed was $1.62 \times 10^7(1/T^2) + 118{,}000(1/T) - 195 = \ln K_a$.
[b] cal.
[c] e.u.

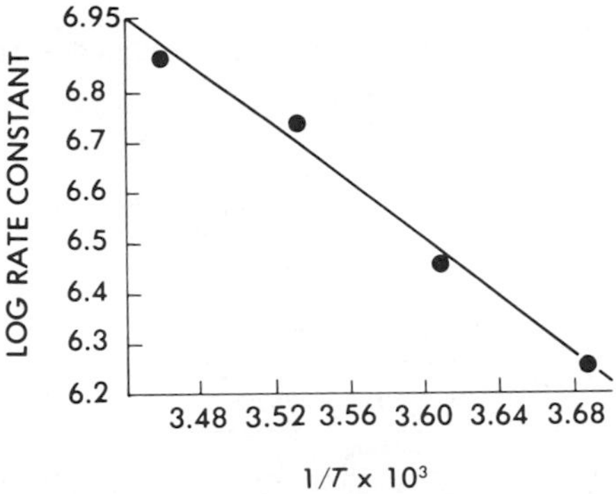

Fig. 7. Plot of the log of the association rate constant versus $1/T$ (K) for dexamethasone binding to glucocorticoid receptors. From Wolff *et al.* (*116*).

tures were of paramount importance in the transition state, the entropy of activation would be negative rather than positive. It is likely that hydrogen bonding contributes very little to the overall driving force for ligand–protein interactions because the net differences in free energy between hydrogen bonding of ligand to protein and hydrogen bonding of ligand or protein to water in the unbound state are probably small. From a consideration of the relationship of the surface area of proteins to hydrophobic bonding (*57*), the energy of binding is best accounted for if the entire steroid is considered to be enveloped by the receptor: the steroid appears as a "hamburger patty" enveloped on both sides by the "hamburger bun" of the receptor. Similar conclusions were reached by Zeelen (*121*) for the progesterone receptor.

From a comparison of the binding of 22 corticoids the approximate free-energy increments of each substituent group were calculated (Table IX). These free-energy group increments can be added to estimate the binding constants of steroids whose binding constants are unknown. Thus the free energy of binding of fluocinolone to the rat hepatoma tissue culture (HTC) receptor over and above progesterone was calculated (Table X). This calculation predicts that fluocinolone would bind to the receptor with a free energy of -1.32 kcal/mol over and above the value for progesterone, in fair agreement with the experimental value of -1.65 kcal/mol. These free-energy increments may be compared with the pharmacologic enhancement factors of Fried and Borman (*39*) (Section III,C,1) (see Table VIII). There is little correlation between the two parameters, indicating again that other variables such as the inhibition of metabolic destruction are of major importance. Similar free-energy increments were subsequently determined for the steroid–corticosterone binding globulin

TABLE IX
Free-Energy Contribution to Binding to the Glucocorticoid Receptor Per Substituent of Progesterone

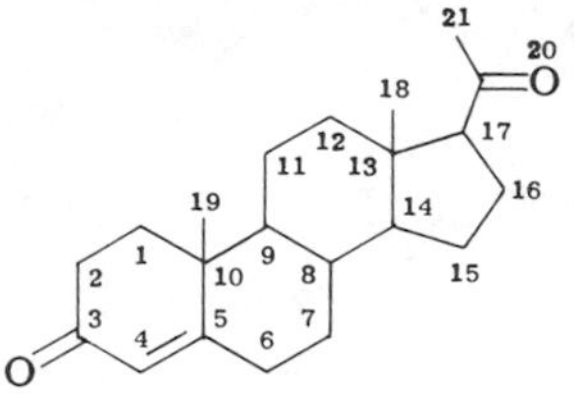

Substituent	Free energy (kcal/mol)[a]	Fried enhancement factor[b]
Δ^1	0.29	3–4
6α-F	−0.36	–
6α-Me	−1.09	2–3
9α-F	−0.57	10
9α-Cl	−0.71	3–5
9α-Br	+1.89	0.4
9α-Methoxy	+2.21	—
11β-OH	−0.89	—
11β-OH → 11-keto	+2.23	—
11-Keto	+1.67	—
16α-Me	−0.11	—
16β-Me	−0.21	0.4
16α-OH + acetonide	−0.35	0.4
17α-OH	+0.49	1–2
21-OH	−0.56	4–7

[a] Data taken from Wolff *et al.* (*116*).
[b] Data taken from Fried and Borman (*39*).

(CBG) system by Mickelson and Westphal (*75*). The receptor present in the cytosol of rat HTC cells appears to have specific sites for hydrogen bonding. The C-3 and C-20 ketone groups are essential; reduction to hydroxyl greatly diminishes binding, suggesting the presence of hydrogen bond donors in the receptor site at the corresonding positions. The C-11 and C-21 hydroxyl groups are important to binding, indicating hydrogen-bond receptors in their proximity. Unlike C-11 and C-21 hydroxyl groups, the C-17 hydroxyl group decreases binding. The receptor either cannot accommodate the size of the group in the position or cannot tolerate the introduction of this polar group into a nonpolar environment. The addition of other relatively nonpolar groups to the steroid molecule generally increases the binding. There is good correspondence between the surface area of the substituent added and the free energy of binding gain.

The conformation of the A ring (*110*), has a pronounced effect on the

TABLE X
Substituents in Fluocinolone in Excess of the Progesterone Skeleton:

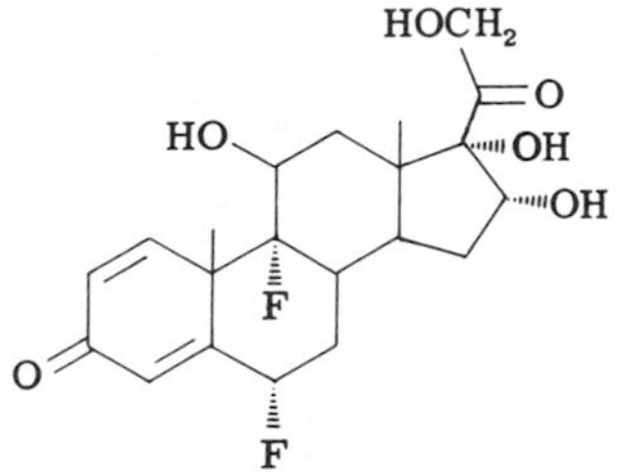

Substituent	ΔG Binding contribution (kcal/mol)
Δ[1]	−0.29
6α-Fluoro	−0.36
9α-Fluoro	−0.57
11β-Hydroxy	−0.89
16α-Hydroxy	+0.86
17α-Hydroxy	+0.49
21-Hydroxy	−0.56
Total	−1.32

binding of the steroid to the receptor. The difference in the C-3–C-17 distance from that of progesterone was employed as a measure of the A-ring conformation, since this distance is strongly influenced by such conformational changes; binding is greater as the distance decreases. A related relationship of the O-3–O-20 distance to biological action has been identified by Dideberg *et al.* (*31*). The inclusion of a fluoro group at C-9 or a double bond at C-1 and C-2 has the greatest effects on the A-ring conformation. Other substituents have varying effects on the direction and magnitude of changes in the A-ring conformation.

The effects of 9α-methoxy and 9α-bromo substituents stand apart in these binding studies. They result in derivatives with low affinities, yet the surface areas are increased due to the respective 9α-substituent. Evidently the size of these substituents prevents the proper engagement of the steroid within the receptor site or induces a conformational change in the receptor such that binding is significantly altered.

To test these relationships multiple regression analysis relating the above four parameters with the logarithm of the dissociation constant was made (Table XI). The surface area (SA) employed for each derivative was the summation of the Bondi (*15*) surface area of each substituent present over that of a progesterone skeleton. The second parameter (P) is a *de*

TABLE XI

K_D Values and Regression Parameters for Binding of Glucocorticoids to the Rat HTC Receptor[a]

Compound	Surface area (Å)^2	Polar interaction	C-3–C-17	9α size	log K_D Observed	log K_D Calculated[b]
6α-Methylprednisolone	50.8	1	−0.26	0	−8.94	−8.65
Dexamethasone	60.9	1	−0.26	0	−8.47	−8.88
Betamethasone	60.9	1	−0.26	0	−8.55	−8.88
9α-Fluorocortisol	47.7	1	−0.18	0	−8.27	−8.46
Dichlorisone	55.3	0	−0.26	0	−8.64	−8.16
Corticosterone	22.7	2	−0.05	0	−8.18	−8.29
9α-Chlorocortisol	58.3	1	0.13	0	−8.24	−8.24
6α-Fluorocortisol	44.2	1	0.05	0	−8.14	−8.04
Prednisolone	28.6	1	−0.26	0	−8.07	−8.15
Cortisol	37.5	1	0.06	0	−7.67	−7.87
11β-Hydroxyprogesterone	11.3	1	0.00	0	−7.51	−7.37
Aldosterone	22.7	1	0.10	0	−7.46	−7.48
Deoxycorticosterone	11.5	1	−0.01	0	−7.36	−7.38

Cortexolone	26.2	0	0.08	0	−7.06	−6.99
Progesterone	0.0	0	0.00	0	−6.85	−6.52
17α-Hydroxyprogesterone	14.8	−1	−0.04	0	−6.48	−6.32
Prednisone	22.4	−2	−0.26	0	−6.18	−6.21
9α-Bromocortisol	62.8	1	0.05	0.3	−6.16	−6.63
Cortisone	31.4	−2	−0.20	0	−6.00	−6.32
9α-Methoxycortisol	73.2	1	−0.02	0.5	−5.90	−5.63
11-Oxoprogesterone	5.2	−2	−0.20	0	−5.51	−5.72
21-Deoxy	49.5	0	−0.26	0	−8.21	−8.03
Paramethasone	57.5	1	−0.26	0	−8.88	−8.80
Fluocinolone	56.6	0	−0.34	0	−8.50	−8.31
Fluocinolone acetonide	89.0	0	−0.34	0	−8.84	−9.04
6α-Fluoro-16α-hydroxycortisol	55.5	0	0.05	0	−7.45	−7.70
Flurandrenolide	87.8	0	0.05	0	−8.74	−8.77
Triamcinolone acetonide	82.4	0	−0.26	0	−8.95	−8.77
6α-fluoroprednisolone	35.2	1	−0.26	0	−8.38	−8.30

[a] From Wolff *et al.* (*116*).
[b] Calculated using Eq. (8).

novo variable representing the interaction of polar groups with the receptor. For each hydroxyl group present in the C-11 and/or C-21 position a value of + 1 is assigned to account for the specific favorable interaction with H-bond donor in the receptor. If no group resides in those positions, a value of 0 is assigned. A value of − 1 is assigned for the presence of each C-17 or C-16 polar group to account for the consequences of placing a polar group in a nonpolar region; and a value of − 2 is given for the presence of the 11-keto functionality to express the conformational change associated with an sp^3 to sp^2 transformation and the undesirable dipole–dipole interaction of the 11-keto group with the hydrogen bond acceptor of the receptor apparently in that position. The total of these values is used for the second parameter denoted as the polar interaction term. The third parameter (*tilt*) expresses the conformation of the A ring through the C-3 to C-17 distance in angstroms. The fourth parameter (X) expresses the size limitation at the 9α-position. The value employed is the maximum of the function (0, $R_X - R_{Cl}$), where R_X is the distance (Å) that a substituent extends radially from the pregnane system. This parameter expresses the size limitation of a 9α-methoxy and bromo derivatives. An excellent correlation was found relating these four parameters to the logarithm of the equilibrium dissociation constant:

$$\log K_D = -0.022 \pm 0.002)SA - (0.59 \pm 0.005)P + (1.50 \pm 0.35)tilt + (6.10 \pm 0.49)X - 6.52 \quad (9)$$

$$n = 29, \quad r = 0.97, \quad s = 0.26$$

For this equation, F, a measure of the significance of the regression, is 106. The value of F indicates that the equation is statistically significant at better than the 0.999 level (*28*). The F statistic for each variable in the equation is SA, 10.4; X, 28.7; *tilt*, 17.8; and P, 67.2. Each parameter is significant at better than the 0.999 level. In a squared correlation matrix of the parameters employed, no coefficient exceeds 0.08, indicating that all of the variables are independent. The percentage of variance (r^2) accounted for by each parameter is: X, 35%; P, 29%, SA, 22%, and *tilt*, 4%. A plot of the calculated versus the observed logarithm of the equlibrium dissociation constant is shown in Fig. 8. The straight line in the graph represents a 1:1 correspondence between observed and calculated K_D values. As can be seen in Fig. 8, the above equation describes the steroid–receptor interactions quantitatively. An examination of the physical significance of Eq. (8) is of interest because it should reflect the thermodynamic contributions of the substituents. Equation (9) represents the effects of substituents on the log K_D of progesterone (**I**) given by the intercept (− 6.52). By multiplying by 2.303RT, the equation is transformed to:

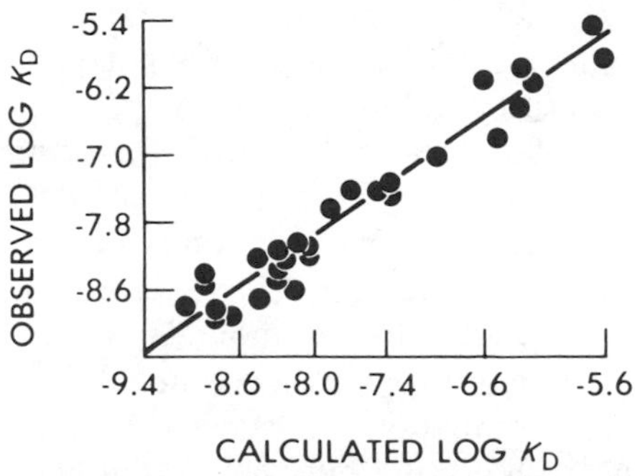

Fig. 8. Plot of calculated (Eq. 1) versus observed logarithm of the equilibrium dissociation constant K_D of antiinflammatory steroids to the rat HTC cell receptor. From Wolff *et al.* (*116*).

$$\Delta G_{\text{assoc}}(\text{cal}) = (-27 \pm 2)SA(\text{cal}/A^2) - (734 \pm 62)P(\text{cal}/P) + (1865 \pm 435)tilt(\text{cal}/A) + (7585 \pm 609)X(\text{cal}/A) - 8143(\text{cal}) \quad (10)$$

giving the thermodynamic equivalent of each parameter. The surface area term shows a contribution of 27 cal/A^2 based on the work of Chothia (*21,22*). The absolute value of 0.76 kcal per P unit agrees well with the values ranging from -0.89 kcal (attractive) to $+0.86$ kcal (repulsive) for hydroxyl groups (Table VIII) and with the figure of -600 cal per hydrogen bond in the binding of trisaccharides to lysozyme (*90*). The huge size of the X term is indicative to the disruptive effect on binding due to the introduction of a group larger than the corresponding "pocket" in the receptor.

A number of other types of steroids have been examined with the hope of obtaining QSAR relationships for receptor binding. Lee *et al.* (*69*) examined the relationship between chemical structure of androst-4-en-3-one derivatives and their affinity for putative progesterone receptors. The binding affinity for 55 derivatives was expressed by Eq. (11):

$$\begin{aligned}\log(\text{relative binding affinity, rabbit receptor}) &= 1.79\\ &+ (0.18 \pm 0.11)\pi_a + (1.45 \pm 0.21)\pi_b\\ &+ (0.010 \pm 0.002)\ \text{surface area in hydrophobic pockets}\\ &- (0.012 \pm 0.003)\ \text{surface area out of hydrophobic pockets}\\ &- (0.99 \pm 0.21)MK\\ &- (0.33 \pm 0.08)\ \text{conformational change} \quad (11)\end{aligned}$$

$$n = 55, \quad r = 0.88, \quad s = 0.54$$

For this equation $F = 29$. In general, any polar group reduced binding. Nonpolar groups enhanced or reduced binding depending on whether the nonpolar group was present in a hydrophobic pocket of the receptor that appears to be near the 6α, 11β, 16α, 17α, 17β, 18, and 21 positions of the rabbit progesterone receptor. By contrast, no such pockets exist near the 7α and 10 positions and hydrophobic groups in those regions interfere with binding. A "misplaced ketone" (*MK*) term is an indicator variable that takes the value 0, except for compounds lacking a ketone at C-3 or possessing a ketone in any ring position other than C-3 in which case it has a value of one. This equation was successful not only in rationalizing the existing data in the literature but was also in harmony with data that appeared subsequent to its formulation. Ponsold *et al.* (*84*) examined the influence of various physicochemical parameters (hydrophobicity, inductive, and steric effects) of 16α-substituted estradiol derivatives on binding (B) to the rat uterus receptor. The best correlation of binding was

$$\log B = -0.346\pi^2 + 0.187\pi - 1.831 \tag{12}$$

$$n = 7, \qquad r = 0.98, \qquad s = 0.072$$

It was concluded that the affinity to the receptor depends on the hydrophobicity of the substituent at the 16α position and that the failure of certain substituents to increase affinity is due to their excessive size. Bergink and Zeelen (*10*) examined the thermodynamics of estrogen association with its receptor and also inferred that hydrophobic binding is of cardinal importance to this process.

B. QSAR of Steroid Pharmacology

In previous sections we considered the application of QSAR methods to individual processes involved in the production of pharmacological effects by steroids. By contrast, in this section we examine attemps to express the gross pharmacological activity of steroids through QSAR methods. Because pharmacological activity depends upon a number of processes, as already noted, a single parameter for a substituent can only represent its average effect on all of these processes. For this reason, QSAR analyses of gross pharmacological activity are usually less precise than those relating to a single process such as drug–receptor binding. But because pharmacological activity is the goal of drug design, considerable interest has been generated in just this approach. Existing studies represent only the beginnings of the correlation of activity with structure and have not led to any particular predictive successes. Yet steroids are relatively rich in molecules in which the effects of structural change are easily understood and therefore represent a fruitful area for investigations in QSAR.

1. Use of *de Novo* Constants

One of the first QSAR analyses of any kind was carried by Fried and Borman (*39*) who examined antiinflammatory steroids obtained through the introduction of halogen, hydroxyl, alkyl, or unsaturation into certain positions of the steroid molecule. It was found that each substituent has an effect on activity that can be given a numerical value: a *de novo* constant or enhancement factor (Table XII). The activity of a final analog is determined by multiplication of the biological activity of a parent compound by the enhancement factors for the substituent groups that it contains. For example, Table XIII illustrates the calculation of the potencies of a sequence of steroids starting with 11β-hydroxyprogesterone and culminating in triamcinolone (**V**). The range obtained are in good agreement with the bioassay figures and their 95% confidence limits. Fried and Borman were unable to derive similar quantitative expressions for salt-retaining activity, although the action of the various substituents on salt retention could be expressed in semiquantitative terms (Table XIII). The effect in this case is additive rather than multiplicative. Additional enhancement factors to those listed in Table XII are found in Table XIV, including those for activity in man.

A Fugita–Ban structure–activity analysis was performed by Justice

TABLE XII
Fried–Borman Enhancement Factors for Various Functional Groups[a]

Functional group	Glycogen deposition rat	Antiinflammatory rat (granuloma)	Effect on urinary sodium[b]
9α-Fluoro	10	7–10	++
9α-Chloro	3–5	3	++
9α-Bromo	0.4[c]	n.d.	+
12α-Fluoro	6–8[d]	n.d.	++
12α-Chloro	4[c]	n.d.	n.d.
1-Dehydro	3–4	3–4	−
6-Dehydro	0.5–0.7	n.d.	+
2α-Methyl	3–6	1–4	++
6α-Methyl	2–3	1–2	−−−
16α-Hydroxyl	0.4–0.5	0.1–0.2	−−−−
17α-Hydroxyl	1–2	4	−
21-Hydroxyl	4–7	25	++
21-Fluoro	2	2	−−

[a] Data from Fried and Borman (*39*). n.d. means no data.
[b] + is retention, − is excretion (on a scale of 1 to 4).
[c] In 1-dehydrosteroids this value is 4.
[d] In the presence of a 17α-hydroxyl group this value is <0.01.

TABLE XIII
Fried–Borman Calculation of Activities of Triamcinolone Using Enhancement Factors[a]

Functional group	Resulting compound	Glycogen deposition		Antiinflammatory (granuloma)		Effect on urinary sodium[b]	
		Calculated	Found	Calculated	Found	Calculated	Found
	11β-Hydroxyprogesterone	–	0.1	n.d.	<0.01	n.d.	n.d.
9α-Fluoro	9α-Fluoro-11β-hydroxyprogesterone	1	0.85	<0.1	<0.1	+++	+++
21-Hydroxy	9α-Fluorocorticosterone	4–7	4.6	<2.5	2.7	+++++	+++++
17α-Hydroxy	9α-Fluorocortisol	4–14	11	11	13	++++	+++
1-Dehydro	9α-Fluoroprednisolone	12–56	28	33–44	20	+++	++++
16α-Hydroxy	Triamcinolone	4.8–28	13	3.3–8.8	4	– –	– –

[a] Data from Fried and Borman (*39*). n.d. means no data.
[b] + is Retention; – is excretion.

TABLE XIV
Enhancement Factors for Important Corticoid Substituents[a]

Group	Antiinflammatory (rat)	Antiinflammatory (man)
1-Dehydro	3	4
2α-Ch_3	4.5	0.7
6-Dehydro	0.5	Variable[b]
6α-CH_3	2	1.3
6α-F	8	2.5
9α-F	8	10
16α-CH_3	1.5	2
16β-CH_3	1.8	2.5
16-Methylene	1.5	—
16α-OH	0.2	0.5
16,17-Acetonide	8	1,(oral)[c]
21-F	2	—
21-Deoxy	0.1	<0.1

[a] Taken from Sarrett *et al.* (*90a*).
[b] Usually <1.
[c] Topical effect is high.

(*60*) on 44 steroids having a common pregn-4-ene-3,20-dione structure. The regression accounted for 75% of the total variance and had $r = 0.868$ and $F = 4.69$. The measured biological activity was glycogen deposition in the rat liver relative to the activity of cortisol. The compounds were substituted at positions 2, 6, 9α, 11β, 16α, 17, and 21; substituents at positions 2, 6, and 17 accounted for 60% of the total variance.

2. Linear Free-Energy Regressions

a. Corticoids. Wolff and Hansch (*112*) carried out the first multiparameter regression analysis for steroids in an examination of the antiinflammatory activity (*117,118*) of 9α-substituted cortisol derivatives (*113,115*). A series of seven active compounds, the 9α-F, 9α-Cl, 9α-Br, 9α-I, 9α-OH, and 9α-CH_3 cortisol derivatives, as well as cortisol itself were analyzed and the results were applied to the inactive 9α-OCH_3, 9α-OEt, and 9α-SCN compounds. Activity was correlated with the inductive effect (σ_I), π, and the size of the substituents (molar refractivity, P_E) giving Eq. (13).

$$\log A = 0.76\pi - 0.22 \log P_E + 2.78\sigma_I + 0.07 \qquad (13)$$

$$n = 7, \qquad r = 0.96, \qquad s = 0.33$$

The equation suggests that the activity of the compound rises with increasing electron withdrawal, decreasing size, and increasing hydrophobicity of the 9α-substituent. Moreover, it correctly predicts that the methoxy, ethoxy, and thiocyano compounds have little or no activity. It is of interest that Fried (*38*) had already taken note of the inverse relationship between the magnitude of corticoid activity and the radius of the 9α-halogen atom. But Fried and Borman (*39*) later argued that the low activity of the 9α-hydroxy and 9α-methoxy compounds, which also have relatively small substituents, indicates that it is the electronegativity of the substituent rather than its size that determines its enhancement properties. Significantly, the quantitative multiparameter regression technique demonstrates the inverse relationship with increasing size, even though a qualitative examination of the data led the earlier workers to conclude otherwise. The meaning of the dependence upon π is more difficult to interpret. The observed increase of activity with increasing hydrophobicity could be due to better transport to the site of action for the more lipophilic compounds and/or to hydrophobic interactions at the active site. In a reexamination of this problem Coburn and Solo (*24*) showed that σ_I and a simple steric factor such as molar refractivity (*MR*) provides a good correlation for the activity of these compounds, provided that the 9α-hydroxylated compound is included from the series. They suggested that compounds containing strongly hydrated 9α-substituents would have a larger effective bulk than is found in the unhydrated species and hence a lower predicted activity. Ahmad and Mellors (*3*) in another reexamination showed that molar parachor gives a better fit than π in single-parameter equations but not in a three-parameter equation. Parachor is defined as the product of the molar volume and the fourth root of the surface tension:

$$P = MD^{-1}Y^{1/4} \tag{14}$$

where P is parachor, M is molecular weight, D is density, and Y is surface tension. When the surface tensions of the compounds in a homologous or analogous series are numerically similar, the parachor values of the analogs are a good measure of the relative molecular sizes. Ahmad *et al.* (*1*) used parachor values in order to relate rat liver glycogen deposition (A_g) to parachor for a series of 12 glucocorticoids. They obtained the relationship

$$A_g = 0.807P - 626.408 \tag{15}$$

$$n = 12, \qquad r = 0.91, \qquad s = 200.15$$

For this equation, $F = 49.0$. Some of the limitations in the QSAR approach to whole-animal pharmacology can be seen in this study in which both cortisone and prednisone are included in the data set. Cortisone (**IX**) and prednisone (**X**) are known to be inactive as such and must be converted to their active metabolites, cortisol (**IV**) and prednisolone (**XI**). Another problem is the prediction that a compound of infinite parachor would be infinitely active, according to Eq. (15), whereas general experi-

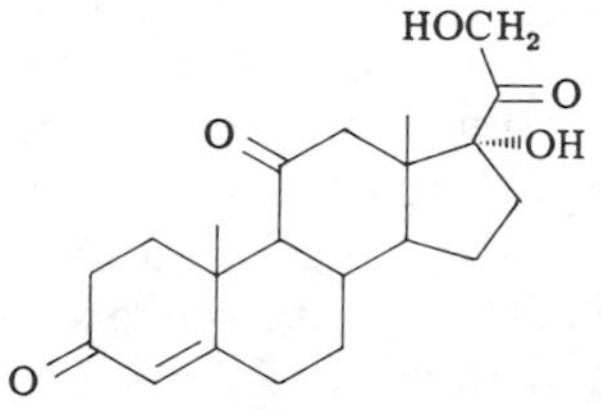

IX

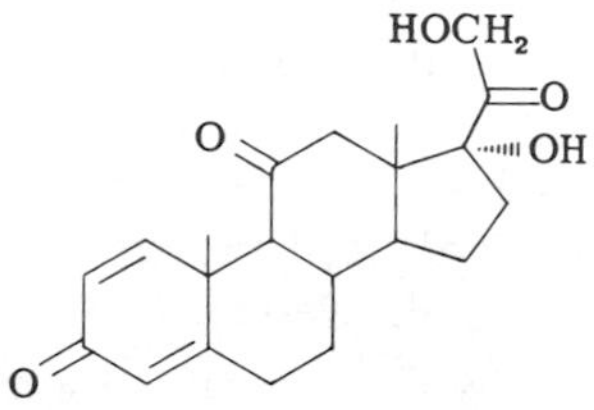

X

ence is that very large substituents of any kind obviate steroid activity. Ahmad *et al.* (*2*) have correlated other steroid activities with parachor.

Rousseau and Schmit have examined new approaches to the problems in this area (*87*).

b. Male Hormone Analogs. Anabolic and androgenic testosterone derivatives have also been investigated through the use of QSAR techniques. Huttenrauch (*49,51*) examined physicochemical factors affecting the activity of steroids and drew a relationship between the energy of hydrophobic binding and anabolic activity. This relationship was expressed in terms of the partition coefficient (*46–48*) and has also been examined by Chaudry and James (*20*). An explanation for the importance of partition coefficient to the activity of such esters is described in Section II,A,1,d.

c. Progestogens. Teutsch *et al.* (*103*) prepared a series of 6-substituted derivatives of 6-dehydro-, 16-methylene-, 17α-acetoxyprogesterone and examined these compounds for progestational (Clauberg) activity. The comparative order of activities of the 6-substituted compounds was found to be 6-Me > 6-Cl > 6-F > 6-Br > 6-N_3 > 6-OCH_3 > 6-SCN > 6-CF_3 > 6-CN > 6-C=NOMe > 6-H > 6-CHO > 6-OC_2H_5 $\simeq$ 6-$OCOCH_3$ > 6-$NHCOCH_3$. In an attempt to relate the steric and electronic characteristics of the C-6 substituents to the progestational (Clauberg) activity, these authors derived steric indexes based on bond lengths and van der Waals radii and used broad estimates of electronic features to conclude that the substituents enhance activity through steric and electronic effects. Their treatment was qualitative and did not consider the partition coefficient of the molecules. Wolff and Hansch (*114*) reexamined these compounds. By omitting two compounds (R = CH_3 and R = C=NOMe) they derived the relationship

$$\log A = (1.14 \pm 0.66)\pi + (0.60 \pm 0.40) \quad (16)$$

$$n = 13, \quad r = 0.751, \quad s = 0.645$$

For this equation $r^2 = 0.564$, and over half the variance in the data is accounted for by the hydrophobic parameter, whereas for similar single-parameter equations involving steric and electronic parameters (the features considered to be most important by Teutsch *et al.*) each individually accounted for less than 20% of the variance. In a third study Topliss and Shapiro (*106*) used the complete data set without omission of any compounds and showed that 58% of the variance in the data was accounted for by π, confirming the findings of Wolff and Hansch. Topliss and Shapiro considered the best equation that accounts for the available data to be

$$\log A = (1.00 \pm 0.57)\pi - (0.05 \pm 0.04)C + (1.32 \pm 0.68) \quad (17)$$

$$n = 14, \quad r = 0.86, \quad s = 0.54$$

where C is a steric measure. This equation accounts for 73% of the variance in the data. As in the glucocorticoids, increased activity is fostered by small, hydrophobic substituents at C-6 and may be explained on the basis of enhanced hydrophobic interactions at the active site.

Van den Broek *et al.* (*107*) synthesized a series of 11β-substituted 17α-ethynyl-19-nortestosterone derivatives (**XII**). First, the 11β-methyl,

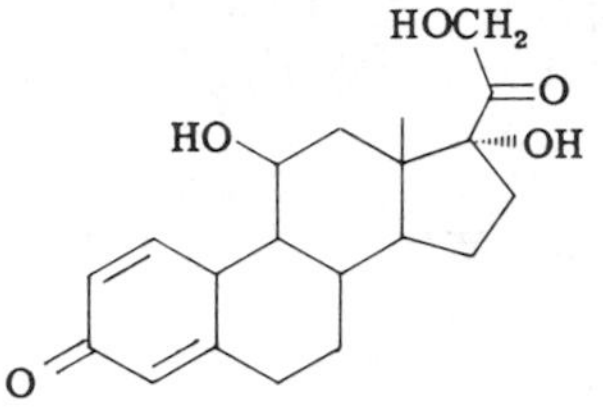

XI

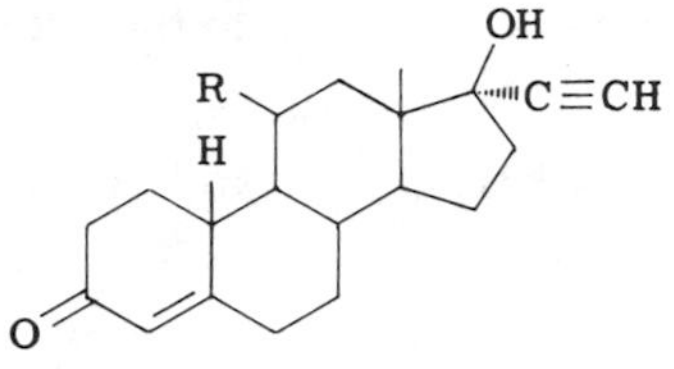

XII

11β-chloro, and 11β-fluoro compounds were synthesized in order to use a variation of the Topliss tree approach (*105*) to examine compounds varying widely in π, the Taft parameter E_S, and σ. A good correlation was observed between progestational or ovulation inhibitory activity and the bulk of the substituent, whereas no correlation was found with σ. Further examination was made by synthesizing an expanded series including the 11β-ethyl, 11β-hydroxy, and 11β-methoxy derivatives to see if a correlation with π existed. In the larger series, the equation

$$\log(\text{relative activity}) = -1.46E_S^X - 0.14M_R + 1.97 \qquad (18)$$

$$n = 7, \quad r = 0.91, \quad s = 0.34$$

was determined. The data are consistent with the notion that high activity in this series is fostered by a 1,3-diaxial interaction between the 11 β-substituent and C-18, as represented by the Taft–Charton parameter E_S^X, whereas it is hindered by bulk, as parameterized by M_R. These results suggest that the effect of the 11β-substituent is to bend the molecule toward the α face in an activity-favoring manner. This work has been further discussed by Zeelen (*123*).

Biagi *et al.* (*13*) examined the relationship between R_M values of corticoids, androgens, and estrogens and their hemolytic action. A parabolic relationship was discerned:

$$\log(1/C) = (0.516 \pm 0.143)R_M(45\%) - (0.514 \pm 0.098)R_M^2(45\%) + (3.933 \pm 0.166) \qquad (19)$$

$$n = 17, \quad r = 0.898, \quad s = 0.281$$

Again, the biological action of testosterone esters as well as protein binding could be correlated with R_M by these workers, who concluded that T_M is a suitable index of lipophilicity for such studies. Such uses of chromatographic hydrophobic parameters in correlation analysis have been reviewed by Tomlinson (*104*).

C. Theoretical Calculations of Factors Affecting Steroid Activity

1. Steric Factors

The conformational mobility of steroids may have profound effects on receptor specificity (*17a,29*). In the following we discuss a number of studies using the techniques of extended Hückel theory and geometry optimization through energy minimization to determine the preferred conformation of steroid molecules. Such energy minimization methods have been developed by Allinger *et al.* (*4,5*), Cohen (*25*), Bucourt *et al.* (*17*), Sedmera *et al.* (*98*), Altona and Hirschmann (*6*), and Profeta *et al.* (*86*). The theoretical results can in some cases be compared to the findings of X-ray crystallography (*34,36,86*). Also discussed are the use of molecular orbital calculations to obtain electronic structure such as those used by Janoschek (*58*), Kollman *et al.* (*65,113*), Repmann (*88*), Sundaram and Mishra (*102*), Schmit and Rousseau (*92,93*), and Gale and Saunders (*40*).

The rigidity of the steroid skeleton depends on structural factors. Thus the introduction of unsaturation into the molecule tends to increase its flexibility. This situation is frequently seen in the antiinflammatory steroids in which the presence of unsaturation at C-4 and C-1 produces compounds that may exist as a range of conformers oscillating over a broad energy minimum, or as several conformers of nearly equal energy separated by a significant barrier (*35*). The estimate of the interatomic distance between such key atoms as O-3 and O-20 and the effect of structural changes on such distances is therefore complicated by the introduction of such flexibility. The effect of variations in orientation of groups at C-3 and C-17 in progestational steroids on biological activity has been discussed (*78*).

A related point of interest is the conformation of the side chain of antiinflammatory steroids and progestational molecules, because this portion of the molecule includes O-20. In principle, a 360° rotation of the side chain is possible, but it is obvious that steric factors will tend to favor only selected conformations. Apart from investigations into this problem, using classical physicochemical and crystallographic methods, quantum mechanical studies (*62*) and energy minimization studies (*92,93*) have been undertaken in this area. Although crystallographic studies (*35*) indicate that O-20 approximately eclipses C-16, the energy minimization calculations of Schmit and Rousseau (*89,92,93*) and Duax *et al.* (*36*) point to significant differences from these results. According to these studies the most important factor influencing the position of the C-20 carbonyl is the presence or absence of a 17α-hydroxyl group. Profeta *et al.* (*86*) found this conflict was due to the use of an inadequate force-field, but crystal packing forces as well as the influence of intermolecular hydrogen bonds could be responsible for other discrepancies between the energy optimized and X-ray diffraction data. Moreover, in certain cases two independent crystallographic structures are observed, indicating that crystallographic data do not necessarily give an unambiguous picture of conformation. A further example of this is seen in the thyroid area (Section III,D,1). Weeks *et al.* (*110*) examined the X-ray structures of six corticosteroids and found that a correlation existed between the bowing of the fused ring system toward the α face with antiinflammatory activity. These changes were brought about by the presence of a C-1 double bond and a 9α-fluoro group. In a related study Schmit and Rousseau (*92,93*) undertook a Free–Wilson analysis of the effect of various substituents on the conformation of the steroid based on their predicted energy minimization structure (not the X-ray structure). As with the X-ray results they found that the curvature of the entire steroid molecule (A/D angle) is increased 30% by a C-1 double bond and 14% by an 11β-hydroxy substituent. It is decreased 14% by a 17α-hydroxy substitution. These results parallel the biological data in rats.

2. Electronic Factors

As discussed in Section II,B,2,a, Fried attempted to explain the effect of steroidal C-9 substituents on antiinflammatory activity through an electronic effect. A closer examination of this question was undertaken by Kollman *et al.* (*65*) using CNDO/2 techniques. It was concluded that the effect on electron density by the 9α-substituent in enhancing the hydrogen-bonding characteristics of the 11β-hydroxyl group is not large enough to account fully for the observed activity differences, and that there must be additional factors explaining the greater antiinflammatory activity of 9α-fluorocortisol relative to cortisol itself.

III. THYROID HORMONES

Thyroid hormones (*59*) are a second class of substances for which extensive QSAR studies have been undertaken. Like the steroids, these compounds also were an early focus of interest, but the bulk of more recent studies has been the extensive study of E. C. Jorgensen and co-workers.

A. Biological Activity and Receptor Binding

Dietrich *et al.* (*32*) examined the relationship between the binding of thyroxine analogs to intact rat hepatic nuclei (*BN*) with antigoiter activity in the rat. This led to the relationship

$$\log(BA) = (0.241 \pm 0.170) + (0.730 \pm 0.134)\log(BN) + (1.116 \pm 0.484)I(4 - \mathrm{H}) \qquad (20)$$

$$n = 29, \quad r = 0.917, \quad s = 0.371$$

where *BA* is the biological activity, *BN* is the nuclear binding, and *I* is an indicator variable for compounds lacking a phenolic hydroxyl group. Similar equations could be derived for the relationship to binding to solubilized hepatic nuclear protein. These high correlations of *in vivo* and *in vitro* activities are in contrast to the situation seen with steroid hormones. They indicate that metabolism, apart from hydroxylation in the 4′ position, does not play a major role in influencing whole animal activity and that, at least in the series examined, all compounds had high intrinsic activity. Thus for thyromimetic compounds, unlike for the steroid drugs, it is possible to extrapolate directly from receptor binding data to gross biological activity.

B. Protein Binding

In a study by Dietrich *et al.* (*32*) the binding of a group of 3,5-diiodothyronines to thyroxine binding globulin (TBG) was correlated with parameters relating to the substituent groups.

$$\log A = 0.563\pi_{3',5'} - 1.100(3' \text{ size} > I) + 2.366\sigma_{3',5'} - 0.098 \qquad (21)$$

$$n = 10, \qquad r = 0.962, \qquad s = 0.355$$

This equation shows that binding is fostered by lipophilic groups up to the size of an iodine atom, and more importantly by the presence of electron-withdrawing groups in the molecule. Presumably electron withdrawal results in more facile formation of the phenoxide ion. It is noteworthy that equations dealing with pharmacological activity of such substances predict increasing activity with electron resulting substituents. Apparently, such substituents decrease ionization of the 4′-hydroxyl group and therefore reduce the affinity for plasma protein leading to increased concentrations of free drug in the plasma.

Andrea *et al.* (*7*) calculated the electrostatic interaction energy of the binding of thyroxine analogs to the plasma protein prealbumin. They concluded that the basis for the higher affinity of L-thyroxine relative to the D isomer resides in a more favorable interaction of the carboxyl group of the L isomer with Lys-15 of the prealbumin. In related work Andrea *et al.* (*9*) obtained the free-energy contributions of substituents to the binding of thyroxine analogs to prealbumin. A complex interplay of forces governs the effects of these substituents on the binding process.

C. Hormone–Receptor Interactions

Andrea *et al.* (*8*) carried out theoretical electronic structure calculations on the binding of small molecules to macromolecules are applied to the affinity of thyroxine analogs for plasma proteins and the nuclear receptor. The results pointed to interactions of the 4′-OH and the 3′- and 5′-substituents with the nuclear receptor. Substituent group interactions were examined by Bolger and Jorgensen (*14*). Crippen (*27*) defined the thyroxine binding site using distance geometry.

D. QSAR of Pharmacological Activity

In a remarkable study that antedated the development of the Hansch approach, Bruice *et al.* (*16*) derived equations relating thyroxine-like activity in amphibia and mammalia of the type:

$$\log(\%\ \text{thyroxine-like activity}) = K \sum F + C \tag{22}$$

where ΣF = the sum of empirical constants for the substituents in the thyroxine analog. Not only were correlations attempted in this way, using empirically derived constants in a manner reminiscent of the Free–Wilson approach, but a more deterministic model employing the dipole moment of the substituent was undertaken. It is noteworthy that these workers did not attempt to use any kind of function relating to distribution coefficient even though the importance of this parameter on drug activity had been known from the time of Meyer (*74*) 50 years earlier. It remained for Hansch and Fujita (*44*) to do this 8 years later, when in one of the first applications of the Hansch approach they developed Eq. (23).

$$\begin{aligned} \log A = & -1.134(\pi_{3',5'})^2 + 7.435\pi_{3',5'} \\ & - 16.323\sigma_{3',5'} - 0.287 \end{aligned} \tag{23}$$

$$n = 9, \quad r = 0.884, \quad s = 0.660$$

This equation predicted activity to be optimal for moderately lipophilic electron-donating 3′- and 5′-substituents and later led to the more extensive investigation of the thyromimetic activities of 3′- and 5′-alkyl-substituted analogs. In 1976 Kubinyi (*67*) and Kubinyi and Kehrhahn (*68*) reported the development of a large series of equations for thyromimetic activity in the rat, using both linear free-energy parameters as well as Free–Wilson type parameters for particular groups. These equations also predict that *in vivo* thyromimetic activity is proportional to the sum of the lipophilicities of the 3′- and 5′-substituents and is increased by electron-donating substituents. In addition they indicate that groups larger than an iodine atom reduce activity. One problem in connection with these studies is that the use of three to five variables to account for the variance of 10 to 23 compounds diminishes the significance of the correlations. Dietrich *et al.* (*32*) developed equations for predicting the *in vivo* rat antigoiter activities of 36 thyromimetic agents, using as many as six variables. They concluded on the basis of three studies that activity is enhanced by bulky lipophilic 3′- and 5′-substituents, up to the limit of substituents the size of an iodine atom, and is also enhanced by electron-donating 3′- and 5′-substituents.

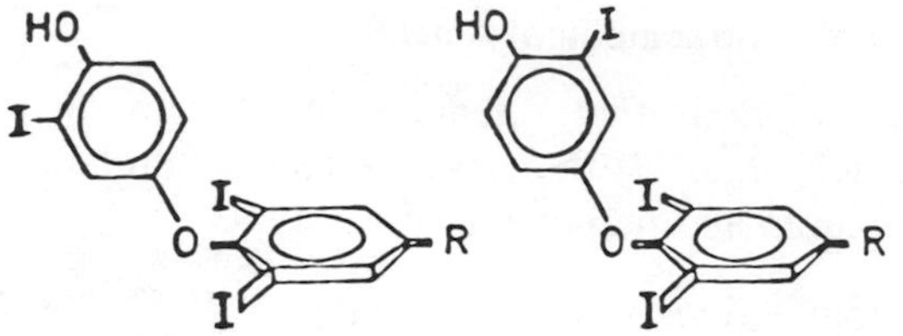

Fig. 9. Distal (left) and proximal (right) conformations of triiodothyronine derivatives. From Jorgensen (*59*), with permission.

E. Steric Factors

Zenker and Jorgensen (*124*) proposed that a perpendicular orientation of the planes of the aromatic rings of 3,5-diiodothyronines would be favored in order to provide minimal interactions between the bulky 3,5-iodines and the 2,6-hydrogens. In this conformation the 3′-iodine of triiodothyronine can be oriented either distally or proximally to the alanine-bearing ring (Fig. 9). Theoretical support for these conclusions was found in the molecular orbital calculations of Kier and Hoyland (*63*) and Kollman *et al.* (*66*) notwithstanding a study (*19*) using the Extended Hückel theory in which it was concluded that the proximal configuration is favored. The 3′-distal conformation of triiodothyronine is presumed to be the hormonally active form.

IV. PEPTIDE HORMONES

The peptide hormones comprise a large group of substances (*73*). The theoretical conformational analysis of portions of even large hormones is being attempted (*87*). QSAR studies (*79*) have been carried out on a number of these products, although in many cases only a single study has been undertaken. These will be discussed in the following section.

A. ACTH

ACTH is a linear polypeptide consisting of 39 amino acid residues. Because a large number of ACTH analogs have been synthesized, Keider and Greven (*61*) used the Fujita–Ban modification of the Free–Wilson analysis to calculate the *de novo* group contribution of each amino acid in the analogs. It was assumed that the contribution of each amino acid residue of the ACTH analogs was independent of the other amino acid residues in the molecule. The biological test involved was the conditioned avoidance response (CAR) in a pole jumping test for rats. In order to estimate the contribution of the various residues, the peptide chain was divided into eight segments. The first seven segments correspond to positions 4–10 in ACTH. Because the last segment contained only one modification, it was treated as a single segment even though it contained six amino acids. In general, good agreement was found between the calculated and observed potencies, indicating that the contributions of each amino acid are indeed independent. In common with all Free–Wilson methods, the calculation gave rise to little information of predictive value because predictions can be made only for compounds with combinations of groups already included in the analysis.

B. Oxytocin

Oxytocin is a nonapeptide. Its conformation has been analyzed by theoretical methods (*80*). As in the case of ACTH, oxytocin has also been analyzed by means of the Free–Wilson approach (*83*). This analysis resulted in a set of segment contributions for the amino acid in positions 1 and 2 (Cys and Tyr, respectively, in the natural hormone). These contributions were strongly correlated with σ. It was concluded that resonance effects of para substitutions on the Tyr-2 have considerable effect on binding, whereas no apparent correlations were found with the lipophilicity at positions 1 and 2. The thermodynamics of binding of oxytocin analogs to neurophysins has been examined (*82*).

C. Angiotensin II

Angiotensin II is an octopeptide producing potent vasopressor action in man. Large numbers of analogs of this material have been prepared. The investigation of the conformation of angiotensin II by George and Kier (*42*) suggested that the principal role played by the residue in the 5 position is the stereochemical control of the adjacent residues relative to each other. The relative contributions to the pressor activity of the lipophilic and aromatic character of the phenyl ring of position 8 was studied by Hsieh *et al.* (*45*). The benzyl side chain of phenylalanine was replaced by a variety of normal or branched aliphatic and substituted aromatic residues. In the absence of aromatic character higher lipophilicity of the analogs resulted in higher pressor activity, as shown by an almost linear correlation with the π value. However, aromatic substituents fell off the line and, therefore, aromaticity is more important than the lipophilic character for full activity.

D. LH–RH

The conformations of luteinizing hormone–releasing hormone (LH–RH) (*76*) and its analogs (*77*) have been calculated and correlated with changes in biological activity.

E. Gastrin Tetrapeptide

Using semiempirical molecular orbital theory, Kier and George (*64*) calculated the conformation of the amino acid residues in gastrin tetrapeptide and estimated the conformation of the peptide itself. A relationship to biological activity was explored.

F. Parathyroid Hormone

The structure of parathyroid hormone has been investigated, using theoretical techniques (*125*).

V. SUMMARY

QSAR studies on hormones were initiated almost 30 years ago and have been continued with increasing frequency in the intervening years. Because hormones have been extensively examined for their detailed mechanism of action, it has been possible to attempt QSAR investigations on absorption, distribution, receptor affinity, and gross pharmacological action. The techniques employed include the elaboration of *de novo* constants, the Free–Wilson method, and the Hansch approach. In addition, molecular orbital calculations have given insight into the conformation and electronic characteristics of these important molecules.

REFERENCES

1. P. Ahmad, C. A. Fyfe, and A. Mellors, *Biochem. Pharmacol.* **24,** 1103 (1975).
2. P. Ahmad, C. A. Fyfe, and A. Mellors, *Can. J. Biochem.* **10,** 1047 (1975).
3. P. Ahmad and A. Mellors, *J. Steroid Biochem.* **7,** 19 (1976).
4. N. L. Allinger and F. Wu, *Tetrahedron* **27,** 5093 (1971).
5. N. L. Allinger, M. T. Tribble, and Y. Yuh, *Steroids* **26,** 398 (1975).
6. C. Altona and H. Hirschmann, *Tetrahedron* **26,** 2173 (1970).
7. T. A. Andrea, E. C. Jorgensen, and P. A. Kollman, *Int. J. Quantum Chem.* **5,** 191 (1978).
8. T. A. Andrea, S. W. Dietrich, W. J. Murray, P. A. Kollman, and E. C. Jorgensen, *J. Med. Chem.* **22,** 221 (1979).

9. T. A. Andrea, R. R. Cavalieri, I. D. Goldfine, and E. C. Jorgensen, *Biochemistry* **19,** 55 (1980).
10. E. W. Bergink and F. J. Zeelen, *Workshop Proc., Diepenbrek, Belg.* 1, (1979).
11. G. L. Biagi, M. C. Guerra, and A. M. Barbaro, *J. Med. Chem.* **13,** 944 (1970).
12. G. L. Biagi, A. M. Barbaro, and M. C. Guerra, *Experientia* **27,** 918 (1971).
13. G. L. Biagi, A. M. Barbaro, O. Gandolfi, M. C. Guerra, and G. Cantelli-Forti, *J. Med. Chem.* **18,** 873 (1975).
14. M. B. Bolger and E. C. Jorgensen, *J. Biol. Chem.* **255,** 10271 (1980).
15. A. Bondi, *J. Phys. Chem.* **68,** 441 (1964).
16. T. C. Bruice, N. Kharasch, and R. J. Winzler, *Arch. Biochem. Biophys.* **62,** 305 (1956).
17. R. Bucourt, N. C. Cohen, and G. Lemoine, *Bull. Soc. Chim. Fr.* p. 903 (1975).
17a. B. Busetta, C. Courseille, G. Preciqoux, and M. Hospital, *J. Steroid Biochem.*, **8,** 63 (1977).
18. T. M. Bustard, *J. Med. Chem.* **17,** 777 (1974).
19. N. Camerman and A. Camerman, *Science* **175,** 764 (1972).
20. M. A. Q. Chaudry and K. C. James, *J. Med. Chem.* **17,** 157 (1974).
21. C. Chothia, *Nature* (*London*) **254,** 304 (1975).
22. C. Chothia, *Nature* (*London*) **248,** 338 (1974).
23. K. C. Chu, *in* "Burger's Medicinal Chemistry" (M. E. Wolff, ed.), 4th ed., Part I, p. 394. Wiley, New York, 1980.
24. R. A. Coburn and A. J. Solo, *J. Med. Chem.* **19,** 748 (1976).
25. N. C. Cohen, *Tetrahedron* **27,** 789 (1971).
26. R. E. Counsell and R. Brueggemeir, *in* "Burger's Medicinal Chemistry" (M. E. Wolff, ed.), 4th ed., Part II, p. 873. Wiley, New York, 1979.
27. G. M. Crippen, *J. Med. Chem.* **24,** 198 (1981).
28. F. E. Croxton and D. J. Cowdon, "Applied General Statistics." Prentice-Hall, Englewood Cliffs, New Jersey, 1955.
29. J. Delettre, J. P. Mornow, G. Lepicard, T. Ojasoo, and J. P. Raynaud, *J. Steroid Biochem.* **13,** 45 (1980).
30. C. H. Demos, V. A. Place, and J. M. Ruegsegger, *Abstr., Int. Congr. Endocrinol., 1st, Copenhagen* p. 759 (1960).
31. O. Dideberg, L. Dupont, and H. Campsteyn, *J. Steroid Biochem.* **7,** 757 (1976).
32. S. W. Dietrich, M. B. Bolger, P. A. Kollman, and E. C. Jorgensen, *J. Med. Chem.* **20,** 863 (1977).
33. J. Draffehn, B. Schonecker, and K. Ponsold, *J. Chromatogr.* **205,** 113 (1981); in press, (1982).
34. W. L. Duax and D. A. Norton, "Atlas of Steroid Structure," Vol. 1. IFI/Plenum, New York, 1975.
35. W. L. Duax, C. M. Weeks, D. C. Rohrer, Y. Osawa, and M. E. Wolff, *J. Steroid Biochem.* **6,** 195 (1975).
36. W. L. Duax, J. F. Griffin, and D. C. Rohrer, *J. Am. Chem. Soc.* **103,** 6705 (1981).
37. G. L. Flynn, *J. Pharm. Sci.* **60,** 345 (1971).
38. J. Fried, *Cancer* (*Philadelphia*) **10,** 752 (1957).
39. J. Fried and A. Borman, *Vitam. Horm.* (*N.Y.*) **16,** 303 (1958).
40. M. M. Gale and L. Saunders, *Biochim. Biophys. Acta* **248,** 466 (1971).
41. O. Gandolfi, A. M. Barbaro, and G. L. Biagi, *Experientia* **29,** 689 (1973).
41a. M. Ganguly, R. H. Carnighan, and U. Westphal, *Biochemistry,* **6,** 2803 (1967).
42. J. M. George and L. B. Kier, *J. Theor. Biol.* **46,** 111 (1974).
43. D. Gould, L. Finckenor, E. B. Hershberg, J. Cassidy, and P. L. Perlman, *J. Am. Chem. Soc.* **79,** 4472 (1956).

44. C. Hansch and T. J. Fujita, *J. Am. Chem. Soc.* **86,** 1616 (1964).
45. K.-H. Hsieh, E. C. Jorgensen, and T. C. Lee, *J. Med. Chem.* **22,** 1038 (1979).
46. R. Hüttenrauch and K. Matthey, *Arch. Pharm. Ber. Dtsch. Pharm. Ges.* **300,** 1007 (1967).
47. R. Hüttenrauch and I. Keiner, *Arch. Pharm. Ber. Dtsch. Pharm. Ges.* **301,** 641 (1968).
48. R. Hüttenrauch and I. Keiner, *Arch. Pharm. Ber. Dtsch. Pharm. Ges.* **301,** 856 (1968).
49. R. Hüttenrauch, *Pharmazie* **24,** 118 (1969).
50. R. Hüttenrauch and I. Scheffler, *J. Chromatogr.* **50,** 529 (1970).
51. R. Hüttenrauch, *Pharmazie* **28,** 84 (1973).
52. K. C. James, *Experientia* **28,** 479 (1972).
53. K. C. James, G. T. Richards, and T. D. Turner, *J. Chromatogr.* **69,** 141 (1972).
54. K. C. James, P. J. Nicholls, and G. T. Richards, *J. Pharm. Pharmacol.* **25,** Supl., 135P (1973).
55. K. C. James, P. J. Nicholls, and G. T. Richards, *Eur. J. Med. Chem.—Chim. Ther.* **10,** 55 (1975).
56. K. C. James, *J. Pharm. Pharmacol.* **28,** 929 (1976).
57. J. Janin and C. Chothia, *J. Mol. Biol.* **100,** 197 (1976).
58. R. Janoschek, *Eur. Biophys. Congr., Proc., 1st, Baden near Vienna* **6,** 55 (1971).
59. E. C. Jorgensen, *in* "Burger's Medicinal Chemistry" (M. E. Wolff, ed.), 4th ed., Part III, p. 103. Wiley, New York, 1980.
60. J. B. Justice, Jr., *J. Med. Chem.* **21,** 465 (1978).
61. J. Keider and H. M. Greven, *Recl. Trav. Chim. Pays-Bas* **98,** 168 (1979).
62. L. B. Kier, *J. Med. Chem.* **11,** 915 (1968).
63. L. B. Kier and J. R. Hoyland, *J. Med. Chem.* **13,** 1182 (1970).
64. L. B. Kier and J. M. George, *J. Med. Chem.* **15,** 384 (1972).
65. P. A. Kollman, D. G. Giannini, W. L. Duax, S. Rothenberg, and M. E. Wolff, *J. Am. Chem. Soc.* **95,** 2869 (1973).
66. P. A. Kollman, W. J. Murray, M. E. Nuss, E. C. Jorgensen, and S. Rothenberg, *J. Am. Chem. Soc.* **95,** 8518 (1973).
67. H. Kubinyi, *J. Med. Chem.* **19,** 587 (1976).
68. H. Kubinyi and O.-H. Kehrhahn, *J. Med. Chem.* **19,** 578 (1976).
69. D. L. Lee, P. A. Kollman, F. J. Marsh, and M. E. Wolff, *J. Med. Chem.* **20,** 1139 (1977).
70. A. W. McKenzie and R. M. Atkinson, *Arch. Dermatol.* **89,** 741 (1964).
71. S. B. Malkinson and M. B. Kirchenbaum, *Arch. Dermatol.* **88,** 427 (1963).
72. H. G. Mautner, *in* "Burger's Medicinal Chemistry" (M. E. Wolff, ed.), 4th ed., Part I, p. 274. Wiley, New York, 1980.
73. J. Meinhofer, *in* "Burger's Medicinal Chemistry" (M. E. Wolff, ed.), 4th ed., Part II, p. 751. Wiley, New York, 1979.
74. H. H. Meyer, *Arch. Exp. Pathol. Pharmakol.* **42,** 109 (1899).
75. K. E. Mickelson and U. Westphal, *Biochemistry* **19,** 585 (1980).
76. F. A. Momany, *J. Am. Chem. Soc.* **98,** 2990 (1976).
77. F. A. Momany, *J. Am. Chem. Soc.* **98,** 2996 (1976).
78. J.-P. Mornan, J. Delettre, G. Lepicard, R. Bally, E. Sourcouf, and P. Bondot, *J. Steroid Biochem.* **8,** 51 (1977).
79. L. Nadasdi and K. Medzihradszky, *Biochem. Biophys. Res. Commun.* **99,** 451 (1981).
80. G. V. Nikiforovich, V. I. Leonova, S. Galaktinov, and G. I. Chipens, *Int. J. Pept. Protein Res.* **13,** 363 (1979).
81. G. A. Overbeek, J. van der Vies, and J. de Visser, *J. Am. Med. Women's Assoc.* **24,** 54 (1969).

82. A. F. Pearlmutter and E. J. Dalton, *Biochemistry* **19,** 3550 (1980).
83. V. Pliska, *Experientia* **34,** 1190 (1978).
84. K. Ponsold, J. Draffehn, and B. Schonecker, *Pharmazie* **32,** 596 (1977).
85. T. L. Popper and A. S. Watnick, *in* "Antiinflammatory Agents" (R. A. Scherer and M. W. Whitehouse, eds.), Vol. 1, p. 245. Academic Press, New York, 1974.
86. S. Profeta, P. A. Kollman, and M. E. Wolff, *J. Am. Chem. Soc.* **104,** 3745 (1982).
87. C. Renneborg-Squilbin, *Int. J. Pept. Protein Res.* **15,** 20 (1980).
88. H. Repmann, *Theor. Chim. Acta* **17,** 396 (1970).
89. G. G. Rousseau and J. P. Schmit, *Ann. Endocrinol.* **41,** 247 (1980).
90. J. A. Rupley, L. Butler, M. Gerring, F. J. Hartedeger, and R. Pecoraro, *Proc. Natl. Acad. Sci. U.S.A.* **57,** 1083 (1967).
90a. L. H. Sarrett, A. A. Patchett, and S. Steelman, *in* "Progress in Drug Research" (E. Jucker, ed.), Vol. 5, pp. 13–153. Birkhauser Verlag, Basel, 1963.
91. H. T. Schedl and J. A. Clifton, *Gastroenterology* **41,** 491 (1961).
92. J. P. Schmit and G. G. Rousseau, *J. Steroid Biochem.* **9,** 909 (1978).
93. J. P. Schmit and G. G. Rousseau, *J. Steroid Biochem.* **9,** 921 (1978).
94. J. J. Schneider and M. L. Lewbart, *J. Chromatogr.* **35,** 287 (1968).
95. R. D. Schoenwald and R. L. Ward, *J. Pharm. Sci.* **67,** 786 (1978).
96. W. Scholtan, *Arzneim.-Forsch.* **18,** 505 (1968).
97. W. Scholtan, K. Schlossmann, and H. Rosenkranz, *Arzneim.-Forsch.* **18,** 767 (1968).
98. P. Sedmera, A. Vitek, and Z. Samek, *Collect. Czech. Chem. Commun.* **37,** 3828 (1972).
99. W. R. Slaunwhite, Jr., G. N. Lockie, N. Back, and A. A. Sandburg, *Science* **135,** 1062 (1962).
100. H. E. Smith, R. G. Smith, D. O. Toft, J. R. Neergard, E. T. Burrows, and B. W. O'Malley, *J. Biol. Chem.* **249,** 5924 (1974).
101. G. K. Suchowsky, *in* "Evaluation of Drug Activities: Pharmacometrics" (D. H. Laurence and A. L. Bacharach, eds.), Vol. 2, p. 711. Academic Press, New York, 1964.
102. K. Sundaram and R. K. Mishra, *Biochim. Biophys. Acta* **94,** 601 (1965).
103. G. Teutsch, L. Weber, G. Page, E. L. Shapiro, H. L. Herzog, R. Neri, and E. J. Collins, *J. Med. Chem.* **16,** 1370 (1973).
104. E. Tomlinson, *J. Chromatogr.* **113,** 1 (1975).
105. J. G. Topliss, *J. Med. Chem.* **15,** 1006 (1972).
106. J. G. Topliss and E. L. Shapiro, *J. Med. Chem.* **18,** 621 (1975).
107. A. J. Van den Broek, A. I. A. Broess, M. J. van den Heuvel, H. P. de Jongh, J. Leehuis, K. H. Schonemann, J. Smits, J. de Visser, N. P. van Vliet, and F. J. Zeelen, *Steroids* **30,** 481 (1977).
108. J. Van der Vies, *Acta Endocrinol.* (*Copenhagen*) **64,** 656 (1970).
109. M. Waelbroeck, E. Van Obberghen, and P. De Meyts. *J. Biol. Chem.* **254,** 7736 (1979).
110. C. M. Weeks, W. L. Duax, and M. E. Wolff, *J. Am. Chem. Soc.* **95,** 2865 (1973).
110a. U. Westphal, *J. Am. Oil Chemists' Soc.* **41,** 481 (1964).
111. U. Westphal, "Steroid–Protein Interactions," p. 110. Springer-Verlag, Berlin and New York, 1971.
112. M. E. Wolff and C. Hansch, *Experientia* **29,** 1111 (1973).
113. M. E. Wolff, C. Hansch, P. A. Kollman, D. G. Giannini, and W. L. Duax, *in* "Quantitative Structure–Activity Relationships," p. 31. Akadémiai Kiadó, Budapest, 1973.
114. M. E. Wolff and C. Hansch, *J. Med. Chem.* **17,** 898 (1974).
115. M. E. Wolff, C. Hansch, D. G. Giannini, P. A. Kollman, W. L. Duax, and J. Baxter, *J. Steroid Biochem.* **6,** 211 (1975).

116. M. E. Wolff, J. D. Baxter, P. A. Kollman, D. L. Lee, I. D. Kuntz, E. Bloom, D. T. Matulich, and J. Morris, *Biochemistry* **17,** 3201 (1978).
117. M. E. Wolff, *in* "Glucocorticoid Hormone Action" (J. D. Baxter and G. G. Rousseau, eds.), p. 97. Springer-Verlag, Berlin and New York, 1979.
118. M. E. Wolff, *in* "Burger's Medicinal Chemistry" (M. E. Wolff, ed.), 4th ed., Part III, p. 1273. Wiley, New York, 1980.
119. O. Wrange, J. Carlstedt-Duke, and J.-A. Gustafsson, *J. Biol. Chem.* **254,** 9284 (1979).
120. F. J. Zeelen, *Abstr. Pap., Int. Symp. Med. Chem., 4th, Noordwikerhout, Neth.* p. 61 (1974).
121. F. J. Zeelen, *in* "Biological Activity and Chemical Structure" (J. A. Keveling, ed.), p. 147. Elsevier, Amsterdam, 1977.
122. F. J. Zeelen, *Abh. Ahad. Wiss. DDR, Abt. Math., Naturwiss., Tech.* 333–336 (1978). [*Chem. Abstr.* **91,** 68774q (1979)].
123. F. J. Zeelen, *Proc. Congr. Hung. Pharmacol. Soc., 3rd, Budapest, 1979,* **3,** 43–49 (1980).
124. N. Zenker and E. C. Jorgensen, *J. Am. Chem. Soc.* **81,** 4643 (1959).
125. J. E. Zull and N. B. Lev, *Proc. Natl. Acad. Sci. U.S.A.* **77,** 3791 (1980).

10

Chemicals Affecting Insects and Mites

PHILIP S. MAGEE

I. INTRODUCTION

Though the fields of application seem far apart, there are much closer relations between pesticides and drugs than generally realized. Drugs are administered deliberately to control problems in specific patients and there may be unfortunate side effects that define a risk–benefit relation. Similarly, pesticides are applied deliberately to control problems in specific crops and there may be unfortunate side effects that also define a risk–benefit relation. In fact, there may be several stages of risk as a drug or pesticide proceeds from the laboratory through manufacturing and to the applicator before reaching the general public. Different criteria are used at each stage to match the estimated risk of those exposed. In both fields, the common by-product of using chemicals to control the human problems of illness, sanitation, and food protection is unwanted toxicity. Thus as toxicants expressing a bewildering variety of special effects on the human system, drugs and pesticides become objects of equal concern to the public and, in turn, to government regulation.

QUANTITATIVE STRUCTURE–ACTIVITY
RELATIONSHIPS OF DRUGS

ISBN 0-12-695150-0

There are varying degrees of common overlap in the areas of actual use. Many of the known bactericides and fungicides used in medicine, sanitation, and crop protection have major uses in one area and minor uses in another. Thus, streptomycin is used in both medicine and agriculture, whereas captan, an agricultural fungicide, has been used to control dandruff in a commercial preparation (Sebb) and by agricultural chemists to control athlete's foot and ringworm. There are very few commercial bactericides and fungicides that do not express activity on both medicinal and crop problems. Similarly, many carbamate and phosphate insecticides that are best known for crop protection find additional uses as sanitary chemicals for disease vector control, as animal medicinals and even, occasionally, in a direct drug use. Propoxur (Baygon) and dimethoate (Cygon) are used to control flies and other pests around homes, recreation areas, food-processing plants, and warehouses. The insecticide naled (Dibrom) is important in mosquito vector control and displays phenomenal activity when applied by air as an undiluted fog of 30–80 μm droplets. A single pound will control mosquitos covering 10–20 acres. Having a low mammalian toxicity, naled can be sprayed directly on farm animals or incorporated in their feed to control both external and internal pests. Some insecticides used on or in livestock, such as ronnel (Dow Chemical), are provided in both agricultural grade (Korlan) and drug grade (Trolene). As an example of direct drug use in humans, paraoxon, the metabolically activated form of parathion, is marketed by Bayer as Mintacol, an acetylcholinesterase inhibitor used to pinpoint the pupils.

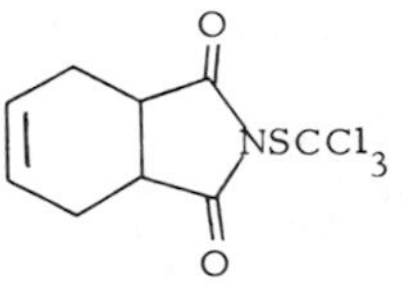

Captan

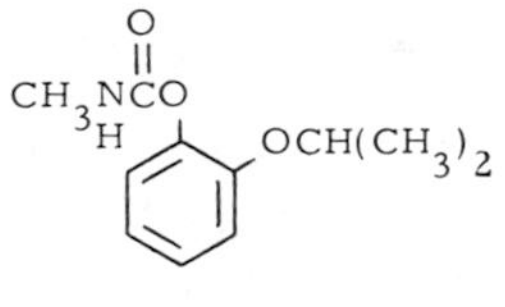

Propoxur

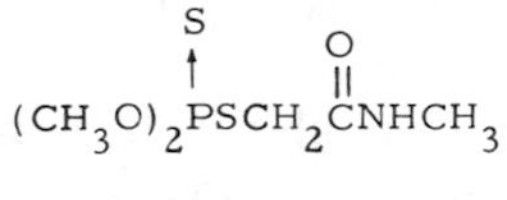

Dimethoate

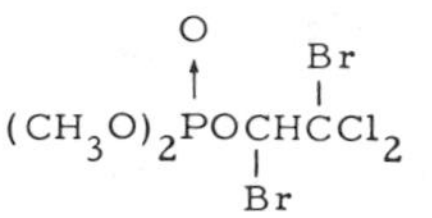

Naled

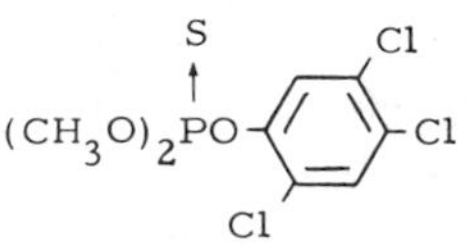

Ronnel

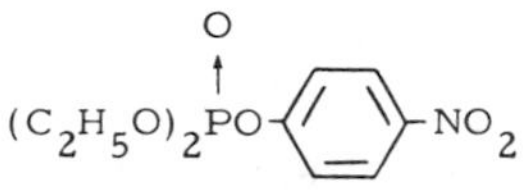

Paraoxon

From a mechanistic viewpoint, there are major areas of common behavior between drugs and pesticides as well as some truly notable differences. Transport phenomena, metabolic activation and degradation, active site binding, and reactivity in cases of irreversible inhibition are common to both classes and depend on similar molecular factors. Unique to pesticides are such matters as fumigant action in soil, xylem and phloem transport in plants, weathering and ultraviolet degradation on leaves, and cuticular penetration into various insects. With these considerations in mind, we can now examine the major chemicals affecting insects and mites.

II. CHEMICALS AFFECTING INSECTS AND MITES

A. General Considerations

Insects are the most numerous and most successful of all forms of life (about 3 million species). At any time about 10^{18} individuals are alive and some have incredible capacity to multiply into uncontrollable hordes. History has been altered many times by insects. Eight emperors have died of diseases carried by fleas and a half million of Napoleon's troops were victims of the body lice vector (*92*). Fortunately for man, only about 0.3% of the insect population destroy agricultural produce or act as vectors for human and animal disease. In 1969 our undersecretary of agriculture estimated that 10,000 species of insects and 1,500 species of nematodes and microscopic worms were enemies of man (*10*). About 600 of the insect species are considered to be serious problems. The mobility of insects and mites from their place of origin and their ability to develop resistance to conventional insecticides are problems that seriously compound man's efforts at control. Thus among the 35 major pest arthropods in the United States, 21 are exotic species and 21 have developed resistance to one or more insecticides. Insects such as European corn borer, Mediterranean fruit fly, and Japanese beetle are familiar to most Americans.

Although insects and mites appear together in agriculture and in human or animal health, there are vast differences between these classes. Insects have six legs, antennae, compound eyes, segmented bodies, and may have wings. Mites and other arachnids have eight legs, no antennae, simple eyes (sometimes in sets), no wings, and one or two fusions of head, thorax, and abdomen. More importantly, they are different biochemically and respond differently to toxicants. Both insects and mites can be killed by acetylcholinesterase (AChE) inhibitors and CNS poisons that interfere with axonal transmission. However, mites are also susceptible to oxidative phosphorylation (OXPHOS) inhibitors and a variety of other chemicals of unknown mode, few of which have any affect on insects. Nematodes are also susceptible to AChE inhibitors, but are additionally controlled by various noninsecticidal nematocides.

In the midst of these variables is the truly difficult problem of selective control. From the mammalian viewpoint, we need to control insects and mites but not farmers, farm animals, and birds that coexist in the same space. Even more difficult is the problem of selective insect control: the honey bee and useful insect predators that provide some measure of biological control must be considered. The bee problem is especially serious, and conflicts between the need to protect crops of great value and the bees that pollinate these and other crops are many. No perfect solution has been found, though many procedures to minimize the problem are in use.

The physicochemical aspects of insecticidal action have been nicely summarized by Fukuto (*27*). Although the posioning process and subsequent events leading to death are quite complex, the major controlling factors are penetration and translocation, metabolic activation and degradation, and target site interaction. Of these, penetration, transport, and target site interaction are frequently relatable by physicochemical analysis especially within restricted classes of compounds having known modes of action. Metabolic events involving activation (delay factor) or degradation (loss of activity) can upset correlations if they proceed differentially within the set under study. In some cases of rapid degradation, order can be restored by the simultaneous use of synergists that suppress oxidative metabolism.

In applying multiple regression analysis and other related techniques to data in this field, there is a natural progression of experimental error that determines the strength of correlation. Direct inhibition of important enzymes such as AChE or studies on the responses of isolated neurons have the highest precision. In whole animal studies, topical applications are most precise followed by the microspray application. Least precise are various feeding tests for sucking and chewing species, which involve leaf dipping followed by infestation, or application to a remote leaf, the stem, or a soil drench to observe systemic activity. Naturally, the more remote the application from the target site, the more diffuse the data become in terms of residual error. Nevertheless, such data can be correlated with physicochemical parameters if the set is of sufficient size and the span of bioactivity is adequate. The beauty of statistical procedures is the ability to sort facts from random error. There is nothing wrong with an explained variance of 50–70%, and the extracted factors can be of immeasurable importance in understanding mode of action or in designing an improved insecticide.

B. Mechanistic Considerations

1. Transport and Other Physical Factors

Transport implies the movement of an insecticide from the point of application to the target site. Agriculture has many situations and boundaries that tend to diversify the transport process. As one example, transport through soil to reach the larvae of soil insects can occur either by solid–liquid phase partitioning or by fumigant action (volatility). Systemic insecticides may be applied to the soil for root uptake or directly to the foliage. In the latter case, many leaves have waxy layers that provide a special barrier for penetration to the vascular system. Once inside the plant, most systemics transport passively by a physical partitioning process, a majority of the compound following the transpiration stream in the xylem. In a few rare cases penetration of the phloem system may occur, permitting downward as well as upward transport. This can be highly desirable for some applications. Mobility in the phloem or living tissue is especially important in forest applications where concealed insects feed on the tender growing parts of trees (*14*). The xylem tissue is so large relative to the phloem that excessive amounts of conventional systemics are necessary to achieve control. The general objective of developing systemic insecticides is to poison the plant against sucking and chewing insects.

Contact insecticides must achieve entry into the insect by cuticle penetration, a different type of physical problem. Contact may occur over the entire body in a direct spray and by fumigant action or perhaps only by leg contact in walking over a previously sprayed surface. Inasmuch as the spray may be solid or liquid with a wide range of viscosities and droplet size, a great variety of microscopic contact processes are possible.

Despite the variety of barriers and special situations, the majority of these processes are passive in nature involving physical partitioning between phases as the major driving force. The weight of experience now tells us that most of these complex translocations tend to correlate well with the easily measured *n*-octanol–water partition ($\log P$). This enormous simplification tells us nothing about the complex sequential details of the transport process. In multiple regression analyses, however, it frequently permits us to segregate this behavior from important details occurring at the target site.

The movement of a series of *N*-alkyl phosphoramidothioates in the cotton leaf petiole provides a relevant example of agricultural transport behavior (*50*). The series under study is related to the commercial systemic insecticide methamidophos (*62*). *n*-Octanol–water partitions were measured to develop π values for each of the *N*-alkyl groups. The rate of systemic movement ($\log k_{tr}$) was found to give a smooth curvilinear plot against the alkyl π values with optimum behavior near *n*-propyl. Regression of $\log k_{tr}$ against π and π^2 gave a highly significant correlation (Eq. 1) (*50*). Although this relation and many others gave good parabolic regressions (*42*), it should not be concluded that the behavior is truly parabolic.

While this particular case appears curvilinear, Kubinyi (*58*) has described a large number of cases where a bilinear model gave a superior fit to the data. At this time it is not clear whether the bilinear response of Kubinyi's examples were related to transport or to the subsequent binding step.

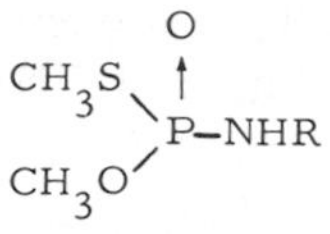

R = CH_3, C_4H_9, C_6H_{13}, C_8H_{17}

$$\log k_{tr} = 2.32\pi - 0.97\pi^2 - 0.75 \quad (1)$$

$$n = 6, \quad r = 0.999$$

Bioconcentration is a log P related problem that can adversely affect the buildup of pesticides in the food chain, leading to unexpectedly high levels in terminal members of the chain. These problems are expecially severe for DDT and other highly lipophilic insecticides, a point to be discussed in more detail under CNS poisons. From a simplistic point of view, the problem is best illustrated by studies involving fish, an ideal live organic phase that cannot get out of the water. Linear free-energy relations are found in both rate and equilibrium studies. The rate of dieldrin uptake in ppb/day by reticulate sculpin has been shown to be an accurate log–log relation (Eq. 2) (*68*).

Dieldrin:

$$\log C = (1.23 \pm 0.14) \log k - 2.84 \quad (2)$$

$$n = 6, \quad r = 0.997, \quad s = 0.089$$

where C is the concentration in ppb and k is the uptake in ppb/day.

In equilibrium studies of eight lipophilic chemicals, Neely *et al.* (*73*) determined the bioconcentration between trout muscle and the exposure water. Although these chemicals are not insecticidal, their log P range (2.64–7.62) includes the range in which bioconcentration of chlorocarbon insecticides occurs. A relationship linking log P to log(bioconcentration factor) was established (Eq. 3) (*73*).

$$\log(BF) = 0.54 \log P + 0.12 \quad (3)$$

$$n = 8, \quad r = 0.948, \quad s = 0.342$$

where BF is the bioconcentration factor in trout muscle.

It is interesting to note that environmental problems have been largely associated with DDT and other chlorinated hydrocarbons, whereas the more polar, readily degraded phosphates are considered relatively safe. There are exceptions, however, as shown by the log *P* studies of Freed *et al.* (*21*). The insecticide leptophos, which has been implicated in delayed neurotoxicity of the CNS in humans, has a log *P* of 6.31, slightly above that of DDT. In solubility terms, the DDT problem can be stated as approximately 10% solubility in fat (100,000 ppm) and 12 ppb solubility in water. Let us return now to the effects of toxicants in fish as a function of log *P*. In a study on loaches, a common fish in Taiwan, Yang and Sun

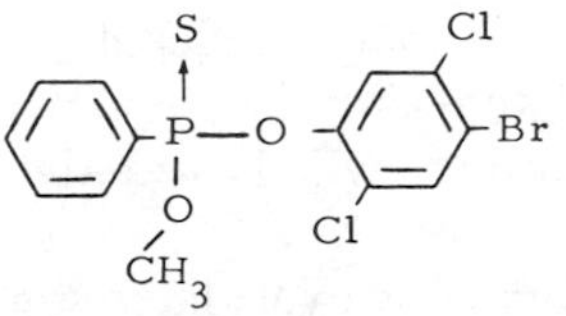

Leptophos
$\log P = 6.31$

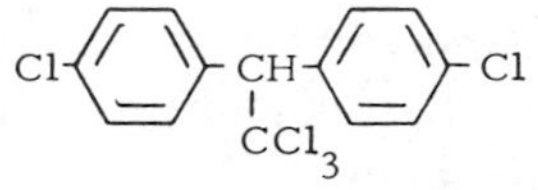

DDT
$\log P = 6.19$

(*100*) found that monocrotophos was 4–9 times as toxic as dieldrin and DDT by injection, consistent with their acute oral toxicities to rats. By absorption from water, however, DDT and dieldrin were found to be 150 and 220 times more toxic than monocrotophos. This extreme result is derived from the huge difference between the distribution of the highly lipophilic dieldrin and DDT and that of the highly hydrophilic monocrotophos. We have no log *P* measurement for monocrotophos but it is miscible with water in all proportions, indicating a negative log *P*. The difference between partitioning of DDT and monocrotophos is at least seven orders of magnitude. Yang and Sun also quoted another interesting ex-

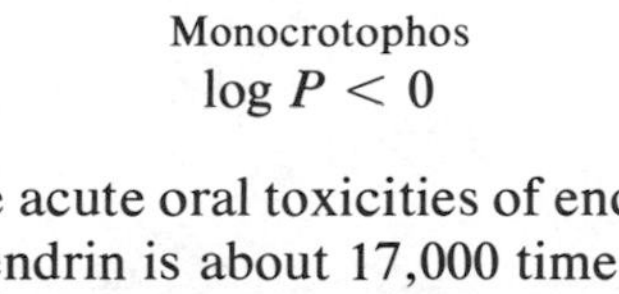

Monocrotophos
$\log P < 0$

ample, namely, that the acute oral toxicities of endrin and monocrotophos are similar in rats but endrin is about 17,000 times more toxic to rainbow trout. The rainbow trout is a member of the salmon family, has much fatty tissue, and is exceptionally sensitive to lipophilic insecticides. It is frequently used as an environmental standard for toxicity problems.

Mode of entry into insects is our next concern. How does a contacted insecticide actually reach the nervous system of an insect? The review on penetration and distribution of insecticides by Brooks (*7*) and a symposium paper by Noble–Nesbitt (*76*) on the structural aspects of penetration through insect cuticles are recommended for the interested reader. Of primary interest to us are the mode of entry studies carried out by Gerolt (*28,29*) who presented evidence to show that penetration could be a complex, indirect process. For both lipophilic and hydrophilic insecticides, Gerolt found that penetration rates of isolated housefly integument were too low to account for the observed toxic action. Entry into the insect appeared to occur by partial penetration of the integument followed by rapid lateral transport through an internal layer without significant penetration to the hemolymph system. Gerolt postulated that insecticides enter the ganglia via the integument of the tracheal system, which is contiguous with that of the body wall.

Not everyone agrees with Gerolt's theory, however; later studies tend to favor classical direct penetration to the hemolymph system. A study on the American cockroach by Moriarty and French (*67*) suggested that dieldrin was not distributed by lateral movement in the cuticle. Also working with American cockroach, Olson (*78*) interpreted his work with dieldrin to support the direct hemolymph route but does not eliminate translocation via the tracheal system. Finally, Winter *et al.* (*98*) showed by electrophoresis that DDT binds to proteins in cockroach hemolymph and discussed the involvement of this factor in the transport process. Obviously, there is controversy over mode of entry among different competent workers and it will take time to sort out the access modes of many different insecticides on many different insects. It seems probable that there is more than one way for a contact insecticide to enter an insect. In terms of direct penetration, there is a remarkable similarity between cockroach cuticle and human skin despite the vast structural differences. Penniston *et al.* (*80*) found the ideal lipophilicity for penetration of human skin by simple phosphates to be $\log P = -1.58$. For penetration of cockroach cuticle by various insecticides including some phosphates, the optimum lipophilicity was $\log P = -1.46$. $\text{Log } P$ values were measured in olive oil and water.

2. Active Site Binding

Binding of insecticides to active enzyme sites is a highly specific process that needs to be considered in some detail. In some cases of binding to proteins it is possible to observe a nonspecific process that is largely independent of the details of structure. Thus Vandenbelt *et al.* (*93*) observed a simple linear dependence on $\log P$ for a variety of classes in reversible binding to albumin (Eq. 4).

$$\log(1/C) = (0.67 \pm 0.10) \log P + (2.60 \pm 0.22) \quad (4)$$

$$n = 25 \text{ (6 classes)}, \quad r = 0.945, \quad s = 0.242$$

This appears to be a case of nonspecific, hydrophobic binding in which the details of structure are less important than general lipophilicity. It is interesting that a number of these compounds have the capacity for strong hydrogen bonds or dipolar interactions, but these potentials are not expressed. Skalsky and Guthrie (*83*) have also found that binding of DDT, dieldrin, carbaryl, and parathion to human serum proteins is of low affinity and hyrophobic in nature. No specific binding sites were demonstrated.

In a structurally related series, a regular dependence on log P of binding or of transport with binding is frequently observed. Hansch and coworkers (*41,42*) have documented 129 cases of linear dependence and 167 cases of curvilinear dependence, whereas Kubinyi (*58*) has reported many examples that are best described as bilinear. The frequent dependence of binding on log P or on the derived parameter π may be partly related to the preponderance of the homologous series brought under study. When substituents are expanded to include highly dipolar groups, other binding forces (Keesom, Debye) can come into play as discussed by McFarland (*63*). In some of these cases, binding may depend on polarizability as expressed by molar refraction (MR) of the whole molecule or of the substituent on a parent structure. Inasmuch as transport and binding can display independent maxima in log P and MR, it is clear that analyses of transport, binding, and reactivity can be very complex in some cases.

Even in the simplest example of nonspecific binding, it is incorrect to think in terms of partitioning from solution "into" a macromolecular phase to account for the log P behavior. The very act of binding has mechanistic implications that extend beyond phase partitioning. Rotations are frozen, conformations are established, and mutual deformation may occur. In more complex cases, strong hydrogen bonds or dipolar interactions may lead to overall binding that approaches the strength of some of the weaker chemical bonds. As Page (*79*) points out in his analysis of enzyme reactivity, a large fraction of the rate acceleration is directly due to the substrate–enzyme binding energy. Binding is basically a weak chemical reaction and it is well to remember that some inhibitions depend only on binding with no subsequent reaction at the active site. A relevant example is the inhibition of acetylcholinesterase by quaternary ammonium ions (*57*). Inhibition is by reversible ion pairing with the anionic site. The esteratic site, 5 Å away, is not involved. Another example that appears to involve hydrophobic binding without subsequent reaction is the interaction of DDT and its analogs with neural membranes (*47*). Steric factors are involved in the binding and will be considered in more detail later.

In specific enzymatic binding, conformation and stereochemistry can be of critical importance. Enzymatic sites are asymmetric and highly sensitive to molecular shape. Jacobson and co-workers are making a substantial contribution to the understanding of minimum energy conformations through their studies on crystalline insecticides [Lapp and Jacobson (*59*), and earlier citations]. Over a dozen commercial carbamate and phosphate insecticides have been described by three-dimensional X-ray analysis. Close examination of these structures can reveal many features that are not readily predictable. As one example, the carbamate group in methiocarb (Mesurol) and, probably in other carbamates, is noncoplanar with the aryl ring (*86*). The methylthio group is also rotated out of plane, as expected, by the 3,5-dimethyl grouping. To explore the effect of chiral centers on AChE inhibition, Wustner and Fukuto (*99*) have synthesized all four optical isomers of a known inhibitor. In this example, both the

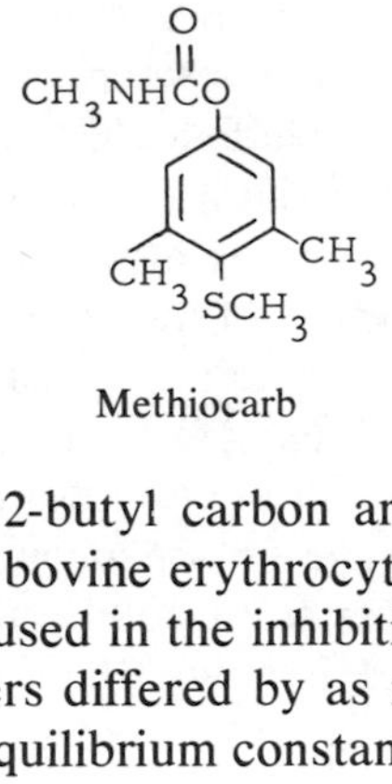

Methiocarb

phosphorus atom and the 2-butyl carbon are chiral centers. Two true AChEs (housefly head and bovine erythrocyte) and one pseudocholinesterase (horse serum) were used in the inhibition studies. Bimolecular inhibition constants of isomers differed by as much as 10,000-fold. When dissected into the affinity equilibrium constant (K_a) and the phosphoryla-

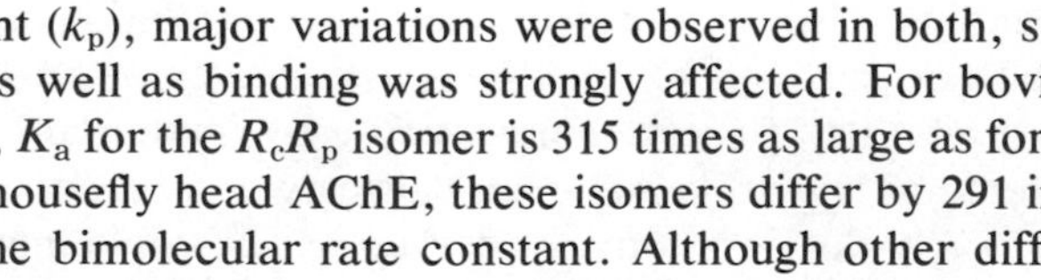

tion constant (k_p), major variations were observed in both, showing that reactivity as well as binding was strongly affected. For bovine erythrocyte AChE, K_a for the R_cR_p isomer is 315 times as large as for the S_cS_p isomer. For housefly head AChE, these isomers differ by 291 in K_a and by 10,300 in the bimolecular rate constant. Although other differences are small, there are only a few cases where the constants are similar. It is clear from this study that asymmetric binding and reactivity are very sensitive functions of stereochemistry. Many commercial insecticides are racemates with one or more chiral centers. The bioactivity of these compounds is an average of that of the isomers, one of which may be almost inactive. Without citation we can also state that *E* and *Z* isomers of vinyl phosphates and oxime carbamates also display major differences in AChE inhibition and presumably in binding affinity.

3. Reactivity Factors

In cases where reaction follows binding, this final step is considered to be a physical organic process not unlike solution reactions that are more readily studied. This analogy implies the possiblity of correlating reactivity with the same electronic and steric parameters used in solution. Early support for this premise was provided by Hansch *et al.* (*35*) in their regression studies on enzyme activities. Enzymatic hydrolyses of substituted phenyl glucosides and homologous 4-nitrophenyl esters were nicely correlated by linear combinations of π with ordinary electronic and steric parameters. Other enzyme reactions, such as acetylation of amines and transacetylation, were also correlated with common solution parameters. It is now a common assumption that electronic and steric parameters generated from simple reactions in solution apply equally well to complex enzyme reactions in test tubes and also in whole living systems. Under this assumption, let us examine these parameters as they apply to chemicals affecting insects and mites.

Like drugs and other biocides, insecticides and miticides possess aromatic and aliphatic structures that can be modified within certain restrictions without departing from the active class. Electronic effects in aliphatic structures correlate best with Taft's σ_I or Charton's rescaled σ_L parameters based on the pK_a values of substituted acetic acids. Taft's σ^* values cannot be recommended because they are poorly separated from the alkyl steric effect (*5*). For aromatic substituents, the Hammett σ and σ^- parameters remain the choice for 3- and 4-substituted systems. These are frequently important in aromatic phosphate and carbamate insecticides where AChE inhibition involves a phenolate leaving group. Ortho substituents need to be treated individually for each bioactive series. Charton has demonstrated that most ortho-substituent effects are electrical in nature but have different mixes of induction and resonance than σ_p (*12*). When segregated from the meta and para cases, they can usually be handled by correlation with σ_I and σ_R or σ_L and σ_D. Use of the limited set of σ_o parameters is not recommended nor is the frequent assumption that $\sigma_o = \sigma_p$ useful due to the variablity of electronic effects from one case to the next. The extended Hammett equation ($a\sigma_I + b\sigma_R$) appears to be the only valid approach to correlating the effects of ortho substituents.

For the specific class of aryl carbamate insecticides, Hetnarski and O'Brien (*43–46*) have developed a charge–transfer parameter, C_T, based on association constants between substituted aryl carbamates and tetracyanoethylene (TCNE) in 1,2-dichloroethane. We will consider the correlations obtained in a later section. These constants have not come into general use, apparently because they do not fill a need. Charton has shown that the extended Hammett equation correlates substituent effects in many charge–transfer associations (*11*).

Steric effects can be handled equivalently with Taft's E_s or Charton's U parameters. Both are kinetically evaluated parameters based on acid-catalyzed hydrolysis of esters. The two sets are highly colinear (r = 0.995) and will provide correlations of equal strength. However, Charton's set is scaled to the van der Waals radii of hydrogen, the halogens, and the symmetrical CX_3 groups. This makes the kinetic size of each group obvious at a glance. The kinetic size expressed by E_s or U is that of a small nucleophile (H_2O) reacting with a dioxocarbocation (protonated ester group) attached to the steric group. This procedure evaluates the steric effect from a simple directional approach, roughly perpendicular to the substituent bond. To the extent that enzyme reactions are like solution reactions, these parameters should give good correlations with inhibition rate constants. However, when steric effects are expressed in the equilibrium association constant (binding), other directional approaches are involved and these kinetic sets may fail to account for the variance. In this respect, Verloop's STERIMOL parameters (L, $B1$–$B5$), based on multidimensional physical measurements of each substituent, may perform better. We shall consider applications of these dimensional parameters in the following sections. No physical chemistry or kinetic studies are required to measure the STERIMOL parameters. Any group can be processed through the STERIMOL computer program (*94*), giving these parameters the unique advantage of being a complete set.

In sets where some of the substituents are hydrogen-bond donors or acceptors, correlations are frequently difficult to obtain because large selective effects on binding and reactivity are present. No one has as yet developed a true hydrogen-bond parameter that varies with the strength of the bond. However, Fujita *et al.* (*23*) and Nishioka *et al.* (*75*) have made effective use of an *HB* indicator variable in analyzing sets containing bonding and nonbonding substituents. The *HB* variable was assigned the value of $HB = 1$ for derivatives having OR, NO_2, NMe_2, CN, or acyl on a ring position and $HB = 0$ for other substituents. Significant correlations were obtained despite the simplicity of approach, which treats the hydrogen bond as present or absent. Differentiating between donor and acceptor groups and incorporating some measure of group basicity and acidity is a job for the future. Unless the measurement of biodata become much more precise, a more sophisticated approach may be meaningless.

Other parameters have been used to express reactivity but have not gained general acceptance. Neely *et al.* (*70*) and Fukuto and Metcalf (*24*) have used infrared stretching vibrations (cm^{-1}) of reacting bonds to correlate rates of AChE inhibition. Neely (*71*) also used molecular orbital calculations of net electron charge to help account for the behavior of some phosphate and carbamate AChE inhibitors. Perhaps the most novel approach to *in vivo* correlations is the use of an *in vitro* pI_{50} as an independent variable by Durden (*15*). Durden's application is related to insecticide correlations (pI_{50} for AChE), but the idea is broader than this and may help bring difficult cases into line.

C. Lethal Chemicals

By lethal chemicals we mean those that enter the insect or mite body by some route and inhibit a function critical to life, resulting in death when a sufficient amount of toxicant is absorbed. Such chemicals may attack the central nervous system, inhibit AChE, uncouple oxidative phosphorylation, or act through a mechanism not yet defined. The major reason for studying series of active insecticides and miticides is to relate molecular structure with bioactivity through some logical procedure. The goals are the same as in drug studies, namely, optimization of activity and mechanistic understanding. Statistical procedures such as regression or factor analysis can certainly aid optimization of activity. However, it should be clearly stated that statistical procedures cannot prove mechanism of action though they can provide support for a working hypothesis. In the sections that follow we will select QSAR analyses that tend to clarify the mode of action.

1. CNS Poisons

Known poisons of the central nervous system of insects and mites will be divided into DDT analogs, other chlorinated hydrocarbons, and pyrethroids. Because of their historical impact and unique structure, DDT and its direct analogs will be treated separately from other chlorinated hydrocarbons.

Chlorinated hydrocarbon insecticides, including DDT, are covered extensively by Brooks (*6*) in a major review. This is a good reference to the early structure–activity studies and to many details regarding toxic action. At about the same time, Metcalf (*66*) published a compact but extensive review of DDT and its close analogs in which he reviews the evidence for nerve poisoning, insect resistance, and environmental problems. Although the exact mechanism of DDT action remains a subject for study, the site of action and the effects it produces are clear. A nerve poison in both insects and mammals, it produces symptoms of intoxication marked by hyperexcitability, tremors leading to convulsions, prostration, and death. The tremors are a result of uncontrolled repetitive discharges in the nerve such that a single impulse from a sensory nerve in the insect produces a prolonged series of impulses. The effects are believed to result from specific inhibition of ion transport through the nerve axon membrane. It has been suggested that DDT has the appropriate size and shape to enter the interstices of cylindrical lipoprotein strands forming the membrane lattices of the nerve axon. This concept has led to several theories based on molecular shape to explain both activity and inactivity of some analogs (*66*). The most modern concept is that of Holan (*47*) who visualizes DDT as a molecular wedge fitting into a dimensionally restricted site that is probably a sodium ion gate. He points out that the CCl_3 apex of the wedge is similar in size to the major axis of a hydrated sodium ion, strongly suggesting a gate blocking mechanism.

Regression analysis has been extremely useful in support of the steric fit model and in revealing other details of DDT action. Uchida *et al.* (*89*) examined the neuroexciting activity of 20 DDT analogs on the isolated nerve cord of American cockroach (*Periplaneta americana*) in comparison with convulsive activity in the live insect. The minimum concentrations to produce repetitive discharge in the nerve cord were highly colinear with those causing convulsive activity in the roach (Eq. 5a) (*89*). This observation directly relates the events occurring on the nerve cord to the observed result in the live insect. Stimulation of cockroach nerve cord also proved to be a good descriptor of lethal effects in an unrelated insect, the Azuku bean weevil (*C. chinensis*) (Eq. 5b) (*89*).

American cockroach:

$$-\log(MEC_{\mathrm{CA}}) = -(0.91 \pm 0.14)\log(MEC_{\mathrm{RD}}) - (2.95 \pm 0.72) \quad (5a)$$

$$n = 14, \quad r = 0.971, \quad s = 0.126$$

Azuki bean weevil:

$$\log(1/LD_{50}) = -(1.19 \pm 0.22)\log(MEC_{\mathrm{RD}}) - (3.50 \pm 1.12) \quad (5b)$$

$$n = 11, \quad r = 0.972, \quad s = 0.180$$

where MEC_{CA} is the minimum effective concentration for convulsive activity
MEC_{RD} is the minimum effective concentration for repetitive discharge

This supports the working hypothesis of similar action in different species. In a test of steric fit theories, Fahmy *et al.* (*18*) studied the variations in bioactivity of 25 DDT analogs against houseflies and mosquito larvae. In all cases the predominant parameter correlating the data was Taft's steric value, E_s. In addition, E_s^2 was also important showing the presence of an optimum steric fit in agreement with Holan and earlier theories. Houseflies synergized with piperonyl butoxide to inhibit the mixed-function oxidase (mfo) system gave a satisfactory correlation against the steric parameter alone (Eq. 6a) (*18*). Mosquito larvae (Eq. 6b) (*18*) tested against a smaller set of analogs also showed an electronic dependence that suggested the possibility of a subsequent reaction of the bound analog.

Synergized houseflies:

$$\log(1/LD_{50}) = -(1.85 \pm 0.22) \sum E_s - (0.85 \pm 0.11) \sum E_s^2 - (2.69 \pm 0.25) \qquad (6a)$$

$$n = 25, \quad r = 0.874, \quad s = 0.31$$

Mosquito larvae:

$$\log(1/LD_{50}) = -(4.90 \pm 0.92) \sum E_s - (0.76 \pm 0.16) \sum E_s^2 - (1.76 \pm 0.43) \sum \sigma^* - (5.29 \pm 1.06) \qquad (6b)$$

$$n = 14, \quad r = 0.889, \quad s = 0.29$$

Calling on the same data, Verloop *et al.* (*94*) found satisfactory regressions with his STERIMOL parameters L and $B4$. In each case the squared term, $(\Sigma L)^2$ or $(\Sigma B4)^2$, was important, reaffirming the existence of an optimum steric fit. Studies by Goodford *et al.* (*33*) on a large set of methoxychlor analogs also suggested an optimum fit (Eq. 7). Their choice of MR as a major parameter was unusual, but it is size related for common groups and the appearance of $(MR)^2$ again suggested an optimum. Similarly, Lee *et al.* (*60*) found steric optima in 19 of 22 regression studies of DDT-related Prolan analogs. Conventional steric parameters such as E_s

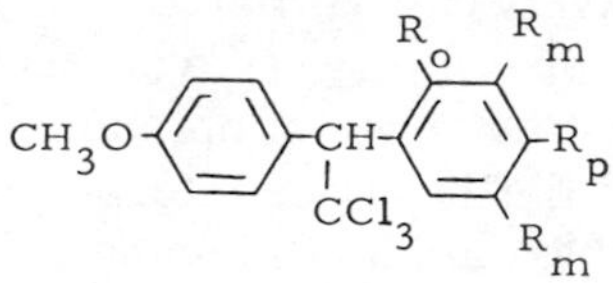

versus Synergized houseflies

$$\log(MW/1000LD_{50}) = (1.51 \pm 0.29)\pi - (2.66 \pm 0.67)R - (0.44 \pm 0.08)MR_o + (0.011 \pm 0.004)(MR_o)^2 - (0.19 \pm 0.03)MR_{m,p} - 0.085 \quad (7)$$

$$n = 14, \qquad r = 0.889$$

were used as well as the STERIMOL parameters and volume related values such as MR and MA (molar attraction). All of these parameters displayed optimum behavior. Their study was somewhat unconventional in using LD_{30} values directly, thus accounting for the unusual regression coefficients and intercept. Although one of their equations containing volume related parameters is shown (Eq. 8) (*60*), they concluded that E_s was the simplest and most practical parameter for studies of this type. All of the foregoing analyses support the general concept of a flexible receptor site of definite dimensions.

One of the most impressive studies of the dimensional requirements of DDT analogs was carried out by Coats *et al.* (*13*) using a simple plotting technique. Eight series of DDT-related insecticides were examined graphically by plotting LD_{50} against the van der Waals volumes of the vari-

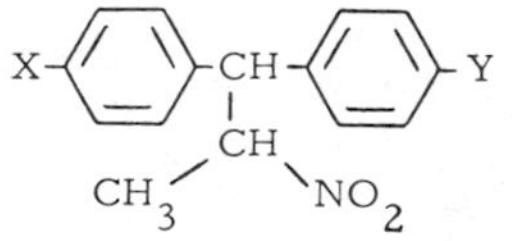

versus Synergized houseflies

$$LD_{50} = -(1.64 \pm 0.25)\sum MA + (6.63 \times 10^{-4}) \pm (1.05 \times 10^{-4})\left(\sum MA\right)^2 + (41.2 \pm 7.40)\sum MR - (0.50 \pm 0.09)\left(\sum MR\right)^2 + (92.6 \pm 24.6)\sum \sigma_p + (223.8 \pm 33.8) \quad (8)$$

$$n = 37, \qquad r = 0.938$$

able groups. In four of the series, variations were made in the ring para positions while holding the aliphatic portion constant. In the other four series the reverse was true. The pattern of insecticidal behavior as a function of substituent volume (V_w) was clear in every case. From a low activity region where substituents are too small there is a very steep descent to a broad region of high activity (low LD_{50}). As the region of optimum size is exceeded, activity rapidly diminishes and the LD_{50} rises steeply with increasing V_w. Although there is considerable variation in some of the data sets, the LD_{50} versus V_w plots are dramatically clear in expressing the concept of optimum steric fit for both the aromatic and aliphatic portions of the structures. A common mechanism for all eight sets is beyond question. More recent work from the same laboratories has confirmed the fact that the bulk of the functional groups is the primary factor controlling DDT analog behavior (*8*).

Most of the structure–activity studies of chlorinated hydrocarbons other than DDT analogs have been carried out on lindane analogs. Insects intoxicated by lindane or dieldrin show violent tremors of the body and legs due to neuroexcitatory action. This behavior is similar to that observed in the case of DDT. However, in a study on isolated abdominal ganglia, Uchida *et al.* (*90*) established the fact that lindane and dieldrin attack a different site than does DDT, producing high levels of acetylcholine. Inhibition by DDT is associated with the noncholinergic region of the ganglia, while lindane probably acts on presynaptic membranes to cause the excess release of acetylcholine. The importance of distribution (log P) in lindane activity was demonstrated by Uchida *et al.* (*88*). Lindane and three isomers were included with a number of unrelated alcohols, phenols, and other neutral compounds in some inhibitory studies. Nearly perfect linear log P correlations were obtained for inhibition of (Na^+,K^+)-ATPase, cockroach nerve conduction, and yeast growth (Eqs. 9a–c) (*88*).

(Na^+,K^+)-ATPase inhibition:

$$pI_{50} = (0.77 \pm 0.08) \log P + (0.53 \pm 0.23) \qquad (9a)$$

$$n = 14, \quad r = 0.988, \quad s = 0.237$$

Saccharomyces cerevisiae inhibition:

$$pI_{50} = (0.92 \pm 0.04) \log P + (0.53 \pm 0.11) \qquad (9b)$$

$$n = 12, \quad r = 0.998, \quad s = 0.101$$

Periplaneta americana nerve conduction:

$$\log(1/MIC) = (0.91 \pm 0.08) \log P + (0.19 \pm 0.19) \qquad (9c)$$

$$n = 12, \quad r = 0.993, \quad s = 0.162$$

As the compounds are unrelated, the critical step common to each is governed by the hydrophobicity of the molecule. Stereochemistry of the four lindane isomers does not play any role as such.

In order to study specific effects of structural changes in the symmetrical lindane structure, Nakajima *et al.* (*69*) synthesized a large number of analogs. Lindane itself has a very simple meso structure with three equatorial and three axial chlorine atoms. Thus, any substitution disrupts the symmetry and can result in an equilibrium mixture of conformations. In general, the meso-type analogs (3- and 3,6-substitution) are more active than the (±) types (1-substitution) and some are almost as active as lindane, especially against mosquitoes.

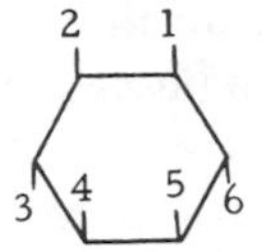

Lindane is 1,2,3,4,5,6-hexachloro

1-Substitutions: F, Br, CH_3, OCH_3, OC_2H_5, H, I, CN, $CONH_2$, COOH, CH_2OH
3-Substitutions: Br, OCH_3, SCH_3 I, OH, OAc
Others: 3,6-diBr; 1,2-F,Br; 1,2-diBr; 1,6-diBr; 1,2,3-triBr; 1,4-diCH_3; hexa-OCH_3

Using a selected series of lindane itself, one lindane isomer and 13 substitution analogs, the minimum concentration required to induce successive afterdischarges in American cockroach nerve cord was measured [$\log(1/MEC_{AD})$]. Convulsive activities [$\log(1/MEC_{CA})$] and minimum lethal doses [$\log(1/MLD)$] for the cockroach were also measured. No regressions were performed and none were needed as each log–log plot is clearly colinear and parallel. The neuroexciting effect on isolated nerve cord is thus directly related to convulsant activity and the terminal lethal effect of these analogs. A dosage of 2–4 times that of the MEC_{CA} was generally fatal to the cockroach. The work on these 15 lindane analogs was extended somewhat by Uchida *et al.* (*91*) who compared the effects of these analogs with those of six aryl *N*-methylcarbamate insecticides. The carbamates cause acetylcholine accumulation by a different mechanism than the lindane analogs, namely, by AChE inhibition. Nevertheless, in plotting convulsive activity [$\log(1/MEC_{CA})$] against neuroexcitatory activity [$\log(1/MEC_{AD})$], the carbamates fall on the same line as the lindane analogs. This is consistent with the idea that acetylcholine, however generated, is responsible for the afterdischarges and the related convulsive activity. It is interesting to note that in plotting lethal activity [$\log(1/MLD)$] against neuroexcitatory activity [$\log(1/MEC_{AD})$] the carbamates fall on a separate, higher activity line than the lindanes. Inasmuch as lindane analogs are not AChE inhibitors, it is probable that some of the neuroexciting acetylcholine is destroyed by the lindane-poisoned insect before it can function.

In a later study by the same research group, Kiso *et al.* (*54*) examined the parametric relations in 38 lindane analogs by regression analyses. Conformational equilibria were measured for the unsymmetrical analogs but these values were not used in the analysis, equal activity of conformers being assumed as a first approximation. A symmetry factor (log 2) was subtracted from the $\log(1/LD_{50})$ values for lindane and the meso-type analogs having a bisecting plane. This procedure was important when meso- and (±) types were analyzed together. As stated earlier, the meso analogs are substantially more active than the (±)-and mixed-type isomers. Thus the 3-SCH_3 and 3,6-diBr analogs are about 1300 times as active as the 1-SCH_3 and 2,3-diBr isomers. Activity data against 3- to 5-day-old female mosquitoes (*Culex pipiens pallens*) were evaluated against several sterically related parameters and log P. The steric parameters were referenced against the chlorine atom: van der Waals radius (Δr_v), van der Waals volume (ΔV_w), and molar refraction (ΔMR). Although it was possible to develop an equation combining meso and (±) analogs, they proved to have different dependencies and were best treated separately (Eq. 10a,b) (*54*). The meso analogs correlated only with Δr_v, which is basically a distance or contact parameter. The mono- and disubstituted (±) analogs showed a group volume dependence with an optimum, similar to the DDT-analog regressions. These data gave an excellent parabolic plot [$\log(1/LD_{50})$ versus ΔV_w]. The different dependencies suggest that steric fit with a specific cavity wall is important with the more active meso analogs. The less active (±) analogs are probing a different direction where group volume rather than distance is more important. Neither set shows an explicit log P dependence though both sets contain low active or inactive members with hydroxylic or carboxylic related groups. This suggests that a minimum hydrophobicity may be required for activity, but above that minimum there is no strong dependence.

Meso analogs:

$$\log(1/LD_{50}) = (1.66 \pm 0.67)\,\Delta r_v + (3.53 \pm 0.19) \tag{10a}$$

$$n = 9, \qquad r = 0.911$$

(±) Analogs (mono- and disubstituted):

$$\log(1/LD_{50}) = -(0.10 \pm 0.03)\,\Delta V_w - (0.02 \pm 0.006)(\Delta V_w)^2 + (3.09 \pm 0.31) \tag{10b}$$

$$n = 16, \qquad r = 0.920, \qquad s = 0.350$$

Other approaches to an understanding of lindane activity are also possible. Block and Newland (*4*) carried out molecular orbital calculations (CNDO/2) on lindane and three of its much weaker configurational isomers. Most important of their results was the finding that lindane has a substantially larger dipole moment than the other isomers (>1 Debye larger). This clearly has implications with respect to binding at polar sites, and lindane does, in fact, bind more strongly to cell membranes than do its less active isomers.

Natural and synthetic pyrethroids are among the most active pesticides known. The superiority of modern synthetic pyrethroids, typified by permethrin and fenvalerate, over a natural pyrethroid such as pyrethrin I is one of the great success stories in pesticide synthesis. Bioactivity has been improved into the incredible range of grams per acre. In addition, sufficient photostability has been developed through structure modification to make field use a practical reality. Natural pyrethroids are ineffective in the field due to rapid light catalyzed degradation, their main use being for household sprays. Pyrethroids are often combined with other insecticides in household sprays because they exhibit the phenomenon of rapid knockdown (paralysis). Ultimate death may result from the slower acting ingredient but rapid knockdown is a satisfying feature in a home aerosol spray. Pyrethroids attack the central nervous system in a manner

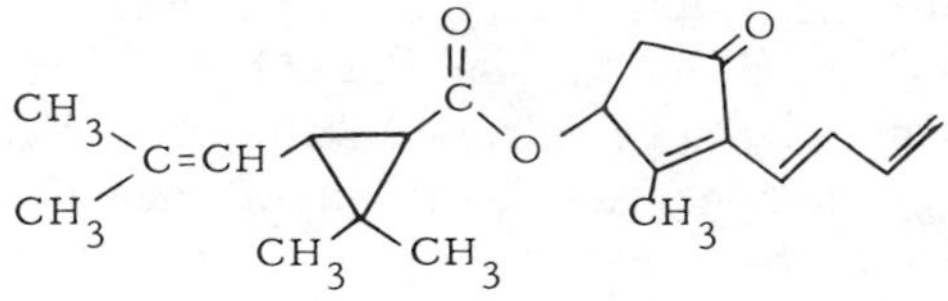

Pyrethrin I

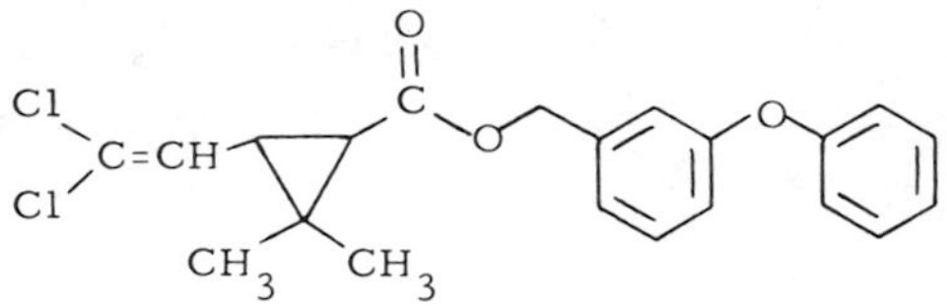

Permethrin

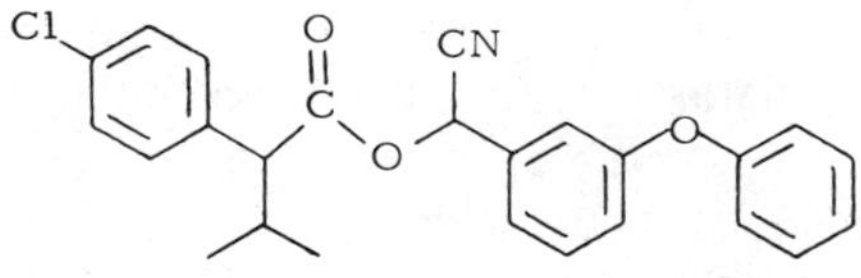

Fenvalerate

similar to DDT with probable interference of sodium ion transport. Based on this concept, Holan *et al.* (*48*) successfully devised active insecticides incorporating features of both DDT and pyrethroids. They found these compounds to have neurophysiological properties qualitatively similar to the pyrethroids.

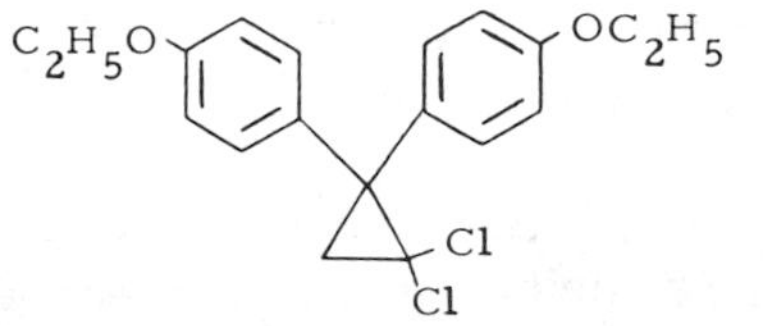

LD_{50}(housefly) = 0.13μg/insect

A study reported by Nishimura and Narahashi in 1978 (*74*) provides a sensitive method for pyrethroid evaluation by measuring direct action on an isolated nerve cord. Their most relevant measurement appears to be the concentration required to increase the frequency of spontaneous discharge to 200% of the control. This *in vitro* method has great promise for future structure–active studies much as direct AChE inhibitions have led to a greater understanding of phosphate and carbamate insecticides. It is interesting to note that afterdischarges in the isolated nerve did not correlate well with pyrethroid insecticidal activity. This is also true for direct AChE inhibition and phosphate or carbamate activities. It simply means that other factors are involved in whole insect toxicity and does not detract from the value of the *in vitro* study.

Only one systematic QSAR study of closely related pyrethroid series has been published though others have been discussed at meetings. This excellent study by Ford (*20*) deals with two relatively weak pyrethroid series based on chrysanthemumic acid. By regression analysis against standard parameters and indicator variables representing special effects, Ford obtained several satisfactory results correlating the log of relative toxicity and knockdown time. Although π/log P was the most frequently observed factor, dependence on electronic and steric effects were also observed in some cases. Unfortunately, the structures under analysis were quite different from more active synthetic pyrethroids, making extrapolation of the results uncertain. Plummer and Pincus (*81*) also report a significant dependence on π/log P for a series of related pyrethroids acting on southern armyworm.

Using a more general approach, Elliott and Janes (*16*) have discussed structure–activity features of the entire class by separating it into seven fragments and treating structural variations in each. Two major factors appear to dominate the expression of activity, namely, distribution and molecular shape. They pointed out that most of the potent pyrethroids have log *P* values near six, similar to DDT. This is characteristic of chemicals attacking the central nervous system, the large log *P* aiding efficient distribution into the phospholipid membrane. The second major factor is molecular shape as described in detail by Elliott and Janes (*16*) and also by Hopfinger and Battershell (*49*). Cis–trans isomerism about the cyclopropane ring is important with large activity differences between isomers. Chirality is also important, particularly when two or more chiral centers are present, greatest potency occurring when each has the "best" configuration. These factors and many more discussed by both teams lead us to picture pyrethroids as shape-dependent molecules that bind to a chiral but flexible cavity in the neuron. The site flexibility has permitted broad variations in structure without losing pyrethroid activity. However, these variations must be made within certain structural limits and some rules may not be broken. In chrysanthemum ester analogs, the gem-dimethyl grouping is essential for high activity, the ester may not be reversed, and the oxygen attachment must be a sp^3 carbon. In these analogs the introduction of the dihalovinyl group in combination with certain synthetic alcohols (e.g., *m*-phenoxybenzyl) has led to the greatest advances in activity and photostability. Until the advent of fenvalerate the chrysanthemum acid structure was considered an essential starting point for new pyrethroid synthesis. Experimental compounds with noncyclic structures and some that are not esters at all are appearing more frequently now. Research work is strongly focused on this field and fundamentally new structures with pyrethroid activity can be expected.

2. AChE Inhibitors

Any discussion of acetylcholinesterase inhibitors should begin with acetylcholinesterase itself. Because of its prevalence in animal systems we must be concerned with a variety of AChEs and even some of the nonneural butyryl- or pseudocholinesterases (ChE). Studies of the effects on bovine erythrocyte AChE and human plasma ChE of insecticides are almost as common as those on insect target AChEs. Inhibition of AChE in humans, animals, and insects can all result in death though the subsequent events following inhibition are different. There are many complex effects of AChE poisoning in mammals; most of the familiar signs, such as pupil contraction, salivation, and lachrymation, result from interference with the autonomic nervous system, (i.e., excessive parasympathetic stimulation). More important, however, are the effects on the neuromuscular junctions in the somatic system, such as fasciculation of the voluntary muscles and final paralysis, of special importance in the respiratory system. Asphyxiation is the ultimate cause of death in mammals. The best evidence for this is that artificial respiration prolongs or even saves life from normally fatal doses. Conversely, the cause of death in an insect is not as clear. Insects have an autonomic nervous system that controls the heart, gut, and spiracles, but there does not seem to be an opposing system as in mammals. The single system is described as the sympathetic or visceral system. However, there is no analogy to the mammalian ganglia, which contain peripheral synapses of the sympathetic system. It appears that the AChE in insects is confined to the central nervous system and that neuromuscular junctions are mediated by other transmitters. In addition, the insect neuromuscular junctions differ greatly from mammalian junctions. Whole muscles are activated by only a few axons, which branch freely, allowing several branches to enter each muscle fiber. There is no single-axon end plate as found in mammalian motor neurons. Another feature that must be appreciated is the difficulty of killing an insect through surgery. It is possible to separate the abdomen from the thorax (bisection) and insert a glass tube to circulate the gut contents. The head may be removed (decapitation) and replaced by a piece of wax to prevent dehydration. As might be expected after these two statements, the heart can also be excised and life goes on. Insects breathe by diffusion and many can live on metabolic water. Some of their own procedures are almost as drastic as the surgeries described. Some mites, chiggers for example, lack a suitable system for defecation and do so by splitting their sides when the need arises. The body repairs itself after each scission. With these facts in mind, let us return to AChE poisoning in the insect. Although the exact mechanism is unclear, the insect is believed to die from prolonged paralysis of the central nervous system due to accumulation of acetylcholine. The symptoms are sequential and predictable: increased irritability followed by hyperexcitability, then tremors in the whole body especially in the extremities, convulsions, loss of coordination, paralysis, and death. Flies undergo a characteristic spinning movement early in the sequence. In studies designed to follow AChE inhibition, the sequence of events can be related to the degree of inhibition. The exact cause of the terminal event is unknown but is probably not due to respiration failure as in the mammal.

Acetylcholinesterase as a class of enzymes is described in excellent detail by Engelhard *et al.* (*17*). This is substantially extended in a later review by O'Brien (*77*). The key role of AChE is to hydrolyze acetylcholine in a microsecond process following its discharge across the synaptic gap. This is a critical part of reestablishing the original state of the neural membrane before a second impulse can be transmitted. The now acetylated AChE must also be returned to its active state by a subsequent rapid hydrolysis step. The entire cycle, which includes resynthesis of acetylcholine from choline and acetic acid (choline acetylase), occurs within milliseconds. To achieve rates of this magnitude the anionic site of AChE is of critical importance. Situated about 5 Å from the esteratic site and believed due to a glutamic acid residue, this site assures diffusion-controlled ion pairing with acetylcholine in the binding step. The esteratic site consists of a serine residue activated by an imidazole group (histidine) and possibly further assisted by a hydrogen-bonding tyrosine hydroxyl.

In all cases of inhibition by insecticidal phosphates or carbamates the rate of reaction of AChE with these neutral compounds is much slower than that with the charged acetylcholine. Moreover, whereas acetylated AChE is regenerated in a millisecond process, carbamoylated AChE requires hours and phosphorylated AChE requires days. In addition, phosphorylated AChE undergoes a subsequent aging reaction (dealkylation), which results in permanently inhibited enzyme. This forces the animal or insect system into the very slow process of synthesizing new AChE under gene control. Workers who are partially inhibited by carbamates can return to work after a few hours of rest. The inhibition is fully reversible. Those inhibited by phosphates are generally segregated from further possible contact for a month or more until their AChE level has returned to normal. It is interesting to note that in humans the classical symptoms do not appear until most of the AChE has been inhibited. This is the reason behind the regular monitoring of AChE in apparently healthy pesticide scientists and other workers exposed to phosphate inhibitors. Any significant lowering of true AChE or pseudo ChE requires immediate reassignment to other work. An inhibited individual is highly vulnerable to a normally nonlethal dose of an AChE poison.

In addition to the esteratic and anionic sites, there appears to be a large hydrophobic area adjacent to the anionic site. According to binding studies by Steinberg *et al.* (*85*), this is a conformationally flexible, hydrophobic area that tends to assume a near planar form. Another study by Abou-Donia *et al.* (*2*), using acetylcholine analogs, supports this concept and indicates a planar or slightly curved surface area with a radius greater than 10 Å. They also support the presence of two hydrophobic areas within the anionic site. Excellent insecticides with dimensions much greater than the natural substrate acetylcholine are good evidence that strong hydrophobic binding occurs beyond the anionic site. In fact, the multiplicity of available binding sites may eventually account for a structural anomaly of aromatic phosphates and carbamates. Substituted phenyl phosphates behave as if binding to a very restricted cavity and only small meta and para groups are accommodated. Phenyl carbamates, on the other hand, behave as though there is plenty of room and may have rather large substituents, especially in the meta position. This would be quite acceptable if the aryl rings were binding in slightly different sites. Carbamate substituents are either electronically neutral or only slightly polar. Binding should be of the nonspecific hydrophobic type. Phosphate substituents are strongly polar and may force the ring to bind in a more constrained position to take advantage of dipolar interactions.

No AChE important to agriculture has been highly purified and sequenced, so exact structure in the sense of α-chymotrypsin, which displays a similar mechanism, is unavailable. Because of the presence of not one, but several AChE isozymes in many insects, the problem is formidable. Thus Tripathi and O'Brien (*87*) isolated four AChE isozymes from the head and three from the thorax of the common housefly by gel electrophoresis. Each of the seven isozymes was different kinetically and responded differently to a set of standard phosphate inhibitors. Thoracic isozymes were more sensitive to inhibition than head isozymes in agreement with studies showing that knockdown and death correlate best with thoracic inhibition. A later study by Zettler and Brady (*102*) showed five electrophoretic bands having cholinesterase activity in thoracic homogenates from the housefly. Thus the overall mechanistic problem is quite complex.

Structure–activity studies on cholinergic insecticides date back to 1956, and much of the early data on the direct *in vitro* inhibition of AChE is treated ably by Hansch and Deutsch (*37*). Many studies have since been carried out and we will select those that provide the most relevant bearing on mechanism. Three main classes will be considered: phosphates and phosphonates together, phosphoramidates, and carbamates. Each of these is a broad class with enormous experimental variations covering aliphatic, aromatic, and heterocyclic types. In the direct inhibition studies reviewed by Hansch and Deutsch, the insecticide must be in the active form, i.e., the oxon form for phosphates, phosphonates, and phosphoramidates. Unmodified *N*-methylcarbamates are also direct inhibitors. In studies on living insects, the insecticides may be in the thion form or any other proinsecticide form that the target can activate metabolically.

The early *in vitro* study of paraoxon analogs by Fukuto and Metcalf (*24*) was a mechanistic breakthrough in the understanding of AChE inhibition, forming the pattern for many later studies. Plotting Hammett's σ constant against the rate of hydrolysis and also against the pI_{50} for inhibition of fly-head AChE, they observed a similar response to the electronic effect. It was clear that a phenolate leaving group was involved in both reactions, establishing hydrolysis by hydroxide ion is a simple model for nucleophilic attack by the serine hydroxyl. There was considerable scatter in the pI_{50} versus σ plot and this was correctly attributed to steric effects. A later study of these data by Hansch (*39*) quantified and refined the observations of Fukuto and Metcalf (Eq. 11) (*39*). The strong dependence on

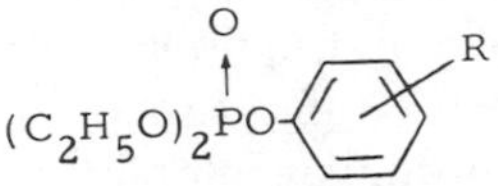 versus Flyhead AChE

$$pI_{50} = (2.45 \pm 0.54)\sigma^- - (0.56 \pm 0.20)E_s + (4.82 \pm 0.41) \quad (11)$$
$$n = 13, \quad r = 0.962, \quad s = 0.408$$

σ^-, a more appropriate electronic factor for phenolate leaving groups, is modified by a smaller steric effect. The observed steric effect is clearly related to molecular fit in the enzyme–inhibitor complex, because the meta and para groups are too distant to affect phosphorylation of the esteratic site. No dependence on π/log *P* was observed, indicating that these substituents do not bond hydrophobically to the enzyme. In a complementary study of some paraoxon-related phosphonates, Fukuto *et al.* (*25*) evaluated data that were later shown by Hansch and Deutsch (*37*) to reveal a steric effect at the reaction center (Eq. 12). Although the electrophilicity of the phosphorus atom was of major importance, the electronic spread in the R group was very small and only the steric effect was observed. When

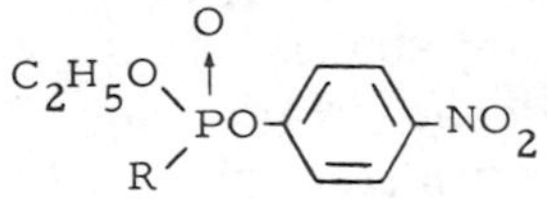 versus Flyhead AChE, bimolecular rate constants

R = alkyl, phenyl

$$\log k_e = 3.74E_s + 7.54 \quad (12)$$
$$n = 13, \quad r = 0.901, \quad s = 0.749$$

coupled with the leaving group correlation of the paraoxon set, this analysis greatly strengthens our mechanistic view of the inhibition. As in the paraoxon study, hydrophobic binding was not a significant factor. In living insects, however, it is possible to observe a dependence on π/log *P*, probably in relation to transport. A recent study of fire ant toxicity by a homologous series of carboalkoxyparathion analogs revealed a π dependence as the only significant factor (*19*) (Eq. 13).

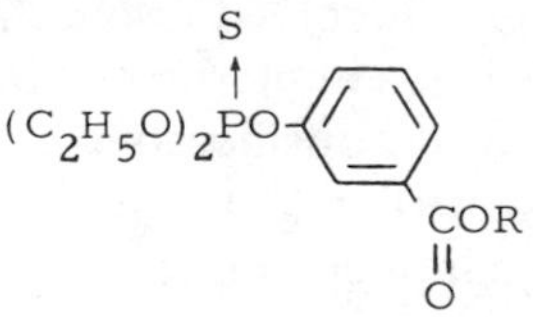 versus Imported fire ant

$$\log(\%\ \text{kill}) = (-0.17 \pm 0.08)\pi + 2.07 \tag{13}$$

$$n = 7, \quad r = 0.928, \quad s = 0.08$$

Phosphoramidate insecticides with phenolic leaving groups show factors in common with the paraoxon class. Thus, Neely *et al.* (*70*) found an excellent linear relation between the bimolecular log k for AChE inhibition and the vibrational frequency of the P—O—Ar stretch for ring substituted phosphoramidates (Eq. 14). No regression was performed but the plot is nearly perfect except for two *tert*-butyl-substituted analogs that appear to fall on a separate, parallel line. Because stretching frequency often correlates with σ constants, this correlation strongly suggests an electronic effect operating on the phenoxy leaving group, similar to that in the paraoxon series. It is interesting to note that Fukuto and Metcalf (*24*) found a similar relation between pI_{50} and CM^{-1} (POAr) in addition to the $pI_{50}-\sigma$ relation for paraoxons. It seems clear then that electronic effects on the leaving groups of both systems are operating in parallel. If the aryl group is held constant, the aliphatic RO and R_2N groups attached to phos-

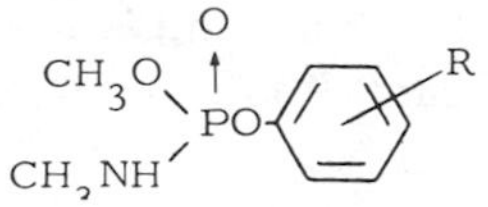

versus Flyhead AChE, bimolecular rate constant

$$\log k = a(CM)^{-1}(\text{POAr}) + b \tag{14}$$

$$n = 10\ (2\ \text{outliers}), \quad r > 0.95$$

phorus can be systematically varied. Variations in the RO group are of limited interest. In nearly all known cases, R = CH_3 or C_2H_5 are the two most active analogs. Activity may still be high when R = n-C_3H_7 or i-C_3H_7 but drops to low levels for larger groups. Because of the very short sets, regression analysis is usually not performed. For some reason substitution of the identically placed RNH or R_2N group is a more forgiving process, the larger groups and longer sets having good activity. Neely and Whitney (*72*) provided some valuable insight by varying the alkyl group in some RNH-phosphoramidates while holding all other structures constant. Rather than use aliphatic electronic and steric constants, they determined the reactivity factor as the rate of hydrolysis in 0.1N NaOH at 50°C. This factor, as log k_h, was regressed sucessfully with π against the bimolecular rate constant for flyhead AChE inhibition (Eq. 15) (*72*). Because we now know that the alkyl groups have essentially identical electronic effects, it is clear that the main factor in log k_h is steric. This can be seen by a simple scrutiny of the log k_h data, which range from 1.78 (R = H) to −1.0 (R =

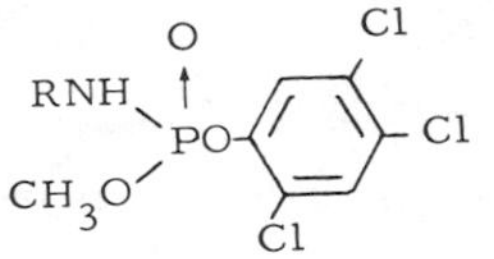

versus Flyhead AChE, bimolecular rate constant

$$\log k = 0.91\pi + 1.17 \log k_h + 3.21 \qquad (15)$$

$$n = 9, \quad r = 0.96, \quad s = 0.315$$

t-Bu). All other points have values between these two extremes. These results are supported and extended by a similar data set collected by Fukuto *et al.* (*26*) and analyzed by Hansch and Deutsch (*37*). The data set is nearly identical, having two fewer RNH groups but including $(CH_3)_2N$ as a single disubstitution example. The best equation found by Hansch and Deutsch (*37*) includes E_s and σ^* together (Eq. 16). At the time, this was interpreted as an expected combination of steric and electronic effects operating to shield the phosphorus atom and simultaneously vary its electrophilicity in the nucleophilic attack by serine hydroxyl. This is quite logical as both effects should be present in the bimolecular reaction. However, we now know that σ^* is highly colinear with E_s due to a poor

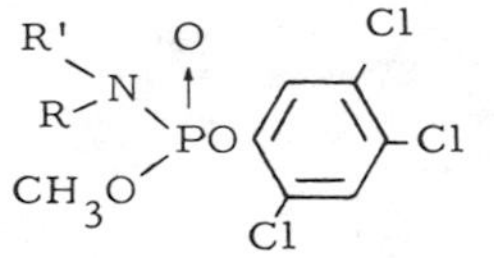

versus Flyhead AChE, bimolecular rate constant

$$\log k = 2.36E_s - 3.91\sigma^* + 4.95 \qquad (16)$$

$$n = 8, \quad r = 0.939, \quad s = 0.438$$

separation of steric and electronic effects. Alkyl groups are almost electroneutral, and no significant electronic span is present in these data. Because the steric dependence on E_s accounts for most of the variance ($r = 0.875$), the best interpretation may be to accept the lower correlation with E_s alone. Steric effects in phosphoramidate insecticides are quite consistent from one class to another. Zerba and Fukuto (*101*) have recently studied some phosphoramidate insecticides related to phoxim. Inhibition studies against housefly AChE and bovine erythrocyte AChE both reveal a primary dependence on the steric size of the R_2N group (Eq. 17) (*101*). All of these regressions indicate that the same mechanistic factors are operating as in the paraoxon phosphates and phosphonate sets. The leaving group depends on electron delocalization while direct attack on phosphorus involves steric and probably small electronic

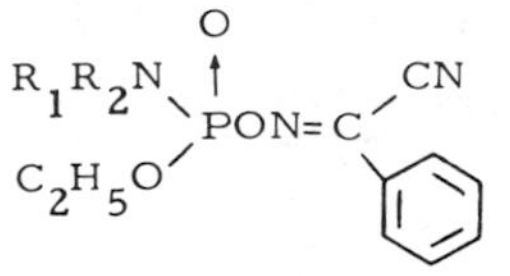

versus Flyhead AChE, bimolecular rate constants

$$\log k = (1.33 \pm 0.65)E_s + 5.23 \quad (17)$$

$$n = 7, \qquad r = 0.923$$

effects. These effects are all consistent with current theory on the mechanism of AChE inhibition.

Recent studies of aromatic *N*-methylcarbamate insecticides in large sets have revealed some surprising complexities not observed in earlier work. For this reason we will treat the earlier studies (1964–1966) separately from the later work (1974–1979). In the earliest work on para-substituted xylenyl carbamates, Metcalf *et al.* (*64*) defined an essential difference between phenyl carbamates and phenyl phosphates. They observed a completely different electronic dependence of pI_{50} (FHAChE) over a broad range of para substituents (Eq. 18) (*64*). Although a reasonably linear plot of pI_{50} versus σ was obtained, the slope was negative rather than positive as found in the paraoxon series. This means that strong electronegative groups such as NO_2, CN, and CH_3SO_2 produced the least active compounds, whereas electropositive groups such as CH_3

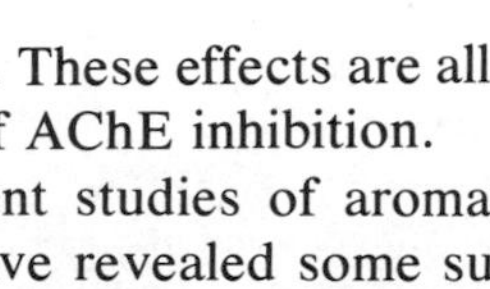

versus Flyhead AChE, I_{50}

$$pI_{50} = -0.83\sigma_p + 6.41 \quad (18)$$

$$n = 12, \qquad r \doteq 0.9$$

and CH_3O produced the most active. Thus we have the first major difference between carbamates and phosphates. Follow-up studies on ortho-, meta-, and para-substituted phenyl *N*-methylcarbamates by Metcalf and Fukuto (*65*) provided data for regression analyses by Hansch and Deutsch (*37*). In a foretaste of later studies, Hansch and Deutsch (*37*) found that whereas the π dependence was similar, the sensitivity to the electronic factor was quite different in the meta and para positions (Eqs. 19a,b). In addition, their correlations of the carefully measured pI_{50} values were rather poor, indicating that other factors were still to be found. In most cases pI_{50} values for enzyme inhibitions are highly reproducible. If the correct factors are selected, correlations with $r > 0.95$ should be achieved. Failure to do so is good evidence for the presence of unsuspected factors. The presence of the hydrophobic binding parameter was

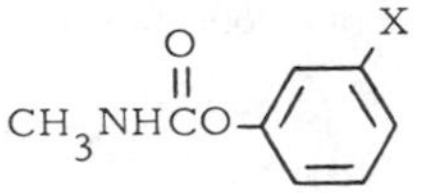

versus Flyhead AChE

$$pI_{50} = (0.78 \pm 0.20)\pi - (1.41 \pm 0.72)\sigma + 4.62 \quad (19a)$$

$$n = 30, \quad r = 0.845, \quad s = 0.508$$

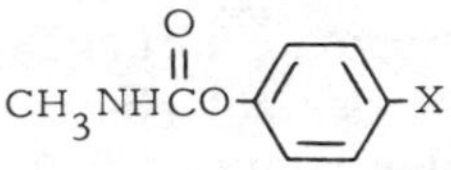

versus Flyhead AChE

$$pI_{50} = (0.71 \pm 0.20)\pi - (0.87 \pm 0.54)\sigma + 3.49 \quad (19b)$$

$$n = 23, \quad r = 0.839, \quad s = 0.399$$

clearly verified in an enzyme inhibition study by Kohn *et al.* (*56*) in which the electronic factor was suppressed. Regression analysis by Magee (*62a*) showed excellent optimal behavior (Eq. 20) (*56,62a*). However, the data

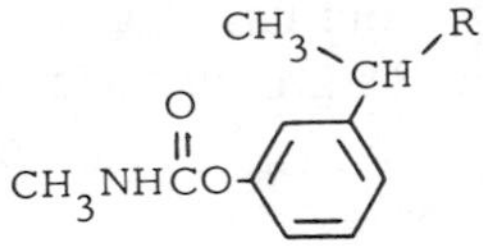

versus bovine erythrocyte AChE, I_{50}

R = CH_3—C_8H_{17}

$$pI_{50} = (1.19 \pm 1.07)\pi - (0.38 \pm 0.23)\pi^2 + 0.83 \quad (20)$$

$$n = 8, \quad r = 0.954, \quad s = 0.290$$

were of sufficient quality that a plot of pI_{50} versus π showed smooth curvilinear but distinctly nonparabolic behavior. Thus the binding properties of this compound set may be unique. It is interesting to note that the optimum falls near R = C_3H_7, corresponding to the commercial corn root-worm insecticide Bux (bufencarb).

The later work by Fujita and co-workers (1974–1979) permits a more detailed description of carbamate insecticide behavior. In preparation for these studies, Fujita *et al.* (*22*) estimated the electronic and hydrophobic substituent parameters of ortho-, meta-, and para-substituted phenyl *N*-methylcarbamates through the base-catalyzed hydrolysis rates and the octanol–water partition coefficient. Particular emphasis was placed on ortho-substituted carbamates, some of which are very potent insecticides.

An excellent linear correlation was obtained between the bimolecular hydrolysis constant and the ionization constant of the corresponding phenol (Eq. 21) (*23*). In addition, an excellent correlation of log k_2 with Ham-

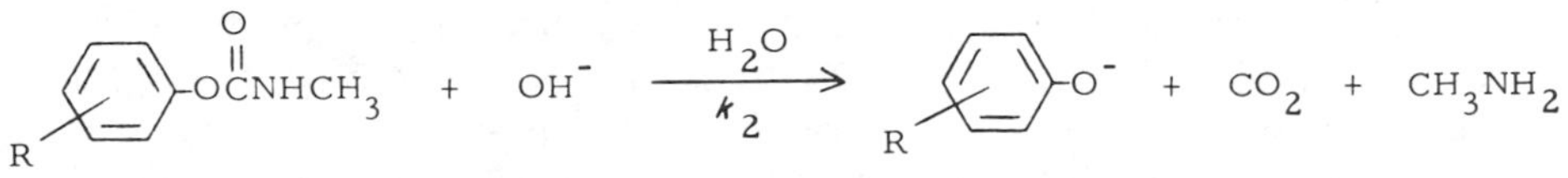

$$\log k_2 = (1.24 \pm 0.07) \log K_A + (14.62 \pm 0.62) \qquad (21)$$

$$n = 26, \quad r = 0.992, \quad s = 0.173$$

mett's σ and σ^- constants was obtained for the meta- and para-substituted carbamates. In an unpublished study of these data by Magee (*62a*), the ortho-substituted carbamates were shown to correlate poorly with σ_p^-, but very nicely with Charton's σ_L and σ_D constants (Eq. 22) (*62a*). Incorporation of Charton's steric constants was not significant, indicating that steric effects are minimal. What is most unusual about the ortho cases is the low resonance contribution (% R = 21.0). A similar factoring of the para cases shows over 50% resonance. This divergence between ortho- and para-substituted carbamates explains the failure of σ_p^- to correlate the ortho set.

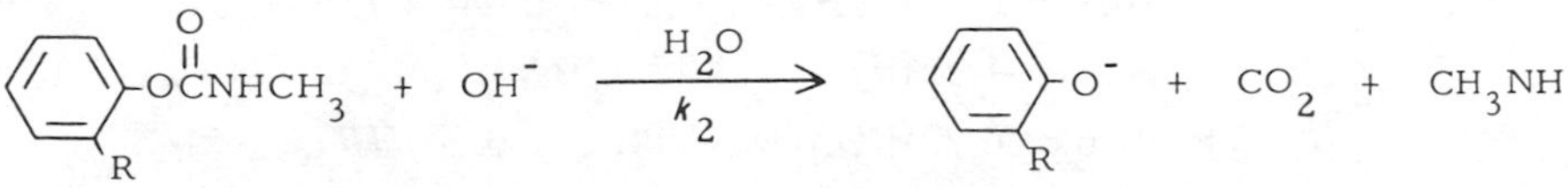

$$\log k_2 = (5.05 \pm 0.57)\sigma_L + (1.34 \pm 0.50)\sigma_D + 1.81 \qquad (22)$$

$$n = 15, \quad r = 0.987, \quad s = 0.263$$

In later work, Fujita *et al.* (*23*) and Nishioka *et al.* (*75*) studied the inhibition of AChE by 53 ortho-, meta-, and para-substituted phenyl *N*-methylcarbamates. The association constants ($1/K_d$) for bovine erythrocyte AChE varied 1000-fold while the carbamoylation constants were rather insensitive to a wide range of structural variation. Correlation of the association constant data, $\log(1/K_d)$, revealed a number of complex features in the binding step. Position dependent values and the introduction of an indicator variable (*HB*) to correct for specific hydrogen bonding of some groups (OR, NO_2, NMe_2, CN, and acyl) were necessary to reduce the variance in the data. In addition, a biphasic electronic effect with $\rho > 0$ and $\rho < 0$ was proposed to account for two distinct mechanisms leading to the same tetrahedral intermediate in the carbamoylation step.

Despite these complexities, their analysis of the data is consistent with the body of evidence supporting the mechanism of AChE inhibition. Extending these concepts to live insects allowed Kamoshita *et al.* (*51,52*) to analyze the insecticidal activity of these carbamates against housefly and the smaller brown planthopper. Satisfactory correlations were obtained involving position-dependent values, hydrogen-bonding constant (*HB*) for special groups, and biphasic electronic effects. In brief, the same factors observed for *in vitro* inhibition of AChE were also found in the studies of live insects.

Goldblum *et al.* (*32*) has formulated a structure–activity relation for a set of 269 *N*-methylcarbamates that inhibit flyhead acetylcholinesterase. This massive study included single and multiple substitutions of nearly every possible type in a single expression. The twelve descriptive parameters included binding (*MR*), steric, and electronic factors, as well as indicator variables for charged and hydrogen-bonding substituents (Eq. 23) (*32*). In all, these variables accounted for 80% of the variance in the data and predicted the pI_{50} within 0.5 log unit or a factor of ± 3 for a concentration range of 1 million. The equation is exceptionally robust with over 22 data points/variable.

$$
\begin{aligned}
pI_{50} = {} & (0.56 \pm 0.08)MR_{3,4,5} + (1.56 \pm 0.20)MR_2 \\
& - (0.61 \pm 0.09)E_s - (0.94 \pm 0.19)\left(\sum \sigma^-_{o,p} + \sigma_m\right) \\
& + (1.43 \pm 0.31)CHG - (0.23 \pm 0.04)(MR_2)^2 \\
& - (5.24 \pm 1.27)F^2_{2,6} + (3.47 \pm 0.90)F_{2,6} \\
& + (0.66 \pm 0.22)RGMR - (0.62 \pm 0.22)HB \\
& - (0.052 \pm 0.02)(MR_3)^2 - (0.56 \pm 0.29)E_{S_2}E_{S_6} \\
& + (3.46 \pm 0.21) \qquad (23)
\end{aligned}
$$

$$n = 269, \quad r = 0.892, \quad s = 0.485$$

A conclusion of the relation impinging on future design is the need for electroneutral substitution ($\Sigma\ \sigma = 0$), either strong attracting or releasing substituents making weaker inhibitors.

A completely different approach to AChE inhibition by aryl carbamates has been taken by Hetnarski and O'Brien (*43–46*). Working with simple para-substituted phenyl *N*-methylcarbamates (*43*), they observed a linear relationship between association constants with tetracyanoethylene (TCNE) and the pI_{50} for inhibition of bovine erythrocyte AChE. This was strengthened by a related study involving para-substituted benzyl *N*-methylcarbamates (*44*), leading to the concept that a charge–transfer complex (CTC) was involved in AChE binding of carbamate insecticides. Hetnarski and O'Brien defined a charge–transfer constant (C_T =

$\log K_X - \log K_H$) where K_X is the association constant for CTC formation with TCNE of the substituted, and K_H is that for the unsubstituted carbamate (*46*). The definition is identical in form to that of the Hammett σ constant. In a parallel paper, they used the C_T constant with the hydrophobic constant (π) to correlate K_d values for inhibition of bovine erythrocyte AChE (*45*) (Eqs. 24a,b). The success of these correlations for binding of simple aryl carbamates to AChE does not necessarily require the charge–transfer complex as an event inasmuch as CTCs are known to correlate with simple electronic and steric factors. Nevertheless, the correlations are highly provocative and certainly deserve more extensive study.

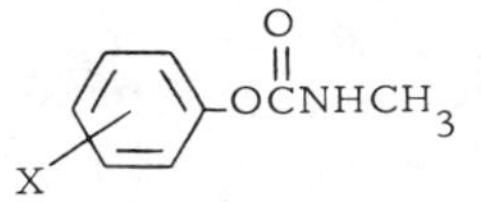

versus Bovine erythrocyte AChE

$$X = \text{para}, \quad K_d = (-3.48 \pm 0.36)C_T - (2.65 \pm 0.22)\pi + 5.88 \tag{24a}$$
$$n = 11, \quad r = 0.989, \quad s = 0.367$$
$$X = \text{meta}, \quad K_d = (-1.23 \pm 0.36)C_T - (1.96 \pm 0.27)\pi + 2.44 \tag{24b}$$
$$n = 9, \quad r = 0.958, \quad s = 0.322$$

Most phosphate, phosphoramidate, and carbamate insecticides that inhibit AChE and pseudo-ChE are also effective as inhibitors of related esterases. The inhibition of insect aliesterase can be more rapid than that of AChE but does not appear to have life threatening consequences. Thus Khasawinah *et al.* (*53*) found complete inhibition of aliesterase in houseflies by methamidophos in 1.5 h, during which time over 90% of the AChE remained intact. Knockdown and mortality were observed nearly 8 h after an LD_{50} treatment, correlating with complete inhibition of thoracic AChE. Hammock *et al.* (*34*) have isolated three esterase fractions from cockroach hemolymph that are active in cleaving juvenile hormone (JH III, terminal epoxy of methyl farnesoate). They observed that phosphates, carbamates, and especially phosphoramidates were strong inhibitors of the JH esterase fractions. It is clear from these observations that the use of AChE inhibitors as insecticides can lead to multiple target effects.

3. OXPHOS Inhibitors

Oxidative phosphorylation provides a mechanism for conserving part of the exotherm from the oxidation of glucose to CO_2 and water. In the transfer of electrons from the Krebs cycle through reduced NAD to oxygen, several of the steps have coupled reactions that absorb free energy by converting ADP and phosphate ion to ATP (*82*). Inhibition or "uncoupling" of these reactions is a life-threatening event due both to thermal imbalance and the loss of ATP required to drive much of the sustaining biochemistry. When an uncoupler is fed to a rat, its respiratory rate increases and its body temperature rises as would be expected if oxidation energy is not conserved as ATP but is lost as heat. Because of the generality of the effect, many uncouplers are toxic to mammals, plants, fungi, bacteria, mites, and some insects. We shall concern ourselves with mite and insect toxicity.

Although organophosphate and carbamate insecticides are often equally toxic to insects and mites, many of the OXPHOS inhibitors that are highly toxic to mites show only low to moderate insect toxicity (*55*). There also appear to be more chemical classes that kill mites than those that kill insects. One might argue that mites are more primitive animals than insects. This may be true but they are sophisticated enough biochemically to develop resistance to all of the known insecticidal and miticidal classes. Unfortunately, not many QSAR studies have been carried out on mites, in particular, for the important class of dinitrophenols. For this reason, we need to rely on the study of a simpler system in order to deduce some of the mechanistic details. Fortunately, Hansch *et al.* (*36*) have done regression studies on a series of phenols that inhibit phosphorylation in yeast. They concluded that pK_a and lipophilicity were the most important variables correlating the data. There was no evidence of a steric effect. The equation shown was reworked by Magee who found the π^2 term to be significant (Eqs. 25a,b) (*36,62a*). When this equation is converted to its equivalent σ form ($-0.57pK_a = 1.14\sigma$), it is seen to be very similar to an equation relating phenol toxicity to *Aspergillus niger* (Eq. 26) (*40,62a*). The similarity of the regression coefficients strongly suggests that the fungus is killed by uncoupling of oxidative phosphorylation.

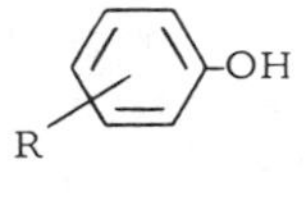

Inhibition of phosphorylation in yeast

$$\log(1/C) = (1.14 \pm 0.49)\sum \pi - (0.37 \pm 0.27)\overline{\sum \pi^2} - (0.57 \pm 0.11)pK_a + 7.73 \quad (25a)$$

$$\log(1/C) = (1.14 \pm 0.49)\sum \pi - (0.37 \pm 0.27)\overline{\sum \pi^2} + (1.14 \pm 0.21)\sum \sigma + 7.73 \quad (25b)$$

$$n = 14, \quad r = 0.968, \quad s = 0.304$$

The history of the dinitrophenols is relevant to their dependence on lipophilicity for high activity. In 1892, 2,4-dinitro-6-methylphenol was first

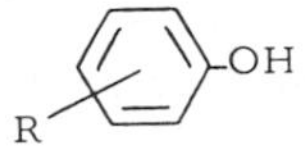

versus *Aspergillus niger*

$$\log(1/C) = (1.44 \pm 0.42) \sum \pi - (0.25 \pm 0.12) \overline{\sum \pi^2} + (1.01 \pm 0.63) \sum \sigma + 2.25 \quad (26)$$

$$n = 18, \quad r = 0.963, \quad s = 0.196$$

used as the potassium salt for control of the nun moth in Europe (*84*). The sodium salt was also used as a herbicide. By 1945 the ortho-methyl group was replaced by *sec*-butyl producing a compound (dinoseb) of superior contact and stomach activity on insects and mites. Dinoseb is also a potent weed killer and is limited to dormant use on fruit trees. From 1946 to 1965 increasingly lipophilic phenol esters were developed that showed high fungicidal as well as herbicidal and miticidal properties. The most impressive of these is dinocap (Karathane), a dinitrophenyl crotonate with a *sec*-octyl group on the ring. Dinocap is a mixture of isomers (2,4- and 2,6-dinitro) one of which is shown below. The progression to more lipo-

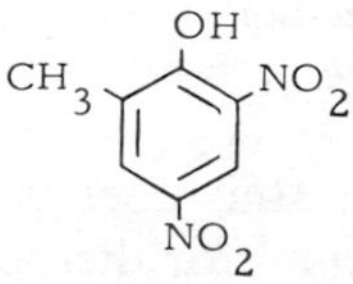

1892

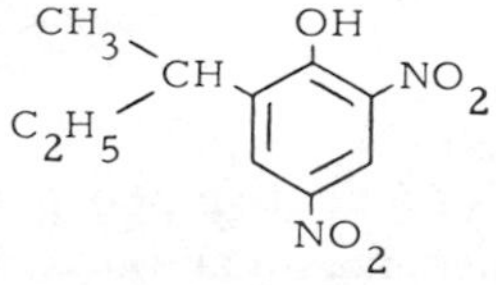

1946

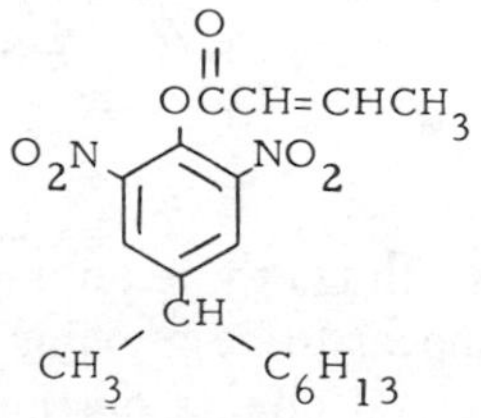

1947

philic compounds with superior activity is an example of gradual optimization in a period when structure–activity relations were not understood.

The uncoupling activity of a large set of miticidal hydrazones was subjected to regression analysis by Büchel and Draber (*9*) in an effort to determine mechanistic factors. Unfortunately, miticidal activity was not reported along with the pI_{50} data on rat liver mitochondria. Despite the size of the set ($n = 60$), the entire pI_{50} range was only 2.13, and 50 of the members fell within 1.0 pI_{50} unit. Nevertheless, by using position dependent parameters, they were able to show that electronic (σ) and binding (π) factors were of prime importance but that steric effects made a minor contribution. These are the same factors operating in the dinitrophenols and like the phenols, ionization of the NH group is important. A linear relation was found between acidity in 50% ethanol–water and σ (r =0.969) for 20 of the meta, para-substituted hydrazones. These obser-

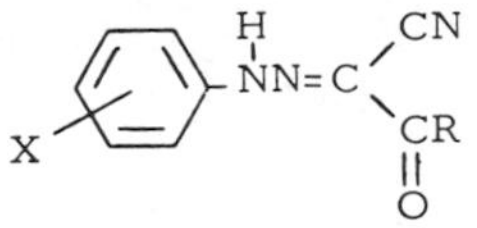

versus Rat liver mitochondria

X = CH_3, CHF_2, Cl, CN, NO_2, SCF_3, SO_2R (R = CH_3, C_2H_5, CF_3)
R = CH_3, $C(CH_3)_3$, OCH_3, OC_2H_5

vations strongly support a mechanistic link between the hydrazones and phenols as OXPHOS inhibitors.

4. Other Types

Chlordimeform (Galecron) is a novel miticide, ovicide, and larvicide. It shows excellent activity against susceptible and phosphate-resistant mites. It is especially effective in controlling larvae of the rice stem borer and is more effective against lindane-resistant than against lindane-susceptible strains. Although reported by Abo-Khatwa and Hollings-

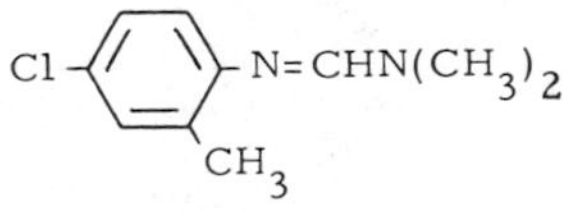

Chlordimeform (Galecron)

worth (*1*) to be an uncoupler of oxidative phosphorylation, this does not appear to be a major lethal mechanism and does not account for the observed effects on the central nervous system. A study by Beeman and Matsumura (*3*) shows that chlordimeform inhibits monoamine oxidase from combined cockroach heads and ventral nerve cords (I_{50} = 4.43 × 10^{-4} M). The authors suggest the possibility that uncoupling may contribute to chlordimeform toxicity but point out that the symptoms of poisoning in cockroaches differ from those induced by dinitrophenols. Their experiments strongly suggest a relation between MAO inhibition and cockroach toxicity. The arguments are weakened, however, by the current lack of understanding of the biochemistry of MAO in insects.

The most interesting study of the chlordimeform mode of action was carried out by Lund *et al.* (*61*) who examined behavioral effects of sublethal doses in tobacco hornworm larvae. When placed on tomato plants previously sprayed with chlordimeform, the initial feeding response was normal. After a few minutes, however, a fine tremor appeared near the head and the larvae crawled or fell off the leaf. Recovery occurred in an hour, and the cycle of brief feeding, tremors, and departure was repeated. The overall result was a considerable reduction in plant consumption at doses far below that needed for direct kill.

Similar responses were observed when applied to tobacco budworm, alfalfa looper, and cabbage looper. For five related chlordimeform analogs excellent linear relations were found between reduced leaf feeding (AC_{50}), tremors (TD_{50}), and the CNS excitation threshold (mol/liter). All correlations were better than $r = 0.95$. The authors make the point that these and certain other behavioral actions are ultimately fatal. Thus the distinction between "lethal" and "behavioral" doses is not sharply defined. They illustrate this by correlating the LD_{50} values of ten formamidines to adult spider mites with the CNS excitation threshold measured on the abdominal ganglion of tobacco hornworm, a set of values strongly related to tremors and reduced leaf feeding. An excellent log–log correlation was obtained ($r = 0.99$), demonstrating a close relationship between the lethal dose of one species and the behavioral dose of another. Studies on the isolated abdominal ganglion of tobacco hornworm support the concept that chlordimeform acts on noncholinergic synapses of the central nervous system.

D. Insecticide Synergists

In combining two or more insecticides to cover a broader spectrum of crop protection, it is frequently found that performance of one of the insecticides is substantially magnified. This synergistic effect results when one insecticide is a better substrate for a degrading enzyme than the other and thus permits more of the synergized compound to reach the target. Although these effects are often observed and can be used to advantage, we will concern ourselves with pure synergists that have no insecticidal activity when applied alone. Most of the known synergists inhibit the microsomal oxidase system (mfo) and are especially active when combined with the easily degradable aryl *N*-methylcarbamates. In general, synergist combinations with carbamates can be highly effective in topical applications and direct contact sprays. However, they do not fare as well in most field applications, possibly because the lipophilic synergists tend to be chromatographed apart from the more polar insecticides in plant tissue.

An extensive study on the structural requirements of 1,3-benzodioxole synergists was carried out by Wilkinson *et al.* (*95*). Some of their data were analyzed by Hansch (*38*) in an attempt to identify the mechanistic features of the action. Using housefly toxicity of carbaryl synergized by a related series of benzodioxoles, Hansch (*38*) was able to establish both binding and electron factors (Eq. 27). Binding showed optimum behavior corresponding to log P_o of 3.8 for the ideal lipophilic character of a synergist for carbaryl on flies. The electronic factor proved unusual and strongly indicative of a radical intermediate. Correlations with several standard σ sets (σ_p, σ_I, σ_p^+) were poor but a special set derived from the homolytic phenylation of benzene derivatives ($\sigma^\cdot$) correlated very well. The two most activating substituents for 1,3-benzodioxoles were nitro and methoxy, groups that normally have opposite effects except in some homolytic reactions. Because replacement of the dioxole hydrogens with deuterium reduced synergistic activity, the formation of a stabilized radical on the dioxomethylene group was strongly implied. Hansch suggested that this relatively stable and lipophilic radical could remain bound to the site that normally oxidizes and desorbs the carbamate insecticide.

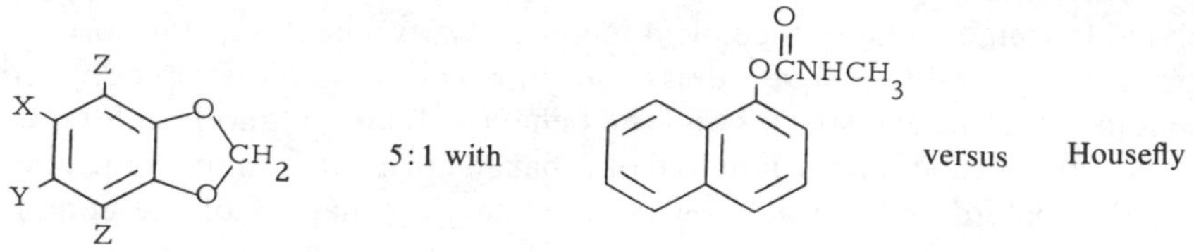

$$SR = (\mathrm{LD}_{50}\ \text{carbaryl})/(\mathrm{LD}_{50}\ \text{carbaryl} + \text{synergist})$$

$$\log(SR) = 0.67\pi - 0.20\pi^2 + 1.32\sigma^\cdot + 1.61 \qquad (27)$$

$$n = 13, \qquad r = 0.929, \qquad s = 0.171$$

Studies by Wilkinson *et al.* (*96,97*) showed substituted imidazoles to be potent inhibitors of microsomal epoxidation, hyroxylation, and N-demethylation in enzyme preparations from rat liver and armyworm gut. In the paper with Hetnarski and Hicks (*97*) measurements of the inhibitory activity of forty-seven 1-, 2-, and 4(5)-aryl-substituted imidazoles against the microsomal preparations were reported. Many of the 1- and 4(5)-substituted compounds were among the most potent inhibitors of microsomal epoxidase and hydroxylase yet reported ($I_{50} = 10^{-7}$ to 10^{-8} *M*). Spectral studies show that aryl imidazoles bind strongly to cytochrome P-450, the suspected site of oxidative activity. As synergists for carbaryl against houseflies, the 4(5)-arylimidazoles proved inactive. Several of the 1-arylimidazoles, however, were extremely active synergists. The most active compound (aryl = 2,3-dimethylphenyl) was one of the strongest synergists yet described. In a related study of homologous 1-alkylimidazoles, Wilkinson *et al.* (*96*) found optimal behavior both *in vitro* (pI_{50}) and *in vivo*. Using carbaryl against houseflies, the synergistic ratio (SR) was measured for imidazole and 12 homologous 1-alkylimidazoles. A satisfactory correlation with π and π^2 was obtained accounting for 85%

of the variance in the data (Eq. 28) (*96*). Although the correlation is acceptable, an examination of the plotted data indicates a complex curvilinear dependence.

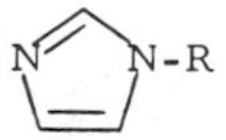

5:1 with

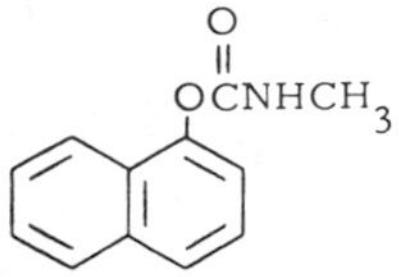

versus Housefly

R = H, $CH_3—C_{12}H_{25}$

$$\log(SR) = 0.49\pi - 0.038\pi^2 + 0.44 \qquad (28)$$

$$n = 13, \quad r = 0.922, \quad s = 0.243$$

An extensive series of 1,2,3-benzothiadiazoles was evaluated by Gil and Wilkinson (*30,31*) as carbaryl synergists and as inhibitors of microsomal preparations from rat liver and armyworm. Fifty-six analogs were tested with carbaryl on houseflies (*30*) and 24 of these showed synergistic ratios ranging from 111 to 454. The most active compounds were 5,6-disubstituted, particularly the 5,6-dichloro, 5-methyl-6-chloro and 5-methoxy-6-chloro (*SR* = 345, 385, 454). Regression analysis was limited to compounds substituted in the 5, 6, and 5,6 positions in order to avoid steric factors that might arise from 4 and 7 substitution. The main objective was to identify the binding and electronic factors. These proved to be π and $\sigma^{\cdot}$, the σ constant related to homolytic phenylation of substituted benzenes (Eq. 29)(*30*). This, of course, is the same unusual factor observed by Hansch (*38*) with the benzodioxole synergists. Gil and Wilkinson drew the analogous conclusion that synergistic activity of the 1,2,3-benzodiazoles depends on both their lipophilic character and their ability to form radicals. Their related study of 47 analogs as inhibitors of

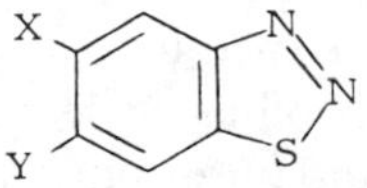

5:1 with

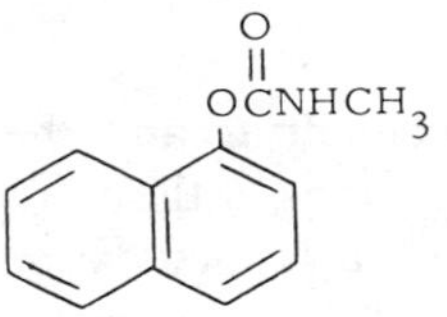

versus Housefly

$$\log(SR) = 0.45\pi + 0.92\sigma^{\cdot} + 1.78 \qquad (29)$$

$$n = 14, \quad r = 0.882, \quad s = 0.117$$

enzyme preparations from rat liver and armyworm gut took a somewhat different turn (*31*). Binding and electronic terms were present as expected but the correlation of pI_{50} values for armyworm gut were defined much better by Hammett's σ than by $\sigma^{\bullet}$ (Eq. 30) (*31*). This suggests a probable difference in synergistic mechanism between housefly and armyworm, a subject worthy of further research. Despite the difference in elec-

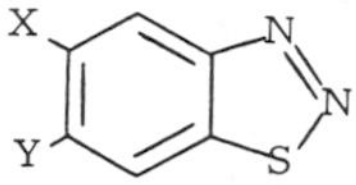

versus Armyworm gut enzyme

$$pI_{50} = (0.76 \pm 0.33)\pi - (0.25 \pm 0.30)\pi^2 - (0.46 \pm 0.34)\sigma - (3.83 \pm 0.15) \quad (30)$$

$$n = 20, \quad r = 0.942, \quad s = 0.212$$

tronic response there is a reasonably good correlation between the pI_{50} values of army worm and the log(*SR*) values for carbaryl against houseflies. The correlation is aided by the fact that π is the dominant parameter in both data sets.

In bringing this review to an end, it seemed appropriate to finish with synergists—chemicals that inhibit the breakdown of direct toxicants. Other topics were considered for inclusion where excellent QSAR studies have been performed. Among these were juvenile hormones and their mimetics, insect growth regulators that inhibit cuticle formation, and various others that prevent normal transition from one development stage to the next. Also considered were behavioral chemicals that affect mating and can be used to lure insects into a toxic trap. In each of these cases the biochemistry and physiology was judged to be too great a departure from our main theme of direct toxicity and thus they were not included.

III. SUMMARY

The relation between drugs and chemicals affecting insects and mites is not immediately apparent, although some AChE inhibitors are useful in medicine and many insecticides are of value in controlling disease vectors. In the area of direct toxicity, desired for insects and mites but not animals and humans, there are many related mechanisms in AChE, MAO, OXPHOS, and CNS inhibition. There are also unique mechanisms that apply only to insects and mites such as knockdown, synergism, juvenilization, sexual responses, antifeeding, and other behavioral effects. At the microscopic level, we find that transport through living tissue correlates with the same parameters in insects and mites as it does for man and other vertebrates. As a physical process, penetration of human skin and cockroach cuticle are remarkably similar. At the molecular level we find that the same parameters correlate binding and reactivity for insect and mite enzymes as for those of higher animals. There are, of course, situations in agriculture such as soil fumigation and transpiration-driven xylem flow that do not overlap the animal world. However, the mechanistic similarities are greater than the differences.

Approaches to correlation of insect and mite data are nearly identical with those of typical drug studies. The parametric approach (Hansch Method) is most frequently applied, but factor analysis, quantum chemical, and pattern recognition approaches have also been effective. In general, the objectives are the same, namely, support for a working hypothesis that can assist the search for improved drugs and pesticides. Both fields generate data that range from highly precise to rather diffuse in terms of measurement error. The best data correlate well in both fields while the worst provide difficult to insoluble problems. There is nothing to suggest that one field has an easier time or a better success-to-failure ratio in QSAR studies. The same factors operate in both, and success depends largely on the quality of the data and the experimental design.

There is one relevant area where drug studies are more than a decade beyond pesticide research. Over a hundred enzymes critical to medicine have been fully sequenced and characterized in three dimensional space, allowing enzyme–substrate and enzyme–inhibitor complexes to be studied in great detail. By contrast, no enzyme of vital importance to agriculture has been sequenced or defined by X-ray crystallography. The situation is complicated in insects and mites by the presence of isozymes having nearly identical physical properties. However, the real difference in the state of enzyme understanding is the level of research funding. When our food supply becomes as important as the cancer problem, a time rapidly approaching, the necessary studies will be quickly done. Agriculture is poised for a great leap forward, a change of pace that will greatly advance QSAR and mechanistic insight for both pesticide and drug action.

REFERENCES

1. N. Abo-Khatwa and R. M. Hollingsworth, (1973). *Pestic. Biochem. Physiol.* **3,** 358 (1973).
2. M. B. Abou-Donia, G. M. Rosen, and J. Paxton, *Int. J. Biochem.* **1,** 371 (1976).
3. R. W. Beeman and F. Matsumura, *Pestic. Biochem. Physiol.* **4,** 325 (1974).
4. A. M. Block and L. W. Newland, *Pestic., Lect. IUPAC Int. Congr. Pestic. Chem., 3rd, Helsinki, 1974* p. 569 (1975).

5. F. G. Bordwell and H. E. Fried, *Tetrahedron Lett.* p. 1121 (1977).
6. G. T. Brooks, *in* "Drug Design" (E. J. Ariëns, ed.), Medicinal Chemistry, Vol. 11-IV, p. 379. Academic Press, New York, 1973.
7. G. T. Brooks, *in* "Insecticide Biochemistry and Physiology" (C. F. Wilkinson, ed.), p. 3. Plenum, New York, 1976.
8. D. D. Brown, R. L. Metcalf, J. G. Sternburg, and J. R. Coats, *Pestic. Biochem. Physiol.* **15,** 43. (1981).
9. K. H. Büchel and W. Draber, *in* "Biological Correlations—The Hansch Approach" (W. Van Valkenburg, ed.), Advances in Chemistry Series, No. 114, p. 141. Am. Chem. Soc., Washington, D.C.
10. J. C. Campbell, *Natl. Agric. Chem. Assoc. News Pestic. Rev.* **28,** 14 (1969).
11. M. Charton, *J. Org. Chem.* **31,** 2996 (1966).
12. M. Charton, *J. Am. Chem. Soc.* **91,** 615, 6649 (1969).
13. J. R. Coats, R. L. Metcalf, and I. P. Kapoor, *J. Agric. Food Chem.* **25,** 859 (1977).
14. C. E. Crisp, C. E. Richmond, N. L. Gillette, M. Look, and B. A. Lucas, *Pestic., Lect. IUPAC Int. Congr. Pestic. Chem., 3rd, Helsinki, 1974* Abst. No. 534 (1975).
15. J. A. Durden, Jr., paper presented at *Int. Congr. Pestic. Chem., 4th, Zurich, 1978.*
16. M. Elliott and N. F. Janes, *Chem. Soc. Rev.* **7,** 473 (1978).
17. N. Engelhard, K. Prchal, and M. Nenner, *Angew. Chem., Int. Ed. Engl.* **6,** 615 (1967).
18. M. A. H. Fahmy, T. R. Fukuto, R. L. Metcalf, and R. L. Holmestead, *J. Agric. Food Chem.* **21,** 585 (1973).
19. T. H. Fisher, W. E. McHenry, E. G. Alley, and H. W. Chambers, *J. Agric. Food Chem.* **28,** 731 (1980).
20. M. G. Ford, *Pestic. Sci.* **10,** 39 (1979).
21. V. H. Freed, D. Schmedding, R. Kohnert, and R. Haque, *Pestic. Biochem. Physiol.* **10,** 203 (1979).
22. T. Fujita, K. Kamoshita, T. Nishioka, and M. Nakajima, *Agric. Biol. Chem.* **38,** 1521 (1974).
23. T. Fujita, T. Nishioka, and M. Nakajima, *J. Med. Chem.* **20,** 1071 (1977).
24. T. R. Fukuto and R. L. Metcalf, *J. Agric. Food Chem.* **4,** 930 (1956).
25. T. R. Fukuto, R. L. Metcalf, and M. Winton, *J. Econ. Entomol.* **52,** 1121 (1959).
26. T. R. Fukuto, R. L. Metcalf, M. Y. Winton, and R. B. March, *J. Econ. Entomol.* **56,** 808 (1963).
27. T. R. Fukuto, *In* "Insecticide Biochemistry and Physiology" (C. F. Wilkinson, ed.), p. 397, Plenum, New York, 1976.
28. P. Gerolt, *Pestic. Sci.* **1,** 209 (1970).
29. P. Gerolt, *Pestic. Sci.* **3,** 43 (1972).
30. D. L. Gil and C. F. Wilkinson, *Pestic. Biochem. Physiol.* **6,** 338 (1976).
31. D. L. Gil and C. F. Wilkinson, *Pestic. Biochem. Physiol.* **7,** 183 (1977).
32. A. Goldblum, M. Yoshimoto, and C. Hansch, *J. Agric. Food Chem.* **29,** 277 (1981).
33. P. J. Goodford, A. T. Hudson, G. C. Sheppey, R. Wooton, M. H. Black, G. J. Sutherland, and J. C. Wickham, *J. Med. Chem.* **19,** 1239 (1976).
34. B. D. Hammock, T. C. Sparks, and S. M. Mumby, *Pestic. Biochem. Physiol.* **7,** 517 (1977).
35. C. Hansch, E. W. Deutsch, and R. N. Smith, *J. Am. Chem. Soc.* **87,** 2738 (1965).
36. C. Hansch, K. Kiehs, and G. L. Lawrence, *J. Am. Chem. Soc.* **87,** 5770 (1965).
37. C. Hansch and E. W. Deutsch, *Biochim. Biophys. Acta* **126,** 117 (1966).
38. C. Hansch, *J. Med. Chem.* **11,** 920 (1968).
39. C. Hansch, *J. Org. Chem.* **35,** 620 (1970).
40. C. Hansch and E. J. Lien *J. Med. Chem.* **14,** 653 (1971).

41. C. Hansch and W. J. Dunn, *J. Pharm. Sci.* **61,** 1 (1972).
42. C. Hansch and J. M. Clayton, *J. Pharm. Sci.* **62,** 1 (1973).
43. B. Hetnarski and R. D. O'Brien, *Pestic. Biochem. Physiol.* **2,** 132 (1972).
44. B. Hetnarski and R. D. O'Brien, *Biochemistry* **12,** 3883 (1973).
45. B. Hetnarski and R. D. O'Brien, *J. Agric. Food Chem.* **23,** 709 (1975).
46. B. Hetnarski and R. D. O'Brien, *J. Med. Chem.* **18,** 29 (1975).
47. G. Holan, *Pestic. Lect., IUPAC Int. Congr. Pestic. Chem. 3rd, Helsinki, 1974* p. 359 (1975).
48. G. Holan, D. F. O'Keefe, K. Rihs, R. Walser, and C. T. Virgona, *Adv. Pestic. Sci. Plenary Lect. Symp. Pap.*, Part 2, *Int. Congr. Pestic. Chem. 4th, Zurich, 1978* p. 201 (1979).
49. A. J. Hopfinger and R. D. Battershell, *Adv. Pestic. Sci. Plenary Lect. Symp. Pap.*, Part 2, *Int. Congr. Pestic. Chem., 4th, Zurich, 1978* p. 196 (1979).
50. M. Hussain, T. R. Fukuto, and H. T. Reynolds, *J. Agric. Food Chem.* **22,** 225 (1974).
51. K. Kamoshita I. Ohno, T. Fujita, T. Nishioka, and M. Nakajima, *Pestic. Biochem. Physiol.* **11,** 83 (1979).
52. K. Kamoshita I. Ohno, K. Kasamatsu, T. Fujita, and M. Nakajima, *Pestic. Biochem. Physiol.* **11,** 104. (1979).
53. A. M. A. Khasawinah, R. B. March, and T. R. Fukuto, *Pestic. Biochem. Physiol.* **9,** 211 (1978).
54. M. Kiso, T. Fujita, N. Kurihara, M. Uchida, K. Tanaka and M. Nakajima, *Pestic. Biochem. Physiol.* **8,** 33 (1978).
55. C. O. Knowles, *in* "Pesticide Selectivity" (J. C. Street, ed.), p. 155. Dekker, New York, 1975.
56. G. K. Kohn, J. N. Ospenson, and J. E. Moore, *J. Agric. Food Chem.* **13,** 232 (1965).
57. R. M. Krupka, *Biochemistry* **3,** 1749 (1964).
58. H. Kubinyi, *J. Med. Chem.* **20,** 625 (1977).
59. R. L. Lapp and R. A. Jacobson, *J. Agric. Food Chem.* **28,** 755 (1980).
60. A.-H. Lee, R. L. Metcalf, J. W. Williams, A. S. Hirwe, J. R. Sanborn, J. R. Coats, and T. R. Fukuto, *Pestic. Biochem. Physiol.* **7,** 426 (1977).
61. A. E. Lund, R. M. Hollingsworth, and L. L. Murdock, *Adv. Pestic. Sci., Plenary Lect. Symp. Pap.*, Part 3, *Int. Congr Pestic. Chem., 4th, Zurich, 1978* p. 465 (1979).
62. P. S. Magee, U.S. Patent No. 3,309,266 (1967).
62a. P. S. Magee, unpublished observations (1976).
63. J. W. McFarland, *Prog. Drug Res.* **15,** 123 (1971).
64. R. L. Metcalf, T. R. Fukuto, and M. Frederickson *J. Agric. Food Chem.* **12,** 231 (1964).
65. R. L. Metcalf and T. R. Fukuto, *J. Agric. Food Chem.* **13,** 220 (1965).
66. R. L. Metcalf, *J. Agric. Food Chem.* **21,** 511 (1973).
67. F. Moriarty and M. C. French, *Pestic. Biochem. Physiol.* **1,** 286 (1971).
68. F. Moriarity, "Organochlorine Insecticides," p. 56. Academic Press, New York, 1975.
69. M. Nakajima, T. Fujita, N. Kurihara, Y. Sanemitsu, M. Uchida, and M. Kiso, *Pestic. Lect. IUPAC Int. Congr. Pestic. Chem., 3rd, Helsinki, 1974* p. 370 (1975).
70. W. B. Neely, I. Unger, E. H. Blair, and R. A. Nyquist, Biochemistry **3,** 1477 (1964).
71. W. B. Neely, *Mol. Pharmacol.* **1,** 137 (1965).
72. W. B. Neely and W. K. Whitney, *J. Agric. Food Chem.* **16,** 571 (1968).
73. W. B. Neely, D. R. Branson, and G. E. Blau, *Environ. Sci. Technol.* **8,** 1113 (1974).
74. K. Nishimura and T. Narahashi, *Pestic. Biochem. Physiol.* **8,** 53 (1978).
75. T. Nishioka. T. Fujita, K. Kamoshita, and M. Nakajima, *Pestic. Biochem. Physiol.* **7,** 107 (1977).

76. J. Noble-Nesbitt, *Pestic. Sci.* **1,** 204 (1970).
77. R. D. O'Brien, *in* "Insecticide Biochemistry and Physiology" (C. F. Wilkinson, ed.), p. 271. Plenum, New York, 1976.
78. W. P. Olson, *Pestic. Biochem. Physiol.* **3,** 384 (1973).
79. M. I. Page, *Angew. Chem., Int. Ed. Engl.* **16,** 449 (1977).
80. J. T. Penniston, L. Beckett, D. L. Bentley, and C. Hansch, *Mol. Pharmacol.* **5,** 333 (1969).
81. E. L. Plummer and D. S. Pincus, *Prepr. Pap. Natl. Meet., 178th, Div. Pestic. Chem. Am. Chem. Soc.,* Abstr. 28 (1979).
82. G. Schatz, *Angew. Chem., Int. Ed. Engl.* **6,** 1035 (1967).
83. H. L. Skalsky and F. E. Guthrie, *Toxicol. Appl. Pharmacol.* **43,** 229 (1978).
84. E. Y. Spencer, (1973). "Guide to the Chemicals Used in Crop Protection," 6th ed., pp. 225, 228, 243. Res. Branch Agric. Can. Ottowa.
85. G. M. Steinberg, M. L. Mednick, J. Maddox, and R. Rice, *J. Med. Chem.* **18,** 1056 (1975).
86. F. Takusagawa and R. A. Jacobson, *J. Agric. Food Chem.* **25,** 329 (1977).
87. R. K. Tripathi and R. D. O'Brien, *Pestic. Biochem. Physiol.* **2,** 418 (1973).
88. M. Uchida, N. Kurihara, T. Fujita, and M. Nakajima, *Pestic. Biochem. Physiol.* **4,** 260 (1974).
89. M. Uchida, H. Naka, Y. Irie, T. Fujita, and M. Nakajima, *Pestic. Biochem. Physiol.* **4,** 451 (1974).
90. M. Uchida, Y. Irie, T. Fujita, and M. Nakajima, *Pestic Biochem. Physiol.* **5,** 253 (1975).
91. M. Uchida, Y. Irie, N. Kurihara, T. Fujita and M. Nakajima, *Pestic. Biochem. Physiol.* **5,** 258 (1975).
92. Union Carbide Corporation, "For a World of Plenty," Bull. F-41044, New York, N.Y.
93. J. M. Vandenbelt, C. Hansch, and C. Church, *J. Med. Chem.* **15,** 787 (1972).
94. A. Verloop, W. Hoogenstraaten, and J. Tipker, *in* "Drug Design" (E. J. Ariëns, ed.), Medicinal Chemistry, Vol. 11-VII, p. 165. Academic Press, New York, 1976.
95. C. F. Wilkinson, R. L. Metcalf, and T. R. Fukuto, *J. Agric. Food Chem.* **14,** p. 73 (1966).
96. C. F. Wilkinson, K. Hetnarski, G. P. Cantwell, and F. J. DiCarlo, *Biochem. Pharmacol.* **23,** 2377 (1974).
97. C. F. Wilkinson, K. Hetnarski, and L. J. Hicks, *Pestic. Biochem. Physiol.* **4,** 299 (1974).
98. C. E. Winter, O. Giannotti, and E. L. Holzhacker, *Pestic. Biochem. Physiol.* **5,** 155 (1975).
99. D. A. Wustner and T. R. Fukuto, *Pestic. Biochem. Physiol.* **4,** 365 (1974).
100. C.-F. Yang and Y.-P. Sun, *Arch. Environ. Contam. Toxicol.* **6,** 325 (1977).
101. E. Zerba and T. R. Fukuto, *J. Agric. Food Chem.* **26,** 1365 (1978).
102. J. L. Zettler and U. E. Brady, *Pestic. Biochem. Physiol.* **5,** 471 (1975).

11

Absorption, Distribution, and Metabolism of Drugs

V. AUSTEL AND E. KUTTER

I. THE SIGNIFICANCE OF QUANTITATIVE RELATIONSHIPS BETWEEN STRUCTURE AND PHARMACOKINETIC PROPERTIES OF CHEMICAL COMPOUNDS

Organisms are composed of a multitude of biological systems each of which has a specific function. A highly organized interplay of these functions guarantees the stability of the organism and protects it from adverse environmental influences. Defects in these functions or their interplay put the organism into a diseased state. Such states can be reverted or their symptoms alleviated by influences from the environment, e.g., by drugs. In order to achieve the desired effect, it is not sufficient that the drug be principally able to interact with the target system(s) in an appropriate

ISBN 0-12-695150-0

manner. Rather, the drug must not interfere with the properly functioning systems (selectivity), and it must be affected by the protective mechanisms of the organism in a predefined manner that depends on the respective therapeutic aim. In a wider sense, all pharmacokinetic factors, such as metabolism, distribution, excretion, and diffusion barriers, belong to such mechanisms. For example, a drug that is required to be orally active and free of central nervous effects, and whose action should last for several hours, ought to pass easily through the intestinal wall but should be held back by the blood–brain barrier. Moreover, metabolism and excretion processes should affect the drug at such a rate that blood levels are maintained above a certain limit for several hours. This situation is not only relevant for the biological evaluation of potential new drugs but also has repercussions on the medicinal chemist's strategy in drug design.

What role can quantitative relationships between structure and pharmacokinetic properties play within such a strategy?

Originally it was hoped that QSAR generally would open up the possibility of predicting the structures of compounds exerting the optimal biological properties, thus allowing new drugs to be searched for in a targeted manner. In practice, however, QSAR have with few exceptions failed to meet these expectations. In our experience the most promising compounds have always been found in very early stages of drug development before any meaningful QSAR could have been derived. Is QSAR therefore only of academic interest? Probably not. There are two ways by which QSAR can contribute to the development of new drugs:

1. Directly by revealing structural factors that govern the biological properties of chemical compounds, and
2. Indirectly by giving insights into the mechanisms that underlie the interactions of chemical compounds with biological systems and vice versa.

The first type of application allows new drugs to be developed systematically. Systematic drug design is aimed at minimizing the experimental expense that is necessary to obtain a certain amount of structure–activity information. This aspect is outlined in detail in references *2–4* and *85* in which a corresponding procedure based on the theory of sets is described.

The knowledge about mechanisms of action can on the one hand help to estimate the therapeutic value of a drug and may on the other hand lead the way to structures with improved biological properties. The practical significance of known QSAR depends on the range of structures for which they are valid and on the extent to which general conclusions can be drawn from them. Because the biological systems that govern pharmacokinetic behavior act on all compounds regardless of their pharmacodynamic properties, known quantitative structure–pharmacokinetic property relationships should have the greatest generalization potential and therefore be of particular utility in prospective drug development.

II. QUANTITATIVE RELATIONSHIPS BETWEEN CHEMICAL STRUCTURE AND PHARMACOKINETIC PROPERTIES

A. General Considerations

In order to derive QSAR, two types of approaches have been applied (*82,107,109,136*):

1. Linear regression analysis (including squared and cross product terms) of biological data with respect to structural and physicochemical properties (empirical QSAR), and
2. Data fitting to theoretically derived models.

In both cases the reliability of the results is usually examined from the point of view of statistical theory. For most practical purposes it is unrealistic to put too much emphasis on such criteria, because every QSAR derived in the course of practical drug design procedures is subject to errors that can be more serious than statistical inaccuracies. Such errors comprise the scatter in the experimental data as well as the fact that the structural (including physicochemical) factors of relevance are generally not completely known. Therefore, QSAR can only be viewed as experimentally more or less supported hypotheses that provide guidelines for the design of additional experiments (e.g., test compounds). More important than the problem of their statistical significance is the question of the prospective value of a QSAR, i.e., the degree to which it is valid in different drug design problems. In this respect model-based QSAR can offer advantages over those empirically derived depending, of course, on the relevance of the model for the biological effect(s) under consideration.

Empirically obtained QSAR, however, frequently serve as a basis for models and thereby gain predictive value beyond the structural area from which they were derived. Generally, the predictive power of any QSAR depends on the range of structures and physicochemical properties that are covered by the underlying test compounds. (This is also true for model-based equations, as the applicability of a model to a certain structural area can only be checked experimentally.) Therefore, QSAR in drug absorption, distribution, and metabolism will be reviewed here in terms of types of chemical structures investigated as well as of relevant

TABLE I
Quantitative Structure–Absorption Relationships

Example number	Types of compounds in the test set	Species	Biological parameter	Relevant factors	Physicochemical parameter	Range of parameter in the test set	Type of dependence	References
Gastric Absorption								
1.	Barbiturates	Rat	$\log k_a$[a]	Lipophilicity	$\log P_{CHCl_3/w}$	−0.14–2.84	Linear	(*67,91*)
2.	Barbiturates	Rat	$\log k_a$[a]	Lipophilicity	ΔR_m[b]	−0.954–0	Linear	(*121*)
3.	4-Aminobenzene-sulfonamides	Rat	$\log k_u$[c]	Lipophilicity	$\log P_{i\text{-amOAc/w}}$	−2.52–1.94	Linear	(*91*)
4.	*O*-Alkyl-, *O*-aryl-carbamates	Rat	$\log k_a$[a]	Lipophilicity	$\log P_{o/w}$ (buffer pH 7.4)	−0.66–2.85	Linear	(*57,58*)
5.	Barbiturates, 4-aminobenzene-sulfonamides	Rat	$\log k_u$[c]	Lipophilicity	$\log P_{i\text{-amOAc/w}}$	−2.52–3.23	Linear	(*91*)
6.	Barbiturates, benzoic acids, phenols	Rat	log(% abs)	Lipophilicity	$\log P_{o/w}$	0.65–2.50	Parabolic $\log P_o = 1.97$	(*88*)
7.	Anilines, anilides, pyrazolones, xanthines	Rat	log(% abs)	Basicity	pK_a	0.3–5.0	Linear	(*88*)
Intestinal Absorption								
8.	4-Aminobenzene-sulfonamides	Rat[e]	$\log k_u M^{1/2}$[c]	Lipophilicity (molar weight)	$\log P_{CHCl_3/w}$ (*MW*)	−2.00–1.49	Parabolic $\log P_o = 1.54$[d]	(*92*)
9.	Aliphatic amides	Rat[e]	log(% abs in 10 min)	Lipophilicity	$\log P_{o/w}$	−4.10 to −1.64	Linear	(*92*)
10.	Steroids	Rat[e]	log(% abs/100 g)	Lipophilicity	$\text{Log } P_{C_6H_6\text{-aq MeOH}}$	−0.85–1.20	Linear	(*92*)
11.	Diarylpropylamines (pheniramine derivatives)	Rat[e]	$t_{1/2}$ (min)	Lipophilicity	$\log P_{heptane/w}$ (buffer pH 6.0)	0.01–0.16	Linear	(*141*)

12.	Aliphatic alcohols, steroids, benzene	Rat[e]	$\log P_{perm}$[f]	Lipophilicity	$\log P_{o/w}$ (buffer pH 6.0)	−0.66–3.90 0.28–3.74	Linear Linear	(98)
	Phenols, aliphatic, aromatic and araliphatic acids, prostaglandins			Molar weight	$\log MW$	1.51–2.60[g] 1.95–2.55	Linear (−)[h] Linear (−)	
13.	Anilines, anilides, pyrazolones	Rat[e]	log(% abs)	Lipophilicity	$\log P_{o/w}$	−0.78–2.65	Parabolic $\log P_o = 1.39$	(88)
				Basicity	pK_a	0.3–10.3	Linear (−)	
	Xanthines, arylethanolamines, quinolines, imidazolines	Rat[e]	log(% abs)	Lipophilicity	$D_{pH\ 5.3}$[i]	−2.74–1.39	Linear	(130)
14.	Xanthines	Rat (*in vitro*)	$\log R$[j]	Lipophilicity	$\log P_{o/w}$ (buffer pH 7.4)	−0.85–1.35	Linear	(127)
15.	Cardiac glycosides	Cat	$Q_{R'}$, S'_{60}, C'_{10}[k]	Lipophilicity	$\log P_{o/w}$[l] R_m[m]	−2.0–2.95	Positive rank correlation	(52)
16.	*O*-Alkyl, *O*-aryl-carbamates	Rat	$\log k_a$[a]	Lipophilicity	$\log P_{o/w}$ (buffer pH 7.4)	−0.66–2.85	Parabolic (Bilinear) $\log P_o = 0.62$	(57) (58)
17.	*O*-Alkyl, *O*-aryl *N*-methyl-carbamates	Rat	$\log k_a$[a]	Lipophilicity	$\log P_{o/w}$ (buffer pH 7.4)	−0.05–2.66	Parabolic $\log P_o = 1.54$	(58)
18.	Sulfanilamides, Un-ionized, Ionized	Rat	$\log k_a$[a]	Lipophilicity	$\log P_{o/w}$ $\log P_{CHCl_3/w}$[n] $\log P_{c-L}$	−0.959–2.186 −1.390–2.144 −2.230–0.056	Linear Linear	 (115)
19.	Barbiturates	Rat[0]	log(% abs)	Lipophilicity	$\log P_{CHCl_3/w}$	−0.15–2.29	Linear	(93)

(*continued*)

TABLE I *(Continued)*

Example number	Types of compounds in the test set	Species	Biological parameter	Relevant factors	Physicochemical parameter	Range of parameter in the test set	Type of dependence	References
20.	Benzoic acids, phenols, barbiturates, pyrazolindiones	Rat[o]	log(% abs)	Lipophilicity, Acidity	$\log P_{o/w}$ pK_a	1.46–3.22 2.3–9.9	Linear Linear	(94)
			log(% abs) $\log k_a$[a]	Lipophilicity	$\log D_{pH\ 6.8}$[i]	−2.52–2.44	Parabolic $\log D_o = 1.49$[p] $\log D_o = 1.63$[q]	(130)
21.	Anilines, anilides, pyrazolones, arylethanolamines, quinolines, imidazolines, levorphan[r]	Rat[0]	log(% abs)	Lipophilicity	$\log P_{o/w}$	0.23–2.65	Parabolic $\log P_o = 1.32$	(94)
				Basicity	pK_a	0.3–10.3	Linear (−)	
				Lipophilicity	$\log D_{pH\ 6.8}$[i]	−1.24–1.39	Linear	(130)
22.	Amino acids	Rabbit[s]	$\log(1/k_1)$[t]	Lipophilicity	π	−1.01–2.64	Linear[u]	(145)
23.	Phenylalanine derivatives	Rabbit[s]	$\log(1/k_1)$[t]	Lipophilicity	π	−1.23–1.12	Linear	
				Electronic properties	σ	−0.66–0.78	Linear	(145)
Buccal Absorption								
24.	Benzoic acids, phenylacetic acids	Human	$\log k$[v]	Lipophilicity	$\log P_{n\text{-heptane/w}}$	0.03–0.88	Linear[w]	(7)

25.	Amphetamines, phenfluramines	Human	log (*abs*/*unabs*)[x]	Lipophilicity	$\log P_{n\text{-heptane/w}}$	0.54–3.95	Linear[y]	(*6*)
Absorption through skin								
26.	Alkyl phosphates	Human	$\log k_p$[z]	Lipophilicity	$\log P_{o/w}$	−0.52–3.98	Parabolic linear (−); $\log P_o = -1.58$	(*120*)
27.	Aliphatic alcohols	Human	$\log k_p$[z]	Lipophilicity	$\log P_{o/w}$	−0.16–2.84	Linear	(*89*)
28.	Steroids	Human	$\log k_p$[z]	Lipophilicity	$\log P_{\text{amylcaproate/w}}$	0.11–1.75	Linear	(*89*)
29.	Phenylboronic acids	Human	$\log C$[aa]	Lipophilicity	$\log P_{o/w}$	0.43–2.38	Linear	(*90*)
					$\log P_{\text{benzene/w}}$	−2.53 to −0.09		
30.	Corticosteroids	Human	log(1/C)[aa,bb]	Lipophilicity	$\log P_{\text{Et}_2\text{O/w}}$	0.00–1.11	Linear	(*90*)
				Water solubility	$\log S$	−4.46 to −2.79	Linear	
31.	Nicotinic acid	Human	log(1/*C*)[cc]	Lipophilicity	$\log P_{\text{Et}_2\text{O/w}}$	−1.66–1.92	Linear	(*90*)
	Alkyl nicotinates			Water solubility	$\log S$	−5.05 to −2.72	Linear	
32.	Alkyl halides, aliphatic alcohols, polyalcohols, ureas, thioureas	Rabbit	$\log k_p$[z]	Lipophilicity	$\log P_{o/w}$	−3.29–2.00	Linear	
				Molecular weight	$\log MW$	1.51–2.26	Linear (−)	(*90*)
Corneal Absorption								
33.	Alkyl 4-amino-benzoates	Rabbit	log *CMP*[dd]	Lipophilicity	*n*[ee]	1–6	Parabolic $n_o = 3$	(*116*)
34.	Corticosteroids	Rabbit	$\log P_{\text{perm}}$[f]	Lipophilicity	$\log P_{o/w}$	1.1–3.8	Parabolic[ff] $\log P_o = 2.9$	(*131*)
35.	Ureas, aliphatic; alcohols; thiourea	Rabbit[gg]	$\log k$[hh]	Lipophilicity	$\log P_{\text{Et}_2\text{O/w}}$	−3.30–0.28	Parabolic $\log P_o = 0.55$	(*120*)

(*continued*)

[a] k_a is the absorption rate constant.
[b] Toluene–acetic acid–water 10:5:4 on paper.

TABLE I *(Continued)*

[c] k_u is the absorption rate constant of undissociated form.
[d] $\log P_{o,o/w} = 2.56$.
[e] Small intestine.
[f] P_{perm} is the permeability coefficient (cm/sec).
[g] The molar weight term accounts for dependence of permeation on the diffusion coefficient. Frequently this dependence does not become apparent because of insufficient variance in molar weight.
[h] (−) denotes negative correlation.
[i] D is the distribution coefficient, where $D = ([\text{ionized}]_{org} + [\text{un-ionized}]_{org})/([\text{ionized}]_w + [\text{un-ionized}]_w)$. If $[\text{ionized}]_{org} \ll [\text{un-ionized}]_{org}$, we obtain $\log D = \log P + \log[1/(1 + 10^{pH-pK_a})] = \log P + C_D$ for acids, and $\log D = \log P + \log[1/(1 + 10^{pK_a-pH})] = \log P + C_D$ for bases, where C_D is a correction term for dissociation, which can be neglected if $pK_a \gg pH$ for acids and $pH \gg pK_a$ for bases.
[j] R is the cumulative transfer rate.
[k] Q_R is the % abs during 60 min, S'_{60} is the AUC for blood level of radioactivity in portal vein between 0 and 60 min, and C'_{10} is the portal vein level of radioactivity after 10 min.
[l] Buffer pH 7.
[m] Octanol coated silica gel—H_2O–CH_3OH R^0_m: −0.17–1.87; silicon coated silica gel—H_2O–acetone R^0_m: 0.18–3.59.
[n] Partition coefficient of the ionized form between lecithin–chloroform and water.
[o] Colon.
[p] For % abs.
[q] For $\log k_a$.
[r] In Scherrer and Howard (*130*).
[s] Ileum.
[t] Binding constant of the amino acid to the transport system.
[u] Methionine is an outlier; probably factors other than lipophilicity also play a role.
[v] Absorption rate constant–buffer pH 4.0.
[w] Considering lipophilicity and acidity, Lien found a parabolic dependence of log(% abs) on $\log P$ (range 1.30–4.92) ($\log P_o = 4.19$) and a positive linear correlation with pK_a (range 2.89–4.89) (*89*). A plot of $\log P_{n\text{-heptane/w}}$ (range < −2.0–1.98) against log(abs/unabs) (under conditions where 10% of the acid is un-ionized) give a linear dependence (*6*).
[x] When 10% un-ionized.
[y] Lien *et al.* derived a parabolic relationship with $\log P$ ($\log P_o = 5.52$) (*89*).
[z] k_p is the permeability constant.
[aa] C is the molar concentration measured or required to cause standard biological response.
[bb] Standard response: vasoconstriction.
[cc] Standard response: induction of erythema.
[dd] CMP is the corneal membrane permeability in cm/sec.
[ee] n is the chain length.
[ff] The drop in permeability coefficient for the most lipophilic compound (progesterone) was shown not to be due to limited solubility.
[gg] Penetration into aqueous humor of the eye.
[hh] k is the permeation rate constant.

physicochemical properties including the range covered by the corresponding parameters.

B. Empirically Derived Relationships

1. Drug Absorption

For most therapeutic purposes, drugs ought to be orally effective and must therefore be absorbed buccally or gastrointestinally. Penetration into and through skin is an important factor in topical application. Quantitative investigations on drug absorption in terms of physicochemical properties are listed in Table I.

Apparently the most important factor that determines absorption is lipophilicity. Its most favorable range for gastrointestinal absorption seems to lie between log $P_{o/w} = 0.5–2.0$ (for ionizable compounds log $D_{o/w}$). For buccal absorption, Lien *et al.* (*89*) derived optimal log *P* values between 4 and 5.5 (for un-ionized forms), which under test conditions correspond to a distribution coefficient of one order of magnitude lower. For dermal absorption, the favorable lipophilicity also seems to extend above log $P = 2$. Another determining factor, water solubility, is less well documented by the data but was shown to be, as expected, positively correlated with dermal absorption. It is interesting to see that there is a substantial difference in the optimal lipophilicity for intestinal absorption between *N*-methylated and nonmethylated carbamates (Examples 16 and 17, Table I). This difference can be attributed to an additional factor, hydrogen bonding, which may be especially important in cases where water solubility becomes the rate-limiting step in drug absorption (*58*). The nonlinear relationship between log k_a and log *P* in Example 16 is, however, not due to limitation in solubility (precipitation of the compounds) (*164*). In considering solubilities as a separate factor, one must bear in mind that there is a linear relationship between lipophilicity and aqueous solubility for liquid (*44,169*) and crystalline compounds [in this case the melting point also determines solubility (*169,171*)]. The same applies to pK_a (electronic properties), which frequently only determines changes in lipophilicity due to ionization. This is nicely demonstrated by Examples 13, 20, and 21 (Table I) in which intestinal absorption can be described either by log *P* and pK_a (*88,94*) or alternatively by a lipophilicity term only, the distribution coefficient log *D* (*130*). As long as drugs are absorbed by passive diffusion, one would also expect a dependence on molecular weight. Normally the influence of this factor is hard to detect because in many cases the compounds in a series have very similar molecular weights.

TABLE II
Quantitative Structure–Protein Binding Relationships

Example number	Types of compounds in the test set	Type of protein	Biological parameter	Relevant factors	Physicochemical parameter	Range of parameter in the test set	Type of dependence	References
1.	Barbiturates	BSA[a]	$\log K_n^b$	Lipophilicity	$\log P_{o/w}$	0.65–2.30	Linear	(*32*)
2.	4-Aminobenzenesulfonamides	BSA HSA[c]	$\log K_n^b$	Lipophilicity	π^d	0.00–2.61	Linear	(*32*)
3.	4-Aminobenzenesulfonamides (subset of 2)	BSA	$\log K_n^b$	Lipophilicity	π^d	0.39–2.61	Linear	
			$\log K_i^e$	Lipophilicity				(*32*)
			$\log K^f$	Acidity	$\Delta\log K_a^g$	3.07–5.83	Linear (−)	
4.	4-Acetylaminobenzenesulfonamides	BSA HSA	$\log K_n^b$	Lipophilicity	π^d	0.00–2.61	Linear	(*32*)
5.	Benzenesulfonylaminopyrimidines	Serum albumin	log(% free)	Lipophilicity	R_m^h	0.28–1.92	Linear (−)	(*134*)
6.	Benzenesulfonamides	HSA	$\log K$	Lipophilicity	$\log P_{i\text{-BuOH/w}}$ (buffer pH 7.4)	−2.0–1.46	Linear	(*132*)
7.	Aryl sulfonamides (incl. sulfonylureas and sulfanilamides)	HSA	$\log (1/C)^i$	Lipophilicity	$\log P_{o/w}$	0.13–3.21	Parabolic $\log P_o = 1.10$	(*21*)
8.	Aryl sulfonamides (incl. sulfonylureas and sulfanilamides)	HSA	$\log D^j$	Lipophilicity	$\log P_{o/w}$	−1.22–3.21	Parabolic $\log P_o = 1.60$	(*22*)
9.	Sulfanilamides	Human and rabbit plasma, rabbit and rat blood	log(bound/free)	Molecular weight	*MW*	172.2–314.4	Linear	(*115,172*)
10.	4-Aminobenzoic acids	HSA	log(% bound)	Lipophilicity	π	−1.14–1.53	Linear	(*135*)

11.	Carboxylic acids (incl. aromatic, alkanoic, phenoxyacetic, cycloalkanoic, quinoline carboxylic)	HSA	$\log(1/C)^{i}$	Lipophilicity	$\log P_{o/w}$	0.77–6.31	Parabolic $\log P_o = 5.48$	(*21*)
12.	Benzoic acids, pyridine carboxylic acids	BSA	$\log K$	Acidity	pK_a	3.8–5.3	Linear $(-)^{k}$	(*113*)
13.	Phenylaminocarbonyl-guanidines	Hemoglobin (horse)	$\log(R/D)^{l}$	Lipophilicity	π $\log P_{o/w}$	−0.12–1.97 0.56–2.39	Linear[m]	(*33*)
14.	2,2-Diaryl-4-amino-butyramides[n]	Human plasma	log(bound/free)	Lipophilicity	$\log P_{o/w}$ (buffer pH 7.4)	−1.31–1.57	Linear	(*12*)
15.	Acetanilides[o]	BSA	$\Delta H, \Delta S$ for binding	Electronic properties	σ	−0.66–0.78	Linear ΔH (−), ΔS (+)	(*17*)
16.	Penicillins[p]	HSA	log(bound/free)	Lipophilicity	$\Sigma \pi^{s}$	−0.48–4.69	Linear	(*10*)
17.	Penicillins	HSA	$\log K$	Lipophilicity	$\log P_{i\text{-BuOH/w}}$ (buffer pH 7.4)	−0.23–1.06	Linear	(*132*)
18.	Penicillins[q]	HSA	$\log(C'/C)^{r}$	Lipophilicity Electronic properties	$\Sigma \pi$ $\Sigma \sigma^{t}$	−0.79–3.44 −0.27–1.43	Parabolic $(-)^{u}$ Linear (−)	(*36*)
19.	Tetracyclines	Plasma	$\log(1/f_u)^{v}$	Lipophilicity	$\log P_{o/w}$ (buffer pH 7.5)	−1.60–0.04	Linear	(*150*)
20.	Tetracyclines	HSA	$\log K$	Lipophilicity	$\log P_{i\text{-BuOH/w}}$ (buffer pH 7.4)	−1.0– −0.43	Linear	(*132*)
21.	Steroids[w]	HSA	$\log K$	Lipophilicity	$\log P_{i\text{-BuOH/w}}$ (buffer pH 6.0)	0.89–1.95	Linear	(*132*)
22.	Steroids[x]	HSA	$\log K$	Lipophilicity	$\log P_{i\text{-BuOH/w}}$ (buffer pH 6.0)	1.74–2.40	Linear	(*132*)

(*continued*)

TABLE II *(Continued)*

Example number	Types of compounds in the test set	Type of protein	Biological parameter	Relevant factors	Physicochemical parameter	Range of parameter in the test set	Type of dependence	References
23.	Steroids[y]	HSA	log K	Lipophilicity	log $P_{i\text{-BuOH/w}}$ (buffer pH 6.0)	0.31–1.65	Linear	*(132)*
24.	Acridines	HSA	log K	Lipophilicity	log $P_{i\text{-BuOH/w}}$ (buffer pH 7.4)	2.07–2.81	Linear	*(132)*
25.	Phenothiazines	BSA	log K_B^z	Lipophilicity	R_m^{aa}	2.17–4.51	Linear	*(59)*
26.	Phenothiazines	BSA	$\log(\beta/\alpha)^{bb}$	Lipophilicity	log $P_{o/w}$ (buffer pH 7.4)	1.58–3.39	Linear	*(75)*
27.	Phenothiazines	BSA	log K	Lipophilicity	log $P_{dodecane/w}$	1.62–2.60	Linear	*(117)*
28.	Benzodiazepines[cc]	Human plasma	% bound	Lipophilicity	$\Sigma \pi^{cc}$	−2.39–0.74	Parabolic $(\Sigma \pi)_o = 0.08$	*(100)*
				Electronic properties	$\Sigma \sigma^{cc}$	−0.66–0.78	Parabolic $(\Sigma \sigma)_o = 0.31$	
29.	Oxazepam esters	Mouse serum HSA	ln(bound/free)	Lipophilicity	R_m^{dd}	−0.15–0.64	Linear[ee]	*(104)*
30.	Phenothiazines, dibenzo[*b*,*f*]azepines, dibenzo[*a*,*d*]cycloheptadienes, dibenzo[*b*,*d*]thiacycloheptadienes (all with aminoalkyl side chains)	BSA	log(bound/free)	Lipophilicity	log $P_{o/w}$	2.16–3.39	Linear	*(34)*
31.	Imidazoles[ff]	HSA	ln(% bound)	Electronic properties	q_r^{ff}	0.0655–1.2487	Linear	*(126)*
32.	Polycyclic hydrocarbons	HSA	log K	Lipophilicity	log $P_{o/w}$	2–8	Linear	*(25)*

33.	Benzyldimethylalkylammonium chlorides	BSA	log K	Lipophilicity	n[gg]	2–16	Parabolic $n_o = 17$	(97)
34.	4-Aminobenzenesulfonamides, anilines, aromatic ketones, phenols, naphthalenes, quinolines, biphenyls, benzofurans, benzoic acids	BSA	$\log(1/C)$[hh]	Lipophilicity	$\log P_{o/w}$	−0.78–3.45	Linear	(154)
35.	Phenols, anilines, naphthalenes, biphenyls, aryl ketones, nitrobenzenes, azobenzenes	Bovine hemoglobin	$\log(1/C)$[hh]	Lipophilicity	$\log P_{o/w}$	1.37–3.58	Linear	(70)
36.	Phenols, benzonitriles, benzyl alcohols, nitrobenzenes, aliphatic alcohols, anilines, naphthylamines, methoxy benzenes, anilides, aliphatic and aromatic ketones, carbamates, thioureas, indoles, naphthalenes, azobenzene	BSA	$\log(1/C)$[hh]	Lipophilicity	$\log P_{o/w}$	0.78–3.82	Linear[ii,jj]	(47)
37.	Sulfapyridines	Rat serum	log K	Lipophilicity	ΔR_m	0.00–1.11	Linear[kk]	(137)
				Acidity	pK_a	5.56–9.21	Linear (−)	

(continued)

TABLE II *(Continued)*

Example number	Types of compounds in the test set	Type of protein	Biological parameter	Relevant factors	Physicochemical parameter	Range of parameter in the test set	Type of dependence	References
38.	Isatin derivatives	Human serum albumin	log(% bound)	Lipophilicity	R_m^{ll}	−0.088–1.031	Linear	*(111)*
39.	Chlorobiocin analogs[mm]	HSA	log(bound/free)	Lipophilicity	log $P_{o/w}$ (buffer pH 7.4)	0.72–2.89	Linear[nn]	*(15)*

[a] Bovine serum albumin.
[b] K_n is the binding constant of the neutral form.
[c] Human serum albumin.
[d] $\pi = \log P - \log P_{\text{sulfanilamide}}$.
[e] K_i is the binding constant of the ionized form.
[f] K is the overall binding constant.
[g] $\Delta\log K_a = pK_a(\text{sulfanilamide}) - pK_a$.
[h] Reversed phase TLC, paraffin oil coated silica gel, buffer pH 7 phosphate–acetone extrapolated to zero acetone.
[i] C is the molar concentration of drug required to displace 50% of albumin-bound 5-dimethylaminonaphthalene-1-sulfonamide.
[j] D is the % decrease in fluorescence of 5-dimethylaminonaphthalene-1-sulfonamide–albumin complex.
[k] *o*-Hydroxy acids are outliers. Low but significant correlations were also obtained between pK_a and BSA binding for sulfanilamides *(114)*; such a correlation was also found with other sulfonamides *(133)*.
[l] R is the number of drug molecules bound per mole of protein; D is the concentration of free drug.
[m] The 3-chloro-4-nitrophenyl derivative is an outlier.
[n] Disopyramide derivatives.
[o] 4-Substituted.
[p] General structure:

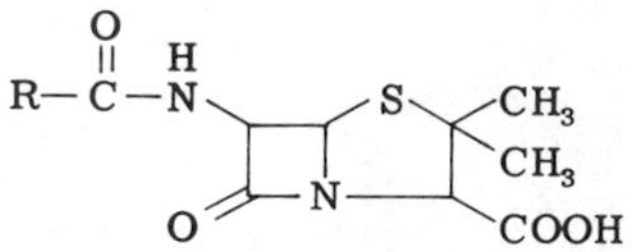

R includes H, alkyl, alkoxyalkyl, aminoalkyl, variously substituted phenyl, phenylalkyl (variously substituted in the alkyl and aryl parts), phenoxyalkyl (substituted in the phenyl part), naphthyl (also substituted), naphthyloxyalkyl, thienylalkyl (substituted in both parts), and quinolinyl (also substituted).

[q] General structure:

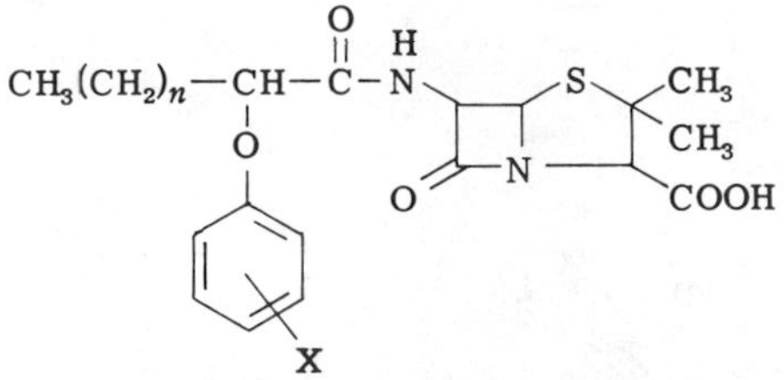

[r] C, C' is the minimum inhibitor constant with and without the presence of HSA.

[s] $\Sigma\ \pi$ refers to the substituents in the phenyl ring and to the alkyl chain.

[t] $\Sigma\ \sigma$ refers to the substituents in the phenyl ring.

[u] Positive correlation with π^2 and negative correlation with π. A parabolic relationship between lipophilicity expressed by R_m (see footnote *a*, Table VI) and serum binding was found by Biagi *et al.* (9) (positive R_m term, negative R_m^2 term).

[v] f_u is the fraction unbound.

[w] Cardiac glycosides and their aglycons.

[x] Progesterone derivatives.

[y] Bisguanylhydrazones.

[z] $\log K_B = \log K + \log[(K_a + [H^+])/K_a]$, where K_B is the binding constant of the free base and K the effective binding constant.

[aa] Reversed phase chromatography, oleyl alcohol impregnated kieselguhr–methanol–water.

[bb] β is the % bound and α is the % free.

[cc] General structure:

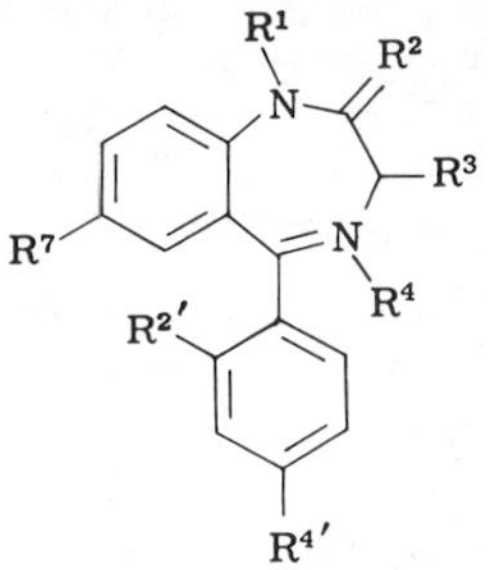

$\Sigma\ \pi$ includes positions 1, 2, 3, 4, 5, and 7; $\Sigma\ \sigma$ includes positions 1, 3, and 7.

(*continued*)

TABLE II *(Continued)*

[dd] Reversed phase TLC, from Maksay *et al.* (*103*).
[ee] Correlation for mouse serum was not as good as for HSA.

[ff] General structure:

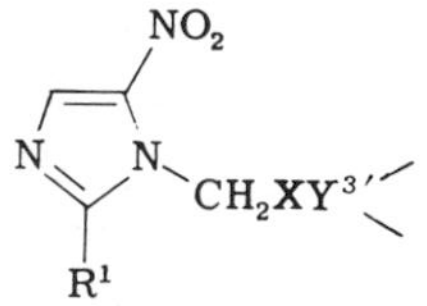

q_r is the frontier electron density at the heteroatom in the 3′ position as calculated by CNDO.
[gg] n is the length of alkyl chain in number of carbon atoms.
[hh] C is the molar concentration necessary to produce a 1:1 complex.
[ii] Linear relationships with log P have also been found for the formation of 2:1, 3:1, and 4:1 complexes (*51*).
[jj] Linear relationships between serum albumin binding and lipophilicity (log P) have been found for phenols (*38*) and barbiturates (*41*) alone.
[kk] Inclusion of ortho-substituted derivatives gives rather poor correlations unless this substitution is accounted for by an indicator variable (negative correlation). See also Seydel and Wempe (*133*).
[ll] Reversed phase TLC, paraffin impregnated silica gel, phosphate buffer-(pH 7.4)–acetone.

[mm] General structure:

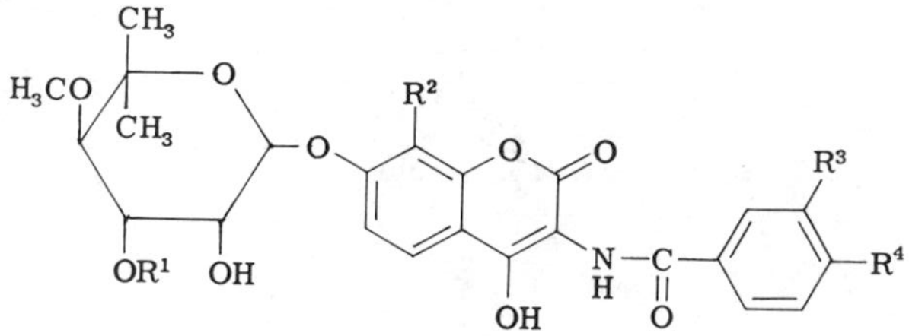

[nn] Specific binding seems to play a role.

In Table I the negative contribution of molecular weight becomes apparent in the case of rabbit whole-skin absorption of various types of compounds (Example 32, Table I) and is accounted for in the biological parameter of Example 8.

Finally, structural features such as shape may play a role in some cases. Thus the great difference in epidermal absorption rate between aliphatic alcohols (Example 27, Table I) and steroids (Example 28) was attributed to the difference in shapes between these two types of compounds (*89*).

2. Protein Binding

Not all of the absorbed drug is available for diffusion into various compartments and for receptor or enzyme binding, but only the fraction that is not bound to proteins. Protein binding must therefore be considered in the design of potential new drugs. QSAR work in this field is summarized in Table II.

Again, lipophilicity is the major determinant, whereby binding increases with increasing lipophilicity. In most cases the relationship is linear even when log *P* values of more than three are reached within the test sets. The optimal log *P* values in parabolic cases vary considerably (1.10–5.48). This suggests a strong dependence of protein binding on

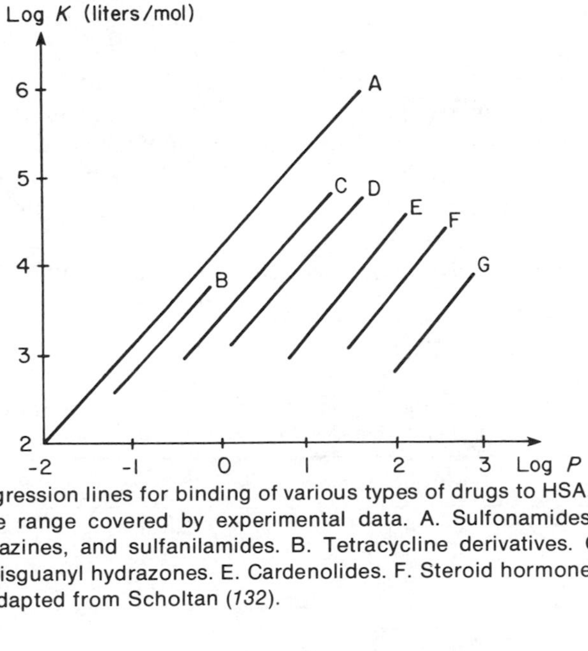

Fig. 1. Regression lines for binding of various types of drugs to HSA. The lines are drawn for the range covered by experimental data. A. Sulfonamides, sulfapyrimidines, sulfadiazines, and sulfanilamides. B. Tetracycline derivatives. C. Penicillins. D. Steroidal bisguanyl hydrazones. E. Cardenolides. F. Steroid hormones. G. Acridine derivatives. Adapted from Scholtan (*132*).

structural features. Thus a plot of log K (binding constant to human serum albumine, HSA) against log P for various types of drugs does not give a single regression line but several parallel lines (Fig. 1).

Even compounds that contain the same basic skeleton (steroid) differ with respect to the log P dependence of protein binding (D, E, and F in Fig. 1). All the compounds can, however, be fitted to a single equation (Eq. 1) in which log k_p, a group specific constant, represents all other factors that may govern protein binding, such as ionic interactions, steric effects, and hydrogen bonding (*132*).

$$\log K = \log k_p + a \log P \tag{1}$$

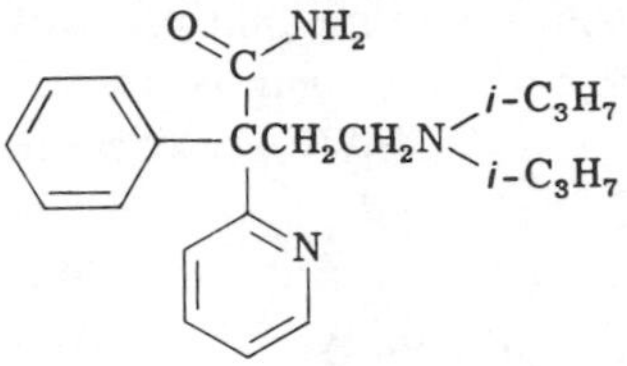

I

The structural dependence of protein binding also becomes evident from the series of disopyramide (**I**) and its derivatives (Example 14, Table II) (*12*). In this case both the intercept and the slope of the regression line vary if structural changes are introduced in different parts of the molecule (Table III). Omission of the basic side chain, leading to an increase in log P by about one unit (at pH 7.4), does not change protein binding. There are two possible explanations for this phenomenon: (1) the side chain does not participate in the binding, which means that local lipophilicity rather than overall lipophilicity may be the decisive factor; or (2) there is a polar interaction between the (protonated) amino group and the protein. Loss of this interaction on omission of the side chain can be compensated by the increase in lipophilicity. The latter hypothesis is sup-

TABLE III

Dependence of the Slope and the Intercept of Regression Lines for Protein Binding on the Site of Structural Variation in Disopyramide Derivatives

Site of variation	Regression coefficient	Intercept	Range of log P_{app}
Carbonamide	0.473	−0.303	−0.752–1.568
Phenyl ring	0.641	−0.369	−1.310–0.603
Pyridyl ring	0.734	−0.476	−0.182–1.393

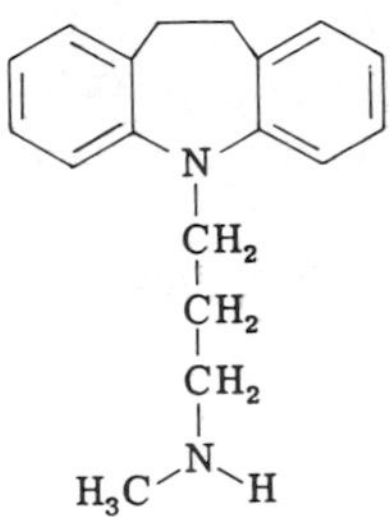

II

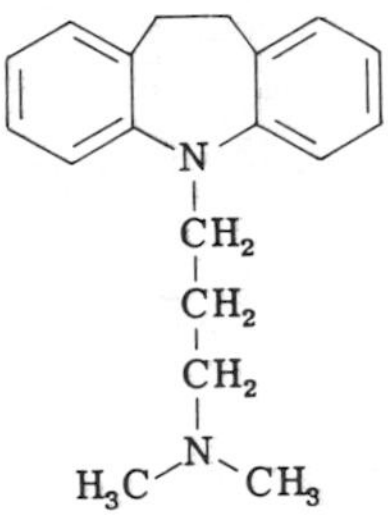

III

ported by the observation that desipramine (**II**), even though less lipophilic than imipramine (**III**), is bound equally strongly to protein. Desipramine is a stronger base (pK_a = 10.2) than imipramine (pK_a = 9.5) and could therefore form stronger ionic bonds with the protein (*34*).

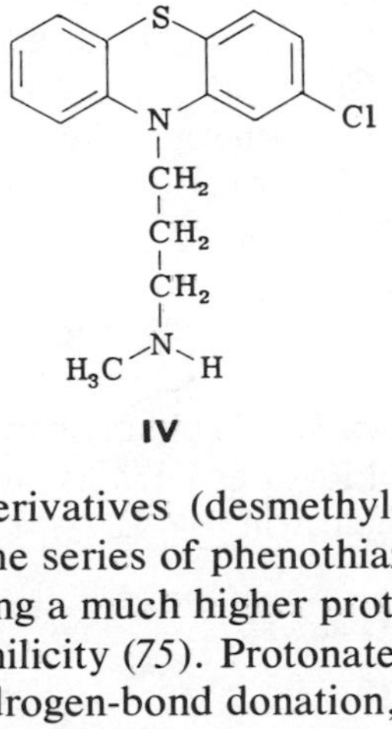

IV

Similarly, desmethyl derivatives (desmethylchlorpromazine, **IV**, and desmethylpromazine) in the series of phenothiazines (Example 26, Table II) were outliers by showing a much higher protein binding than could be expected from their lipophilicity (*75*). Protonated amino groups may also bind to the protein via hydrogen-bond donation, which would explain the observation that protein binding decreases with increasing basicity in disopyramid derivatives with variously substituted amino moieties (*13*).

Polar interactions that are governed by pK_a were detected for certain carboxylic acids (Example 12, Table II) (*113*), whereas the pK_a dependence in Example 3 reflects the change in lipophilicity due to ionization (*32*). Sulfonamides can bind to proteins in the anionic form (*23,124,133*) as demonstrated by the negative correlation of protein binding and pK_a in Example 37 (Table II).

Compounds with strong intramolecular steric interactions are sometimes outliers or give a rather poor fit to protein binding–log P regressions. Such effects were noted with the 2′-substituted benzodiazepines of Example 28 (Table II) (*100*) with sulfonamides (Example 37) (*133,137*) and in Example 13 in which the 3-chloro-4-nitrophenyl derivative is an outlier probably due to twisting of the nitro group out of the plane of the ring (*33*).

In summary, QSAR have shown that within a series of closely related compounds protein binding increases with lipophilicity. Differences between individual structural types are not well explained and cannot be predicted.

3. Distribution

The concentration of a drug that is available to a receptor is not only dependent on absorption and protein binding but also on distribution away from or into the tissue that contains the receptor. In this connection distribution into CNS is of particular interest. Examples in which this and other distribution processes have been investigated by QSAR are given in Table IV.

Penetration into the brain seems to be governed by lipophilicity only [in the case of penetration rate constants, an additional term in molecular weight may be detectable (see Example 4, Table IV) provided the test set varies enough in this factor]. With regard to log P_0, which has been found for various types of centrally acting drugs, and under the premise that lipophilicity governs mainly the diffusion of these drugs into brain, Lien (*95*) considered a range of log $P_{\mathrm{pH}\,7.4}$ of 1.4–2.7 ideal for CNS-active compounds. The values in Examples 2, 3, and 5 (Table IV) fall within this range (note that a log $P_{\mathrm{o,heptane/w}}$ of 0.2 is equivalent to a log $P_{\mathrm{o,o/w}}$ of 1.4), the value in Example 1 does not. Probably penetration into brain can also depend on other structural features such as molecular shape. Perhaps future QSAR work in this field will reveal such additional factors.

4. Elimination of Drugs

Drugs are eliminated either by metabolic transformation or by direct or biliary excretion.

a. Metabolic Transformation. Metabolic transformation is a composite process in which at least three steps are involved: (1) binding of the drug to the enzyme; (2) chemical modification of the drug molecule, which in turn can be a multistep reaction (e.g., Examples 34 and 35, Table V); and (3) desorption of the metabolite from the enzyme. Examples for quantitative treatment of single steps and the overall reaction are collected in Table V. (Enzymatic reactions that are not directly involved in drug metabolism are not generally included.) As can be expected from protein binding studies, the main determinant of enzyme binding is lipophilicity, which is positively correlated (Examples 1, 3, 13, 14, 17, 20, 28, 30, and 33, Table V).

Lipophilicity was expressed in terms of log P or lipophilic substituent constants or molar refractivity (MR). In the case of Example 13 (Table V), however, a substitution of MR by π yielded poorer correlations. Therefore, binding of a compound may also be governed by its polarizability (due to interaction via dispersion forces). The finding (Example 20) that, contrary to para-substituted derivatives, no dependence on lipophilicity was observed for meta derivatives may be an indication of the importance of local rather than global lipophilicity. This is not surprising because metabolic transformation by an enzyme requires specific binding, which ought to be primarily dependent on local physicochemical properties. This fact is again documented in Example 13 in which local polarizabilities (MR, MR_2, and MR_3) must be introduced separately into the regression equation. The three molar refractivities are attributed to the groups that are assumed to occupy different binding spaces (ρ_1, ρ_2, and ρ_3) of the molecule (Fig. 2).

Consequently, molecular shape and steric properties must be considered important factors for enzyme binding. Thus the binding of D-isomers of the compounds in Fig. 2 was only poorly correlated with MR_2, probably because R^2 in these isomers cannot bind to ρ_2 space (*50*). The importance of steric factors becomes clear from the necessity of introducing an extra indicator variable for valine derivatives in which R^2 is a bulky isopropyl group. Contributions from steric factors were also found in Examples 3 and 28 (Table V). In the latter case, branched-chain alkylamines are bound over 100 times less strongly than those with straight chains. In Example 30 the isopropyl ether was an outlier. Examples 13, 14, 17, and 20 reveal the possible importance of electronic properties (σ^*, σ^-).

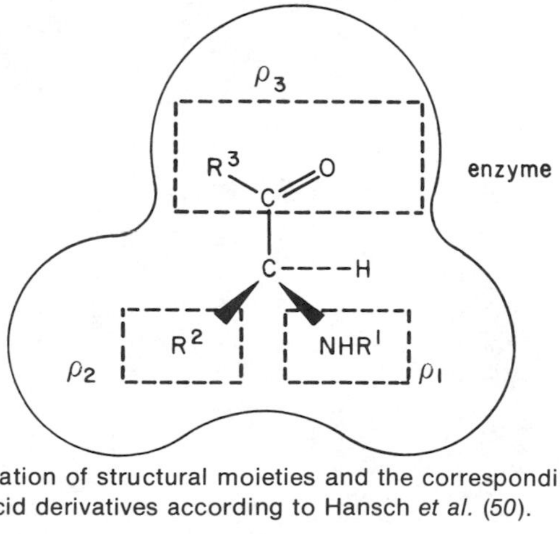

Fig. 2. Specification of structural moieties and the corresponding binding spaces for *N*-acylamino acid derivatives according to Hansch *et al.* (*50*).

TABLE IV
QSAR for Distribution of Drugs

Example number	Types of compounds in the test set	Species	Biological parameter	Relevant factors	Physicochemical parameter	Range of parameter in the test set	Type of dependence	References
1.	Phenylethylamines	Man (brain)	log (halucinogenic activity)	Lipophilicity	log $P_{o/w}$ (buffer pH 7.4)	1.00–4.31	Parabolic log $P_o = 3.14$	*(11)*
2.	Arylaminoimidazolines (clonidine derivatives)	Rat (brain)	$\log(C_{brain}/C_{iv})^a$	Lipophilicity	log $P_{o/w}$ (buffer pH 7.4)	−1.92–2.24	Parabolic log $P_o = 2.11$	*(148)*
3.	Morphine derivatives, 4-arylpiperidines, aralkylamines	Rabbit (brain)	$\log(C_{i.ventr}/C_{iv})^b$	Lipophilicity	log $P_{heptane/w}$ (buffer pH 7.4)	−5.00–1.29	Parabolic[d] log $P_o = 0.2$	*(84)*
			$\log(C_{brain}/C_{plasma})^c$				Linear	
4.	Various compounds[e]	Rat (brain)	log P_c^f	Lipophilicity	log $P_{o/w}$	−3.67–3.19	Linear[g]	*(86)*
				Molecular weight	log MW	1.78–2.60	Linear (−)	
5.	Phenylboronic acids	Mouse (brain)	log C^h	Lipophilicity	$\Sigma\, \pi$ (log P)	−3.50–1.79	Parabolic $\pi_o = 0.7$ log $P_o = 2.3$	*(40)*
6.	Carbohydrates, barbiturates, phenyl- and phenoxyalkyl-	Guinea pig (atria)	$\log(T/M)^i$	Lipophilicity	log $P_{o/w}$	−3.67–3.62	Linear[j]	*(101)*

amines, quaternary ammonium compounds, piperidine derivatives, coumarins, pyrazoles, steroids, aromatic amides, arylacetic acids

[a] C_{brain} is the brain concentration (ng/g brain tissue, wet weight) reached at maximum decrease in blood pressure following dose C_{iv} (μg/kg body weight).

[b] $C_{iv} = 1/ED_{iv}$, where ED_{iv} is the iv dose that gives a threshold response at the time of maximum effect. $C_{i\ ventr} = 1/ED_{i\ ventr}$, where $ED_{i\ ventr}$ is the intraventricular dose that gives a threshold analgesic effect.

[c] C_{brain} is the brain concentration at a standard response, and C_{plasma} is the plasma concentration at a standard response.

[d] The log P term is not statistically warranted. Omitting this term, Jacobson *et al.* (*65*) derived an equation that contains only a $(\log P)^2$ term. The log P_o value of 0.0 is, however, not significantly different from the one reported in Kutter *et al.* (*84*).

[e] NaCl, urea, glycerol, creatinine, 5-fluorouracil, dianhydrogalactitol, metronidazole, ascorbate, galactidol, misonidazole, ftorafur, BCNU, procarbazine, CCNU, pyrimethamine, PCNU, DDMP, DDEP, dibromodulcitol, spirohydantoin mustard, sucrose, Baker's antifol, adriamycin, epipodophylotoxin, vincristine, and bleomycin. (The last four compounds have molecular weights of >400 and did not fit the regression line; they were excluded from the regression analysis.)

[f] P_c is the brain capillary permeability coefficient in cm/sec.

[g] A positive linear correlation between $\log P_c$ and $\log (P(MW)^{-1/2})$ (the latter of which equals $\log P - 0.5 \log MW$) was found. The term in molecular weight accounts for its influence on the diffusion coefficient. The regression does not seem to hold for compounds with $MW > 400$.

[h] C is the concentration of boron (μg/g brain) at 15 min.

[i] T/M tissue to medium ratio.

[j] The equation also contained a linear term in log(bound/free) for atrial homogenate, $\log(B/F_{hom})$, which was positively correlated. Replacing $\log(B/F_{hom})$ by a term in $\log(B/F_{HSA})$ (protein binding) gave an inferior correlation. $\text{Log}(B/F_{hom})$ and $\log(B/F_{HSA})$ were linearly correlated with log P but only 64% and 50%, respectively, of the variance was explained by the regression equation, indicating the importance of structural factors.

TABLE V
Quantitative Structure—Metabolism Relationships

Example number	Type of compounds in the test set	Type of metabolic reaction	Biological parameter	Relevant factors	Physicochemical parameter	Range of parameter in the test set	Type of dependence	References
1.	4-Aminobenzene-sulfonamides	N⁴-acylation[a]	$\log V^{b}_{\max}$	Lipophilicity	π^{c}	0.00–2.61	Linear (−)[e]	(*32*)
				Acidity	$\Delta\log K^{d}_{a}$	0.00–5.83	Linear (−)	
		N⁴-acylation[f]	$\log(1/K_{m})^{g}$	Lipophilicity	π	0.00–2.61	Linear[i]	(*31*)
			$\log k^{h}$	Lipophilicity	π^{c}	0.00–2.61	Linear[j]	
2.	Anilines	Acetyltransferase catalyzed acetylation[k]	$\log A^{l}_{x}$	Lipophilicity	π	−1.16–1.13	Linear	(*37*)
				Electronic properties	σ^{-} or ϵ^{m}	−0.17–1.27	Linear (−)[n]	
						1.827–1.853	Linear	
3.	Barbiturates[o]	Metabolism in rat association with liver microsomal cytochrome *P*-450, and hepatic clearance		Lipophilicity	$f_{subt}{}^{r}$	3.46–6.62	Parabolic[t] $f_{subt_o} = 5.39$	
			$\log K^{p}_{s}$	Steric Properties (molar volume)	V^{s}_{1}	13.67–40.77	Linear	(*146*)
			$\log RHC^{q}$	Lipophilicity	f_{subt}	3.46–6.62	Parabolic $f_{subt_o} = 6.05$	
4.	5-Ethyl-5-alkyl barbiturates	Cytochrome *P*-450 binding	$1/K^{p}_{s}$	Lipophilicity	$\log P_{o/w}$	1.7–4.1	Parabolic $\log P_{o} = 3.0$	(*173*)
5.	Barbiturates	Metabolism by rabbit liver microsomes	$\log mr^{u}$	Lipophilicity	$\log P_{o/w}$	0.46–2.19	Linear	(*68*)
6.	Barbiturates	Metabolic elimination (intact rat and perfused rat liver)	$k_{cl}(\text{rel})^{v}$	Lipophilicity	$\log P_{o/w}$	0.87–4.13	Parabolic[w] $\log P_{o} = 3.54$	(*174*)

7.	Barbiturates	Metabolic elimination (intact rat)	k_{cl}^{x}	Lipophilicity	$\log P_{CCl_4/w}$ (buffer pH 7.4)	−1.7–1.3	Linear[y]	(99)
8.	Barbiturates	Metabolic change	log(% excreted unchanged)	Lipophilicity	$\log P_{o/w}$	0.65–2.45	Linear (−)[z]	(43)
		In vitro liver metabolism				1.15–2.15		
			log(% metabolized)	Lipophilicity	$\log P_{o/w}$		Linear	
		In vivo metabolism (mouse)				0.65–2.15		
9.	Oxazepamesters	Hydrolysis by mouse liver microsomes	$\log(V_R/V_{CH_3})^{aa}$	Steric properties	E_s	−2.0–0.0	Linear (−)[bb]	(102)
10.	4-Nitrophenyl esters of alkanoic acids	Hydrolysis by human serum esterase	$\log A_x^l$	Steric properties	E_s	−1.54–0.00	Linear[cc]	
				Lipophilicity	π	0.50–2.00	Linear	(37)
				Electronic properties	σ^*	−0.19–0.00	Linear (−)	
		Hydrolysis by chymotrypsin	$\log k_3^{dd}$	Electronic properties	σ^*	−0.30–1.05	Linear	
				Steric properties	E_s	1.54–1.24	Linear	(49)
				Lipophilicity	π	0.00–4.13	Linear	
11.	4-Nitrophenyl esters of benzoic acids	Hydrolysis by chymotrypsin	$\log k_2^{ee}$	Electronic properties	$\Sigma \sigma^*$	−0.78–0.79	Linear	(50)
				Lipophilicity or dispersion forces or size	ΣMR^{ff}	0.19–2.06	Linear	

(*continued*)

TABLE V (*Continued*)

Example number	Type of compounds in the test set	Type of metabolic reaction	Biological parameter	Relevant factors	Physicochemical parameter	Range of parameter in the test set	Type of dependence	References
12.	4-Nitrophenyl esters of aliphatic[gg] and aromatic carboxylic acids	Hydrolysis by chymotrypsin	$\log k_3^{dd}$	Electronic properties	σ^*	−0.30–1.14	Linear	
				Steric properties	E_s	−2.58–1.24	Linear[hh]	(50)
				Lipophilicity or dispersion forces or size	MR^{ff}	0.10–4.57	Linear	
13.	*N*-Acylamino acid esters[ii]	Ester hydrolysis by chymotrypsin	$\log(1/K_{mapp})^{jj}$	Lipophilicity or dispersion forces or size	$MR_1^{ff,kk}$	1.49–5.01	Linear[ll]	
					MR_2	0.56–4.23	Linear	(50)
					MR_3	0.79–3.78	Linear	
				Electronic properties	σ^*	−0.21–1.14	Linear cross term $MR_1MR_2MR_3$ (−)	
14.	*N*-Acylglycine esters[mm]	Ester hydrolysis by chymotrypsin	$\log(1/K_{mapp})^{jj}$	Lipophilicity or dispersion forces or size	$MR_1^{ff,kk}$	1.49–4.52	Linear	
					MR_3	0.79–3.78	Linear	(50)
				Electronic properties	σ^*	−0.21–1.14	Linear	
15.	*N*-Acylamino acid esters[nn]	Ester hydrolysis by chymotrypsin	$\log k_2^{ee}$	Lipophilicity or dispersion forces or size	$MR_1^{ff,kk}$	1.49–3.46	Linear (−)[oo]	(50)
					MR_2	0.56–3.18	Linear	
16.	*N*-Acylamino acid ester (D and L)[pp]	Ester hydrolysis by chymotrypsin	$\log k_3^{dd}$	Lipophilicity or dispersion forces or size	$MR_2^{ff,kk}$	0.56–3.18	Linear[qq]	(50)

17.	Nicotinoylalanine esters[rr]	Ester hydrolysis by chymotrypsin	$\log(1/K_m)$[g]	Electronic properties	σ^*[ss]	−0.30–1.32	Linear[tt]	(35)
				Lipophilicity or dispersion forces or size	MR[ff,ss]	0.79–3.22	Linear	
18.	Phenyl acetates	Hydrolysis by butylcholin esterase	k_{rel}[uu]	Electronic properties	f_5[vv]	0.42–0.50	Linear[ww]	(64)
19.	Alkyl *p*-nitrobenzoates	Ester hydrolysis (mouse cutaneous homogenates)	$\log RH$[xx]	Lipophilicity	f[yy]	0.701–2.258	Linear	(119)
				Steric factors	I[zz]	1–3	Linear (−)	
20.	Phenyl β-D-glycosides	Hydrolysis by emulsin	$\log(k_1/k_2)$[aaa]	Electronic properties	σ^-	−0.26–1.27	Linear[bbb]	
							Linear	
			$\log k'_3$	Lipophilicity	π	−0.33–1.78	Linear	(37)
							Linear (−)	
21.	Aliphatic amines (primary)[ccc]	Oxidative deamination[ddd]	$\log mr$[eee]	Lipophilicity	$\log P_{o/w}$	0.39–3.44	Parabolic[fff] $\log P_o = 2.50$	(42)
				Basicity	pK_a	9.34–10.70	Linear	
22.	Aliphatic amines[ccc] (secondary)	Oxidative deamination[ddd]	$\log mr$	lipophilicity	$\log P_{o/w}$	0.20–3.46	Parabolic[fff] $\log P_o = 2.54$	(42)
23.	Aliphatic amines (primary, *n*-alkyl)	Oxidative deamination[ggg]	$\log mr$	Lipophilicity	$\log P_{o/w}$	−0.69–2.81	Parabolic[fff] $\log P_o = 1.71$	(42)
24.	Aliphatic amines[hhh] (primary)	Oxidative deamination[iii]	$\log mr$	Lipophilicity	$\log P_{o/w}$	−0.32–2.44	Parabolic[fff] $\log P_o = 1.74$	(42)
				Basicity	pK_a	9.34–10.63	Linear	
		Oxidative deamination[iii]	$\log mr$	Lipophilicity	$\log P_{o/w}$	−0.32–2.44	Parabolic $\log P_o = 1.74$	(42)
25.	Benzylamines (*m*- and *p*-substituted)	Oxidative deamination[jjj]	$\log mr$[kkk]	Lipophilicity	$\log P_{o/w}$	0.60–2.35	Linear[mmm]	(42)
				Steric properties	E_s[lll]	−0.75–1.24	Linear	

(*continued*)

TABLE V (*Continued*)

Example number	Type of compounds in the test set	Type of metabolic reaction	Biological parameter	Relevant factors	Physicochemical parameter	Range of parameter in the test set	Type of dependence	References
26.	*N*-Methylamines[nnn] (tertiary)	Oxidative demethylation by microsomes	log *RBR*[ooo]	Lipophilicity	log $P_{o/w}$	1.50–4.20	Linear	(*39,48*)
				Basicity	ΔpK_a^{ppp}	−2.40–2.40	Parabolic[qqq] (−) (−)	
27.	*N*-Substituted amphetamines	N-deamination (human)	log *DEA*[rrr]	Lipophilicity	log $P_{heptane/w}$ (buffer pH 7.4)	−1.51–3.83	Linear	
					or Σf^{sss}	1.17–4.52	Linear	(*147*)
				Steric properties	V_R	13.67–56.07	Linear (−)	
28.	Aliphatic amines	Binding to rabbit liver microsome *P*-450	$\log(1/K_1)^{ttt}$	Lipophilicity	n^{uuu}	3–12	Linear[vvv]	(*66*)
29.	*N*,*N*-Dimethyl-amines[www]	*N*-Oxide formation by microsomal mixed function oxidase	$\log k_{ox}^{xxx}$	Lipophilicity	log $P_{o/w}$	0.27–8.77	Parabolic[yyy] log P_o = 5.69	(*149*)
30.	4-Nitrophenylalkyl ethers	Oxidative dealkylation by rat liver microsomal *P*-450	$\log K_s^{zzz}$	Lipophilicity	log $P_{o/w}$ (buffer pH 7.4)	2.0–3.6	Linear (−)[aaaa]	(*1*)
31.	Phenols	Conversion of microsomal *P*-450 to *P*-420	$\log(1/C)^{bbbb}$	Lipophilicity	$\Sigma \pi$	−1.29–4.39	Linear	(*48,63*)
32.	Anilines				(log $P_{o/w}$)	−0.73–0.98	Linear	(*48,63*)

33.	Aromatic dimethylamines, barbiturates, morphine derivatives, xanthines, phenylethylamines, indole derivatives	Oxidation by rat liver microsomal NADPH-oxidase	$\log(1/K_{m\ corr})^{cccc}$	Lipophilicity	$\log P_{o/w}$	−0.07–3.55	Linear	(*48,105*)
34.	2-Substituted anilines	4-Hydroxylation by microsomes	$\log RBR^{dddd}$	Electronic properties	$\mathbf{R}^{eeee}$	−0.20–0.16	Linear $(-)^{ffff}$	(*48*)
				Lipophilicity	$\log P_{o/w}$	0.90–2.09	Linear	
35.	3-Substituted anilines			Steric properties	E_s	−1.28–1.24	Linear	(*48*)
				Lipophilicity	$\log P_{o/w}$	1.30–3.16	Linear	
36.	4-Alkoxy-acetanilides	N-Hydroxylation by mouse liver microsomes[gggg]	log rate[hhhh]	Lipophilicity	n^{iiii}	1–4	Linear[jjjj]	(*69*)
37.	Benzoic acids (4-subst.)	Glucuronide formation (rabbit)	$\log mr^{kkkk}$	Lipophilicity	$\log P_{o/w}$	1.06–2.99	Parabolic $\log P_o = 2.34$	(*42*)
38.	Primary aliphatic alcohols	Glucuronide formation (rabbit)	$\log mr^{llll}$	Lipophilicity	$\log P_{o/w}$	−0.16–3.34	Parabolic[nnnn] $\log P_o = 2.29$	(*42*)
39.	Secondary aliphatic alcohols			Steric properties	ΣE_s^{mmmm}	1.35–2.48	Linear (−)	
				Lipophilicity	$\log P_{o/w}$	0.14–2.61	Parabolic[oooo] $\log P_o = 1.75$	(*42*)
40	Phenols	Glucuronidation by rat liver microsomes[pppp]	$\log(1/K_m)$	Lipophilicity	$\log P_{o/w}$	1.34–3.31	Linear[rrrr]	(*127a*)
			$\log A^{qqqq}$	Lipophilicity	$\log P_{o/w}$	1.34–2.59	Linear[ssss]	

(*continued*)

TABLE V *(Continued)*

Example number	Type of compounds in the test set	Type of metabolic reaction	Biological parameter	Relevant factors	Physicochemical parameter	Range of parameter in the test set	Type of dependence	References
41.	Benzoic acids (4-substituted)	Hippuric acid formation (rabbit)	log mr^{tttt}	Lipophilicity	log $P_{o/w}$	1.06–2.99	Parabolic log $P_o = 2.37$	*(42)*
42.	2-Sulfapyridines	Metabolic clearance (rat)	log Cl_M^{uuu}	Lipophilicity Electronic properties	ΔR_m^{vvv} pK_a	0.00–1.17 5.78–9.74	Linear $(-)^{wwww}$ Linear	*(137)*
43.	Various compounds[xxxx]	Various[xxxx] processes	$R_{(r/s)}^{yyyy}$	Lipophilicity	log $P_{o/w}$	0.76–6.92	Linear	*(87)*

[a] Pigeon liver acetyltransferase.
[b] V_{max} is the maximum acetylation velocity.
[c] $\pi = \log P - \log P_{sulfanilamide}$.
[d] $\Delta \log K_a = pK_{a\ sulfanilamide} - pK_a$.
[e] Correlated with $\log V_{max} - \log[(K_a + [H^+])/[H^+]]$.
[f] Rat, rabbit, and human.
[g] K_m is the Michaelis constant.
[h] $\text{Log } k = \log k_{Ac} + \log[(K_a + [H^+])/[H^+]]$; k_{Ac} is the acylation rate constant (h^{-1}); the second term expresses the dissociation effect of the free drug.
[i] Correlated with $\log(1/K_m) + \log[(K_a + [H^+])/[H^+]]$.
[j] Terms in ΔpK_a played a significant role only in a correlation with $\log k_{Ac}$ (negative correlation), which was, however, considerably poorer than the correlation with $\log k$.
[k] Acetylaminophenylazobenzenesulfonic acid was used as acetyl donor.
[l] A_x is the reaction rate.
[m] ϵ is the electron density on amino nitrogen as obtained from quantum mechanical calculations.
[n] Acetyl transfer to aminophenylazobenzene sulfonic acid from various acetyl donors was positively correlated with π and σ^-.
[o] General structure:

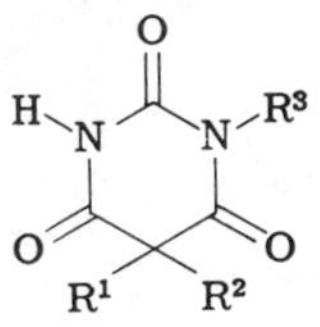

R^1 is the substituent with the smaller volume, R^2 is the substituent with the larger volume, and R^3 is H or CH_3.

[p] K_s is the spectral dissociation constant.
[q] *RHC* is the relative hepatic clearance (heptabarbital = 1.00).
[r] f_{subt} is the sum of hydrophobic fragment constants for R^1, R^2, and R^3.

[s] V_1 is the volume (ml/mol) of R^1, and V_2 is the volume of R^2.

[t] In addition, the regression equation contains a (positively correlated) indicator variable I, which is 1 for $R^3 = CH_3$. An improvement of the fit is obtained when a term in V_2 (range 34.13–95.51) is added. However, V_2 is highly correlated with f_{subt} so that an equally good fit is obtained with V_1, V_2, and I in which the dependence on V_2 is parabolic ($V_{2_o} = 73.6$). Thus the equations do not allow the question to be answered as to whether barbiturate binding to the enzyme is governed by lipophilicity or steric properties or both. The contribution of I may point to steric or hydrogen-bonding interactions.

[u] *mr* is the *in vitro* metabolic rate constant (nmol/min/g wet weight of liver).

[v] k_{cl} (rel) is the relative clearance rate (reference heptabarbital).

[w] Allyl and bromoallyl derivatives are outliers, possibly because of differences in metabolism.

[x] k_{cl} is the clearance rate (per min) from a two-compartment model.

[y] Thiopental is an outlier.

[z] Signifying a positive linear dependence of metabolic change rate on lipophilicity.

[aa] Relative rate of hydrolysis.

[bb] A dependence on electronic factors (σ^*, linear) could also be detected. Substrate binding (K_m) increases with lipophilicity (number of carbon atoms, n) up to a maximum ($n_o = 4$). The subsequent decrease is explained by steric hindrance becoming the dominating factor.

[cc] The variance in E_s accounts for 90% of the variance in hydrolysis rate.

[dd] k_3 is the deacylation rate of the enzyme.

[ee] k_2 is the rate of acylation of the enzyme.

[ff] *MR* values are scaled by 0.1.

[gg] Unsubstituted and substituted by halogen and acylamino.

[hh] Aromatic acids needed to be represented by an additional indicator variable (negatively correlated). It is concluded that E_s alone did not account sufficiently for the influence of the phenyl ring on deacylation of the enzyme.

[ii] Acyl groups: aliphatic, aromatic, heteroaromatic, alkoxycarbonyl, and alkylsulfonyl. Ester groups: aliphatic and aromatic.

[jj] $K_{mapp} = (k_{-1} + k_2)/k_1$, in which the constants are defined on the basis of the following reaction scheme: $\text{E-CH}_2\text{OH} + \text{RCOOR}' \underset{k_{-1}}{\overset{k_1}{\rightleftharpoons}} \text{E-CH}_2\text{OH} \cdot \text{RCOOR}' \xrightarrow{k_2} \text{HOR}' + \text{E-CH}_2\text{OCOR} \xrightarrow[\text{H}_2\text{O}]{k_3} \text{E-CH}_2\text{OH} + \text{RCOOH}$. E-$CH_2OH$ stands for the enzyme and its catalytic serin moiety.

[kk] MR_1, MR_2, MR_3, and σ^* refer to $NHCOR^1$, OR^3, and R^3, respectively, in the following general structure:

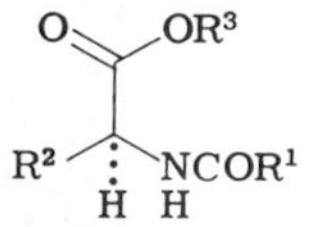

[ll] Using π instead of *MR* gave poorer correlations, which suggests that the binding is not a typically hydrophobic interaction but may be due to dispersion forces that are better correlated with polarizability. The expected involvement of configurational properties could be demonstrated by an analysis of the D isomers for which $\log(1/K_{mapp})$ was only poorly correlated with MR_2 (R^1 and R^3 were kept constant). This means that in these isomers, R^2 does not contribute significantly to binding. Valine derivatives fitted the regression only when accounted for by an indicator variable (negatively correlated), indicating the possible importance of steric factors. Similar results were obtained from an analysis of chymotrypsin binding of *N*-acylamino acid amides of the following general structure:

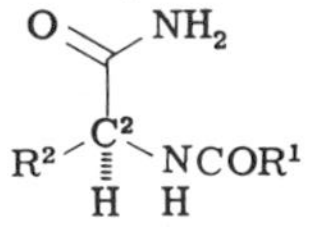

In this case molar refractivities *MR*-L and *MR*-S were used, which refer to the larger and the smaller substituent in position 2, regardless of the configuration at this carbon atom (*175*). For related work, see also Hansch and Coats (*46*).

(*continued*)

[mm] Acyl group: aliphatic, aromatic, and heteroaromatic.
[nn] Acyl group: aliphatic and aromatic; ester group: aliphatic.
[oo] Valine derivatives had to be accounted for by a negatively correlated indicator variable. No significant contribution from R^3 was present. This may, however, be due to insufficient variation of R. The negative regression coefficient of MR_1 was explained by a possible desorption of this part of the molecule from the enzyme in the transacylation step.
[pp] Acyl group: aliphatic, aromatic, heteroaromatic, and benzyloxycarbonyl; ester group: aliphatic and 4-nitrophenyl.
[qq] D isomers and valine derivatives had to be represented by additional (negatively correlated) indicator variables. MR_1 did not contribute significantly. A regression equation was also derived for the overall hydrolysis (log K_{cat}). This equation is composed of terms in MR_2 and MR_2^2 (there is an optimal size for R^2), an indicator variable for valine (negative correlation) and a (negatively correlated) cross term $MR_1MR_2MR_3$. The latter was interpreted as R^1 playing a constant negative role in the ester hydrolysis.
[rr] Ester group: variously substituted alkyl.

[ss] σ^* refers to R, MR to OR in the following general structure:

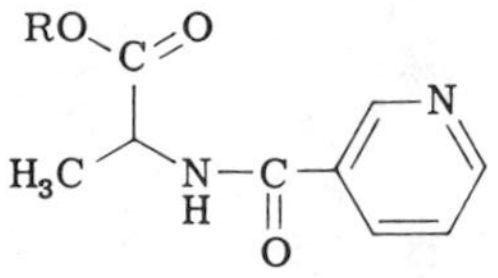

[tt] The test compounds were chosen so as to reduce colinearity between π and MR in comparison with Example 13. Adding the MR term to the correlation with σ^* gave a significant improvement, whereas π did not. This result supports the conclusions drawn in Hansch (*49*).[ll] The MR term may reflect conformational changes in the enzyme due to the interaction with the substrate. Combining the data with those used in Example 13 gave a good correlation with regression coefficients close to those obtained there.
[uu] k_{rel} is the relative rate of hydrolysis (unsubstituted = 100%).

[vv] f_5 is the frontier electron density at position 5 and S_8 is the superdelocalizability at position 8.

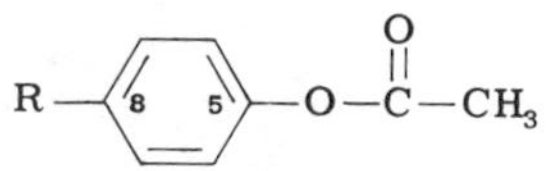

[ww] A slight correlation was found between the relative rate of hydrolysis by acetylcholinesterase and S_8^{vv}.
[xx] RH is the initial rate of hydrolysis (μmol/g tissue/min).
[yy] f is the hydrophobic fragment constant of the alkyl group.
[zz] I is the indicator variable for α-branching of the alkyl group.
[aaa] $k_1/k_2 = 1/K_m$; it is the absorption constant. k_3' is the constant for product formation and release from the enzyme–substrate complex and enzyme–product complex, respectively.
[bbb] Two steps of the hydrolysis were considered individually: (1) formation of the enzyme–substrate complex, $\log(k_1/k_2)$ and (2) formation and release of product, $\log k_3'$. When ortho meta, and para derivatives were examined separately, the following results were obtained. (1) In both the first and the second step lipophilicity was an important factor for para substituted derivatives but did not contribute significantly to the hydrolysis of meta derivatives. Setting $\pi_m = 0$, meta and para derivatives could be combined in one good correlation. (2) With ortho substituents both electronic properties and lipophilicity played a role, but the regression accounted for only 61% ($\log[k_1/k_2]$) and 55% ($\log k_3'$) of the variance in the biological data, respectively, which can be attributed to contributions from steric effects. For meta and para derivatives, a good correlation between the overall reaction ($\log[k_1/k_2]k_3'$) and σ^- (positive) was obtained, but lipophilicity did not play a significant role. This result is to be expected considering the absence of lipophilic influence for meta derivatives and the opposing contributions from this factor to the first (positive) and second step (negative).

[ccc] Alkyl, aralkyl, acylalkyl, and hydroxyalkyl.

[ddd] Rabbit liver amine oxidase.

[eee] *mr* is the relative metabolic rate (reference: 2-phenylethylamine).

[fff] Primary and secondary amines had to be treated separately. In both cases the optimal lipophilicity is the same, but with secondary amines no significant contribution from pK_a (range 9.60–10.98) could be detected. Considering the confidence limits, sets 21–24 show that optimal lipophilicity for these reactions is not dramatically species dependent. Unexplained variance was attributed to steric factors. This conclusion is supported by the fact that corresponding α-alkyl or α-aryl substituted amines and tertiary amines are not substrates of the enzyme.

[ggg] Cattle liver amine oxidase.

[hhh] Alkyl, aralkyl, and hydroxyalkyl.

[iii] Cattle (first row) and cat (second row) liver extract.

[jjj] Beef liver mitochondria.

[kkk] $mr = Q_{ox}$ value (microequivalents O_2/h/g mitochondria).

[lll] For the para substituent.

[mmm] The meta derivatives give a high correlation with log P alone, which is not improved by additional terms. Replacing E_s by a molar volume term leads to a less satisfactory correlation. The meta derivatives alone show a different slope in log P (0.452) as compared with the whole set (0.623), indicating a difference in hydrophobic effect between meta and para derivatives. The difference in the type of structural dependence to that found for sets 21–24 is explained in terms of conformational differences of the enzyme in its natural environment and in isolation.

[nnn] Straight chain and branched alkyls, also substituted by phenyl, acetylenic, hydroxy, and acyloxy groups.

[ooo] *RBR* is the amount of formaldehyde produced from a fixed amount of amine.

[ppp] $\Delta pK_a = pK_a - 9.5$.

[qqq] Both the linear and the squared term in ΔpK_a are negatively correlated. The squared term indicates that metabolic demethylation proceeds maximally at an optimal electron density on the nitrogen atom corresponding to $pK_{a_0} = 9.5$.

[rrr] *DEA* is the rate constant for first dealkylation.

[sss] f is the hydrophobic fragment constant of the two nitrogen substituents; V_R is the volume of substituent cleaved by *N*-dealkylation.

[ttt] K_1 is the dissociation constant for type *b* binding (pH 7.4).

[uuu] n is the chain length.

[vvv] Above $n = 8$ the $\log(1/K_1)$ versus n curve leveled off. On a log P representation of lipophilicity benzylamine also fitted into the regression. Branched chain alkylamines bind over 100 times less strongly.

[www] Alkyl, aryl, phenothiazines, and morphine derivatives.

[xxx] k_{ox} is the oxidation rate of substrate dependent NADPH (mol/min/mg protein).

[yyy] Addition of a pK_a term did not improve the correlation significantly.

[zzz] K_s is the spectral dissociation constant.

[aaaa] The isopropyl ether is an outlier (K_s too low), α-deuterated alkyl ethers fit the regression; a poor (negative) correlation was also found between log K_m and log P.

[bbbb] C is the molar concentration for 50% reduction.

[cccc] $K_{m\ corr}$ is the Michaelis constant corrected for the concentration of the neutral form of the molecule.

[dddd] *RBR* is the percentage of the 2-chloroaniline 4-hydroxylation.

[eeee] **R** is the Swain and Lupton resonance parameter.

[ffff] The transformation is a multistep reaction: (1) epoxide formation, (2) nucleophilic opening of the epoxide by water, and (3) elimination of one hydroxy group.

[gggg] Untreated as well as induced with 2,3,7,8-tetrachlorodibenzo-*p*-dioxin (TCDD).

[hhhh] Reaction rate refers to formation of metabolite (nmol/min/nmol P-450).

(continued)

TABLE V *(Continued)*

[iiii] n is the chain length.

[jjjj] The correlation is based on only three points. O-dealkylation was unaffected by chain length.

[kkkk] mr is the rate of glucuronide formation.

[llll] mr is the % glucuronide formation.

[mmmm] ΣE_s is taken over all substituents on the carbinol carbon atom (including H).

[nnnn] Primary and secondary alcohols had to be treated separately because of differences in the rate of the competing oxidation, which is more efficient with primary alcohols. The negative term in E_s is regarded as a reflection of steric hindrance of oxidation whereby glucuronidation, which seems to be less sensitive to steric effects, can compete more efficiently.

[oooo] Addition of terms in E_s or σ^* does not improve the correlation (insufficient variance in E_s?).

[pppp] Treated with Triton X-100.

[qqqq] A = glucuronidation activity (ng/min/mg microsomal protein).

[rrrr] For 4-substituted phenols, a linear correlation was also obtained for a set of mono- and disubstituted (including ortho substituted) phenols. Terms for electronic (σ^-) and steric (E_s) properties did not improve the equations.

[ssss] For 3- and 4-substituted phenols; ortho substituted phenols did not show any correlation between log A and log P or E_s or both.

[tttt] mr is the hippuric acid formation.

[uuuu] Cl_M is the metabolic clearance (ml/min).

[vvvv] ΔR_m values were determined by reversed phase TLC on paraffin oil coated silica gel, buffer pH 5.0.

[wwww] A separate study on acylation rate by rat liver preparations showed similar dependence on lipophilicity and acidity.

[xxxx] Benzopyrene (aromatic hydroxylation), chlorpromazine (sulfur oxidation), zoxazolamine (aromatic hydroxylation), *p*-nitrobenzoic acid (reduction of NO_2), L-amphetamine (deamination), hexobarbital (aliphatic hydroxylation), codeine (O-dealkylation), acetanilide (aromatic hydroxylation), and aminopyrine (*N*-demethylation).

[yyyy] $R_{(r/s)}$ is the ratio of enzymatic activity in rough and smooth microsomal subfraction.

For the last step, desorption, inverse dependencies on the factors governing enzyme binding can be expected. This may explain the negative correlation between the overall reaction rate and lipophilicity in Example 1 (Table V) as well as the hardly significant contribution of lipophilicity to the overall glycoside hydrolysis in Example 20. In the latter case the positive influence on binding is canceled by the opposite effect on desorption (negative correlation between the rate of product formation from the enzyme–substrate complex and lipophilicity).

The actual transformation step(s) depend(s), as expected, on electronic (expressed by pK_a, various σ constants, resonance constants, electron densities) and steric properties [expressed by E_S or indicator variables (e.g., Example 15, Table V)], but lipophilicity (probably local) may also play a role (e.g., Examples 1, 10, and 20).

All the factors that can determine the individual steps of metabolic transformation, i.e., lipophilic, electronic, steric properties, and structural features must also be considered for the overall reaction. The significance of structural features is shown in Example 6 (Table V) where allyl and bromoallyl barbiturates do not fit the regression line, probably because of different metabolism (*174*). In Example 7 thiopental is an outlier. Some of these properties may not, however, appear in correlations with the overall metabolic rate because (1) the influences that a certain factor exerts on individual steps cancel (Example 20, Table V), and (2) one reaction step becomes rate limiting for the overall process. Thus the dependence of the oxidation processes in Examples 31 and 32 on only lipophilicity is due to absorption being the rate-limiting step (*48*).

b. Excretion. Both net biliary and renal excretion result from two counteracting processes, actual excretion and reuptake. The reuptake process depends on the same factors as absorption (see Section II,B,1). Literature data on quantitative treatment of excretion are scarce; some examples are summarized in Table VI.

From these examples two factors, lipophilicity and electronic properties (acidity), emerge as relevant. An additional important factor is molecular weight. Thus renal excretion (glomerular filtration) is limited to molecules with a molecular weight of less than 5000. Biliary excretion becomes significant only above molecular weights of about 300. In addition, the presence of a polar group (structural factor) such as carbohydrate moieties or ionizable (at physicological pH) groups can become an important factor. If these groups are only weakly basic or acidic, biliary excretion should become dependent on pK_a (electronic factor) as shown in Example 2 (Table VI) for sulfathiazoles, which are weak acids and which show a negative dependence of biliary excretion on pK_a. (Weaker acids

TABLE VI
Quantitative Structure–Excretion Relationships

Example number	Type of compounds in the test set	Route of excretion	Biological parameter	Relevant factors	Physicochemical parameter	Range of parameter in the test set	Type of dependence	References
1.	Penicillins	Biliary (rat)	log(% excr 0–4 h)	Lipophilicity	$\log P$	1.06–3.24	Parabolic (−)[b] $\log P_o = 2.99$	(*96*)
					R_m[a]	0.07–1.62	Linear	(*125*)
2.	Sulfathiazoles	Biliary (rat)	log(% excr)	Lipophilicity	$\text{Log } P_{o/w}$	−0.98–1.53	Parabolic $\log P_o = 0.6$	(*96*)
				Electronic properties	pK_a	2.86–7.23	Linear (−)	
3.	Sulfapyridines	Renal (rat)	$\log Cl_R$[c]	Lipophilicity	ΔR_m	0.00–1.17	Linear (−)	(*137*)
				Electronic properties	pK_a	5.78–9.74	Linear	
4.	4-Aminobenzene-sulfonamides	Renal (rat, rabbit, human)	$\log k$[d]	Lipophilicity	π	0.00–2.61	Linear[f]	
				Electronic properties	ΔpK_a[e]	0.00–5.05	Linear	(*31*)
5.	N-Substituted amphetamines	Renal (human)	$\log PEU$[g]	Lipophilicity	$\log P_{\text{heptane/w}}$ (buffer pH 7.4)	−2.26–3.83	Parabolic[i] (−) (−) $\log P_o = -2.24$	(*147*)
			$\log EXC$		Σf[h]	0.94–4.52	Linear (−)	

[a] Reversed phase TLC (silicon impregnated silica gel), mobile phase sodium acetate–veronal buffer, pH 7.4 + acetone (*9*).
[b] Biliary excretion of cephalosporins in rats has been found to increase progressively with molecular weight from a threshold of 450 and up (*165*).
[c] Cl_R is the renal clearance (ml/min).
[d] $\log k = \log k_{Ex} - \log[(K_A + [H^+])/[H^+]]$, where K_{Ex} is the excretion rate constant; the second term accounts for the dissociation of the compound at urinary pH.
[e] Difference to pK_a of sulfanilamide.
[f] In rabbits the pK_a is negatively correlated, which is attributed to species differences; in humans, terms derived from chloroform–buffer pH 7.4 partition coefficients gave a much better correlation. A very poor correlation was obtained for $\log_{Ex}$ alone.
[g] *PEU* is the percent excreted unchanged and *EXC* is the excretion rate constant.
[h] f is the hydrophobic fragment constant for substituents on nitrogen.
[j] Both the terms in $\log P$ and $(\log P)^2$ are negatively correlated.

are ionized to a lesser degree and therefore excreted comparatively more slowly.) The significance of competing reabsorption (enterohepatic circulation) is documented by the negative dependence of net excretion on lipophilicity in Example 1 (Table VI). The negative correlation between net renal clearance and lipophilicity in Example 3 can be explained either by increased tubular reuptake (which ought to be positively correlated with lipophilicity) or by increased protein binding (only the free drug in plasma is subject to glomerular filtration).

c. Duration of Effect. The duration of pharmacological effects of drugs is influenced not only by elimination processes and distribution phenomena (including protein binding) but also by the biological properties of metabolites (e.g., if these are also active). Therefore, duration of effect can in principle depend on all the factors that govern these biological properties. Unless one of these processes becomes dominating, simple regression analysis will generally not be able to explain the variance in duration of effects. For the same reason the type of dependence on structural or physicochemical properties varies from test set to test set. Thus in Example 1 (Table VII) the duration of the effect is negatively correlated with lipophilicity whereas in example 2 the opposite is observed. In Example 4 only compounds with a lipophilicity of less than $\Sigma\ \pi = -0.5$ are long acting. As demonstrated in Examples 3 and 4, structure–activity classifications (e.g., discriminant or cluster analysis) can become a valuable tool in the analysis of those biological measurements that result from a superposition of several effects.

C. Model-Based Relationships

The empirical regression analysis dealt with in the preceding paragraph assumes that biological activities of drugs can be described by linear combinations of free-energy related descriptors of chemical structures. Deviations from linearity are accounted for by the introduction of squared terms or cross products. From a theoretical point of view, this approach is unsatisfactory as long as no physical significance can be attributed to these additional terms. Therefore, models have been developed that could it is hoped, give a more meaningful and more exact explanation of the variance in the biological data.

1. Absorption Models

Koizumi *et al.* (*71*) and Wagner and Sedman (*155*) applied a relatively simple model to describe buccal and gastrointestinal absorption. The model consists of two aqueous phases separated by a lipid membrane.

TABLE VII
Quantitative Relationships between Structure and Duration of Biological Effects

Example number	Type of compounds in the test set	Biological measurement	Parameter	Relevant factors	Physicochemical parameter	Range of parameter in the test set	Type of dependence	References
1.	2-Propenyl barbiturates	Duration of action ip adm (mice)	$\log T^a$	Lipophilicity	$\log P_{o/w}$	1.15–2.65	Linear (−)	(*48*)
2.	Testosterone esters	Time of maximum effect	$\log T^b$	Lipophilicity	R_m^c	−0.60–0.96	Linear	(*8*)
3.	Barbiturates	Duration of effect ip or subcutaneous (mice, rats, rabbits)	T^d	Structural properties	Atom-, bond-structural descriptors, molecular connectivity		Location of group in parameter space (discriminant analysis)	(*142*)
4.	2-Arylimidazo [4,5-*b*]pyridines	Duration of effect iv cat)	T^e	Lipophilicity	$\Sigma \pi$	−1.60–0.94	Location of group in lipophilicity space	(*85*)

[a] Hours.
[b] Days.
[c] Reversed phase TLC, 54% acetone in mobile phase.
[d] In minutes; groups were formed according to certain ranges of duration.
[e] Two groups were formed: (1) duration of effect 30 min on 2 mg/kg iv or 60 min on 4 mg/kg iv; and (2) duration of effect below these limits.

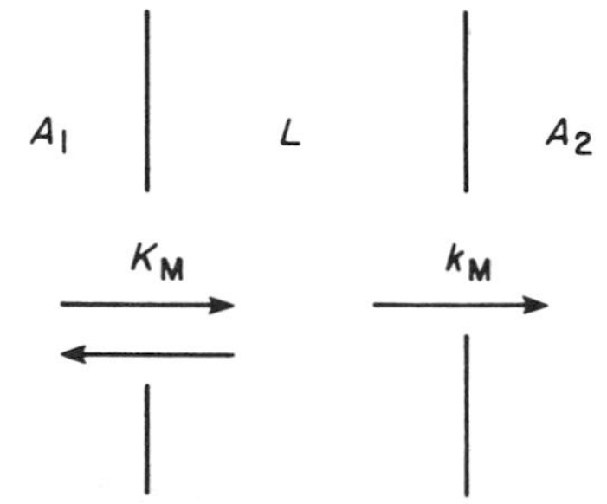

Fig. 3. Absorption model according to Wagner and Sedman. A_1: first aqueous phase (representing buccal or gastrointestinal fluid). A_2: second aqueous phase (representing blood serum). K_M: partition coefficient between buccal or gastrointestinal fluid and membrane. k_M: first-order rate constant for transport of the drug out of the membrane. L: lipid membrane (representing buccal or gastrointestinal wall).

Wagner and Sedman assume that equilibrium partitioning of a solute between the first aqueous phase and the membrane takes place rapidly in comparison with diffusion from the lipid phase into the second aqueous phase (Fig. 3). The first and the second aqueous phases represent gastrointestinal or buccal fluid and blood serum, respectively. The lipid membrane stands for gastrointestinal or buccal walls. Back diffusion from blood into membrane is considered negligible.

From this model Eq. (2) can be derived for k_{app}, the apparent first-order rate constant for disapearance of the drug from the gastrointestinal or buccal lumen.

$$k_{app} = k_m K_m/(1 + K_m) \tag{2}$$

In Eq. (2) k_m signifies the first-order rate constant for drug transport out of the membrane, and K_m is the partition coefficient between buccal or gastrointestinal fluid and the corresponding walls. K_m is related to the intrinsic partition coefficient P between these fluids and the membrane by Eq. (3), in which V_m and V_w refer to the volume of the membrane and the fluid, respectively.

$$K_m = (V_m/V_w)P_m \tag{3}$$

P_m can be expressed in terms of measured partition coefficients P between water and organic phases (e.g., *n*-octanol) via the Collander equation (*14*) (Eq. 4), in which a and b are constants.

$$P_m = bP^a \tag{4}$$

Koizumi *et al.* (*71*) assume that transfer from the membrane into blood is determined by the diffusion rate through the membrane, in which case k_m can be expressed by Eq. (5).

$$k_m = eAD \tag{5}$$

A is the interface area between the lipid and the aqueous phase (assumed to be equal on both sides), D is the diffusion coefficient, and e is a constant. Because D is inversely proportional to the square root of the molecular weight (M) and because for a given experimental series A is a constant, Eq. (5) can be transformed into Eq. (6). For test sets, the members of which do not differ significantly in molecular weight, k_m can be considered constant.

$$k_m = CM^{-1/2} \tag{6}$$

Assuming that, for many common partition systems, b in Eq. (4) will not differ much from unity, Koizumi *et al.* (*71*) derived Eq. (7), which relates absorption rate constants for un-ionized molecules to lipophilicity (P) and molecular weight.

$$k_{app} = C'PM^{-1/2}/(1 + C''P) \tag{7}$$

where C' and C'' are constants.

At low lipophilicities ($K_m \ll 1$) Eq. (2) predicts a linear increase of drug absorption rate with increasing lipophilicity (eq. 8), whereas at high lipophilicity a plateau is reached at $k_{app} = k_m$ (provided k is constant for the whole series under investigation).

$$\log k_{app} = a \log P + c \tag{8}$$

where $c = bk_m(V_m/V_w)$.

For ionizable drugs Eq. (2) must be replaced by Eq. (9) if only the nonionized molecules can enter the lipid membrane and by Eq. (10) otherwise.

$$k_{app} = \frac{k_{mu} f_u K_{mu}}{1 + f_u K_{mu}} \tag{9}$$

$$k_{app} = \frac{k_{mu} f_u k_{mu} + k_{mi}(1 - f_u)K_{mi}}{1 + f_u K_{mu} + (1 - f_u)K_{mi}} \tag{10}$$

In these equations k_{mu} and k_{mi} are the first order rate constants for the transport of the un-ionized and the ionized form of the drug, respectively, out of the membrane into the second aqueous phase. The terms K_{mu} and K_{mi} refer to the partition coefficients of the un-ionized and ionized species, respectively, and f, the fraction un-ionized, is given by Eq. (11).

$$f_u = 1/(1 + 10^{\mathrm{pH}-\mathrm{p}K_a}) \quad \text{for mono basic acids}$$

$$f_u = 1/(1 + 10^{\mathrm{p}K_a-\mathrm{pH}}) \quad \text{for mono acidic bases} \tag{11}$$

Using Eq. (2), Wagner (*156*) has derived equations that relate drug absorption to measured lipophilicities. For drugs in which only the unionized form is absorbed, Eqs. (12) and (13) refer to reversed phase and normal thin layer or paper chromatography, respectively, whereas Eq. (14) relates to partition coefficients. The terms d and n are constants, which like k_{mu} can be obtained by iterative curve fitting.

$$k_{app} = \frac{k_{mu}\,[(1 - R_f)/R_f]^n}{(d/f_u)^{n-1} + [(1 - R_f)/R_f]^n} \tag{12}$$

$$k_{app} = \frac{k_{mu}[R_f/(1 - R_f)]^n}{(d/f_u)^{n-1} + [R_f/(1 - R_f)]^n} \tag{13}$$

$$k_{app} = \frac{k_{mu}P^n}{(d/f_u) + P^n} \tag{14}$$

The model has been successfully applied to buccal absorption of n-alkanoic acids in man (dependence on lipophilicity as represented by chain length) (*155*) and gastric absorption of barbiturates in the rat (reversed-phase R_f, paper chromatography R_f, and octanol–water partition coefficients) (*156*). In 1980 Plá-Delfina *et al.* (*122*) reported a comparison of the Wagner–Sedman model with a linear or parabolic regression analysis. They measured the first-order absorption rate constant (rat gut *in situ*) of sulfanilamides. Lipophilicity was determined by reversed-phase thin layer chromatography. The R_f values ranged from 0.124 to 0.800. It was found that the Wagner–Sedman model gave a considerably better fit than linear or parabolic equations. Koizumi *et al.* applied Eq. (7) to small intestinal (*72*) and the gastric (*71*) absorption of sulfonamides in rats. In the latter case some members with low molecular weight and low lipophilicity were absorbed much faster than expected from the model. Diffusion of these compounds through aqueous pores was considered as a possible explanation. The same authors also treated renal excretion (tubular reuptake) (*73*).

The contribution to drug absorption of passage through aqueous pores was investigated by Plá-Delfina and Moreno (*123*). On the basis of the Wagner–Sedman extraction theory, the authors derived equations for the absorption rate constant as a function of partition coefficients. These equations describe the absorption of low and medium molecular weight carbamates and barbiturates by rat gut better than the Wagner–Sedman theory. The latter was, however, suitable for the absorption of a series of sulfanilamides. However, all of these compounds have molecular weights higher than 250 and may therefore no longer be able to pass through aqueous pores. For barbiturates and N-methylcarbamates, a threshold

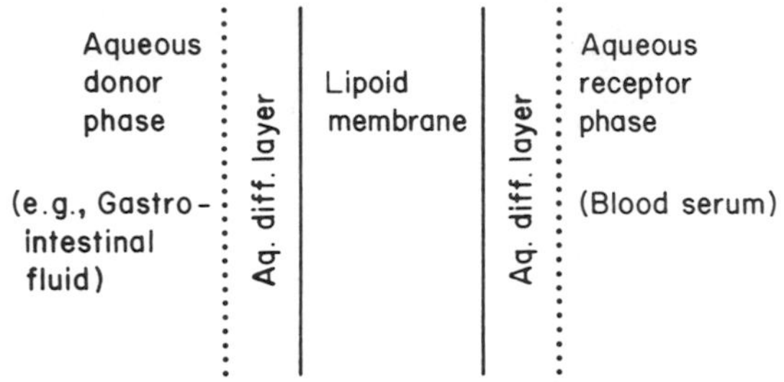

Fig. 4. Absorption model according to Stehle and Higuchi.

value for the molecular weight of 250 was found, above which diffusion through aqueous pores becomes negligible. The corresponding value for straight chain-substituted carbamates was 200.

Another model, proposed by Stehle and Higuchi (*139,140*), assumes stationary aqueous diffusion layers at the interfaces between the donor and receptor aqueous phases and the membrane (Fig. 4). This model predicts a linear increase in the logarithm of the transport rate into the receptor phase with log P at low lipophilicities, which for high lipophilicities asymptotically approaches an optimum. Under these latter conditions diffusion of the solute through the stationary aqueous layer between donor phase and membrane becomes rate limiting. The model can also be applied to ionizable compounds.

On the basis of extended theoretical treatment of this model (*143*), Suzuki *et al.* (*144*) discussed four particular models in which the bulk aqueous donor phase and the diffusion layer was followed by one of the following: (1) a lipid phase, (2a) a lipid and a subsequent aqueous phase (diffusion layer) (Fig. 5), (2b) an aqueous and a subsequent lipid phase, (3) a heterogeneous phase (lipid + aqueous), or (4) a lipid and a subsequent

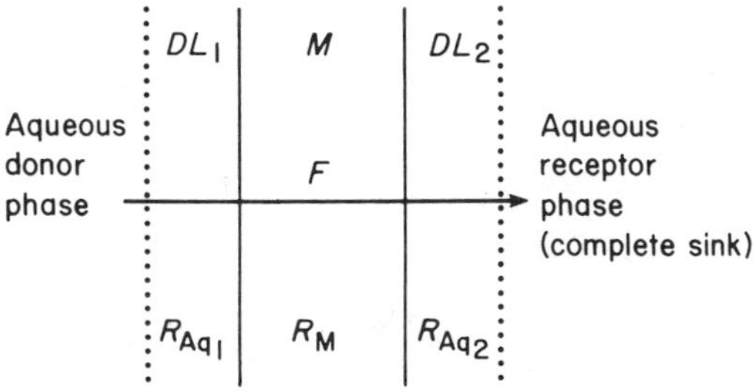

Fig. 5. Three-phase absorption model (model 2a). M: lipid membrane. DL_1, DL_2: aqueous diffusion layers. R_{AQ_1}, R_{AQ_2}: resistance of the diffusion layer to drug penetration. R_M: resistance of the membrane to drug penetration. F: flux of the drug.

heterogeneous phase. The whole sequence was in each case followed by a complete sink. The models were applied to gastrointestinal absorption data for sulfonamides and barbiturates. A good correlation between measured and calculated absorption rate constants was found with models (1), (2a), and (3) for sulfonamides and with model (1) for barbiturates. Model (2a) was also found successful in describing the buccal absorption of straight-chain alkanoic acids with four to eight carbon atoms (*55*). In order to account for the possibility that a drug molecule is not only absorbed by passive diffusion through a lipid membrane but can also pass through aqueous pores, Ho *et al.* (*56*) used model (3) with the premise that all molecular species (ionized and un-ionized) can pass through the aqueous pores under the influence of osmotic and hydrostatic flow and that the lipid component of the heterogeneous phase is only accessible to the un-ionized species.

Both models, with and without diffusion layer, are able to explain the so-called pH shift without having to assume transport of the ionized species. The term *pH shift* refers to the observation that the fraction absorbed is higher than expected from the pH–partition hypothesis, which states that unless there is a significant contribution from the ionized species, the transport rate of a compound is proportional to the fraction of the un-ionized form.

Both models predict that the pH shift increases with the lipophilicity of the compound. In addition, from the diffusion layer model a dependence of the pH shift on the thickness of this layer is to be expected. Tsuji *et al.* (*152*) checked this prediction for β-lactam antibiotics in an *in vitro* two-phase transport study and indeed found a right shift of the pH–absorption curves when the agitation of the system became slower. *In situ* gastrointestinal absorption of β-lactams was also investigated by Tsuji *et al.* (*153*) whereby they expanded the absorption model by a decomposition process taking place in the donor aqueous phase (*151,153*). They found that monobasic penicillins are mainly absorbed from the small intestine via passive diffusion of the un-ionized species, whereas gastric absorption and transport of the ionic species play only a minor role.

In order to explain the pH shift, Winne (*163*) proposed a model that consists of a bulk aqueous phase followed by a barrier and the blood phase. The barrier was assumed to consist of alternating aqueous and lipid layers, the first of which is the stationary aqueous diffusion layer. The model was applied to the absorption of barbital and sulfaethidole by rat small intestines and to the buccal absorption of *p*-toluic acid.

On the basis of equations from references *143*, *144*, and *163*, Schaper (*128*) derived an equation that relates first-order absorption rate constants to the partition coefficients of the un-ionized and the ionized forms of a chemical compound as well as to pH. This equation could be reasonably well fitted to the buccal absorption of alkanoic and phenylacetic acids.

Drug absorption can also be limited by solubility. Using model (2a) (Fig. 5), Flynn and Yalkowsky (*24,166–168,170*) derived equations for drug transport through membranes. Thus (for steady-state conditions) Eq. (15) describes the dependence of drug transport rate (F) upon the concentration difference between the aqueous donor phase and the aqueous receptor phase (ΔC), the resistance of the aqueous diffusion layers ($R_{aq} = R_{aq_1} + R_{aq_2}$) and of the membrane ($R_m$) to drug transport and the lipophilicity (P_m) of the drug (P_m is the membrane–water partition coefficient of the drug).

$$F = \Delta C/[R_{aq} + (R_m/P_m)] \tag{15}$$

If transport through aqueous pores also plays a significant role, the flux can be expressed by Eq. (16), in which R_p is the total resistance of the aqueous pores.

$$F = \Delta C/[R_{aq} + (R_m/P_m)] + \Delta C/R_p \tag{16}$$

Under physiological conditions, the concentration of the drug in the gastric or intestinal lumen (aqueous donor phase) is much greater than in the blood (aqueous receptor phase) so that ΔC can be approximated by the former concentration. The terms R_{aq} and R_m depend upon the thickness of the aqueous diffusion layers and of the membrane, respectively, and upon the diffusion constants of the drug in aqueous and lipid medium. Under fixed experimental conditions and within a series of closely related compounds, R_{aq} and R_m can be considered constant so that at low lipophilicities ($R_{aq} \ll R_m/P_m$) a linear relationship between this property and absorption rate is to be expected. For highly lipophilic compounds, ($R_{aq} \gg R_m/P_m$) the absorption rate approaches a constant value. These conclusions are qualitatively equal to the ones drawn from Eq. (2). Both equations, however, indicate that unless other factors than lipophilicity play a role, no optimum lipophilicity exists. One of these factors is solubility S, which limits the concentration C in the donor phase. The maximum possible flux under these conditions is given by Eq. (17).

$$F_{max} = S/[R_{aq} + (R_m/P_m)] \tag{17}$$

Because lipophilicity influences absorption rate and solubility in opposite ways, an optimum lipophilicity can be expected for a set of structurally related compounds. For homologous series, Yalkowsky and Morozowich (*170*) reported the following equations relating partition coefficient (P) and solubility to chain length (n) in which P_0 and S_0 pertain to the reference congener.

$$\log P = \log P_0 + 0.5n \tag{18}$$

$$\log S = \log S_0 - 0.6n \tag{19}$$

The different chain length–flux relationships that can be obtained by incorporating Eqs. (18) and (19) into Eq. 16 are detailed in references *24* and *166–168*. The model has been applied to the permeation of alkyl 4-aminobenzoates through model membranes (*24*) and of aliphatic alcohols through human stratum corneum *in vitro* (*166*) as well as to some other biological properties of congeneric series.

A model (based on convective diffusion theory), which assumes transport dependence on the penetration through the lipid phase and through an aqueous diffusion layer on the side of the receptor aqueous phase, was proposed by Nelson and Shah (*118,138*) and applied to the diffusion of alkyl 4-aminobenzoates through an artificial membrane (*138*).

2. Distribution Models

Parabolic relationships between biological properties and lipophilicity are not only found with pharmacokinetic but also with pharmacodynamic measurements. Penniston *et al.* (*120*) and Hansch (*45*) explained this observation with a distribution model (Fig. 6), which can also include absorption.

The model assumes that a drug that is administered to and dissolved in an aqueous compartment A_1 must pass through a sequence of alternating lipid and aqueous compartments until it reaches the receptor that has direct access to the last compartment. The model also assumes that the drug is removed from the last compartment by an irreversible process

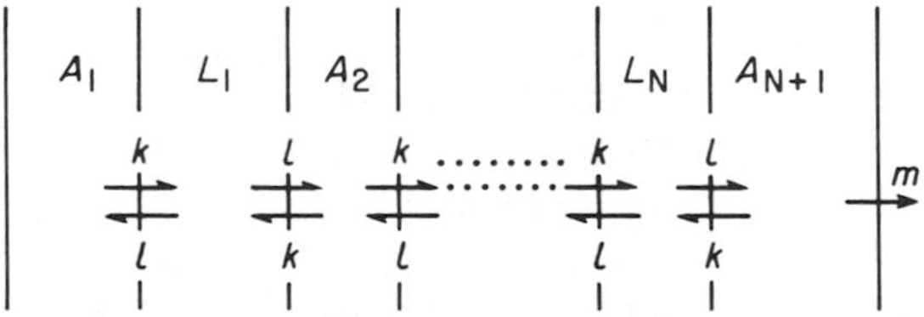

Fig. 6. Distribution model according to Penniston *et al.* (*120*). A_1: aqueous compartment to which the drug is administered. A_2–A_{N+1}: subsequent aqueous compartments. L_1–L_2: lipid compartments. k: rate constant for passage from aqueous to lipid compartments. l: rate constant for passage from lipid to aqueous compartment. m: first-order rate constant for irreversible elimination of the drug from the last compartment.

having rate constant m. The transport through the compartments is governed by the rate constants k for transport from aqueous to lipid phases and l for the reverse transport. The constants k and l are taken to be the same for all phases. The terms k and l determine the partition coefficient ($P = k/l$), and their product is arbitrarily chosen to equal unity ($k \cdot l = 1$). From this model, equations for the time dependence of drug concentration in every single compartment can be derived. Solving these equations for the last compartment of a 20-barrier model, taking time $t = 10$ units and $m = 1$, a series of points in a log P versus log C plot were obtained (C is the concentration in the last compartment) that could be acceptably fitted to a parabolic equation. Because the biological response is proportional to the occupation of the receptors by drug molecules and therefore to the concentration of the drug in the last compartment, a parabolic relationship between biological response and lipophilicity is to be expected.

Fitting experimental data to parabolic equations between biological properties and lipophilicity frequently results in systematic deviations of more hydrophilic congeners. In this area a linear relationship describes the data best. Franke (*26–30*) suggested that these observations can be explained if one assumes that nonlinearity is not due to transport but rather to binding phenomena. Initially, binding (to a receptor or plasma protein) increases linearly with lipophilicity until the parts of the molecule that form hydrophobic bonds with the protein (receptor) become too large to be adapted by the binding site. Consequently, more and more of the free energy that would be gained through increasing lipophilicity is lost through unfavorable steric interactions. Eventually the latter factor becomes dominant, and the biological property versus lipophilicity curve declines with increasing lipophilicity. This situation can be described by Eqs. (20) and (21) and is shown graphically in Fig. 7.

$$Bp = a'lip + b' \qquad \text{for } lip \leq lip_{\mathrm{L}} \tag{20}$$

$$Bp = a''lip^2 + b''lip + c'' \qquad \text{for } lip \geq lip_{\mathrm{L}} \tag{21}$$

In these equations Bp and lip represent linear free-energy related parameters for the biological property and lipophilicity, respectively; lip_{L} is the maximum lipophilicity that is compatible with an easy fit to the hydrophobic part of the receptor site and is given by the intersection of the two functions, Eq. (20) and Eq. (21). Equations (20) and (21) can be combined to give Eq. (22) in which $\delta = 1$ if $lip - lip_{\mathrm{L}} > 0$, and $\delta = 0$ otherwise.

$$Bp = a(lip - lip_{\mathrm{L}})^2\delta + b\ lip + c \tag{22}$$

Franke and Schmidt (*28*) compared this model with the parabolic model of

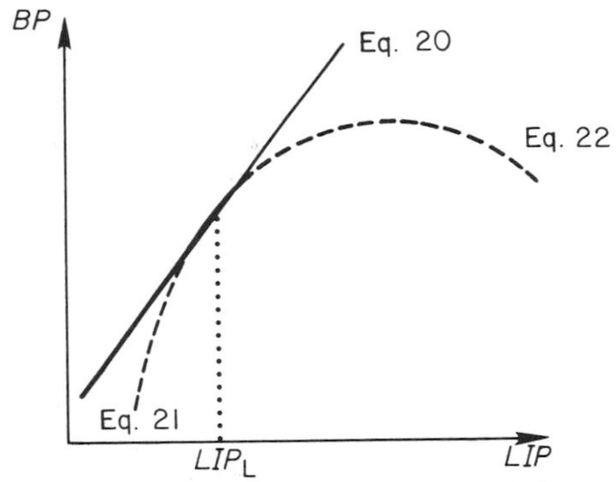

Fig. 7. Dependence of biological properties on lipophilicity according to Franke's protein binding model. *BP, LIP*: linear free-energy related parameters for biological property and lipophilicity. LIP_L: lipophilicity limit for easy fit to the receptor.

Hansch on the basis of literature data. Among others, the following structural types and biological activities were considered: (1) anticonvulsant activity of cyclic imides in mice and rats, (2) antimicrobial activity of phenols, alkylene diamidines and diguanides, and quinine related compounds and (3) narcotic activity of alkanols.

The fit of these data was slightly but not significantly ($p = 0.05$) better than in the Hansch model. In our own work on cardiotonic 2-phenylimidazo[4,5-*b*]pyridines (*5*) an equation containing a $(lip - lip_L)^2\delta$ term explained *in vitro* activity (rat atria) considerably better than an equation with a simple lip^2 term. Although a clear-cut distinction between the two explanations (transport versus receptor or protein binding) for nonlinear relationships between biological properties and lipophilicity could not be achieved, the "protein binding model" is certainly of heuristic value. Probably both transport and binding can in principle be responsible for nonlinearities, but individual contributions are dependent on the nature of the biological experiment. Moreover, in whole animals, deviations from linear relationships can also be brought about by differences in metabolism and excretion that are both insufficiently accounted for by the two models.

McFarland (*112*) used the Hansch model in order to calculate probabilities for a drug molecule, administered to compartment A_1, to reach the subsequent compartments. By plotting the logarithms of this probability against $\log(k/l)$, $\log P$ curves were obtained that could be reasonably approximated by parabolas. For every number of compartments a different curve resulted, but all of them had a maximum at $\log k/l = \log P_o = 0$.

Dearden and Townend (*18–20*) examined the model shown in Fig. 6 more closely, following in principle the procedure of Penniston *et al.* They calculated the concentration in all lipid compartments after $t = 10$ time units and found that the optimal lipophilicity (log P_0) increased with decreasing number of the compartment. Thus log P_0 for compartment L_2 was 1.25, whereas for compartment L_9 a value of 0.25 was obtained. This finding suggests that the experimentally observed log P_0 for a series depends on the nature of the biological test model. Thus log P_0 ought to be higher for simple organisms and *in vitro* preparations than for complex pharmacological models in which there are long random walks to the receptor sites (theoretically log P_0 approaches zero under these conditions). At least qualitative support for this view might come from some observations made on log P_0 for drug actions on biological systems that differ in complexity. Thus for CNS activity in mice, a rather complex system, log P_0 was found to be about 2 for various types of compounds such as barbiturates, acetylenic alcohols, diacylureas, and phenylboronic acids. In simple *in vitro* systems such as isolated bacteria or frog ventricle, however, log P_0 values of about 6 were observed with a number of different chemical structures, e.g., hydrocupreines, phenols, and thiocyanates (*45*). Whereas the curves found at 10 time units quite reasonably resemble parabolas, a definite distortion takes place at 80 time units with a concomitant shift of log P_0 to higher values (e.g., for L_9, Log $P_0 = 0.95$). For very long periods ($t = 640$ units), curves with a minimum near log $P = 0$ are obtained. This is because compounds for which log $P \approx 0$ are readily absorbed but are also most rapidly excreted. Considering the time required to reach maximal concentration, the authors found that it is shortest for compounds for which log $P \approx 0$ and increases for lower and higher lipophilicities (the time versus log P curves increase in steepness with increasing compartment number). This result is very important for the interpretation of biological data that refer to a response measured at a fixed time after administration of the drug. Highly lipophilic or hydrophilic compounds that are active may be overlooked if relatively short test times are applied. As far as the relationship between maximal concentration and log P is concerned, linear curves are obtained for low lipophilicities. The curves level off at higher log P values and approach a maximum asymptotically. In the absence of competing processes, such as metabolism, a very lipophilic drug will eventually give a higher concentration in the compartment adjacent to the receptor than one that is less lipophilic.

Whereas the above models are mainly concerned with distribution kinetics, the distribution model devised by Higuchi and Davis (*54*) is equilibrium based. Such models can be applied to test systems in which the drug rapidly achieves equilibrium or pseudoequilibrium distribution. The biological test system is represented by a number of regions widely differing in their physical properties and therefore their affinities for the added drug species. The biological activity is assumed to be determined by the relative amount of drug distributed to the receptor from the total system. The model consists of an aqueous compartment (*w*) to which the drug is added, *n* accessible additional compartments (e.g., tissue, lipoidal, and protein), and a compartment *r*, which represents the receptor. Thermodynamic equilibrium or pseudoequilibrium exists between all of these compartments with respect to the distribution of the drug (the drug has the same thermodynamic activity in all compartments). The biological response within the investigated series of compounds depends exclusively on the extent to which the receptor is occupied. The amount of receptor bound drug is considered negligible with respect to the total amount of drug (T) in the system. Under equilibrium conditions the drug is distributed over the system according to Eq. (23) in which c refers to the concentration of the drug in a certain compartment of volume V.

$$\mathrm{T} = c_\mathrm{w} V_\mathrm{w} + \sum_{i=1}^{n} c_i V_i \qquad (c_\mathrm{r} V_\mathrm{r} \text{ is negligible}) \tag{23}$$

The concentrations in the compartments i (c_i) relative to the concentration in the aqueous compartment (c_w) are determined by the corresponding partition coefficients P_i (Eq. 24).

$$P_\mathrm{i} = c_\mathrm{i}/c_\mathrm{w} \tag{24}$$

Assuming equal intrinsic activity for the compounds of a series, Eq. (25) can be derived. This equation relates the dose T, which elicits a standard biological response, to the partition properties of the respective compound. The partition coefficient (P_r) for the receptor can be related to the octanol–water partition coefficient by the Collander equation. A constant term is given as c

$$\log(1/T) = \log P_\mathrm{r} - \log(V_\mathrm{w} + \sum_{i=1}^{n} P_i V_i) + c \tag{25}$$

where $c = \log(k/B_\mathrm{p})$.

Equation 25 predicts a linear relationship between $\log(1/T)$ and $\log P$ ($V_\mathrm{w} \gg \Sigma_{i=1}^{n} P_i V_i$) for hydrophilic members of a series. For more lipophilic compounds, where $\Sigma_{i=1}^{n} P_i V_i$ can no longer be neglected, the $\log(1/T)$ versus $\log P$ curve is expected to level off more and more. Eventually an optimum will be reached beyond which a decline in activity is predicted.

Even though the assumption of pseudoequilibrium does not seem to be too realistic, the model can apparently simulate experimentally obtained lipophilicity–activity relationships.

A two-compartment version of the Higuchi–Davis model was used by Hyde (*60,61*) to derive equations for drug activity, represented by $\log(1/T)$, in relation to lipophilicity ($\log P_{o/w}$). The model consists of an aqueous phase (A), a lipid phase (B), and a subsequent receptor. It is assumed that there is an equilibrium between the receptor-bound drug and the free drug in the latter phase. The following relationship is obtained (Eq. 26), which shows an asymptotic approach of activity to a maximum with increasing lipophilicity, assuming equal intrinsic activity for all compounds of the series.

$$\log(1/T) = c - \log(b' + 10^{-a\log P_{o/w}}) \tag{26}$$

Hyde and Lord (*62*) and Kubinyi (*80*) extended this model by inserting a third compartment (C) between the lipophilic phase (B) and the receptor. They showed that an optimal lipophilicity can be expected when the lipophilic character of phase C is intermediate between that of phases A and B. Otherwise a plateau is reached.

The equations that have been derived so far from the equilibrium model only refer to compounds that under the experimental conditions are at least practically un-ionized. In practice, however, many drugs are weak acids or bases, which are more or less ionized at experimental pH. The influence of ionization on absorption and distribution of drugs has been treated theoretically by Martin (*106,108,110*). Two models have been considered.

1. There is an aqueous and a nonaqueous compartment between which the drug is equilibrated. A second equilibrium exists between the receptor-bound drug and the free drug in the aqueous (or alternatively nonaqueous) compartment.
2. There are one or more aqueous compartments in which the compound is ionized to different degrees and one or more nonaqueous compartments. The receptor-bound drug is again in equilibrium with the free drug in one type of compartment.

For every model three cases were calculated, where only the un-ionized, where only the ionized, and where both the ionized and the un-ionized species are bound to the receptor. The models were also extended to cases where additional factors (electronic and steric) play a role in receptor binding or partitioning. $\log(1/C)$ (C is the concentration of drug giving a standard biological response) versus $\log P$ curves were calculated for various degrees of ionization. Usually, linear relationships are obtained that level off at higher $\log P$ values and eventually approach a constant activity except where the polarity of the receptor compartment is intermediate between the lipophilic and the aqueous compartment, in which case an optimal log P exists.

An equilibrium distribution model that consists of three phases, two aqueous and one lipid, was used by Watanabe and Kozaki (*74,157,158*) to account for the volumes of distribution of bases. One of the aqueous phases has a pH of 7.4 and represents blood plasma. It is in equilibrium with an adjoining aqueous phase (signifying various other aqueous compartments in the body that are connected to plasma via aqueous pores) of a different pH. The first aqueous phase also borders the lipid phase. This model predicts that the apparent volume of distribution (V') is independent of lipophilicity for low apparent partition coefficients (P'), whereas at higher lipophilicities a linear relationship exists between log V' and log P'. The model was found to reproduce experimental data quite well for a number of bases in three animal species (rabbits, rats, and dogs). The bases varied considerably both with respect to lipophilicity (log $P_{n\text{-heptane-water}}$ ranges from -5 to $+3$ within the series) and structure (phenethylamines, anilines, phenothiazines, pyrazoles, imidazolines, and quinolines). The experimental values of methylene blue, however, were at variance with those predicted. Abnormal binding to erythrocytes or plasma binding was considered but did not give a satisfactory explanation (*74*).

Using an equilibrium model that consists of a central aqueous phase from which the drug is distributed into a receptor phase (absorbing a negligible amount of the total drug) and a number of equilipophilic loss phases, Davies *et al.* (*16*) discussed the significance of micro partition coefficients. The micro partition coefficients refer to the partition of specific conformers of a drug that are in thermodynamic equilibrium. The idea is that the micro partition coefficients determine the conformer composition in the various phases. As far as micro coefficients can be influenced by structural changes, the design of molecules can be envisioned for which the active conformer has favorable partition properties with respect to the receptor phase.

Both the kinetic and the equilibrium treatment of drug absorption and distribution can be expressed through a bilinear mathematical model, as was shown by Kubinyi (*76–81,83*). The model (Fig. 8) consists of three compartments, an aqueous one (A_1) to which the drug is administered, a lipophilic one (L) (representing a membrane), and a second aqueous compartment (A_2) with an adjoining receptor (R). The assumption is made that compartments A_1 and A_2 can be treated equally with respect to the partitioning of the drug, which therefore has the same concentration c_w in both compartments at equilibrium. For these conditions Eq. (23) can be

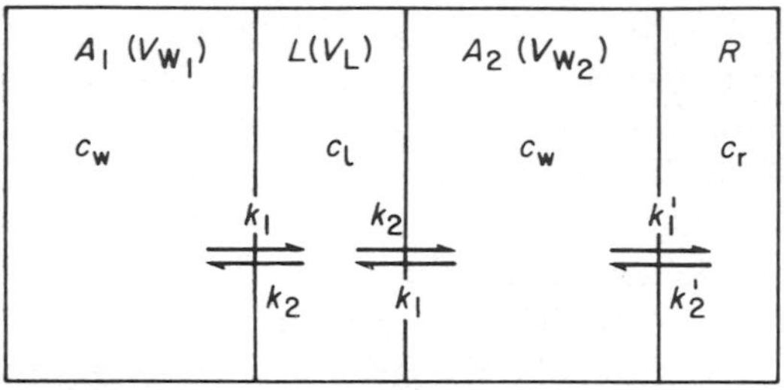

Fig. 8. Three-compartment model from which the bilinear model can be derived (*76*). A_1, A_2: aqueous phases with volumes V_{w_1} and V_{w_2}, respectively. L: lipid phase with volume V_L. R: receptor phase. c_w, c_l, c_r: concentration of the drug in the aqueous, lipid, and receptor phases, respectively, at equilibrium or pseudoequilibrium. k_1, k_1': rate constants for transport of drug molecules from aqueous to lipid and receptor phases, respectively. k_2, k_2': rate constants for transport of drug molecules from lipid or receptor phases, respectively, to aqueous phases. Adapted from Kubinyi (*76*).

rewritten as expressed in Eq. (*27*), in which V_{w_1}, V_{w_2}, and V_l are the volumes of the first and second aqueous and the lipid phase, respectively; c_l is the concentration of the drug in the lipid phase.

$$T = c_w V_{w_1} + c_l V_l + c_w V_{w_2} = c_w V_w + c_l V_l \tag{27}$$

Following the reasoning that led to Eq. (25), Eq. (28) can be derived, in which β is the ratio between the volumes of the lipid and the aqueous phases and a_r, a_l and b_l are constants from Collander equations, which relate octanol–water partition coefficients to receptor–aqueous phase and lipophilic–aqueous phase partition coefficients.

$$\log(1/T) = a_r \log P - \log(\beta b_l P_l^a + 1) + c' \tag{28}$$

If log P is determined in a system that is very similar to the biological system of the model (with respect to partitioning), b_l and a_l will be approximately unity and Eq. (28) is simplified to a bilinear model (Eq. 29).

$$\log(1/T) = a_r \log P - \log(\beta P + 1) + c' \tag{29}$$

A similar expression can be obtained from a kinetic treatment of the model presented in Fig. 8. Assuming that the biological response is proportional to the probability $W_{1,r}$ of a drug molecule added to compartment A_1 to reach the receptor phase R and applying McFarlands probabilistic model, Kubinyi derived Eq. (30), which is very similar to Eq. (29).

$$\log W_{1,r} = a' \log P + b' \log(\beta P + 1) + c'' \tag{30}$$

In a similar manner Kubinyi (*80*) treated other distribution models of various complexity. Several pharmacokinetic processes (*76,80,81*) were treated quantitatively with the bilinear model: the buccal absorption of alkanoic acids, the gastric and intestinal absorption of *n*-alkylcarbamates, the colonic absorption of acids (carboxylic acids, phenols, and acidic *N*-heterocycles), the renal clearance of probenecid analogs, dermal absorption of phorboldiesters, and the distribution of *n*-alkanols from blood into brain. In every case very good agreement between measured and calculated values was found. The same applied to a number of other biological activities (*78*).

Van de Waterbeemd *et al.* (*162a*) examined the transport kinetics implied in the three-compartment model of Fig. 8 for the two limiting conditions $t \rightarrow \infty$ (equilibrium) and $t = 0$ (initial transport process). They showed that whether or not a given system reaches equilibrium (or pseudoequilibrium) within a certain time is not only a matter of lipophilicity, that is, the relative values of the transport rate constants (k_1, k_2), but also depends on their absolute values. At a given time the concentration of a drug in the last compartment is proportional to $k_1^{(n-1)/2} k_2^{(n-1)/2}$ if this phase is aqueous (n is odd) and $k_1^{n/1} k_2^{n-2/2}$ if this compartment is lipophilic (n is even). A dependence of drug transport on lipophilicity (k_1/k_2) alone can be expected only when k_1 and k_2 are exclusively functions of lipophilicity. The two constants (k_1^{obs} for transport from the aqueous into the lipid phase, and k_2^{obs} for the reverse process) were measured by van de Waterbeemd *et al.* (*160,161*) for un-ionizable 4-acylaminobenzenesulfonamides in the system octanol–water. Plotting log k against log P gave curves with linear ascending parts (at low lipophilicities with positive slope for log k_1^{obs} and at high lipophilicities with negative slope for log k_2^{obs}) that leveled off and approached a constant value. These curves were in good agreement with those calculated from a drug transport model proposed by the authors (*162*). This model consists of a stirred aqueous phase followed by a stationary aqueous diffusion layer, a stationary lipid diffusion layer, and a stirred lipid layer. Using their two-phase experimental models the authors have also investigated a set of 15 compounds differing widely in structure and lipophilicity (log $P_{app\ o/w}$ ranges from -2.45 to $+3.15$) (*159*). The log k^{obs} values agreed very well with the proposed drug transport model. Equally good results were obtained when this set was combined with the set of sulfonamides mentioned above. No dependence on molecular size (represented by molecular weight, ranging from 78 to 532 in the set of 15 compounds) was found.

Models for the pH dependence of protein binding and of the log P, pK_a, and pH dependence of competitive displacement of drugs from proteins by other drugs have recently been reported (*53,129*). In the first case propranolol and diethanolamine fusidate have been used as examples (*53*). In the second case the displacement of 4-sulfanilamido-6-methoxypyrimidine from albumin by phenobarbital, pentobarbital, and phenoxymethylpenicillin was studied (*129*).

III. CONCLUSIONS

The quantitative treatment of drug absorption, distribution, and metabolism has strongly supported the view that fundamental relationships between these biological properties and the physicochemical properties of a compound exist. This result is extremely important because it makes systematic drug design feasible. If there were no, or only incidental, correlations between chemical structures and these biological properties, synthetic accessibility would be the only reasonable criterion for designing structures with potentially improved pharmacokinetic properties.

The preceding paragraph, however, also shows the limitations of the QSAR approach very clearly. Thus the factors as well as their influence on a certain pharmacokinetic property vary considerably from test set to test set. This is especially true for complex or composite processes such as metabolism and excretion. It is therefore little wonder that QSAR on properties such as elimination behavior, which are of eminent practical importance (e.g., for the duration of drug effects), have been reported rather seldom (apparently a quantitative description by the customary methods is in most cases not possible). Other important properties, especially absorption phenomena, are now comparatively well understood. In this field QSAR were able to yield some valuable generally applicable concepts such as that of optimal lipophilicity. Thus it was possible to specify the ranges of lipophilicity for which good gastrointestinal (log $P_{o/w}$ = 0.5–2.0) absorption or penetration through the blood–brain barrier (log $P_{o/w}$ = 1.4–2.7) might be expected.

Of course, there will be quite a number of exceptions, but meanwhile so many supporting data have accumulated that these rules can be safely applied by the medicinal chemist, at least as a first working hypothesis.

The increase in computer efficiency made it feasible to develop theoretical models that can describe (and eventually predict) biological properties of compounds. These models have in some examples been shown to explain experimental observations more satisfactorily than linear free-energy based empirical correlations. However, this improvement normally has to be payed for by a larger number of constants that need to be fitted to the data.

This automatically requires the data base, that is, the number of test compounds and/or biological tests, to be increased in order to obtain meaningful results. Because the experimental capacity is a crucial factor in practical drug development, the application of model-based QSAR will be rather limited. Moreover, these theoretical models pertain so far only to comparatively simple processes, such as absorption through a membrane or distribution into a small number of compartments. If such a process is the main determinant of the measured biological signal, a normal regression analysis will in most cases also yield results that are fully satisfactory for practical purposes. If, however, several processes contribute significantly to the biological signal (e.g., in *in vivo* tests) the models are no longer applicable and cannot be expected to give a meaningful fit to the data. Such situations may, however, still be reasonably well handled with classification methods such as cluster analysis, principal component or factor analysis, and discriminant analysis.

These methods only allow determination of locations of groups of biologically similar compounds in chemical and physicochemical parameter space and are therefore less sensitive to factors of secondary importance, which, if unknown, can prevent ordinary regression or model-based analysis from yielding acceptable results. However, the information obtained from classifications is much less precise. Thus classifications cannot answer the question as to which particular compound will give the maximal response. Instead, a smaller or larger set of compounds that surpass a certain level of response is defined. In practical drug design, in which there is a search for compounds that show an overall optimal behavior (not necessarily a maximum with respect to a particular biological property), this information is quite sufficient. In addition, explicit pharmacokinetic data from a greater number of structurally related compounds will always be scarce during a normal drug development procedure. Biological data, which contain pharmacokinetic information implicitly (e.g., from whole-animal models), are, however, usually available in greater quantity. Again, only classification methods are suitable for the analysis of such data. Therefore, in practical drug design, the application of classification methods, especially in the field of pharmacokinetics, will become more and more important. In the very late stages of a development, regression analysis (empirical or based on simple models) may become interesting, whereas complicated models will not play a significant role.

This estimation of the role of QSAR may have to be changed considerably if one is concerned with the mechanistic aspects of drug action. In pharmacokinetics these aspects can refer to such questions as the structure of the active site of metabolizing enzymes, the mode of absorption, distribution or excretion of a drug, or specific versus nonspecific binding to plasma proteins. Such studies require precise data analysis in order to allow detection of relatively small deviations of calculated values from observed values. Such deviations can be decisive criteria for the evaluation of alternative models, and they can also lead to new insights into pharmacokinetic processes. For such purposes regression and especially model-based data analysis may play an increasingly significant role in the future.

REFERENCES

1. K. A. S. Al-Gailany, J. W. Bridges, and K. J. Netter, *Biochem. Pharmacol.* **24,** 867 (1975).
2. V. Austel and E. Kutter, *in* "Arzneimittelentwicklung" (E. Kutter, ed.), p. 135. Thieme, Stuttgart, 1978.
3. V. Austel and E. Kutter, *in* "Drug Design" (E. J. Ariëns, ed.), Medicinal Chemistry, Vol. X, p. 1. Academic Press, New York, 1980.
4. V. Austel and E. Kutter, *Arzneim.-Forsch.* **31,** 130 (1981).
5. V. Austel and E. Kutter, unpublished observations (1979).
6. A. H. Beckett and A. C. Moffat, *J. Pharm. Pharmacol.* **21,** 144 S (1969).
7. A. H. Beckett and A. C. Moffat, *J. Pharm. Pharmacol.* **22,** 15 (1970).
8. G. L. Biagi, A. M. Barbaro, and M. C. Guerra, *Experientia* **27,** 918 (1971).
9. G. L. Biagi, A. M. Barbaro, and M. C. Guerra, *Adv. Chem. Ser.* **114,** 61 (1972).
10. A. E. Bird and A. C. Marshall, *Biochem. Pharmacol.* **16,** 2275 (1967).
11. C. E. Brafknecht, D. E. Nichols, and W. J. Dunn, *J. Med. Chem.* **18,** 208 (1975).
12. Y. W. Chien, H. J. Lambert, and T. K. Lin, *J. Pharm. Sci.* **64,** 961 (1975).
13. Y. C. Chien, M. J. Akers, and P. K. Yonan, *J. Pharm. Sci.* **64,** 1632 (1975).
14. R. Collander, *Acta Chem. Scand.* **5,** 774 (1951).
15. C. J. Coulson and V. J. Smith, *J. Pharm. Sci.* **69,** 799 (1980).
16. R. H. Davies, B. Sheard, and P. J. Taylor, *J. Pharm. Sci.* **68,** 396 (1979).
17. J. C. Dearden and E. Tomlinson, *J. Pharm. Pharmacol.* **22,** 535 (1970).
18. J. C. Dearden and M. S. Townend, *J. Pharm. Pharmacol.* **28,** 13P (1976).
19. J. C. Dearden and M. S. Townend, *in* "Herbicides and Fungicides" (N. R. McFarlane, ed.), Spec. Publ. No. **29,** p. 135. Chem. Soc., London, 1977.
20. J. C. Dearden and M. S. Townend, *in* "Quantitative Structure–Activity Analysis" (R. Franke and P. Oehme, eds.), p. 387. Akademie-Verlag, Berlin, 1978.
21. W. J. Dunn, *J. Med. Chem.* **16,** 484 (1973).
22. W. J. Dunn, *J. Pharm. Sci.* **62,** 1575 (1973).
23. R. Elofsson, S. O. Nilsson, and B. Kluczykowska, *Acta Pharm. Suec.* **8,** 465 (1971).
24. G. L. Flynn and S. H. Yalkowsky, *J. Pharm. Sci.* **61,** 838 (1972).
25. R. Franke, *Bioichim. Biophys. Acta* **160,** 378 (1968).
26. R. Franke, *Acta Biol. Med. Ger.* **25,** 757 (1970).
27. R. Franke, *Acta Biol. Med. Ger.* **25,** 789 (1970).
28. R. Franke and W. Schmidt, *Acta Biol. Med. Ger.* **31,** 273 (1973).
29. R. Franke, *Experientia, Suppl.* No. 23, p. 25 (1976).
30. R. Franke, *Farmaco, Ed. Sci.* **34,** 545 (1979).
31. T. Fujita, *Adv. Chem. Ser.* **114,** 80 (1972).
32. T. Fjuita, *J. Med. Chem.* **15,** 1049 (1972).
33. D. Gilbert, P. J. Goodford, F. E. Norrington, B. C. Weatherley, and S. G. Williams, *Br. J. Pharmacol.* **55,** 117 (1975).

34. H. Glasser and J. Krieglstein, *Naunyn-Schmiedeberg's Arch. Pharmacol.* **265,** 321 (1970).
35. C. Grieco, C. Hansch, C. Silipo, R. N. Smith, A. Vittoria, and K. Yamada, *Arch. Biochem. Biophys.* **194,** 542 (1979).
36. C. Hansch and A. R. Steward, *J. Med. Chem.* **7,** 691 (1964).
37. C. Hansch, E. W. Deutsch, and R. N. Smith, *J. Am. Chem. Soc.* **87,** 2738 (1965).
38. C. Hansch, K. Kiehs, and G. Lawrence, *J. Am. Chem. Soc.* **87,** 5770 (1965).
39. C. Hansch, A. R. Steward, and J. Iwasa, *J. Med. Chem.* **8,** 868 (1965).
40. C. Hansch, A. R. Steward, and J. Iwasa, *Mol. Pharmacol.* **1,** 87 (1965).
41. C. Hansch, *Proc. Int. Congr. Pharmacol., 3d São Paulo 1966,* **7,** 141 (1968).
42. C. Hansch, E. J. Lien, and F. Helmer, *Arch. Biochem. Biophys.* **128,** 319 (1968).
43. C. Hansch, A. R. Steward, S. M. Anderson, and D. Bentley, *J. Med. Chem.* **11,** 1 (1968).
44. C. Hansch, J. E. Quinlan, and G. L. Lawrence, *J. Org. Chem.* **33,** 347 (1968).
45. C. Hansch, *Acc. Chem. Res.* **2,** 232 (1969).
46. C. Hansch and E. Coats, *J. Pharm. Sci.* **59,** 731 (1970).
47. C. Hansch, *Proc. Int. Congr. Pharmacol., 4th, Basel, 1969* **4,** 128 (1970).
48. C. Hansch, *Drug Metab. Rev.* **1,** 1 (1972).
49. C. Hansch, *J. Org. Chem.* **37,** 92 (1972).
50. C. Hansch, C. Grieco, C. Silipo, and A. Vittoria, *J. Med. Chem.* **20,** 1420 (1977).
51. F. Helmer, K. Kiehs, and C. Hansch, *Biochemistry* **7,** 2858 (1968).
52. F. W. Hempelmann, N. Heinz, and H. Flasch, *Arzneim.-Forsch.* **28,** 2182 (1978).
53. J. A. Henry, A. W. Dunlop, S. N. Mitchell, P. Turner, and P. Adams, *J. Pharm. Pharmacol.* **33,** 179 (1981).
54. T. Higuchi and S. S. Davis, *J. Pharm. Sci.* **59,** 1376 (1970).
55. N. F. H. Ho and W. I. Higuchi, *J. Pharm. Sci.* **60,** 537 (1971).
56. N. F. H. Ho, W. I. Higuchi, and J. Turi, *J. Pharm. Sci.* **61,** 192 (1972).
57. J. B. Houston, D. G. Upshall, and J. W. Bridges, *J. Pharmacol. Exp. Ther.* **189,** 244 (1974).
58. J. B. Houston, D. G. Upshall, and J. W. Bridges, *J. Pharmacol. Exp. Ther.* **195,** 67 (1975).
59. A. Hulshoff and J. H. Perrin, *J. Med. Chem.* **20,** 430 (1977).
60. R. M. Hyde, *J. Med. Chem.* **18,** 231 (1975).
61. R. M. Hyde, *Chem. Ind.* (*London*) p. 859 (1977).
62. R. M. Hyde and E. Lord, *Eur. J. Med. Chem.—Chim. Ther.* **14,** 199 (1979).
63. Y. Ichikawa and T. Yamano, *Biochim. Biophys. Acta* **147,** 518 (1967).
64. A. Inuye, Y. Shinagawa, and Y. Takaishi, *Arch. Int. Pharmacodyn.* **144,** 319 (1963).
65. A. E. Jacobson, W. A. Klee, and W. J. Dunn, *Eur. J. Med. Chem.—Chim. Ther.* **12,** 49 (1977).
66. C. R. F. Jefcoate, J. L. Gaylor, and R. L. Calabrese, *Biochemistry* **8,** 3455 (1969).
67. K. Kakemi, T. Arita, R. Hori, and R. Konishi, *Chem. Pharm. Bull.* **15,** 1534 (1967).
68. N. Kaneniwa, M. Hiura, and S. Nakagawa, *Chem. Pharm. Bull.* **27,** 1501 (1979).
69. I. M. Kapetanović, J. M. Strong, and J. J. Mieyal, *J. Pharmacol. Exp. Ther.* **209,** 20 (1979).
70. K. Kiehs, C. Hansch, and L. Moore, *Biochemistry* **5,** 2602 (1966).
71. T. Koizumi, T. Arita, and K. Kakemi, *Chem. Pharm. Bull.* **12,** 413 (1964).
72. T. Koizumi, T. Arita, and K. Kakemi, *Chem. Pharm. Bull.* **12,** 421 (1964).
73. T. Koizumi, T. Arita, and K. Kakemi, *Chem. Pharm. Bull.* **12,** 428 (1964).
74. A. Kozaki and J. Watanabe, *J. Pharm. Dyn.* **2,** 37 (1979).
75. J. Krieglstein, W. Meiler, and J. Staab, *Biochem. Pharmacol.* **21,** 985 (1972).

76. H. Kubinyi, *Arzneim.-Forsch.* **26,** 1991 (1976).
77. H. Kubinyi, *in* "Biological Activity and Chemical Structure" (J. A. Keverling-Buismman, ed.), Pharmacochemistry Library, Vol. II, p. 239. Elsevier, Amsterdam/New York, 1977.
78. H. Kubinyi, *J. Med. Chem.* **20,** 625 (1977).
79. H. Kubinyi and O.-H. Kehrhahn, *Arzneim.-Forsch.* **28,** 598 (1978).
80. H. Kubinyi, *Arzneim.-Forsch.* **29,** 1067 (1979).
81. H. Kubinyi, *Farmaco, Ed. Sci.* **34,** 248 (1979).
82. H. Kubinyi, *Prog. Drug Res.* **23,** 97 (1979).
83. H. Kubinyi, *Prog. Drug. Res.* **23,** 168 (1979).
84. E. Kutter, A. Herz, H.-J. Teschemacher, and R. Hess, *J. Med. Chem.* **13,** 801 (1970).
85. E. Kutter and V. Austel, *Arzneim.-Forsch.* **31,** 135 (1981).
86. V. A. Levin, *J. Med. Chem.* **23,** 682 (1980).
87. E. Lien and C. Hansch, *J. Pharm. Sci.* **57,** 1027 (1968).
88. E. J. Lien, *Drug Intell. Clin. Pharm.* **4,** 7 (1970).
89. E. J. Lien, R. T. Koda, and G. L. Tong, *Drug Intell. Clin. Pharm.* **5,** 38 (1971).
90. E. J. Lien and G. L. Tong, *J. Soc. Cosmet. Chem.* **24,** 371 (1973).
91. E. J. Lien, *in* "Drug Design" (E. J. Ariëns, ed.), Medicinal Chemistry, Vol. V, p. 85. Academic Press, New York, 1974.
92. E. J. Lien, *in* "Drug Design" (E. J. Ariëns, ed.), Medicinal Chemistry, Vol. V, p. 89. Academic Press, New York, 1974.
93. E. J. Lien, *in* "Drug Design" (E. J. Ariëns, ed.), Medicinal Chemistry, Vol. V, p. 92. Academic Press, New York, 1974.
94. E. J. Lien, *in* "Drug Design" (E. J. Ariëns, ed.), Medicinal Chemistry, Vol. V, p. 93. Academic Press, New York, 1974.
95. E. J. Lien, *in* "Drug Design" (E. J. Ariëns, ed.), Medicinal Chemistry, Vol. V, p. 122. Academic Press, New York, 1974.
96. E. J. Lien, *in* "Drug Design" (E. J. Ariëns, ed.), Medicinal Chemistry, Vol. V, p. 106. Academic Press, New York, 1974.
97. E. J. Lien and J. H. Perrin, *J. Med. Chem.* **19,** 849 (1976).
98. E. J. Lien and P. H. Wang, *J. Pharm. Sci.* **69,** 648 (1980).
99. Y.-J. Lin, S. Awazu, M. Hanano, and H. Nogami, *Chem. Pharm. Bull.* **21,** 2749 (1973).
100. R. W. Lucek and C. B. Coutinho, *Mol. Pharmacol.* **12,** 612 (1976).
101. H. Lüllmann, P. B. M. W. M. Timmermans, G. M. Weikert, and A. Ziegler, *J. Med. Chem.* **23,** 560 (1980).
102. G. Maksay, Z. Tegyey, and L. Ötvös, *Hoppe-Seyler's Z. Physiol. Chem.* **359,** 879 (1978).
103. G. Maksay, Z. Tegyey, and L. Ötvös, *J. Chromatogr.* **174,** 447 (1979).
104. G. Maksay, Z. Tegyey, and L. Ötvös, *J. Med. Chem.* **22,** 1443 (1979).
105. Y. C. Martin and C. Hansch, *J. Med. Chem.* **14,** 777 (1971).
106. Y. C. Martin and J. J. Hackbarth, *J. Med. Chem.* **19,** 1033 (1976).
107. Y. C. Martin, "Quantitative Drug Design. A Critical Introduction." Med. Res. Ser. (G. L. Grunewald ed.) Dekker, New York, 1978.
108. Y. C. Martin, "Quantitative Drug Design. A Critical Introduction," Med. Res. Ser. (G. L. Grunewald ed.) p. 139. Dekker, New York, 1978.
109. Y. C. Martin, *in* "Drug Design" (E. J. Ariëns, ed.), Medicinal Chemistry, Vol. VIII, p. 1. Academic Press, New York, 1979.
110. Y. C. Martin, *in* "Drug Design" (E. J. Ariëns, ed.), Medicinal Chemistry, Vol. VIII, p. 59. Academic Press, New York, 1979).
111. D. Maysinger and M. Movrin, *Acta Pharm. Jugosl.* **29,** 175 (1979).

112. J. W. McFarland, *J. Med. Chem.* **13,** 1192 (1970).
113. I. Moriguchi, *Chem. Pharm. Bull.* **16,** 597 (1968).
114. I. Morgiguchi, S. Wada, and T. Nishizawa., *Chem. Pharm. Bull.* **16,** 601 (1968).
115. T. Morishita, M. Yamazaki, N. Yata, and A. Kamada, *Chem. Pharm. Bull.* **21,** 2309 (1973).
116. G. L. Mosher and T. J. Mikkelson, *Int. J. Pharm.* **2,** 239 (1979).
117. N. Nambu and T. Nagai, *Chem. Pharm. Bull.* **20,** 2463 (1972).
118. K. G. Nelson and A. C. Shah, *J. Pharm. Sci.* **66,** 137 (1977).
119. A. Pannatier, B. Testa, and J.-C. Etter, *Int. J. Pharm.* **8,** 167 (1981).
120. J. T. Penniston, L. Beckett, D. L. Bentley, and C. Hansch, *Mol. Pharmacol.* **5,** 333 (1969).
121. J. M. Plá-Delfina, J. Moreno, and A. del Pozo, *J. Pharmacokinet. Biopharm.* **1,** 243 (1973).
122. M. Plá-Delfina, J. Moreno, V. Frías, R. Obach, and A. del Pozo, *J. Pharmacokinet. Biopharm.* **8,** 297 (1980).
123. M. Plá-Delfina and J. Moreno, *J. Pharmacokinet. Biopharm.* **9,** 191 (1981).
124. J. Rieder, *Arzneim.-Forsch.* **13,** 81 (1963).
125. A. Ryrfeldt, *J. Pharm. Pharmacol.* **23,** 463 (1971).
126. D. R. Sanvordeker, Y. M. Chien, T. K. Lin, and H. J. Lambert, *J. Pharm. Sci.* **64,** 1797 (1975).
127. D. R. Sanvordeker, S. Pophristov, and A. Christensen, *Drug Dev. Ind. Pharm.* **3,** 149 (1977).
127a. M. Schaefer, I. Okulicz-Kozaryn, A.-M. Batt, G. Siest, and V. Loppinet, *Eur. J. Med. Chem.—Chim. Ther.* **16,** 461 (1981).
128. K.-J. Schaper, Strategy in Drug Research *2nd, IUPAC-IUPHAR Symp., Noordwijkerhout, Neth. poster* (1981).
129. K.-J. Schaper and J. K. Seydel, Strategy in Drug Research *2nd, IUPAC-IUPHAR Symp., Noordwijkerhout, Neth.* poster (1981).
130. R. A. Scherrer and S. M. Howard, *J. Med. Chem.* **20,** 53 (1977).
131. R. D. Schoenwald and R. L. Ward, *J. Pharm. Sci.* **67,** 786 (1978).
132. W. Scholtan, *Arzneim.-Forsch.* **18,** 505 (1968).
133. J. K. Seydel and E. Wempe, *Arzneim.-Forsch.* **21,** 187 (1971).
134. J. K. Seydel, H. Ahrens, and W. Losert, *J. Med. Chem.* **18,** 234 (1975).
135. J. K. Seydel and W. Butte, *J. Med. Chem.* **20,** 439 (1977).
136. J. K. Seydel and K. J. Schaper, "Chemische Struktur und biologische Aktivität von Wirkstoffen." Verlag Chemie, Weinheim, 1979.
137. J. K. Seydel, D. Trettin, H. P. Cordes, O. Wassermann, and M. Malyusz, *J. Med. Chem.* **23,** 607 (1980).
138. A. C. Shah and K. G. Nelson, *J. Pharm. Sci.* **69,** 210 (1980).
139. R. G. Stehle and W. I. Higuchi, *J. Pharm. Sci.* **56,** 1367 (1967).
140. R. G. Stehle and W. I. Higuchi, *J. Pharm. Sci.* **61,** 1922 (1972).
141. N. R. Strahl and S. Lopez, *J. Pharm. Sci.* **67,** 1041 (1978).
142. A. J. Stuper and P. C. Jurs, *J. Pharm. Sci.* **67,** 745 (1978).
143. A. Suzuki, W. I. Higuchi, and N. F. H. Ho, *J. Pharm. Sci.* **59,** 644 (1970).
144. A. Suzuki, W. I. Higuchi, and N. F. H. Ho, *J. Pharm. Sci.* **59,** 651 (1970).
145. A. W. Tai and E. J. Lien, *Acta Pharm. Jugosl.* **30,** 171 (1980).
146. B. Testa, *Pharm. Acta Helv.* **53,** 143 (1978).
147. B. Testa and B. Salvesen, *J. Pharm. Sci.* **69,** 497 (1980).
148. P. B. M. W. M. Timmermans and P. A. van Zwieten, *J. Med. Chem.* **20,** 1636 (1977).
149. G. L. Tong and E. J. Lien, *J. Pharm. Sci.* **65,** 1651 (1976).

150. S. Toon and M. Rowland, *J. Pharm. Pharmacol.* **31,** Suppl., 43P (1979).
151. A. Tsuji, E. Miyamoto, I. Kagami, H. Sakaguchi, and T. Yamana, *J. Pharm. Sci.* **67,** 1701 (1978).
152. A. Tsuji, E. Miyamoto, N. Hashimoto, and T. Yamana, *J. Pharm. Sci.* **67,** 1705 (1978).
153. A. Tsuji, E. Miyamoto, O. Kubo, and T. Yamana, *J. Pharm. Sci.* **68,** 812 (1979).
154. J. M. Vandenbelt, C. Hansch, and C. Church, *J. Med. Chem.* **15,** 787 (1972).
155. J. G. Wagner and A. J. Sedman, *J. Pharmacokinet. Biopharm.* **1,** 23 (1973).
156. J. G. Wagner, "Fundamentals in Clinical Pharmacokinetics," p. 217. Drug Intelligence Publ. Hamilton, Illinois, 1975.
157. J. Watanabe and A. Kozaki, *Chem. Pharm. Bull.* **26,** 665 (1978).
158. J. Watanabe and A. Kozaki, *Chem. Pharm. Bull.* **26,** 3463 (1978).
159. H. van de Waterbeemd, P. van Bakel, and A. Jansen, *J. Pharm. Sci.* **70,** 1081 (1981).
160. H. van de Waterbeemd, S. van Boeckel, A. Jansen, and K. Gerritsma, *Eur. J. Med. Chem.—Chim. Ther.* **15,** 279 (1980).
161. J. T. M. van de Waterbeemd, A. C. A. Jansen, and K. W. Gerritsma, *Pharm. Weekbl.* **115,** 825 (1980).
162. J. T. M. van de Waterbeemd, C. C. A. A. van Boekel, R. L. F. M. de Sévaux, A. C. A. Jansen, and K. W. Gerritsma, *Pharm. Weekbl.* **116,** 224 (1981).
162a. J. T. M. van de Waterbeemd, A. C. A. Jansen, and K. W. Gerritsma, *Pharm. Weekbl.* **113,** 1097 (1978).
163. D. Winne, *J. Pharmacokinet. Biopharm.* **5,** 53 (1977).
164. S. G. Wood, D. G. Upshall, and J. W. Bridges, *J. Pharm. Pharmacol.* **31,** 192 (1979).
165. W. E. Wright and V. D. Line, *Antimicrob. Agents Chemother.* **17,** 842 (1980).
166. S. H. Yalkowsky and G. L. Flynn, *J. Pharm. Sci.* **62,** 210 (1973).
167. S. H. Yalkowsky, T. G. Slunick, and G. L. Flynn, *J. Pharm. Sci.* **63,** 691 (1974).
168. S. H. Yalkowsky and G. L. Flynn, *J. Pharm. Sci.* **63,** 1276 (1974).
169. S. H. Yalkowsky and M. Morozowich, *in* "Drug Design" (E. J. Ariëns, ed.), Medicinal Chemistry, Vol. IX, p. 149. Academic Press, New York, 1980.
170. S. H. Yalkowsky and M. Morozowich, *in* "Drug Design" (E. J. Ariëns, ed.), Medicinal Chemistry, Vol. IX, p. 123. Academic Press, New York, 1980.
171. S. H. Yalkowsky and S. C. Valvani, *J. Pharm. Sci.* **69,** 912 (1980).
172. M. Yamazaki, N. Kakega, T. Morishita, A. Kamada, and M. Aoki, *Chem. Pharm. Bull.* **18,** 708 (1970).
173. T. D. Yih and J. M. van Rossum, *Biochem. Pharmacol.* **26,** 2117 (1977).
174. T. D. Yih and J. M. van Rossum, *J. Pharmacol. Exp. Ther.* **203,** 184 (1977).
175. M. Yoshimoto and C. Hansch, *J. Org. Chem.* **41,** 2269 (1976).

12

Commentary

JOHN G. TOPLISS

It seems appropriate to end this book with a commentary on the place of QSAR in medicinal chemistry and the contributions it has made to that subject as detailed in the preceding chapters.

There is a widespread tendency to judge QSAR solely as a potential predictive tool for the discovery of medically and commercially viable new drugs. This is particularly true of scientists in the pharmaceutical industry who constitute the majority of medicinal chemists and whose mission is the very practical one of discovery and development of new drug substances. There is no question that the predictive potential of QSAR is its most dramatic and controversial aspect. Doubtless some advocates have fostered overly optimistic hopes in this direction, but this should not be allowed to obscure the many ways that QSAR has been shown to contribute to the development and understanding of the field of medicinal chemistry.

In my view perhaps the single most significant contribution to date has been the development of a systematic and fairly complete understanding in quantitative terms of the role of lipophilicity in drug action. This embraces relative potencies, tissue and organ specificity, differentiation of pharmacological effects, absorption and distribution phenomena, mechanisms, and receptor site interactions. The concept of log P_0, the optimum lipophilicity for maximum drug potency, was established early in the development of QSAR by Corwin Hansch. It has been shown to be of particular importance with regard to CNS drugs (Chapter 8, p. 330 and Chapter 11, p. 469), and partition coefficient ranges for effective entry of compounds into the CNS have been established. The converse of this is also very important where absence of a CNS effect is desired, a point well illustrated in the case of the antiulcer drug pirenzepine (Chapter 6, p. 279).

QUANTITATIVE STRUCTURE-ACTIVITY
RELATIONSHIPS OF DRUGS

ISBN 0-12-695150-0

Another nice demonstration of the use of this idea is in distinguishing between the specific and nonspecific components of antimicrobial drug action (Chapter 2, p. 26). Also, optimal log P_0 values were shown to be very different for activity against gram-negative and gram-positive bacteria, which fits with the fact that gram-negative cell wall contains more lipid and hence may be relatively more effective in slowing down the passage of highly lipophilic molecules (Chapter 2, p. 27). The approach of obtaining log P_0 in a lead series at an early stage, reflecting optimum transport properties, and then optimizing activity with respect to other physicochemical parameters, was used in the design of *m*-AMSA (Chapter 4, p. 166) an anticancer drug in advanced clinical trial in the U.S. and Europe. Also of importance to antitumor agent design is that log P_0 can be expected to be quite different for different tumor types, e.g., log $P_0 = 0$ for *N*-nitrosoureas against ascitic tumors, whereas solid tumors such as Walker 256 respond to more lipophilic drugs with a log P_0 value of about 2 (Chapter 4, p. 173). Optimal oral absorption of a wide spectrum of drug substances, obviously a matter of greater importance in drug design, has been shown to be generally associated with a log P_0 value of 0.5–2.0 (Chapter 11, p. 445).

Relative lipophilicity is a simple and adequate quantitative basis for understanding such things as the activity of anesthetics (Chapter 8, p. 332), the effect of nonspecific agents on membranes relating to certain types of antiarrhythmic agents (Chapter 5, pp. 221–226), the selectivity of many β blockers (Chapter 5, pp. 184, 188), and their nonspecific effects (Chapter 5, pp. 196–197), the topical antiinflammatory activity of steroidal esters (Chapter 9, p. 358), the relative activities of antitumor aziridines and mitomycins (Chapter 4, pp. 149–151), the protein binding of drugs (Chapter 11, p. 453), and the bioconcentration affecting the buildup of pesticides in the food chain (Chapter 10, p. 398).

As pointed out in Chapter 3 (p. 127), the critical role of lipophilicity has been established for the *in vitro* antibacterial activity of certain series of substituted erythromycins, leucomycins, lincomycins, rifamycins, coumermycins, and β-lactams and the *in vivo* antibacterial activity of penicillins.

Information on receptor sites has been gleaned from QSAR studies and has enhanced our knowledge and understanding in this area. Thus from QSAR studies on inhibitors of dihydrofolate reductase (DHFR) crude maps have been inferred for the character of "enzymatic space" in the binding region for dihydrofolate. A hydrophobic pocket is incorporated in a particular region for both mammalian and bacterial enzymes with the pocket larger in the bacterial than in the mammalian enzyme (Chapter 2, pp. 46–47). A good picture of the β receptor is emerging (Chapter 5, pp. 183, 188, 193, 243), and a view of the α receptor is being developed (Chapter 5, pp. 218, 243) from QSAR studies. The receptor binding of steroids has been well visualized in a model arrived at through QSAR studies (Chapter 9, p. 365). Several models of the mode of inhibition of protein synthesis by chloramphenicol, lincomycin, and erythromycin have been proposed (Chapter 3, p. 103). Modeling studies have resulted in a number of proposals for receptor sites for antiinflammatory drugs that provide a better understanding of how these drugs may be acting at the molecular level (Chapter 7, pp. 310–320). A map of the dopamine receptor has been constructed, which has particular relevance to the design of neuroleptic agents (Chapter 8, p. 343). QSAR studies employing regression analysis have shown utility in supporting the stem fit model for DDT action involving a flexible receptor site of definite dimensions.

A substantial amount of useful information has been gathered from QSAR studies concerning the mechanism of action of drugs. A good part of this falls in the field of antiinfective agents. A very good discussion of how QSAR studies can distinguish between specific and nonspecific antimicrobial drug action is provided in Chapter 2 (pp. 25–36). A log P_0 value of about 6 is suggested to be characteristic for structurally nonspecific neutral agents that damage the cell membrane of gram-positive bacteria. Low log P_0 values for quaternary and alkanoic acid series suggested activity of a somewhat more specific kind probably involving anionic and cationic receptors, respectively. A number of QSAR studies support the view that with esters of 4-hydroxybenzoic acid (parabens) the cell membrane is the sensitive site (Chapter 2, pp. 35–36). A QSAR study of the antimicrobial activity of long chain esters of β-alanine has nicely shown the value of QSAR in differentiating specific and nonspecific mechanisms and in demonstrating the critical role of hydrophobic effects with regard to nonspecific action (Chapter 2, p. 36). An interesting concept of hydrophobic and hydrophilic pathways to bacterial receptors has been formulated (Chapter 2, p. 28) relating to different log P values of compounds, which has particular relevance to β-lactam antibiotics.

The use of equation intercepts has allowed close parallels to be drawn between equations for antibacterial activity and hemolytic effects on red blood cells for various series of compounds, which has led to the conclusion that certain series of antifungal agents act by membrane perturbation. Again using intercept information, QSAR studies on a series of 2,4-bis(arylamino)pyrimidines, demonstrating potent broad activity against gram-positive and gram-negative bacteria and fungi, have suggested that a structurally specific drug effect, rather than a membrane perturbing effect, is involved. This is an example of the use of QSAR, within an established framework with similar biological systems, to draw mechanistic conclusions (Chapter 2, p. 29).

QSAR in the form of model based equations led to the conclusion that for nitrophenols the ionic species is approximately 4000 times less potent than the neutral form (Chapter 2, p. 34). Studies using quantum chemical methodology resulted in the conclusion that for lincomycins and clindamycins it is the neutral form that binds to the receptor (Chapter 3, p. 97).

QSAR studies have added considerably to our understanding of the action of antibacterial sulfonamides (Chapter 2, pp. 39–44) and have been used to support and reinforce the suggestion that the antibacterial effect of dapsone on *Mycobacterium leprae* is qualitatively different from its effect and that of related sulfones and sulfonamides on other mycobacteria (Chapter 2, pp. 44–46). Employing the technique of discriminant analysis, pyrimidines have been classified as reversible or irreversible inhibitors of bacterial growth (Chapter 2, pp. 50–51) and QSAR studies using physicochemical parameters have provided strong support for a proposed mechanism of action of the tuberculostatic activity of isoniazid derivatives (Chapter 2, pp. 52–54). QSAR work on griseofulvin analogs suggests that activity may result from reaction of the enone system with a nucleophile such as an SH group in an enzyme involved in fungal metabolism (Chapter 2, p. 58).

In a different therapeutic area an interesting difference between the electronic influence of substituents in aspirins and salicylates with regard to their ulcerogenic effect was demonstrated by QSAR studies, which lends support to the idea that these classes of agents act by different mechanisms (Chapter 7, pp. 296–297).

A very useful concept in the realm of QSAR is that of bioisosterism. A striking example of its use coupled with physicochemical rationales is in the H_2 antagonist field. A successful progression was made from burimamide, a compound having the desired pharmacological profile in humans but with insufficient potency, especially on oral administration, first to metiamide with greatly increased potency and oral activity but unacceptable toxicity, and then to cimetidine, an enormously successful antiulcer drug (Chapter 6, pp. 261–265).

The field of molecular modeling has undergone rapid recent development as a result of the work of Gund, Hopfinger, Marshall, Langridge, and others. Highly sophisticated graphics capability is available that can handle macromolecules of the complexity of DNA or proteins (Chapter 1, pp. 14–15). Perhaps the most impressive success of computer modeling techniques has been in the remarkable simplification of somatostatin from its 14-peptide to a 7-peptide cycle, resulting in an improvement of biological efficacy. A key point here was that many of the active modifications suggested by the modeling would have been contraindicated by the results of single amino acid replacements (Chapter 6, pp. 272–273).

There are numerous examples throughout this book of how QSAR in the form of classic linear free-energy relationship methodology has accounted satisfactorily for quantitative relative activity in a series in terms of readily understandable physicochemical phenomena. This has been a marked advance in medicinal chemistry and represents an important stage in the development of our understanding of the fundamentals of what processes and factors control drug action. We can now frequently do much better than merely stating in a descriptive SAR sense that "chloro is superior to methyl and a methoxy substituent abolishes activity." Not to be overlooked are advances in series design and planning made possible through QSAR methodology, which permits a more rational and economical exploration of a compound series to be made (Chapter 1, p. 13).

Apart from supplying a more fundamental and scientific explanation of changes in activity as structure is varied in a series, QSAR has often provided more practical benefits to the medicinal chemist engaged in new drug discovery work. Thus examination of QSAR equations and the list of compounds already synthesized has resulted in the conclusion that further work in the series is not likely to be productive. In the field of anticancer drugs (Chapter 4) such a conclusion was reached from QSAR studies in connection with separation of activity and toxicity of aromatic nitrogen mustards (p. 146), bis-1-(1-aziridinyl)phosphinylcarbamates (pp. 151–152), triazines (p. 155), and anthracyclines (p. 167).

In a series of colchicine analogs of interest for their anticancer properties it was concluded, after synthesizing only a small number of compounds, that variation in the 7 and 10 positions should be abandoned because of a strong intercorrelation of activity and toxicity and variation in the 4 position undertaken (Chapter 4, p. 171). It was apparent in certain series of antiinflammatory drugs that maximum potency had been reached and that further synthesis was not justified (Chapter 7, p. 324). In a series of triazines of interest as potential antibacterial agents, it was clear that to achieve useful potency log *P* would have to be so high that the compounds would be strongly serum bound *in vivo* and thus there was no scope for development of a useful agent (Chapter 2, pp. 51–52). QSAR studies have lent strong support to the view that the nitro group in nitroimidazoles and related nitroheterocycles is essential and attempts to find an effective replacement are doomed to failure (Chapter 2, p. 68). In a series of erythromycin analogs it was noted that "establishment of regression equations with an opimum log *P* and negative steric effects helped in the decision to terminate the synthesis of further analogs" (Chapter 3, p. 92).

More impressive and useful than just "turning off" synthesis in a series are directions of a more positive kind that can come out of QSAR studies. QSAR studies of diphenhydramines suggest the possibility of discovering a potent antihistamine lacking the ability to cross the blood brain barrier and thus not cause undesirable effects associated with CNS entry such as drowsiness (Chapter 6, pp. 260–261). In a series of aminoxylidides of potential interest as antiarrhythmics, the optimum log *P* for both antiarrhythmic and CNS properties was similar. Therefore it was concluded that the goal of separating these activities would be best approached by the synthesis of more basic compounds (Chapter 5, p. 229). Examples have been noted in the field of antiinflammatory agents where QSAR correlations have been followed by new compound synthesis. Some measure of success was achieved, although in only one case was a significant increase of *in vivo* activity realized (Chapter 7, p. 324). A direction could be deduced for the separation of the antiinflammatory and ulcerogenic properties of aspirins. Thus QSAR studies allow the conclusion that electron-withdrawing 5-substituents, lipophilic enough to produce a log *P* for the molecule in the 2.6–3.0 range, should produce the maximum separation between these two properties (Chapter 7, p. 296). Early QSAR studies on thyroxine analogs led to the more extensive investigation of the thyromimetic activity of 3′,5′-alkyl substituted analogs (Chapter 9, p. 385). The potency of new erythromycin analogs was correctly predicted by a QSAR equation (Chapter 3, p. 91). QSAR studies on an antifungal series from which the compound Cicloperox was chosen for clinical trial confirmed this as a sound choice (Chapter 2, pp. 57–58).

Dramatic increases in potency have been achieved for PCA inhibitors in the antiallergy field using QSAR techniques of the linear free-energy type. In a series of 2-phenyl-8-azapurinones a 100-fold potency enhancement was achieved largely, but not entirely on the basis of QSAR (Chapter 6, pp. 276–277). Even more impressive was a similar potency boost achieved in a series of pyranenamines purely by QSAR methodology (Chapter 6, pp. 274–276). Important aspects here were that new directions in the series were identified through QSAR that were not obvious by traditional approaches and that the synthesis of compounds with highly unusual substituents were inspired, which turned out to be the most potent in the series. This study illustrates, probably better than any other published to date, the inherent potential of QSAR. A highly favorable outcome was experienced in using QSAR (Free–Wilson approach) in a series of antimicrobial quinoxaline 1,4-dioxides. A predicted highly potent compound was synthesized and not only were expectations borne out in terms of *in vitro* potency, but the compound also possessed exceptional *in vivo* activity (Chapter 2, p. 55).

In some cases that have been well studied it is clear that the complexity of the problem has as yet been too much to overcome. A number of credible attempts have been made to unlock the secrets of the chloramphenicol series; however, a clear, comprehensive, and convincing picture of forces controlling relative activity has not emerged to date. The tetracyclines have also received a fair amount of attention, but an added dimension of complexity exists here because several groups are present that can ionize at biological pH values. There is the same problem in the case of the less well-studied aminoglycosides. It is therefore not surprising that QSAR has not registered significant success in these series (Chapter 3, pp. 87, 104).

QSAR studies on the same compound series using different methodologies can produce results that are difficult to account for in that they emphasize different critical factors. A case in point is a series of antihypertensive benzothiadiazines that have been analyzed in five separate studies (Chapter 5, pp. 210–211).

It must also be recognized, as all QSAR practioners know, that many attempted QSAR studies are abandoned and never reported because of lack of any meaningful results. Reasons for this vary but may include inherent complexity of the problem, inaccurate biological data, failure to account for critical activity controlling factors, inadequate spread of biological activity or physicochemical parameter values, or co-variance of parameter values. Failures due to poor experimental design or data, of course, do not reflect on the value of QSAR methodology as such. Criteria that must be met for successful QSAR studies have been reviewed in Chapter 1 (p. 16).

Although an increasing number of suggestions that have been made based on QSAR studies are being tested out in practice, more needs to be done along these lines to be able to better evaluate the value of QSAR-based predictions.

It is interesting to review those cases in which QSAR methodology has played a significant role in the discovery of drugs that have achieved clinical significance. Mention has already been made of cimetidine, an antiulcer drug, for which the concept of bioisosterism was employed (Chapter 6, p. 265) and *m*-AMSA for which linear free energy (LFE) or Hansch based methodology was utilized (Chapter 4, p. 166). Another interesting case is described in Chapter 5 (pp. 190–193) involving the QSAR aided discovery of a new potent, selective and, nondepressive, clinically active β blocker with a unique side chain. A potent diuretic now in advanced clinical trial, muzolimine, was designed with the assistance of a simplified operational scheme QSAR approach (Chapter 5, pp. 205–206). Again in the cardiovascular field, a new cardiotonic agent, AR-L115, also in advanced clinical trials, was discovered, employing a novel QSAR-based method that makes use of the theory of sets (Chapter 5, p. 235).

A major difficulty in QSAR studies is the oversimplification inherent in relating complex pharmacological processes to physicochemical parameters and geometric patterns. A measured pharmacological result or end point represents the sum of a number of processes such as absorption, distribution, metabolism, receptor affinity, and intrinsic activity. Sorting out complex situations is a lengthy process, if it can be accomplished at all, and many compounds must be made to obtain meaningful correlations. In a practical situation in a drug discovery program a clinical candidate may well be selected before enough data has been generated to perform an effective QSAR analysis. Or alternatively, the problem will have been abandoned for other reasons, such as discouraging degree of progress, time constraints, and other more exciting prospects. These are clearly factors that limit the overall role that QSAR can play in new drug discovery. The prospective use of QSAR is most effective when one or two fairly readily identifiable factors are dominant in controlling activity so that this information can be exploited at an early state in the development of a series.

It is clear from surveying QSAR studies reported to date that these have increased our basic understanding of forces at work in determining drug action, potency, and selectivity. Such increased understanding provides an improved basis for future work suggesting potentially fruitful avenues to pursue. It also serves to order the many ideas that medicinal chemists may have for structural modifications of lead compounds in probabilistic terms. Contributions of this type are far more likely than the pinpointing of a compound not even remotely contemplated by the medicinal chemist.

QSAR methods for the most part were not well enough established to be part of the ongoing development of most of today's established drug classes. However, given the current level of acceptance of, and familiarity with, QSAR methodology and its increasing sophistication, it seems likely that QSAR will have a much greater integral role in drug discovery during the decade of the 1980s. It will still, however, be one tool among several and must not be viewed as a potentially magic instrument that will precisely identify the new drug discoveries of the future. Emphasis among the various QSAR methodologies will undoubtedly change and it is apparent that molecular modeling will become much more prominent.

Viewed in broad context it is clear from the work reviewed in this book that QSAR has played an increasing role in the development of medicinal chemistry as a rational science over the past 15 years and in the discovery of new drugs. We may expect that this role will increase over the coming decade.

Index

B

C

Q

R

S

W

X

MEDICINAL CHEMISTRY

A Series of Monographs

EDITED BY

GEORGE DESTEVENS

Department of Chemistry
Drew University
Madison, NJ 07940

Volume 1. GEORGE DESTEVENS. Diuretics: Chemistry and Pharmacology. 1963

Volume 2. RODOLFO PAOLETTI (ED.). Lipid Pharmacology. Volume I. 1964. RODOLFO PAOLETTI AND CHARLES J. GLUECK (EDS.). Volume II. 1976

Volume 3. E. J. ARIENS (ED.). Molecular Pharmacology: The Mode of Action of Biologically Active Compounds. (In two volumes.) 1964

Volume 4. MAXWELL GORDON (ED.). Psychopharmacological Agents. Volume I. 1964. Volume II. 1967. Volume III. 1974. Volume IV. 1976

Volume 5. GEORGE DESTEVENS (ED.). Analgetics. 1965

Volume 6. ROLAND H. THORP AND LEONARD B. COBBIN. Cardiac Stimulant Substances. 1967

Volume 7. EMIL SCHLITTLER (ED.). Antihypertensive Agents. 1967

Volume 8. U. S. VON EULER AND RUNE ELIASSON. Prostaglandins. 1967

Volume 9. G. D. CAMPBELL (ED.). Oral Hypoglycaemic Agents: Pharmacology and Therapeutics. 1969

Volume 10. LEMONT B. KIER. Molecular Orbital Theory in Drug Research. 1971

Volume 11. E. J. ARIENS (ED.). Drug Design. Volumes I and II. 1971. Volume III. 1972. Volume IV. 1973. Volumes V and VI. 1975. Volume VII. 1976. Volume VIII. 1978. Volume IX. 1979. Volume X. 1980.

Volume 12. PAUL E. THOMPSON AND LESLIE M. WERBEL. Antimalarial Agents: Chemistry and Pharmacology. 1972

Volume 13. ROBERT A. SCHERRER AND MICHAEL W. WHITEHOUSE (Eds.). Antiinflammatory Agents: Chemistry and Pharmacology. (In two volumes.) 1974

Volume 14. LEMONT B. KIER AND LOWELL H. HALL. Molecular Connectivity in Chemistry and Drug Research. 1976

Volume 15. Julius A. Vida. Anticonvulsants. 1977

Volume 16. John M. Cassady and John D. Douros (Eds.). Anticancer Agents Based on Natural Product Models. 1980

Volume 17. Federico Arcamone. Doxorubicin. 1981

Volume 18. Erwin Margulies (Ed.). Myocardial Infarction and Cardiac Death. 1983

Volume 19. John G. Topliss (Ed.). Quantitative Structure-Activity Relationships of Drugs. 1983

In preparation

Volume 20. Peter P. Mager. Multidimensional Pharmacochemistry: Design of Safer Drugs. 1983

PJDP. book typos

p 179 Scheme 1 platelets 7th line from bottom ~~cardiomiopathy~~ cardiomiopathy

p 185 eq 3. symbol missing. Also where is reference to eq 3 in text.

p 187 line 3 mean experimental error = ±0.12

Preface 2nd paragraph ... what ...

p 123 5th line from bottom — phenylglycine

p 212 3rd line rats

p240 ~~page~~ (two thirds down page Equation (8[illegible]) [illegible] (8[illegible]).

also —, but clearly Eq (4)? should be Eq 83.

—... the numbers in parenthesis are standard errors (no numbers in parenthesis!)

~~p256~~ p 516 (index) Quantum Chemical Calculation PCILO (256)

p212 next to last line on page Eq 22 ?

p213 structure XYXV is missing.

p208 eq. (35) −0.026 Ti

p323 eq 67 – define meaning of D

p157 next to bottom line analogs of XV in Table I